a LANGE medical book

Pharmacology
Examination
& Board Review

Tenth Edition

Anthony J. Trevor, PhD

Professor Emeritus of Pharmacology and Toxicology
Department of Cellular & Molecular Pharmacology
University of California, San Francisco

Bertram G. Katzung, MD, PhD

Professor Emeritus of Pharmacology
Department of Cellular & Molecular Pharmacology
University of California, San Francisco

Marieke Kruidering-Hall, PhD

Associate Professor & Academy Chair of Pharmacology Education
Department of Cellular & Molecular Pharmacology
University of California, San Francisco

Susan B. Masters, PhD

Professor
Department of Cellular & Molecular Pharmacology
University of California, San Francisco

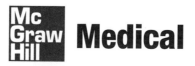

New York   Chicago   San Francisco   Lisbon   London   Madrid   Mexico City
Milan   New Delhi   San Juan   Seoul   Singapore   Sydney   Toronto

Katzung & Trevor's Pharmacology: Examination & Board Review, Tenth Edition

1 2 3 4 5 6 7 8 9 0   QDB/QDB   16 15 14 13

ISBN 978-0-07-178923-3
MHID 0-07-178923-5

Notice

Medicine is an ever-changing science. As new research and clinical experience broaden our knowledge, changes in treatment and drug therapy are required. The authors and the publisher of this work have checked with sources believed to be reliable in their efforts to provide information that is complete and generally in accord with the standards accepted at the time of publication. However, in view of the possibility of human error or changes in medical sciences, neither the authors nor the publisher nor any other party who has been involved in the preparation or publication of this work warrants that the information contained herein is in every respect accurate or complete, and they disclaim all responsibility for any errors or omissions or for the results obtained from use of the information contained in this work. Readers are encouraged to confirm the information contained herein with other sources. For example and in particular, readers are advised to check the product information sheet included in the package of each drug they plan to administer to be certain that the information contained in this work is accurate and that changes have not been made in the recommended dose or in the contraindications for administration. This recommendation is of particular importance in connection with new or infrequently used drugs.

This book was set in Adobe Garamond by Cenveo Publisher Services.
The editors were Michael Weitz and Karen Edmonson.
The production supervisor was Sherri Souffrance.
Project management was provided by Harleen Chopra, Cenveo Publisher Services.
The illustration manager was Armen Ovsepyan.
The text designer was Elise Lansdon; the cover designer was Thomas DePierro.
The cover art shows the action of a beta blocker drug (yellow spheres) as a beta-receptor antagonist at the nerve synapses. It blocks some of the receptors (shown as indentations) that enable the neurotransmitter adrenaline (epinephrine, blue spheres) released from the presynaptic cell (top) to the postsynaptic cell downstream (bottom). *Credit:* David Mack/Photo Researchers, Inc.
The index was prepared by BIM Indexing & Proofreading Services.
Quad/Graphics was printer and binder.

This book is printed on acid-free paper.

INTERNATIONAL EDITION ISBN 978-0-07-181350-1; MHID 0-07-181350-0 Copyright @2013. Exclusive rights by the McGraw-Hill Companies, Inc., for manufacture and export. This book cannot be re-exported from the country to which it is consigned by McGraw-Hill. The International Edition is not available in North America.

Contents

Preface

This book is designed to help students review pharmacology and to prepare for both regular course examinations and board examinations. The tenth edition has been extensively reviewed to make such preparation as active and efficient as possible. As with earlier editions, rigorous standards of accuracy and currency have been maintained in keeping with the book's status as the companion to the *Basic & Clinical Pharmacology* textbook. This review book divides pharmacology into the topics used in most courses and textbooks. Major introductory chapters (eg, autonomic pharmacology and CNS pharmacology) are included for integration with relevant physiology and biochemistry. The chapter-based approach facilitates use of this book in conjunction with course notes or a larger text. We recommend several strategies to make reviewing more effective.

First, each chapter has a short discussion of the major concepts that underlie its basic principles or the specific drug group, accompanied by explanatory figures and tables. The figures are in full color and many are new to this edition. Students are advised to read the text thoroughly before they attempt to answer the study questions at the end of each chapter. If a concept is found to be difficult or confusing, the student is advised to consult a regular textbook such as *Basic & Clinical Pharmacology*, 12th edition.

Second, each drug-oriented chapter opens with an "**Overview**" that organizes the group of drugs visually in diagrammatic form. We recommend that students practice reproducing the overview diagram from memory.

Third, a list of **High Yield Terms to Learn** and their definitions is near the front of most chapters. Make sure that you are able to define those terms.

Fourth, many chapters include a "**Skill Keeper**" question that prompts the student to review previous material and to see links between related topics. We suggest that students try to answer Skill Keeper questions on their own before checking the answers that are provided at the end of the chapter.

Fifth, each of the sixty-one chapters contains upto ten **sample questions** followed by a set of answers with explanations. For most effective learning, you should take each set of sample questions as if it were a real examination. After you have answered every question, work through the answers. When you are analyzing the answers, make sure that you understand why each choice is either correct or incorrect.

Sixth, each chapter includes a **Checklist** of focused tasks that you should be able to do once you have finished the chapter.

Seventh, each chapter ends with a **Summary Table** that lists the most important drugs and includes key information concerning their mechanisms of action, effects, clinical uses, pharmacokinetics, drug interactions, and toxicities.

Eighth, when preparing for a comprehensive examination you should review the list of drugs in **Appendix I: Key Words for Key Drugs**. Students are also advised to check this appendix at the same time that they work through the chapters so they can begin to identify drugs out of the context of a chapter that reviews a restricted set of drugs.

Ninth, after you have worked your way through most or all of the chapters and have a good grasp of the Key Drugs, you should take the comprehensive examinations, each of 100 questions, presented in **Appendices II and III**. These examinations are followed by a list of answers each with a short explanation or rationale underlying the correct choice and the numbers of the chapters in which more information can be found if needed. We recommend that you take an entire examination or a block of questions as if it were a real examination: commit to answers for the whole set before you check the answers. As you work through the answers, make sure that you understand why each distractor is either correct or incorrect. If you need to, return to the relevant chapters(s) to review the text that covers key concepts and facts that form the basis for the question.

Tenth, you can use the strategies in Appendix IV for improving your test performance. General advice for studying and approaching examinations includes strategies for several types of questions that follow specific formats.

We recommend that this book be used with a regular text. *Basic & Clinical Pharmacology*, 12th edition (McGraw-Hill, 2012), follows the chapter sequence used here. However, this review book is designed to complement any standard medical pharmacology text. The student who completes and understands *Pharmacology: Examination & Board Review* will greatly improve his or her performance and will have an excellent command of pharmacology.

Because it was developed in parallel with the textbook *Basic & Clinical Pharmacology*, this review book represents the authors' interpretations of chapters written by contributors to that text. We are grateful to those contributors, to our other faculty colleagues, and to our students, who have taught us most of what we know about teaching.

We welcome the participation of Marieke Kruidering-Hall, PhD, a recipient of the Distinguished Teaching Award of the University of California, San Francisco, as a co-author of this 10th edition of *Pharmacology: Examination & Board Review.*

We very much appreciate the invaluable contributions to this text afforded by the editorial team of Karen Edmonson, Rachel D'Annucci Henriquez, Harleen Chopra, Harriet Lebowitz, and Michael Weitz. The authors also thank Alice Camp for her excellent proofreading contributions to this and earlier editions.

Anthony J. Trevor, PhD
Bertram G. Katzung, MD, PhD
Marieke Kruidering-Hall, PhD
Susan B. Masters, PhD

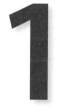

Introduction

Pharmacology is the body of knowledge concerned with the action of chemicals on biologic systems. **Medical pharmacology** is the area of pharmacology concerned with the use of chemicals in the prevention, diagnosis, and treatment of disease, especially in humans. **Toxicology** is the area of pharmacology concerned with the undesirable effects of chemicals on biologic systems. **Pharmacokinetics** describes the effects of the body on drugs, eg, absorption, excretion, etc. **Pharmacodynamics** denotes the actions of the drug on the body, such as mechanism of action and therapeutic and toxic effects. This chapter introduces the basic principles of pharmacokinetics and pharmacodynamics that will be applied in subsequent chapters.

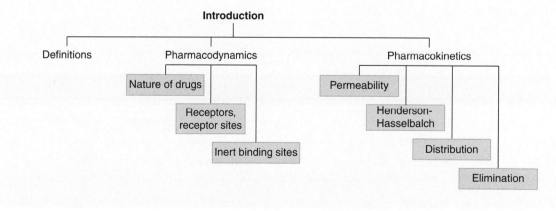

THE NATURE OF DRUGS

Drugs in common use include inorganic ions, nonpeptide organic molecules, small peptides and proteins, nucleic acids, lipids, and carbohydrates. Some are found in plants or animals, but many are partially or completely synthetic. Many biologically important endogenous molecules and exogenous drugs are optically active; that is, they contain one or more asymmetric centers and can exist as enantiomers. The enantiomers of optically active drugs usually differ, sometimes more than 1000-fold, in their affinity for their biologic receptor sites. Furthermore, such enantiomers may be metabolized at different rates in the body, with important clinical consequences.

A. Size and Molecular Weight

Drugs vary in size from molecular weight (MW) 7 (lithium) to over MW 50,000 (thrombolytic enzymes, other proteins). Most drugs, however, have molecular weights between 100 and 1000. Drugs smaller than MW 100 are rarely sufficiently selective in

their actions, whereas drugs much larger than MW 1000 are often poorly absorbed and poorly distributed in the body.

B. Drug-Receptor Bonds

Drugs bind to receptors with a variety of chemical bonds. These include very strong covalent bonds (which usually result in irreversible action), somewhat weaker electrostatic bonds (eg, between a cation and an anion), and much weaker interactions (eg, hydrogen, van der Waals, and hydrophobic bonds).

PHARMACODYNAMIC PRINCIPLES

A. Receptors and Receptor Sites

Drug actions are mediated through the effects of drug molecules on drug **receptors** in the body. Most receptors are large regulatory molecules that influence important biochemical processes (eg, enzymes involved in glucose metabolism) or physiologic processes (eg, neurotransmitter receptors, neurotransmitter reuptake transporters, and ion transporters).

If drug-receptor binding results in activation of the receptor, the drug is termed an **agonist**; if inhibition results, the drug is considered an **antagonist**. Some drugs mimic *agonist* molecules by *inhibiting* metabolic enzymes, eg, acetylcholinesterase inhibitors. As suggested in Figure 1–1, a receptor molecule may have several binding sites. Quantitation of the effects of drug-receptor binding as a function of dose yields **dose-response curves** that provide information about the nature of the drug-receptor interaction. Dose-response phenomena are discussed in more detail in Chapter 2. A few drugs are enzymes themselves (eg, thrombolytic enzymes that dissolve blood clots; pegloticase, which metabolizes

uric acid). These drugs do not act on endogenous receptors but on endogenous substrate molecules.

B. Inert Binding Sites

Because most drug molecules are much smaller than their receptor molecules (discussed in the text that follows), specific regions of receptor molecules often can be identified that provide the local areas for drug binding. Such areas are termed **receptor sites**. In addition, drugs bind to other nonregulatory molecules in the body without producing a discernible effect. Such binding sites are termed **inert binding sites**. In some compartments of the body (eg, the plasma), inert binding sites play an important role in buffering the concentration of a drug because bound drug does not contribute directly to the concentration gradient that drives diffusion. **Albumin** and **orosomucoid** (α_1-acid glycoprotein) are two important plasma proteins with significant drug-binding capacity.

High-Yield Terms to Learn

Drugs	Substances that act on biologic systems at the chemical (molecular) level and alter their functions
Drug receptors	The molecular components of the body with which drugs interact to bring about their effects
Distribution phase	The phase of drug movement from the site of administration into the tissues
Elimination phase	The phase of drug inactivation or removal from the body by metabolism or excretion
Endocytosis, exocytosis	Endocytosis: Absorption of material across a cell membrane by enclosing it in cell membrane material and pulling it into the cell, where it can be released. Exocytosis: Expulsion of material from vesicles in the cell into the extracellular space
Permeation	Movement of a molecule (eg, drug) through the biologic medium
Pharmacodynamics	The actions of a drug on the body, including receptor interactions, dose-response phenomena, and mechanisms of therapeutic and toxic actions
Pharmacokinetics	The actions of the body on the drug, including absorption, distribution, metabolism, and elimination. Elimination of a drug may be achieved by metabolism or by excretion. *Biodisposition* is a term sometimes used to describe the processes of metabolism and excretion
Transporter	A specialized molecule, usually a protein, that carries a drug, transmitter, or other molecule across a membrane in which it is not permeable, eg, Na^+/K^+ ATPase, serotonin reuptake transporter, etc

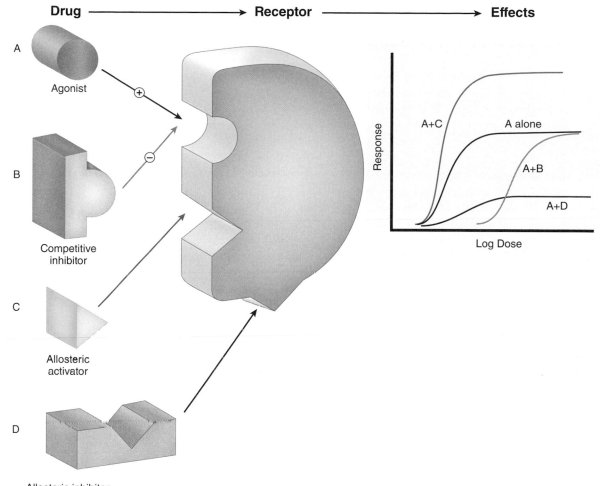

Drug ⟶ **Receptor** ⟶ **Effects**

FIGURE 1–1 Potential mechanisms of drug interaction with a receptor. Possible effects resulting from these interactions are diagrammed in the dose-response curves at the right. The traditional agonist (drug A)-receptor binding process results in the dose-response curve denoted "A alone." B is a pharmacologic antagonist drug that competes with the agonist for binding to the receptor site. The dose-response curve produced by increasing doses of A in the presence of a fixed concentration of B is indicated by the curve "A+B." Drugs C and D act at different sites on the receptor molecule; they are *allosteric* activators or inhibitors. Note that allosteric inhibitors do not compete with the agonist drug for binding to the receptor, and they may bind reversibly or irreversibly. (Reproduced, with permission, from Katzung BG, editor: *Basic & Clinical Pharmacology,* 12th ed. McGraw-Hill, 2012: Fig. 1–3.)

PHARMACOKINETIC PRINCIPLES

To produce useful therapeutic effects, most drugs must be absorbed, distributed, and eliminated. Pharmacokinetic principles make rational dosing possible by quantifying these processes.

THE MOVEMENT OF DRUGS IN THE BODY

To reach its receptors and bring about a biologic effect, a drug molecule (eg, a benzodiazepine sedative) must travel from the site of administration (eg, the gastrointestinal tract) to the site of action (eg, the brain).

A. Permeation

Permeation is the movement of drug molecules into and within the biologic environment. It involves several processes, the most important of which are discussed next.

1. Aqueous diffusion—Aqueous diffusion is the movement of molecules through the watery extracellular and intracellular spaces. The membranes of most capillaries have small water-filled pores that permit the aqueous diffusion of molecules up to the size of small proteins between the blood and the extravascular space.

This is a passive process governed by Fick's law (see later discussion). The capillaries in the brain, testes, and some other organs lack aqueous pores, and these tissues are less exposed to some drugs.

2. Lipid diffusion—Lipid diffusion is the passive movement of molecules through membranes and other lipid structures. Like aqueous diffusion, this process is governed by Fick's law (see later discussion).

3. Transport by special carriers—Drugs that do not readily diffuse through membranes may be transported across barriers by mechanisms that carry similar endogenous substances. A very large number of such transporter molecules have been identified, and many of these are important in the movement of drugs or as targets of drug action. Unlike aqueous and lipid diffusion, carrier transport is not governed by Fick's law and is capacity-limited. Important examples are transporters for ions (eg, Na^+/K^+ ATPase), for neurotransmitters (eg, transporters for serotonin, norepinephrine), for metabolites (eg, glucose, amino acids), and for foreign molecules (**xenobiotics**) such as anticancer drugs.

Selective inhibitors for these carriers may have clinical value; for example, several antidepressants act by inhibiting the transport of amine neurotransmitters back into the nerve endings from which they have been released. After release, such amine neurotransmitters (dopamine, norepinephrine, and serotonin) and some other transmitters are recycled into nerve endings by transport molecules. Probenecid, which inhibits transport of uric acid, penicillin, and other weak acids in the nephron, is used to increase the excretion of uric acid in gout. The family of P-glycoprotein transport molecules, previously identified in malignant cells as one cause of cancer drug resistance, has been identified in the epithelium of the gastrointestinal tract and in the blood-brain barrier.

4. Endocytosis, pinocytosis—Endocytosis occurs through binding of the transported molecule to specialized components (receptors) on cell membranes, with subsequent internalization by infolding of that area of the membrane. The contents of the resulting intracellular vesicle are subsequently released into the cytoplasm of the cell. Endocytosis permits very large or very lipid-insoluble chemicals to enter cells. For example, large molecules such as proteins may cross cell membranes by endocytosis. Smaller, polar substances such as vitamin B_{12} and iron combine with special proteins (B_{12} with intrinsic factor and iron with transferrin), and the complexes enter cells by this mechanism. Because the substance to be transported must combine with a membrane receptor, endocytotic transport can be quite selective. **Exocytosis** is the reverse process, that is, the expulsion of material that is membrane-encapsulated inside the cell from the cell. Most neurotransmitters are released by exocytosis.

B. Fick's Law of Diffusion

Fick's law predicts the rate of movement of molecules across a barrier. The concentration gradient ($C_1 - C_2$) and permeability coefficient for the drug and the area and thickness of the barrier membrane are used to compute the rate as follows:

$$Rate = (C_1 - C_2) \times \frac{Permeability\ coefficient}{Thickness} \times Area \qquad (1)$$

Thus, drug absorption is faster from organs with large surface areas, such as the small intestine, than from organs with smaller absorbing areas (the stomach). Furthermore, drug absorption is faster from organs with thin membrane barriers (eg, the lung) than from those with thick barriers (eg, the skin).

C. Water and Lipid Solubility of Drugs

1. Solubility—The aqueous solubility of a drug is often a function of the electrostatic charge (degree of ionization, polarity) of the molecule, because water molecules behave as dipoles and are attracted to charged drug molecules, forming an aqueous shell around them. Conversely, the lipid solubility of a molecule is inversely proportional to its charge.

Many drugs are weak bases or weak acids. For such molecules, the *pH of the medium* determines the fraction of molecules charged (ionized) versus uncharged (nonionized). If the pK_a of the drug and the pH of the medium are known, the fraction of molecules in the ionized state can be predicted by means of the **Henderson-Hasselbalch** equation:

$$\log\left(\frac{Protonated\ form}{Unprotonated\ form}\right) = pK_a - pH \qquad (2)$$

"Protonated" means *associated with a proton* (a hydrogen ion); this form of the equation applies to both acids and bases.

2. Ionization of weak acids and bases—Weak bases are ionized—and therefore more polar and more water-soluble—when they are protonated. Weak acids are not ionized—and so are less water-soluble—when they are protonated.

The following equations summarize these points:

RNH_3^+	RNH_2	$+$	H^+
protonated weak base (charged, more water-soluble)	unprotonated weak base (uncharged, more lipid-soluble)	proton	(3)

$RCOOH$	$RCOO^-$	$+$	H^+
protonated weak acid (uncharged, more lipid-soluble)	unprotonated weak acid (charged, more water-soluble)	proton	(4)

The Henderson-Hasselbalch relationship is clinically important when it is necessary to estimate or alter the partition of drugs between compartments of differing pH. For example, most drugs

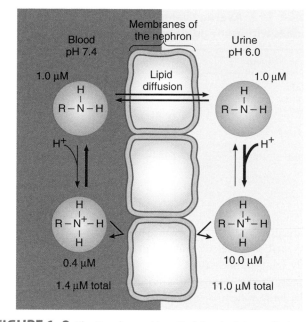

FIGURE 1-2 The Henderson-Hasselbalch principle applied to drug excretion in the urine. Because the nonionized form diffuses readily across the lipid barriers of the nephron, this form may reach equal concentrations in the blood and urine; in contrast, the ionized form does not diffuse as readily. Protonation occurs within the blood and the urine according to the Henderson-Hasselbalch equation. Pyrimethamine, a weak base of pK_a 7.0, is used in this example. At blood pH, only 0.4 μmol of the protonated species will be present for each 1.0 μmol of the unprotonated form. The total concentration in the blood will thus be 1.4 μmol/L if the concentration of the unprotonated form is 1.0 μmol/L. In the urine at pH 6.0, 10 μmol of the nondiffusible ionized form will be present for each 1.0 μmol of the unprotonated, diffusible, form. Therefore, the total urine concentration (11 μmol/L) may be almost 8 times higher than the blood concentration.

TABLE 1-1 Common routes of drug administration.

Oral (swallowed)	Offers maximal convenience; absorption is often slower. Subject to the **first-pass effect**, in which a significant amount of the agent is metabolized in the gut wall, portal circulation, and liver before it reaches the systemic circulation
Buccal and sublingual (not swallowed)	Direct absorption into the systemic venous circulation, bypassing the hepatic portal circuit and first-pass metabolism
Intravenous	Instantaneous and complete absorption (by definition, bioavailability is 100%). Potentially more dangerous
Intramuscular	Often faster and more complete (higher bioavailability) than with oral administration. Large volumes may be given if the drug is not too irritating. First-pass metabolism is avoided
Subcutaneous	Slower absorption than the intramuscular route. First-pass metabolism is avoided.
Rectal (suppository)	The rectal route offers partial avoidance of the first-pass effect. Larger amounts of drug and drugs with unpleasant tastes are better administered rectally than by the buccal or sublingual routes
Inhalation	Route offers delivery closest to respiratory tissues (eg, for asthma). Usually very rapid absorption (eg, for anesthetic gases)
Topical	The topical route includes application to the skin or to the mucous membrane of the eye, ear, nose, throat, airway, or vagina for *local* effect
Transdermal	The transdermal route involves application to the skin for *systemic* effect. Absorption usually occurs very slowly (because of the thickness of the skin), but the first-pass effect is avoided

are freely filtered at the glomerulus, but lipid-soluble drugs can be rapidly reabsorbed from the tubular urine. If a patient takes an overdose of a weak acid drug, for example, aspirin, the excretion of this drug is faster in alkaline urine. This is because a drug that is a weak acid dissociates to its charged, polar form in alkaline solution, and this form cannot readily diffuse from the renal tubule back into the blood; that is, the drug is trapped in the tubule. Conversely, excretion of a weak base (eg, pyrimethamine, amphetamine) is faster in acidic urine (Figure 1–2).

ABSORPTION OF DRUGS

A. Routes of Administration

Drugs usually enter the body at sites remote from the target tissue or organ and thus require transport by the circulation to the intended site of action. To enter the bloodstream, a drug must be absorbed from its site of administration (unless the drug has been injected directly into the vascular compartment). The rate and efficiency of absorption differ depending on a drug's route of administration. In fact, for some drugs, the amount absorbed may be only a small fraction of the dose administered when given by certain routes. The amount absorbed into the systemic circulation divided by the amount of drug administered constitutes its **bioavailability** by that route. Common routes of administration and some of their features are listed in Table 1–1.

B. Blood Flow

Blood flow influences absorption from intramuscular and subcutaneous sites and, in shock, from the gastrointestinal tract as well. High blood flow maintains a high drug depot-to-blood concentration gradient and thus facilitates absorption.

C. Concentration

The concentration of drug at the site of administration is important in determining the concentration gradient relative to the blood as noted previously. As indicated by Fick's law (Equation 1), the concentration gradient is a major determinant of the rate of absorption. Drug concentration in the vehicle is particularly important in the absorption of drugs applied topically.

DISTRIBUTION OF DRUGS

A. Determinants of Distribution

The distribution of drugs to the tissues depends on the following:

1. Size of the organ—The size of the organ determines the concentration gradient between blood and the organ. For example, skeletal muscle can take up a large *amount* of drug because the concentration in the muscle tissue remains low (and the blood-tissue gradient high) even after relatively large amounts of drug have been transferred; this occurs because skeletal muscle is a very large organ. In contrast, because the brain is smaller, distribution of a smaller amount of drug into it will raise the tissue concentration and reduce to zero the blood-tissue concentration gradient, preventing further uptake of drug.

2. Blood flow—Blood flow to the tissue is an important determinant of the *rate of uptake* of drug, although blood flow may not affect the *amount* of drug in the tissue at equilibrium. As a result, well-perfused tissues (eg, brain, heart, kidneys, and splanchnic organs) usually achieve high tissue concentrations sooner than poorly perfused tissues (eg, fat, bone).

3. Solubility—The solubility of a drug in tissue influences the concentration of the drug in the extracellular fluid surrounding the blood vessels. If the drug is very soluble in the cells, the concentration in the perivascular extracellular space will be lower and diffusion from the vessel into the extravascular tissue space will be facilitated. For example, some organs (such as the brain) have a high lipid content and thus dissolve a high concentration of lipid-soluble agents rapidly.

4. Binding—Binding of a drug to macromolecules in the blood or a tissue compartment tends to increase the drug's concentration in that compartment. For example, warfarin is strongly bound to plasma albumin, which restricts warfarin's diffusion out of the vascular compartment. Conversely, chloroquine is strongly bound to extravascular tissue proteins, which results in a marked reduction in the plasma concentration of chloroquine.

B. Apparent Volume of Distribution and Physical Volumes

The apparent volume of distribution (V_d) is an important pharmacokinetic parameter that reflects the above determinants of the distribution of a drug in the body. V_d relates the amount of drug in the body to the concentration in the plasma (Chapter 3). In contrast, the physical volumes of various body compartments are less important in pharmacokinetics (Table 1–2). However,

TABLE 1–2 Average values for some physical volumes within the adult human body.

Compartment	Volume (L/kg body weight)
Plasma	0.04
Blood	0.08
Extracellular water	0.2
Total body water	0.6
Fat	0.2–0.35

obesity alters the ratios of total body water to body weight and fat to total body weight, and this may be important when using highly lipid-soluble drugs. A simple approximate rule for the aqueous compartments of the normal body is as follows: 40% of the body weight is intracellular water and 20% is extracellular water; thus, water constitutes approximately 60% of body weight.

METABOLISM OF DRUGS

Drug **disposition** is sometimes used to refer to metabolism and elimination of drugs. Some authorities use disposition to denote distribution as well as metabolism and elimination. Metabolism of a drug sometimes terminates its action, but other effects of drug metabolism are also important. Some drugs when given orally are metabolized before they enter the systemic circulation. This first-pass metabolism was referred to in Table 1–1 as one cause of low bioavailability. Drug metabolism occurs primarily in the liver and is discussed in greater detail in Chapter 4.

A. Drug Metabolism as a Mechanism of Termination of Drug Action

The action of many drugs (eg, sympathomimetics, phenothiazines) is terminated before they are excreted because they are metabolized to biologically inactive derivatives. Conversion to a metabolite is a form of **elimination**.

B. Drug Metabolism as a Mechanism of Drug Activation

Prodrugs (eg, levodopa, minoxidil) are inactive as administered and must be metabolized in the body to become active. Many drugs are active as administered and have active metabolites as well (eg, morphine, some benzodiazepines).

C. Drug Elimination Without Metabolism

Some drugs (eg, lithium, many others) are not modified by the body; they continue to act until they are excreted.

ELIMINATION OF DRUGS

Along with the dosage, the rate of elimination following the last dose (disappearance of the active molecules from the site of action, the bloodstream, and the body) determines the duration of action for most drugs. Therefore, knowledge of the time course of concentration in plasma is important in predicting the intensity and duration of effect for most drugs. ***Note:*** Drug *elimination* is not the same as drug *excretion:* A drug may be eliminated by metabolism long before the modified molecules are excreted from the body. For most drugs and their metabolites, excretion is primarily by way of the kidney. Anesthetic gases, a major exception, are excreted primarily by the lungs. For drugs with active metabolites (eg, diazepam), elimination of the parent molecule by metabolism is not synonymous with termination of action. For drugs that are not metabolized, excretion is the mode of elimination. A small number of drugs combine irreversibly with their receptors, so that disappearance from the bloodstream is not equivalent to cessation of drug action: These drugs may have a very prolonged action. For example, phenoxybenzamine, an irreversible inhibitor of α adrenoceptors, is eliminated from the bloodstream in less than 1 h after administration. The drug's action, however, lasts for 48 h, the time required for turnover of the receptors.

A. First-Order Elimination

The term *first-order elimination* implies that the rate of elimination is proportional to the concentration (ie, the higher the concentration, the greater the amount of drug eliminated per unit time). The result is that the drug's concentration in plasma decreases exponentially with time (Figure 1–3, left). Drugs with first-order elimination have a characteristic **half-life of elimination** that is constant regardless of the amount of drug in the body. The concentration of such a drug in the blood will decrease by 50% for every half-life. Most drugs in clinical use demonstrate first-order kinetics.

B. Zero-Order Elimination

The term *zero-order elimination* implies that the rate of elimination is constant regardless of concentration (Figure 1–3, right). This occurs with drugs that saturate their elimination mechanisms at concentrations of clinical interest. As a result, the concentrations of these drugs in plasma decrease in a linear fashion over time. This is typical of ethanol (over most of its plasma concentration range) and of phenytoin and aspirin at high therapeutic or toxic concentrations.

PHARMACOKINETIC MODELS

A. Multicompartment Distribution

After absorption into the circulation, many drugs undergo an early distribution phase followed by a slower elimination phase. Mathematically, this behavior can be simulated by means of a "two-compartment model" as shown in Figure 1–4. The two compartments consist of the blood and the extravascular tissues. (Note that each phase is associated with a characteristic half-life: $t_{1/2\alpha}$ for the first phase, $t_{1/2\beta}$ for the second phase. Note also that when concentration is plotted on a logarithmic axis, the elimination phase for a first-order drug is a straight line.)

B. Other Distribution Models

A few drugs behave as if they were distributed to only 1 compartment (eg, if they are restricted to the vascular compartment). Others have more complex distributions that require more than 2 compartments for construction of accurate mathematical models.

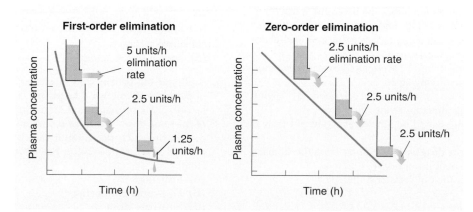

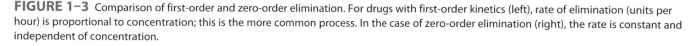

FIGURE 1–3 Comparison of first-order and zero-order elimination. For drugs with first-order kinetics (left), rate of elimination (units per hour) is proportional to concentration; this is the more common process. In the case of zero-order elimination (right), the rate is constant and independent of concentration.

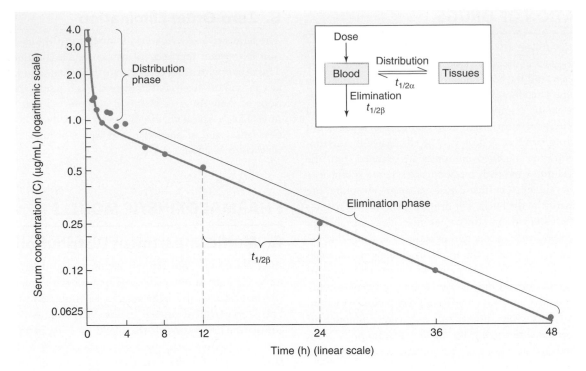

FIGURE 1–4 Serum concentration-time curve after administration of chlordiazepoxide as an intravenous bolus. The experimental data are plotted on a semilogarithmic scale as filled circles. This drug follows first-order kinetics and appears to occupy two compartments. The initial curvilinear portion of the data represents the distribution phase, with drug equilibrating between the blood compartment and the tissue compartment. The linear portion of the curve represents drug elimination. The elimination half-life ($t_{1/2\beta}$) can be extracted graphically as shown by measuring the time between any two plasma concentration points on the elimination phase that differ by twofold. (See Chapter 3 for additional details.) (Modified and reproduced, with permission, from Greenblatt DJ, Koch-Weser J: Drug therapy: Clinical pharmacokinetics. *N Engl J Med* 1975;293:702. Copyright © 1975 Massachusetts Medical Society. All rights reserved.)

QUESTIONS

1. A 3-year-old is brought to the emergency department having just ingested a large overdose of diphenhydramine, an antihistaminic drug. Diphenhydramine is a weak base with a pK_a of 8.8. It is capable of entering most tissues, including the brain. On physical examination, the heart rate is 100/min, blood pressure 90/50 mm Hg, and respiratory rate 20/min. Which of the following statements about this case of diphenhydramine overdose is most correct?
   (A) Urinary excretion would be accelerated by administration of NH_4Cl, an acidifying agent
   (B) Urinary excretion would be accelerated by giving $NaHCO_3$, an alkalinizing agent
   (C) More of the drug would be ionized at blood pH than at stomach pH
   (D) Absorption of the drug would be faster from the stomach than from the small intestine
   (E) Hemodialysis is the only effective therapy

2. Botulinum toxin is a large protein molecule. Its action on cholinergic transmission depends on an intracellular action within nerve endings. Which one of the following processes is best suited for permeation of very large protein molecules into cells?
   (A) Aqueous diffusion
   (B) Aqueous hydrolysis
   (C) Endocytosis
   (D) Lipid diffusion
   (E) Special carrier transport

3. A 60-year-old patient with severe cancer pain is given 10 mg of morphine by mouth. The plasma concentration is found to be only 30% of that found after intravenous administration of the same dose. Which of the following terms describes the process by which the amount of active drug in the body is reduced *after* administration but *before* entering the systemic circulation?
   (A) Excretion
   (B) First-order elimination
   (C) First-pass effect
   (D) Metabolism
   (E) Pharmacokinetics

4. A 12-year-old child has bacterial pharyngitis and is to receive an oral antibiotic. Ampicillin is a weak organic acid with a pK_a of 2.5. What percentage of a given dose will be in the lipid-soluble form in the duodenum at a pH of 4.5?
(A) About 1%
(B) About 10%
(C) About 50%
(D) About 90%
(E) About 99%

5. Ampicillin is eliminated by first-order kinetics. Which of the following statements best describes the process by which the plasma concentration of this drug declines?
(A) There is only 1 metabolic path for drug elimination
(B) The half-life is the same regardless of the plasma concentration
(C) The drug is largely metabolized in the liver after oral administration and has low bioavailability
(D) The rate of elimination is proportional to the rate of administration at all times
(E) The drug is distributed to only 1 compartment outside the vascular system

6. Which of the following statements is most correct regarding the termination of drug action?
(A) Drugs must be excreted from the body to terminate their action
(B) Metabolism of drugs always increases their water solubility
(C) Metabolism of drugs always abolishes their pharmacologic activity
(D) Hepatic metabolism and renal excretion are the two most important mechanisms involved
(E) Distribution of a drug out of the bloodstream terminates the drug's effects

7. Which statement about the distribution of drugs to specific tissues is most correct?
(A) Distribution to an organ is independent of blood flow
(B) Distribution is independent of the solubility of the drug in that tissue
(C) Distribution depends on the unbound drug concentration gradient between blood and the tissue
(D) Distribution is increased for drugs that are strongly bound to plasma proteins
(E) Distribution has no effect on the half-life of the drug

8. The pharmacokinetic process that distinguishes the elimination of ethanol and high doses of phenytoin and aspirin from the elimination of most other drugs is called
(A) Distribution
(B) Excretion
(C) First-pass effect
(D) First-order elimination
(E) Zero-order elimination

9. The set of properties that characterize the effects of a drug on the body is called
(A) Distribution
(B) Permeation
(C) Pharmacodynamics
(D) Pharmacokinetics
(E) Protonation

10. A new drug was administered intravenously, and its plasma levels were measured for several hours. A graph was prepared as shown below, with the plasma levels plotted on a logarithmic ordinate and time on a linear abscissa. It was concluded that the drug has first-order kinetics. From this graph, what is the best estimate of the half-life?

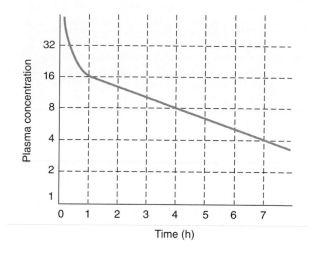

(A) 0.5 h
(B) 1 h
(C) 3 h
(D) 4 h
(E) 7 h

ANSWERS

1. Questions that deal with acid-base (Henderson-Hasselbalch) manipulations are common on examinations. Since absorption involves permeation across lipid membranes, we can in theory treat an overdose by decreasing absorption from the gut and reabsorption from the tubular urine by making the drug *less lipid-soluble*. Ionization attracts water molecules and decreases lipid solubility. Diphenhydramine is a weak base, which means that it is more ionized when protonated, ie, at acid pH. Choice **C** suggests that the drug would be more ionized at pH 7.4 than at pH 2.0, which is clearly wrong. Choice **D** says (in effect) that the more ionized form is absorbed faster, which is incorrect. **A** and **B** are opposites because NH_4Cl is an acidifying salt and sodium bicarbonate an alkalinizing one. (From the point of view of test strategy, opposites in a list of answers always deserve careful attention.) **E** is a distracter. Because an acid environment favors ionization of a weak base, we should give NH_4Cl. The answer is **A**. Note that clinical management of overdose involves many other considerations in addition to trapping the drug in urine; manipulation of urine pH may be contraindicated for other reasons.

2. Endocytosis is an important mechanism for transport of very large molecules across membranes. Aqueous diffusion is not involved in transport across the lipid barrier of cell membranes. Lipid diffusion and special carrier transport are common for smaller molecules. Hydrolysis has nothing to do with the mechanisms of permeation; rather, hydrolysis is one mechanism of drug metabolism. The answer is **C**.

3. U.S. Medical Licensing Examination (USMLE)-type questions often contain a lengthy clinical description in the stem. One can often determine the relevance of the clinical data by scanning the list of answers, see Appendix IV. In this question, the emphasis is clearly on pharmacokinetic principles. "First-pass effect" is the term given to elimination of a drug before it enters the systemic circulation (ie, on its first pass through the portal circulation and liver). The first-pass effect is usually, but not always, due to metabolism in the gut, the portal blood, or the liver. The answer is **C**.

4. Ampicillin is an acid, so it is more ionized at alkaline pH and less ionized at acidic pH. The Henderson-Hasselbalch equation predicts that the ratio changes from 50/50 at the pH equal to the pK_a to 1/10 (protonated/unprotonated) at 1 pH unit more alkaline than the pK_a and 1/100 at 2 pH units more alkaline. For acids, the protonated form is the nonionized, more lipid-soluble form. The answer is **A**.

5. "First-order" means that the elimination rate is proportional to the concentration perfusing the organ of elimination. The half-life is a constant. The rate of elimination is proportional to the rate of administration only at steady state. The order of elimination is independent of the number of compartments into which a drug distributes. The answer is **B**.

6. Note the "trigger" words ("must," "always") in choices **A, B,** and **C,** see Appendix IV. The answer is **D**.

7. This is a straightforward question of pharmacokinetic distribution concepts. From the list of determinants of drug distribution given on page 6, choice **C** is correct.

8. The excretion of most drugs follows first-order kinetics. However, ethanol and, in higher doses, aspirin and phenytoin follow zero-order kinetics; that is, their elimination rates are constant regardless of blood concentration. The answer is **E**.

9. Definitions. Pharmacodynamics is the term given to drug actions on the body. The answer is **C**.

10. Drugs with first-order kinetics have constant half-lives, and when the log of the concentration in a body compartment is plotted versus time, a straight line results. The half-life is defined as the time required for the concentration to decrease by 50%. As shown in the graph, the concentration decreased from 16 units at 1 h to 8 units at 4 h and 4 units at 7 h; therefore, the half-life is 4 h minus 1 h or 3 h. The answer is **C**.

CHECKLIST

When you complete this chapter, you should be able to:

❑ Define and describe the terms receptor and receptor site.

❑ Distinguish between a competitive inhibitor and an allosteric inhibitor.

❑ Predict the relative ease of permeation of a weak acid or base from a knowledge of its pK_a, the pH of the medium, and the Henderson-Hasselbalch equation.

❑ List and discuss the common routes of drug administration and excretion.

❑ Draw graphs of the blood level versus time for drugs subject to zero-order elimination and for drugs subject to first-order elimination. Label the axes appropriately.

CHAPTER 1 Summary Table

Major Concept	Description
Nature of drugs	Drugs are chemicals that modify body functions. They may be ions, carbohydrates, lipids, or proteins. They vary in size from lithium (MW 7) to proteins (MW ≥ 50,000)
Drug permeation	Most drugs are administered at a site distant from their target tissue. To reach the target, they must permeate through both lipid and aqueous pathways. Movement of drugs occurs by means of aqueous diffusion, lipid diffusion, transport by special carriers, or by exocytosis and endocytosis
Rate of diffusion	Aqueous diffusion and lipid diffusion are predicted by Fick's law and are directly proportional to the concentration gradient, area, and permeability coefficient and inversely proportional to the length or thickness of the diffusion path
Drug trapping	Because the permeability coefficient of a weak base or weak acid varies with the pH according to the Henderson-Hasselbalch equation, drugs may be trapped in a cellular compartment in which the pH is such as to reduce their solubility in the barriers surrounding the compartment
Routes of administration	Drugs are usually administered by one of the following routes of administration: oral, buccal, sublingual, topical, transdermal, intravenous, subcutaneous, intramuscular, or rectal, or by inhalation
Drug distribution	After absorption, drugs are distributed to different parts of the body depending on concentration gradient, blood flow, solubility, and binding in the tissue
Drug elimination	Drugs are eliminated by reducing their concentration or amount in the body. This occurs when the drug is inactivated by metabolism or excreted from the body
Elimination kinetics	The rate of elimination of drugs may be zero order (ie, constant regardless of concentration) or first order (ie, proportional to the concentration)

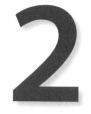

Pharmacodynamics

Pharmacodynamics deals with the effects of drugs on biologic systems, whereas pharmacokinetics (Chapter 3) deals with actions of the biologic system on the drug. The principles of pharmacodynamics apply to all biologic systems, from isolated receptors in the test tube to patients with specific diseases.

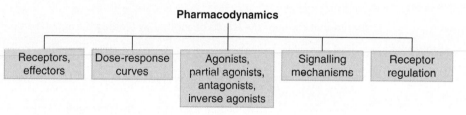

Pharmacodynamics

- Receptors, effectors
- Dose-response curves
- Agonists, partial agonists, antagonists, inverse agonists
- Signalling mechanisms
- Receptor regulation

RECEPTORS

Receptors are the specific molecules in a biologic system with which drugs interact to produce changes in the function of the system. Receptors must be **selective** in their ligand-binding characteristics (so as to respond to the proper chemical signal and not to meaningless ones). Receptors must also be **modifiable** when they bind a drug molecule (so as to bring about the functional change). Many receptors have been identified, purified, chemically characterized, and cloned. Most are proteins; a few are other macromolecules such as DNA. Some authorities consider enzymes as a separate category; for the purposes of this book, enzymes that are affected by drugs are considered receptors. The **receptor site** (also known as the **recognition site**) for a drug is the specific binding region of the receptor macromolecule and has a relatively high and selective affinity for the drug molecule. The interaction of a drug with its receptor is the fundamental event that initiates the action of the drug, and many drugs are classified on the basis of their primary receptor affinity.

EFFECTORS

Effectors are molecules that translate the drug-receptor interaction into a change in cellular activity. The best examples of effectors are enzymes such as adenylyl cyclase. Some receptors are also effectors in that a single molecule may incorporate both the drug-binding site and the effector mechanism. For example, a tyrosine kinase effector is part of the insulin receptor molecule, and a sodium-potassium channel is the effector part of the nicotinic acetylcholine receptor.

GRADED DOSE-RESPONSE RELATIONSHIPS

When the response of a particular receptor-effector system is measured against increasing concentrations of a drug, the graph of the response versus the drug concentration or dose is called a *graded dose-response curve* (Figure 2–1A). Plotting the same data on a semilogarithmic concentration axis usually results in a sigmoid curve, which simplifies the mathematical manipulation of the dose-response data (Figure 2–1B). The efficacy (E_{max}) and potency (EC_{50} or ED_{50}) parameters are derived from these data. The *smaller* the EC_{50} (or ED_{50}), the *greater* the potency of the drug.

GRADED DOSE-BINDING RELATIONSHIP & BINDING AFFINITY

It is possible to measure the percentage of receptors bound by a drug, and by plotting this percentage against the log of the concentration of the drug, a *dose-binding* graph similar to the dose-response

High-Yield Terms to Learn

Receptor	A molecule to which a drug binds to bring about a change in function of the biologic system
Inert binding molecule or site	A molecule to which a drug may bind without changing any function
Receptor site	Specific region of the receptor molecule to which the drug binds
Spare receptor	Receptor that does not bind drug when the drug concentration is sufficient to produce maximal effect; present when $K_d > EC_{50}$
Effector	Component of a system that accomplishes the biologic effect after the receptor is activated by an agonist; often a channel or enzyme molecule, may be part of the receptor molecule
Agonist	A drug that activates its receptor upon binding
Pharmacologic antagonist	A drug that binds without activating its receptor and thereby prevents activation by an agonist
Competitive antagonist	A pharmacologic antagonist that can be overcome by increasing the concentration of agonist
Irreversible antagonist	A pharmacologic antagonist that cannot be overcome by increasing agonist concentration
Physiologic antagonist	A drug that counters the effects of another by binding to a different receptor and causing opposing effects
Chemical antagonist	A drug that counters the effects of another by binding the agonist drug (not the receptor)
Allosteric agonist, antagonist	A drug that binds to a receptor molecule without interfering with normal agonist binding but alters the response to the normal agonist
Partial agonist	A drug that binds to its receptor but produces a smaller effect at full dosage than a full agonist
Inverse agonist	A drug that binds to the inactive state of receptor molecules and decreases constitutive activity (see text)
Graded dose-response curve	A graph of increasing response to increasing drug concentration or dose
Quantal dose-response curve	A graph of the fraction of a population that shows a specified response at progressively increasing doses
EC_{50}, ED_{50}, TD_{50}, etc	In graded dose-response curves, the concentration or dose that causes 50% of the maximal effect or toxicity. In quantal dose-response curves, the concentration or dose that causes a specified response in 50% of the population under study
K_d	The concentration of drug that binds 50% of the receptors in the system
Efficacy, maximal efficacy	The maximal effect that can be achieved with a particular drug, regardless of dose

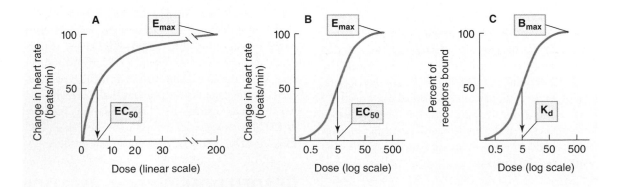

FIGURE 2–1 Graded dose-response and dose-binding graphs. (In isolated tissue preparations, *concentration* is usually used as the measure of dose.) **A.** Relation between drug dose or concentration (abscissa) and drug effect (ordinate). When the dose axis is linear, a hyperbolic curve is commonly obtained. **B.** Same data, logarithmic dose axis. The dose or concentration at which effect is half-maximal is denoted EC_{50}, whereas the maximal effect is E_{max}. **C.** If the percentage of receptors that bind drug is plotted against drug concentration, a similar curve is obtained, and the concentration at which 50% of the receptors are bound is denoted K_d, and the maximal number of receptors bound is termed B_{max}.

curve is obtained (Figure 2–1C). The concentration of drug required to bind 50% of the receptor sites is denoted K_d and is a useful measure of the affinity of a drug molecule for its binding site on the receptor molecule. The smaller the K_d, the greater the affinity of the drug for its receptor. If the number of binding sites on each receptor molecule is known, it is possible to determine the total number of receptors in the system from the $\mathbf{B_{max}}$.

QUANTAL DOSE-RESPONSE RELATIONSHIPS

When the minimum dose required to produce a specified response is determined in each member of a population, the *quantal dose-response relationship* is defined (Figure 2–2). For example, a blood pressure-lowering drug might be studied by measuring the dose required to lower the mean arterial pressure by 20 mm Hg in 100 hypertensive patients. When plotted as the percentage of the population that shows this response at each dose versus the log of the dose administered, a cumulative quantal dose-response curve, usually sigmoid in shape, is obtained. The **median effective (ED_{50}), median toxic (TD_{50})**, and (in animals) **median lethal (LD_{50})** doses are derived from experiments carried out in this manner. Because the magnitude of the specified effect is arbitrarily determined, the ED_{50} determined by quantal dose-response measurements has no direct relation to the ED_{50} determined from

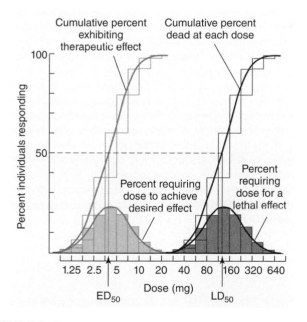

FIGURE 2–2 Quantal dose-response plots from a study of the therapeutic and lethal effects of a new drug in mice. Shaded boxes (and the accompanying bell-shaped curves) indicate the frequency distribution of doses of drug required to produce a specified effect, that is, the percentage of animals that required a particular dose to exhibit the effect. The open boxes (and corresponding sigmoidal curves) indicate the cumulative frequency distribution of responses, which are lognormally distributed. (Modified and reproduced, with permission, from Katzung BG, editor: *Basic & Clinical Pharmacology*, 12th ed. McGraw-Hill, 2012: Fig. 2–2.)

graded dose-response curves. Unlike the graded dose-response determination, no attempt is made to determine the maximal effect of the drug. Quantal dose-response data provide information about the variation in sensitivity to the drug in a given population, and if the variation is small, the curve is steep.

EFFICACY

Efficacy—often called maximal efficacy—is the greatest effect (E_{max}) an agonist can produce if the dose is taken to the highest tolerated level. Efficacy is determined mainly by the nature of the drug and the receptor and its associated effector system. It can be measured with a graded dose-response curve (Figure 2–1) but not with a quantal dose-response curve. By definition, **partial agonists** have lower maximal efficacy than full agonists (see later discussion).

POTENCY

Potency denotes the amount of drug needed to produce a given effect. In graded dose-response measurements, the effect usually chosen is 50% of the maximal effect and the concentration or dose causing this effect is called the **EC_{50}** or **ED_{50}** (Figure 2–1A and B). Potency is determined mainly by the affinity of the receptor for the drug and the number of receptors available. In quantal dose-response measurements, **ED_{50}, TD_{50},** and **LD_{50}** are also potency variables (median effective, toxic, and lethal doses, respectively, in 50% of the population studied). Thus, potency can be determined from either graded or quantal dose-response curves (eg, Figures 2–1 and 2–2, respectively), but the numbers obtained are not identical.

SPARE RECEPTORS

Spare receptors are said to exist if the maximal drug response (E_{max}) is obtained at less than 100% occupation of the receptors (B_{max}). In practice, the determination is usually made by comparing the concentration for 50% of maximal effect (EC_{50}) with the concentration for 50% of maximal binding (K_d). If the EC_{50} is less than the K_d, spare receptors are said to exist (Figure 2–3). This might result from 1 of 2 mechanisms. First, the duration of the activation of the effector may be much greater than the duration of the drug-receptor interaction. Second, the actual number of receptors may exceed the number of effector molecules available. The presence of spare receptors increases sensitivity to the agonist because the likelihood of a drug-receptor interaction increases in proportion to the number of receptors available. (For contrast, the system depicted in Figure 2–1, panels B and C, does not have spare receptors, since the EC_{50} and the K_d are equal.)

AGONISTS, PARTIAL AGONISTS, & INVERSE AGONISTS

Modern concepts of drug-receptor interactions consider the receptor to have at least 2 states—active and inactive. In the

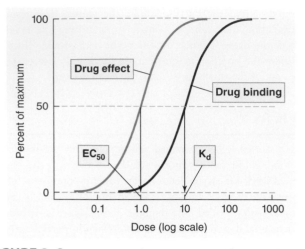

FIGURE 2–3 In a system with spare receptors, the EC_{50} is lower than the K_d, indicating that to achieve 50% of maximal effect, less than 50% of the receptors must be activated. Explanations for this phenomenon are discussed in the text.

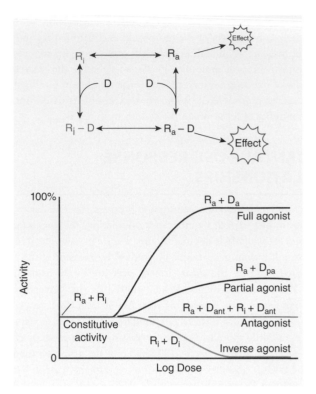

FIGURE 2–4 **Upper:** One model of drug-receptor interactions. The receptor is able to assume 2 conformations, R_i and R_a. In the R_i state, it is inactive and produces no effect, even when combined with a drug (D) molecule. In the R_a state, it activates its effectors and an effect is recorded, even in the absence of ligand. In the absence of drug, the equilibrium between R_i and R_a determines the degree of constitutive activity. **Lower:** A full agonist drug (D_a) has a much higher affinity for the R_a than for the R_i receptor conformation, and a maximal effect is produced at sufficiently high drug concentration. A partial agonist drug (D_{pa}) has somewhat greater affinity for the R_a than for the R_i conformation and produces less effect, even at saturating concentrations. A neutral antagonist (D_{ant}) binds with equal affinity to both receptor conformations and prevents binding of agonist. An inverse agonist (D_i) binds much more avidly to the R_i receptor conformation, prevents conversion to the R_a state, and reduces constitutive activity. (Modified and reproduced, with permission, from Katzung BG, editor: *Basic & Clinical Pharmacology*, 12th ed. McGraw-Hill, 2012: Fig. 1–4.)

absence of ligand, a receptor might be fully active or completely inactive; alternatively, an equilibrium state might exist with some receptors in the activated state and with most in the inactive state ($R_a + R_i$; Figure 2–4). Many receptor systems exhibit some activity in the absence of ligand, suggesting that some fraction of the receptors are always in the activated state. Activity in the absence of ligand is called **constitutive activity**. A **full agonist** is a drug capable of fully activating the effector system when it binds to the receptor. In the model system illustrated in Figure 2–4, a full agonist has high affinity for the activated receptor conformation, and sufficiently high concentrations result in all the receptors achieving the activated state ($R_a – D_a$). A **partial agonist** produces less than the full effect, even when it has saturated the receptors (R_a-D_{pa} + R_i-D_{pa}), presumably by combining with both receptor conformations, but favoring the active state. In the presence of a full agonist, a partial agonist acts as an inhibitor. In this model, **neutral antagonists** bind with *equal* affinity to the R_i and R_a states, preventing binding by an agonist and preventing any deviation from the level of constitutive activity. In contrast, **inverse agonists** have a much higher affinity for the inactive R_i state than for R_a and decrease or abolish any constitutive activity.

ANTAGONISTS

A. Competitive and Irreversible Pharmacologic Antagonists

Competitive antagonists are drugs that bind to, or very close to, the agonist receptor site in a reversible way without activating the effector system for that receptor. Neutral antagonists bind the receptor without shifting the R_a versus R_i equilibrium (Figure 2–4). In the presence of a competitive antagonist, the log dose-response curve for an agonist is shifted to higher doses (ie, horizontally to

the right on the dose axis), but the same maximal effect is reached (Figure 2–5A). The agonist, if given in a high enough concentration, can displace the antagonist and fully activate the receptors. In contrast, an irreversible antagonist causes a downward shift of the maximum, with no shift of the curve on the dose axis unless spare receptors are present (Figure 2–5B). Unlike the effects of a competitive antagonist, the effects of an irreversible antagonist cannot be overcome by adding more agonist. Competitive antagonists increase the ED_{50}; irreversible antagonists do not (unless spare receptors are present). A noncompetitive antagonist that acts at an allosteric site of the receptor (see Figure 1–1) may bind reversibly

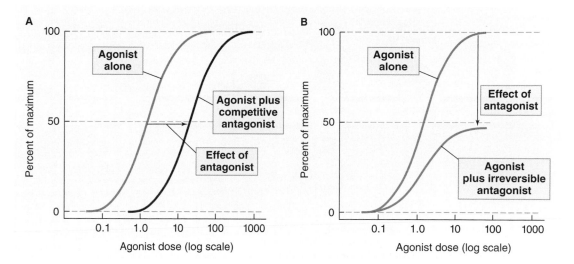

FIGURE 2–5 Agonist dose-response curves in the presence of competitive and irreversible antagonists. Note the use of a logarithmic scale for drug concentration. **A.** A competitive antagonist has an effect illustrated by the shift of the agonist curve to the right. **B.** An irreversible (or noncompetitive) antagonist shifts the agonist curve downward.

or irreversibly; a noncompetitive antagonist that acts at the receptor site binds irreversibly.

B. Physiologic Antagonists

A physiologic antagonist binds to a *different* receptor molecule, producing an effect opposite to that produced by the drug it antagonizes. Thus, it differs from a pharmacologic antagonist, which interacts with the *same* receptor as the drug it inhibits. Familiar examples of physiologic antagonists are the antagonism of the bronchoconstrictor action of histamine by epinephrine's bronchodilator action and glucagon's antagonism of the cardiac effects of propranolol.

C. Chemical Antagonists

A chemical antagonist interacts directly with the drug being antagonized to remove it or to prevent it from binding to its target. A chemical antagonist does not depend on interaction with the agonist's receptor (although such interaction may occur). Common examples of chemical antagonists are dimercaprol, a chelator of lead and some other toxic metals, and pralidoxime, which combines avidly with the phosphorus in organophosphate cholinesterase inhibitors.

> ### SKILL KEEPER: ALLOSTERIC ANTAGONISTS (SEE CHAPTER 1)
>
> *Describe the difference between a pharmacologic antagonist and an allosteric inhibitor. How could you differentiate these two experimentally?*

THERAPEUTIC INDEX & THERAPEUTIC WINDOW

The therapeutic index is the ratio of the TD_{50} (or LD_{50}) to the ED_{50}, determined from quantal dose-response curves. The therapeutic index represents an estimate of the safety of a drug, because a very safe drug might be expected to have a very large toxic dose and a much smaller effective dose. For example, in Figure 2–2, the ED_{50} is approximately 3 mg, and the LD_{50} is approximately 150 mg. The therapeutic index is therefore approximately 150/3, or 50, in mice. Obviously, a full range of toxic doses cannot be ethically studied in humans. Furthermore, factors such as the varying slopes of dose-response curves make this estimate a poor safety index even in animals.

The therapeutic window, a more clinically useful index of safety, describes the *dosage range* between the minimum effective therapeutic concentration or dose, and the minimum toxic concentration or dose. For example, if the average minimum therapeutic plasma concentration of theophylline is 8 mg/L and toxic effects are observed at 18 mg/L, the therapeutic window is 8–18 mg/L. Both the therapeutic index and the therapeutic window depend on the specific toxic effect used in the determination.

SIGNALING MECHANISMS

Once an agonist drug has bound to its receptor, some effector mechanism is activated. The receptor-effector system may be an enzyme in the intracellular space (eg, cyclooxygenase, a target of nonsteroidal anti-inflammatory drugs) or in the membrane or extracellular space (eg, acetylcholinesterase). Neurotransmitter reuptake transporters (eg, the norepinephrine transporter, NET, and the dopamine transporter, DAT, are receptors for many drugs, eg, antidepressants and cocaine. Most antiarrhythmic

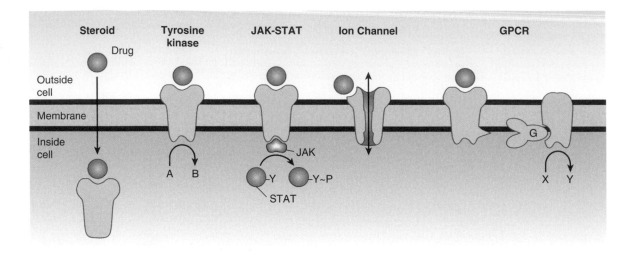

FIGURE 2–6 Signaling mechanisms for drug effects. Five major signaling mechanisms are recognized: (1) transmembrane diffusion of the drug to bind to an intracellular receptor; (2) transmembrane enzyme receptors, whose outer domain provides the receptor function and inner domain provides the effector mechanism converting A to B; (3) transmembrane receptors that, after activation by an appropriate ligand, activate separate cytoplasmic tyrosine kinase molecules (JAKs), which phosphorylate STAT molecules that regulate transcription (Y, tyrosine; P, phosphate); (4) transmembrane channels that are gated open or closed by the binding of a drug to the receptor site; and (5) G protein-coupled receptors, which use a coupling protein to activate a separate effector molecule. (Modified and reproduced, with permission, from Katzung BG, editor: *Basic & Clinical Pharmacology,* 12th ed. McGraw-Hill, 2012: Fig. 2–5.)

drugs target voltage-activated ion channels in the membrane for sodium, potassium, or calcium. For the largest group of drug-receptor interactions, the drug is present in the extracellular space, whereas the effector mechanism resides inside the cell and modifies some intracellular process. These classic drug-receptor interactions involve signaling *across* the membrane. Five major types of transmembrane-signaling mechanisms for receptor-effector systems have been defined (Figure 2–6, Table 2–1).

RECEPTOR REGULATION

Receptors are dynamically regulated in number, location, and sensitivity. Changes can occur over short times (minutes) and longer periods (days).

Frequent or continuous exposure to agonists often results in short-term diminution of the receptor response, sometimes called **tachyphylaxis**. Several mechanisms are responsible for this phenomenon.

TABLE 2–1 Types of transmembrane signaling receptors.

Receptor Type	Description
Steroid-like	Steroids, vitamin D, nitric oxide, and a few other highly membrane-permeable agents cross the membrane and activate intracellular receptors. The effector molecule may be part of the receptor or separate
Membrane-spanning receptor-effector enzymes	Insulin, epidermal growth factor, and similar agents bind to the extracellular domain of molecules that incorporate tyrosine kinase enzyme activity in their intracellular domains. Most of these receptors dimerize upon activation
Membrane receptors that bind intracellular tyrosine kinase enzymes	Many cytokines activate receptor molecules that bind intracellular tyrosine kinase enzymes (Janus kinases, JAKs) that activate transcription regulators (signal transducers and activators of transcription, STATs) that migrate to the nucleus to bring about the final effect
Ligand-activated or modulated membrane ion channels	Certain Na^+/K^+ channels are activated by drugs: acetylcholine activates nicotinic Na^+/K^+ channels, serotonin activates $5\text{-}HT_3$ Na^+/K^+ channels. Benzodiazepines and several other sedative hypnotics allosterically modulate GABA-activated Cl^- channels
G-protein-coupled receptors (GPCRs)	GPCRs consist of 7 transmembrane (7-TM) domains and when activated by extracellular ligands, bind trimeric G proteins and cause the release of activated G_α and $G_{\beta\gamma}$ units. These activated units, in turn, modulate cytoplasmic effectors. The effectors commonly synthesize or release second messengers such as cAMP, IP_3, and DAG. GPCRs are the most common type of receptors in the body

cAMP, cyclic adenosine monophosphate; IP_3, inositol trisphosphate; DAG, diacylglycerol.

First, intracellular molecules may block access of a G protein to the activated receptor molecule. For example, the molecule β-arrestin has been shown to bind to an intracellular loop of the β adrenoceptor when the receptor is continuously activated. Beta-arrestin prevents access of the G_s-coupling protein and thus desensitizes the tissue to further β-agonist activation within minutes. Removal of the β agonist results in removal of β-arrestin and restoration of the full response after a few minutes or hours.

Second, agonist-bound receptors may be internalized by endocytosis, removing them from further exposure to extracellular molecules. The internalized receptor molecule may then be either reinserted into the membrane (eg, morphine receptors) or degraded (eg, β adrenoceptors, epidermal growth factor receptors). In some cases, the internalization-reinsertion process may actually be necessary for normal functioning of the receptor-effector system.

Third, continuous activation of the receptor-effector system may lead to depletion of some essential substrate required for downstream effects. For example, depletion of thiol cofactors may be responsible for tolerance to nitroglycerin. In some cases, repletion of the missing substrate (eg, by administration of glutathione) can reverse the tolerance.

Long-term reductions in receptor number (**downregulation**) may occur in response to continuous exposure to agonists. The opposite change (**upregulation**) occurs when receptor activation is blocked for prolonged periods (usually several days) by pharmacologic antagonists or by denervation.

QUESTIONS

1. A 55-year-old woman with hypertension is to be treated with a vasodilator drug. Drugs X and Y have the same mechanism of action. Drug X in a dose of 5 mg produces the same decrease in blood pressure as 500 mg of drug Y. Which of the following statements best describes these results?
   (A) Drug Y is less efficacious than drug X
   (B) Drug X is about 100 times more potent than drug Y
   (C) Toxicity of drug X is less than that of drug Y
   (D) Drug X has a wider therapeutic window than drug Y
   (E) Drug X will have a shorter duration of action than drug Y because less of drug X is present over the time course of drug action

2. Graded and quantal dose-response curves are being used for evaluation of a new antiasthmatic drug in the animal laboratory and in clinical trials. Which of the following statements best describes *quantal* dose-response curves?
   (A) More precisely quantitated than graded dose-response curves
   (B) Obtainable from the study of intact subjects but not from isolated tissue preparations
   (C) Used to determine the maximal efficacy of the drug
   (D) Used to determine the statistical variation (standard deviation) of the maximal response to the drug
   (E) Used to determine the variation in sensitivity of subjects to the drug

3. Prior to clinical trials in patients with heart failure, an animal study was carried out to compare two new positive inotropic drugs (A and B) to a current standard agent (C). The results of cardiac output measurements are shown in the graph below.

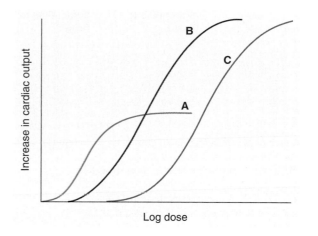

Which of the following statements is correct?
   (A) Drug A is most effective
   (B) Drug B is least potent
   (C) Drug C is most potent
   (D) Drug B is more potent than drug C and more effective than drug A
   (E) Drug A is more potent than drug B and more effective than drug C

4. A study was carried out in isolated, perfused animal hearts. In the absence of other drugs, pindolol, a β-adrenoceptor ligand, caused an increase in heart rate. In the presence of highly effective β stimulants, however, pindolol caused a dose-dependent, reversible decrease in heart rate. Which of the following expressions best describes pindolol?
   (A) A chemical antagonist
   (B) An irreversible antagonist
   (C) A partial agonist
   (D) A physiologic antagonist
   (E) A spare receptor agonist

5. Beta adrenoceptors in the heart regulate cardiac rate and contractile strength. Several studies have indicated that in humans and experimental animals, about 90% of β adrenoceptors in the heart are spare receptors. Which of the following statements about spare receptors is most correct?
   (A) Spare receptors, in the absence of drug, are sequestered in the cytoplasm
   (B) Spare receptors may be detected by finding that the drug-receptor interaction lasts longer than the intracellular effect
   (C) Spare receptors influence the maximal efficacy of the drug-receptor system
   (D) Spare receptors activate the effector machinery of the cell without the need for a drug
   (E) Spare receptors may be detected by the finding that the EC_{50} is smaller than the K_d for the agonist

6. Two cholesterol-lowering drugs, X and Y, were studied in a large group of patients, and the percentages of the group showing a specific therapeutic effect (35% reduction in low-density lipoprotein [LDL] cholesterol) were determined. The results are shown in the following table.

Drug Dose (mg)	Percent Responding to Drug X	Percent Responding to Drug Y
5	1	10
10	5	20
20	10	50
50	50	70
100	70	90
200	90	100

Which of the following statements about these results is correct?
(A) Drug X is safer than drug Y
(B) Drug Y is more effective than drug X
(C) The 2 drugs act on the same receptors
(D) Drug X is less potent than drug Y
(E) The therapeutic index of drug Y is 10

7. Sugammadex is a new drug that reverses the action of rocuronium and certain other skeletal muscle-relaxing agents. It appears to interact directly with the rocuronium molecule and not at all with the rocuronium receptor. Which of the following terms best describes sugammadex?
(A) Chemical antagonist
(B) Noncompetitive antagonist
(C) Partial agonist
(D) Pharmacologic antagonist
(E) Physiologic antagonist

DIRECTIONS: 8–10. Each of the curves in the graph below may be considered a concentration-effect curve or a concentration-binding curve.

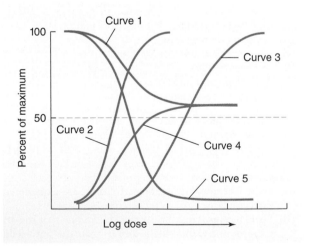

8. Which of the curves in the graph describes the percentage of *binding* of a large dose of full agonist to its receptors as the concentration of a partial agonist is increased from low to very high levels?
(A) Curve 1
(B) Curve 2
(C) Curve 3
(D) Curve 4
(E) Curve 5

9. Which of the curves in the graph describes the percentage *effect* observed when a large dose of full agonist is present throughout the experiment and the concentration of a partial agonist is increased from low to very high levels?
(A) Curve 1
(B) Curve 2
(C) Curve 3
(D) Curve 4
(E) Curve 5

10. Which of the curves in the graph describes the percentage of *binding* of the partial agonist whose *effect* is shown by Curve 4 if the system has many spare receptors?
(A) Curve 1
(B) Curve 2
(C) Curve 3
(D) Curve 4
(E) Curve 5

ANSWERS

1. No information is given regarding the maximal antihypertensive response to either drug. Similarly, no information about toxicity is provided. The fact that a given response is achieved with a smaller dose of drug X indicates that X is more potent than Y in the ratio of 500:5. The answer is **B.**

2. Graded (not quantal) dose-response curves must be used to determine maximal efficacy (maximal response). Quantal dose-response curves show only the frequency of occurrence of a specified response, which may be therapeutically effective (ED) or toxic (TD). The answer is **E.**

3. Drug A produces 50% of its maximal effect at a lower dose than either B or C and thus is the most potent; drug C is the least potent. However, drug A, a partial agonist, is less efficacious than drugs B and C. The answer is **D.**

4. Choices involving chemical or physiologic antagonism are incorrect because pindolol is said to act at β receptors and to block β stimulants. The drug effect is reversible, so choice **B** is incorrect. "Spare receptor agonist" is a nonsense distracter. The answer is **C.**

5. There is no difference in location between "spare" and other receptors. Spare receptors may be defined as those that are not needed for binding drug to achieve the maximal effect. Spare receptors influence the *sensitivity* of the system to an agonist because the statistical probability of a drug-receptor interaction increases with the total number of receptors. They do not alter the maximal efficacy. If they do not bind an agonist molecule, spare receptors do not activate an effector molecule. EC_{50} *less* than K_d is an indication of the presence of spare receptors. The answer is **E.**

6. No information is presented regarding the safety of these drugs. Similarly, no information on efficacy (maximal effect) is presented; this requires graded dose-response curves. Although both drugs are said to be producing a therapeutic effect, no information on their receptor mechanisms is given. Since no data on toxicity are available, the therapeutic index cannot be determined. The answer is **D** because the ED_{50} of drug Y (20 mg/d) is less than that of drug X (50 mg/d).

7. Sugammadex interacts directly with rocuronium and not with the rocuronium receptor; therefore, it is a chemical antagonist. The answer is **A.**

8. The binding of a full agonist *decreases* as the concentration of a partial agonist is increased to very high levels. As the partial agonist displaces more and more of the full agonist, the percentage of receptors that bind the full agonist drops to zero, that is, Curve 5. The answer is **E.**

9. Curve 1 describes the *response* of the system when a full agonist is displaced by increasing concentrations of partial agonist. This is because the increasing percentage of receptors binding the partial agonist finally produce the maximal effect typical of the partial agonist. The answer is **A.**

10. Partial agonists, like full agonists, bind 100% of their receptors when present in a high enough concentration. Therefore, the binding curve (but not the effect curve) will go to 100%. If the effect curve is Curve 4 and many spare receptors are present, the binding Curve must be displaced to the right of Curve 4 ($K_d > EC_{50}$). Therefore, Curve 3 fits the description better than Curve 2. The answer is **C.**

SKILL KEEPER ANSWER: ALLOSTERIC ANTAGONISTS

Allosteric antagonists do not bind to the agonist receptor site; they bind to some other region of the receptor molecule that results in inhibition of the response to agonists (see Figure 1–1). They do not prevent binding of the agonist. In contrast, pharmacologic antagonists bind to the agonist site and prevent access of the agonist. The difference can be detected experimentally by evaluating competition between the binding of radioisotopically labeled antagonist and the agonist. High concentrations of agonist displace or prevent the binding of a pharmacologic antagonist but not an allosteric antagonist.

CHECKLIST

When you complete this chapter, you should be able to:

❑ Compare the efficacy and the potency of 2 drugs on the basis of their graded dose-response curves.

❑ Predict the effect of a partial agonist in a patient in the presence and in the absence of a full agonist.

❑ Name the types of antagonists used in therapeutics.

❑ Describe the difference between an inverse agonist and a pharmacologic antagonist.

❑ Specify whether a pharmacologic antagonist is competitive or irreversible based on its effects on the dose-response curve and the dose-binding curve of an agonist in the presence of the antagonist.

❑ Give examples of competitive and irreversible pharmacologic antagonists and of physiologic and chemical antagonists.

❑ Name 5 transmembrane signaling methods by which drug-receptor interactions exert their effects.

❑ Describe 2 mechanisms of receptor regulation.

CHAPTER 2 Summary Table

Major Concept	Description
Graded vs quantal responses	Responses are graded when they increment gradually (eg, heart rate change) as the dose of drug increases; they are quantal when they switch from no effect to a specified effect at a certain dose (eg, from arrhythmia to normal sinus rhythm)
Graded vs quantal dose response curves	Graded dose response curves plot the increment in physiologic or biochemical response as dose or concentration is increased. Quantal dose response curves plot the increment in the percent of the population under study that responds as the dose is increased
Efficacy vs potency	Efficacy represents the *maximal ability* of a drug to accomplish a particular type of effect, whereas potency reflects the *amount* of drug (the dose) required to cause a specific amount of effect. A drug may have high efficacy but low potency or vice versa
Agonism and antagonism	The ability to activate (agonism) or inhibit (antagonism) a biologic system or effect. Different drugs may have very different effects on a receptor. The effect may be to activate, partially activate, or inhibit the receptor's function. In addition, the binding of a drug may be at the site that an endogenous ligand binds that receptor, or at a different site
Transmembrane signaling	Many drugs act on intracellular functions but reach their targets in the extracellular space. On reaching the target, some drugs diffuse through the cell membrane and act on intracellular receptors. Most act on receptors on the extracellular face of the cell membrane and modify the intracellular function of those receptors by *transmembrane signaling*
Receptor regulation	Receptors are in dynamic equilibrium, being synthesized in the interior of the cell, inserted into the cell membranes, sequestered out of the membranes, and degraded at various rates. These changes are noted as *upregulation* or *downregulation* of the receptor numbers.

Pharmacokinetics

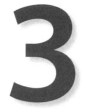

Pharmacokinetics denotes the effects of biologic systems on drugs. The major processes involved in pharmacokinetics are **absorption, distribution,** and **elimination.** Appropriate application of pharmacokinetic data and a few simple formulas makes it possible to calculate **loading** and **maintenance doses.**

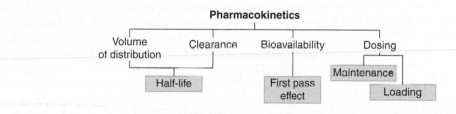

High-Yield Terms to Learn

Volume of distribution (apparent)	The ratio of the amount of drug in the body to the drug concentration in the plasma or blood
Clearance	The ratio of the rate of elimination of a drug to the concentration of the drug in the plasma or blood
Half-life	The time required for the amount of drug in the body or blood to fall by 50%. For drugs eliminated by first-order kinetics, this number is a constant regardless of the concentration
Bioavailability	The fraction (or percentage) of the administered dose of drug that reaches the systemic circulation
Area under the curve (AUC)	The graphic area under a plot of drug concentration versus time after a single dose or during a single dosing interval
Peak and trough concentrations	The maximum and minimum drug concentrations achieved during repeated dosing cycles
Minimum effective concentration (MEC)	The plasma drug concentration below which a patient's response is too small for clinical benefit
First-pass effect, presystemic elimination	The elimination of drug that occurs after administration but before it enters the systemic circulation (eg, during passage through the gut wall, portal circulation, or liver for an orally administered drug)
Steady state	In pharmacokinetics, the condition in which the average total amount of drug in the body does not change over multiple dosing cycles (ie, the condition in which the rate of drug elimination equals the rate of administration)
Biodisposition	Often used as a synonym for pharmacokinetics; the processes of drug absorption, distribution, and elimination. Sometimes used more narrowly to describe elimination

EFFECTIVE DRUG CONCENTRATION

The effective drug concentration is the concentration of a drug *at the receptor site*. In patients, drug concentrations are more readily measured in the blood. Except for topically applied agents, the concentration at the receptor site is usually proportional to the drug's concentration in the plasma or whole blood at equilibrium. The plasma concentration is a function of the rate of input of the drug (by absorption) into the plasma, the rate of distribution, and the rate of elimination. If the rate of input is known, the remaining processes are well described by 2 primary parameters: **apparent volume of distribution (V_d)** and **clearance (CL).** These parameters are unique for a particular drug and a particular patient but have average values in large populations that can be used to predict drug concentrations.

VOLUME OF DISTRIBUTION

The volume of distribution (V_d) relates the amount of drug in the body to the plasma concentration according to the following equation:

$$V_d = \frac{\text{Amount of drug in the body}}{\text{Plasma drug concentration}} \tag{1}$$

(Units = Volume)

The calculated parameter for the V_d has no direct physical equivalent; therefore, it is usually denoted as the *apparent* V_d. A drug that is completely retained in the plasma compartment (Figure 3–1) will have a V_d equal to the plasma volume (about 4% of body weight). The V_d of drugs that are normally bound to plasma proteins such

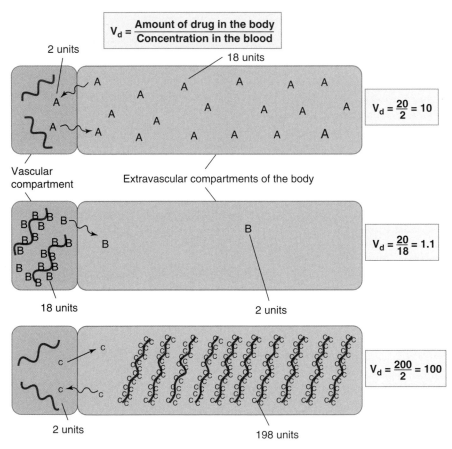

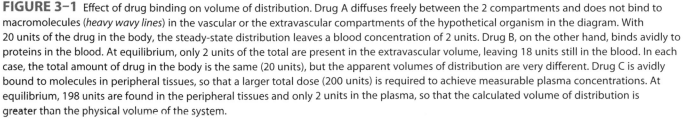

FIGURE 3–1 Effect of drug binding on volume of distribution. Drug A diffuses freely between the 2 compartments and does not bind to macromolecules (*heavy wavy lines*) in the vascular or the extravascular compartments of the hypothetical organism in the diagram. With 20 units of the drug in the body, the steady-state distribution leaves a blood concentration of 2 units. Drug B, on the other hand, binds avidly to proteins in the blood. At equilibrium, only 2 units of the total are present in the extravascular volume, leaving 18 units still in the blood. In each case, the total amount of drug in the body is the same (20 units), but the apparent volumes of distribution are very different. Drug C is avidly bound to molecules in peripheral tissues, so that a larger total dose (200 units) is required to achieve measurable plasma concentrations. At equilibrium, 198 units are found in the peripheral tissues and only 2 units in the plasma, so that the calculated volume of distribution is greater than the physical volume of the system.

as albumin can be altered by liver disease (through reduced protein synthesis) and kidney disease (through urinary protein loss). On the other hand, if a drug is avidly bound in peripheral tissues, the drug's concentration in plasma may drop to very low values even though the total amount in the body is large. As a result, the V_d may greatly exceed the total physical volume of the body. For example, 50,000 liters is the average V_d for the drug quinacrine in persons whose average physical body volume is 70 liters.

CLEARANCE

Clearance (CL) relates the rate of elimination to the plasma concentration:

$$CL = \frac{\text{Rate of elimination of drug}}{\text{Plasma drug concentration}}$$

(2)

(Units = Volume per unit time)

For a drug eliminated with first-order kinetics, clearance is a constant; that is, the ratio of rate of elimination to plasma concentration is the same regardless of plasma concentration (Figure 3–2). The magnitudes of clearance for different drugs range from a small percentage of the blood flow to a maximum of the total blood flow to the organs of elimination. Clearance depends on the drug, blood flow, and the condition of the organs of elimination in the patient. The clearance of a particular drug by an individual organ is equivalent to the extraction capability of that organ for that drug times the rate of delivery of drug to the organ. Thus, the clearance of a drug that is very effectively extracted by an organ (ie, the blood is completely cleared of the drug as it passes through the organ) is

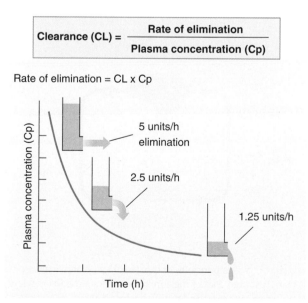

FIGURE 3–2 The clearance of the great majority of drugs is relatively constant over a broad range of plasma concentrations. Since elimination rate is equal to clearance times plasma concentration, the elimination rate will be rapid at first and slow as the concentration decreases.

often *flow-limited*. For such a drug, the total clearance from the body is a function of blood flow through the eliminating organ and is limited by the blood flow to that organ. In this situation, other conditions—cardiac disease, or other drugs that change blood flow—may have more dramatic effects on clearance than disease of the organ of elimination. Note that for drugs eliminated with zero-order kinetics (see Figure 1–3, right), clearance is *not* constant.

HALF-LIFE

Half-life ($t_{1/2}$) is a derived parameter, completely determined by V_d and CL. Like clearance, half-life is a constant for drugs that follow first-order kinetics. Half-life can be determined graphically from a plot of the blood level versus time (eg, Figure 1–4) or from the following relationship:

$$t_{1/2} = \frac{0.693 \times V_d}{CL}$$

(3)

(Units = Time)

One must know both primary variables (V_d and CL) to predict changes in half-life. Disease, age, and other variables usually alter the clearance of a drug much more than they alter its V_d. The half-life determines the rate at which blood concentration rises during a constant infusion and falls after administration is stopped (Figure 3–3). The effect of a drug at 87–90% of its steady-state concentration is clinically indistinguishable from the steady-state effect; thus, 3–4 half-lives of dosing at a constant rate are considered adequate to produce the effect to be expected at steady state with a specified rate of chronic dosing.

BIOAVAILABILITY

The bioavailability of a drug is the fraction (F) of the administered dose that reaches the systemic circulation. Bioavailability is defined as unity (or 100%) in the case of intravenous administration. After administration by other routes, bioavailability is generally reduced by incomplete absorption (and in the intestine, expulsion of drug by intestinal transporters), first-pass metabolism, and any distribution into other tissues that occurs before the drug enters the systemic circulation. Even for drugs with equal bioavailabilities, entry into the systemic circulation occurs over varying periods of time, depending on the drug formulation and other factors. To account for such factors, the concentration appearing in the plasma is integrated over time to obtain an integrated total **area under the plasma concentration curve (AUC,** Figure 3–4).

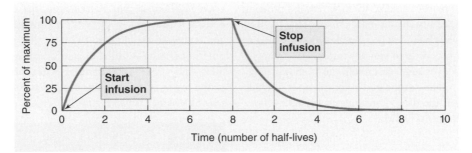

FIGURE 3–3 Plasma concentration (plotted as percentage of maximum) of a drug given by constant intravenous infusion for 8 half-lives and then stopped. The concentration rises smoothly with time and always reaches 50% of steady state after 1 half-life, 75% after 2 half-lives, 87.5% after 3 half-lives, and so on. The decline in concentration after stopping drug administration follows the same type of curve: 50% is left after 1 half-life, 25% after 2 half-lives, and so on. The asymptotic approach to steady state on both increasing and decreasing limbs of the curve is characteristic of drugs that have first-order kinetics.

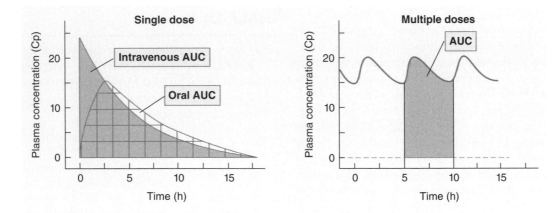

FIGURE 3–4 The area under the curve (AUC) is used to calculate the bioavailability of a drug. The AUC can be derived from either single-dose studies (left) or multiple-dose measurements (right). Bioavailability is calculated from $AUC_{(route)}/AUC_{(IV)}$.

EXTRACTION

Removal of a drug by an organ can be specified as the extraction ratio, that is, the fraction or percentage of the drug removed from the perfusing blood during its passage through the organ (Figure 3–5). After steady-state concentration in plasma has been achieved, the extraction ratio is one measure of the elimination of the drug by that organ.

Drugs that have a high hepatic extraction ratio have a large first-pass effect; the bioavailability of these drugs after oral administration is low.

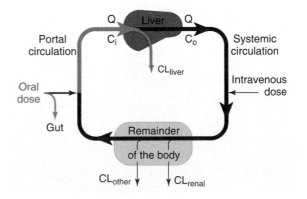

FIGURE 3–5 The principles of organ extraction and first-pass effect are illustrated. Part of the administered oral dose (*blue*) is lost to metabolism in the gut and the liver before it enters the systemic circulation: This is the first-pass effect. The extraction of drug from the circulation by the liver is equal to blood flow times the difference between entering and leaving drug concentration, ie, $Q \times (C_i - C_o)$. CL, clearance. (Modified and reproduced, with permission, from Katzung BG, editor: *Basic & Clinical Pharmacology*, 8th ed. McGraw-Hill, 2001.)

SKILL KEEPER 2: FIRST-PASS EFFECT (SEE CHAPTER 1)

The oral route of administration is the most likely to have a large first-pass effect and therefore low bioavailability. What tissues contribute to this effect? The Skill Keeper Answer appears at the end of the chapter.

DOSAGE REGIMENS

A dosage regimen is a plan for drug administration over a period of time. An optimal dosage regimen results in the achievement of therapeutic levels of the drug in the blood without exceeding the minimum toxic concentration. To maintain the plasma concentration within a specified range over long periods of therapy, a schedule of *maintenance doses* is used. If it is necessary to achieve the target plasma level rapidly, a *loading dose* is used to "load" the V_d with the drug. Ideally, the dosing plan is based on knowledge of both the minimum therapeutic and minimum toxic concentrations for the drug, as well as its clearance and V_d.

A. Maintenance Dosage

Because the maintenance rate of drug administration is equal to the rate of elimination at steady state (this is the definition of steady state), the maintenance dosage is a function of clearance (from Equation 2).

$$\text{Dosing rate} = \frac{\text{CL} \times \text{Desired plasma concentration}}{\text{Bioavailability}} \quad (4)$$

Note that V_d is not involved in the calculation of maintenance dosing rate. The dosing rate computed for maintenance dosage is the average dose per unit time. When performing such calculations, make certain that the units are in agreement throughout. For example, if clearance is given in mL/min, the resulting dosing rate is a per minute rate. Because convenience of administration is desirable for chronic therapy, doses should be given orally if possible and only once or a few times per day. The size of the daily dose (dose per minute × 60 min/h × 24 h/d) is a simple extension of the preceding information. The number of doses to be given per day is usually determined by the half-life of the drug and the difference between the minimum therapeutic and toxic concentrations (see Therapeutic Window, next).

If it is important to maintain a concentration above the minimum therapeutic level at all times, either a larger dose is given at long intervals or smaller doses at more frequent intervals. If the difference between the toxic and therapeutic concentrations is small, then smaller and more frequent doses must be administered to prevent toxicity.

B. Loading Dosage

If the therapeutic concentration must be achieved rapidly and the V_d is large, a large loading dose may be needed at the onset of therapy. This can be calculated from the following equation:

$$\text{Loading dose} = \frac{V_d \times \text{Desired plasma concentration}}{\text{Bioavailability}} \quad (5)$$

Note that clearance does not enter into this computation. If the loading dose is large (V_d much larger than blood volume), the dose should be given slowly to prevent toxicity due to excessively high plasma levels during the distribution phase.

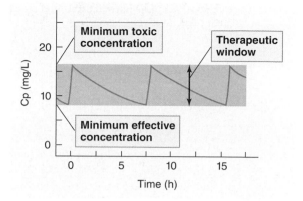

FIGURE 3–6 The therapeutic window for theophylline in a typical patient. The minimum effective concentration in this patient was found to be 8 mg/L; the minimum toxic concentration was found to be 16 mg/L. The therapeutic window is indicated by the blue area. To maintain the plasma concentration (Cp) within the window, this drug must be given at least once every half-life (7.5 h in this patient) because the minimum effective concentration is half the minimum toxic concentration and Cp will decay by 50% in 1 half-life. (**Note:** This concept applies to drugs given in the ordinary, prompt-release form. Slow-release formulations can often be given at longer intervals.)

THERAPEUTIC WINDOW

The therapeutic window is the safe range between the minimum therapeutic concentration and the minimum toxic concentration of a drug. The concept is used to determine the acceptable range of plasma levels when designing a dosing regimen. Thus, the minimum effective concentration usually determines the desired **trough** levels of a drug given intermittently, whereas the minimum toxic concentration determines the permissible **peak** plasma concentration. For example, the drug theophylline has a therapeutic concentration range of 8–20 mg/L but may be toxic at concentrations of more than 15 mg/L. The therapeutic window for a patient might thus be 8–16 mg/L (Figure 3–6). Unfortunately, for some drugs the therapeutic and toxic concentrations vary so greatly among patients that it is impossible to predict the therapeutic window in a given patient. Such drugs must be titrated individually in each patient.

ADJUSTMENT OF DOSAGE WHEN ELIMINATION IS ALTERED BY DISEASE

Renal disease or reduced cardiac output often reduces the clearance of drugs that depend on renal function. Alteration of clearance by liver disease is less common but may also occur. Impairment of hepatic clearance occurs (for high extraction drugs) when liver blood flow is reduced, as in heart failure, and in severe cirrhosis and other forms of liver failure. The dosage in a patient with renal impairment may be corrected by multiplying the average dosage for a normal person times the ratio of the patient's altered creatinine clearance (CL_{cr}) to normal creatinine clearance (approximately 100 mL/min, or 6 L/h).

$$\text{Corrected dosage} = \text{Average dosage} \times \frac{\text{Patient's } CL_{cr}}{100 \text{ mL/min}} \quad (6)$$

This simplified approach ignores nonrenal routes of clearance that may be significant. If a drug is cleared partly by the kidney and partly by other routes, Equation 6 should be applied to the part of the dose that is eliminated by the kidney. For example, if a drug is 50% cleared by the kidney and 50% by the liver and the normal dosage is 200 mg/d, the hepatic and renal elimination rates are each 100 mg/d. Therefore, the corrected dosage in a patient with a creatinine clearance of 20 mL/min will be:

$$\text{Dosage} = 100 \text{ mg/d (liver)} + 100 \text{ mg/d}$$

$$\times \frac{20 \text{ mL/min}}{100 \text{ mL/min}} \text{ (kidney)} \quad (7)$$

$$\text{Dosage} = 100 \text{ mg/d} + 20 \text{ mg/d} = 120 \text{ mg/d}$$

Renal function is altered by many diseases and is often decreased in older patients. Because it is important in the elimination of drugs, assessing renal function is important in estimating dosage in patients. The most important renal variable in drug elimination is glomerular filtration rate (GFR), and creatinine clearance (CL_{cr}) is a convenient approximation of GFR. CL_{cr} can be measured directly, but this requires careful measurement of both serum creatinine concentration and a timed total urine creatinine. A common shortcut that requires only the serum (or plasma) creatinine measurement (S_{cr}) is the use of an equation. One such equation in common use is the Cockcroft-Gault equation:

$$CL_{cr} \text{(mL/min)} = \frac{(140 - \text{Age}) \times \text{body weight (kg)}}{72 \times S_{cr}} \quad (8)$$

The result is multiplied by 0.85 for females. A similar equation for GFR is the MDRD equation:

GFR (mL/min/1.73 m² body surface area)

$$= \frac{175 \times (0.742 \text{ if female}) \times (1.212 \text{ if African American})}{S_{cr}^{1.154} \times \text{Age}^{0.203}} \quad (9)$$

QUESTIONS

Questions 1–2. Mr Jones is admitted to the hospital with cough, shortness of breath, and fever. History, physical examination, and culture of the sputum lead to a diagnosis of pneumonia due to gram-negative bacteria. The antibiotic tobramycin is ordered. The clearance and V_d of tobramycin in Mr Jones are 80 mL/min and 40 L, respectively.

1. What maintenance dose should be administered intravenously every 6 h to eventually obtain average steady-state plasma concentrations of 4 mg/L?
   (A) 0.32 mg
   (B) 19.2 mg
   (C) 115 mg
   (D) 160 mg
   (E) 230 mg

2. If you wish to give Mr Jones an intravenous loading dose to achieve the therapeutic plasma concentration of 4 mg/L rapidly, how much should be given?
   (A) 0.1 mg
   (B) 10 mg
   (C) 115.2 mg
   (D) 160 mg
   (E) None of the above

3. Verapamil and phenytoin are both eliminated from the body by metabolism in the liver. Verapamil has a clearance of 1.5 L/min, approximately equal to liver blood flow, whereas phenytoin has a clearance of 0.1 L/min. When these compounds are administered along with rifampin, a drug that markedly increases hepatic drug-metabolizing enzymes, which of the following is most likely?
   (A) The half-lives of both verapamil and phenytoin will be markedly increased
   (B) The clearance of both verapamil and phenytoin will be markedly decreased
   (C) The clearance of verapamil will be unchanged, whereas the clearance of phenytoin will be increased
   (D) The half-life of phenytoin will be unchanged, whereas the half-life of verapamil will be increased
   (E) The clearance of both drugs will be unchanged

4. A 50-year-old woman with metastatic breast cancer has elected to participate in the trial of a new chemotherapeutic agent. It is given by constant intravenous infusion of 8 mg/h. Plasma concentrations (Cp) are measured with the results shown in the following table.

Time After Start of Infusion (h)	Plasma Concentration (mg/L)
1	0.8
2	1.3
4	2.0
8	3.0
10	3.6
16	3.7
20	3.84
25	3.95
30	4.0
40	4.0

What conclusion can be drawn from these data?
(A) Volume of distribution is 30 L
(B) Clearance is 2 L/h
(C) Elimination follows zero-order kinetics
(D) Half-life is 8 h
(E) Doubling the rate of infusion would result in a plasma concentration of 16 mg/L at 40 h

5. You are the only physician in a clinic that is cut off from the outside world by violent storms and flooding. A 19-year-old woman is brought to the clinic with severe asthmatic wheezing. Because of the lack of other drugs, you decide to use intravenous theophylline for treatment. The pharmacokinetics of theophylline include the following average parameters: V_d 35 L; CL 48 mL/min; half-life 8 h. If an intravenous infusion of theophylline is started at a rate of 0.48 mg/min, how long would it take to reach 93.75% of the final steady-state concentration?
(A) Approximately 48 min
(B) Approximately 7.4 h
(C) Approximately 8 h
(D) Approximately 24 h
(E) Approximately 32 h

6-7. A 74-year-old retired mechanic is admitted with a myocardial infarction and a severe acute cardiac arrhythmia. You decide to give lidocaine to correct the arrhythmia.

6. A continuous intravenous infusion of lidocaine, 1.92 mg/min, is started at 8 AM. The average pharmacokinetic parameters of lidocaine are: V_d 77 L; clearance 640 mL/min; half-life 1.4 h. What is the expected steady-state plasma concentration?
(A) 40 mg/L
(B) 3.0 mg/L
(C) 0.025 mg/L
(D) 7.2 mg/L
(E) 3.46 mg/L

7. Your patient has been receiving lidocaine for 8 h, and the arrhythmia is suppressed. However, there are some signs of toxicity. You decide to obtain a plasma concentration measurement. When the results come back, the plasma level is exactly twice what you expected. How should the infusion rate be modified?
(A) Changed to 0.48 mg/min
(B) Changed to 0.96 mg/min
(C) Halted for 1.4 h and then restarted at 0.96 mg/min
(D) Halted for 1.4 h and then restarted at 1.92 mg/min
(E) No change but the plasma level should be measured again

8. A 63-year-old woman in the intensive care unit requires an infusion of procainamide. Its half-life is 2 h. The infusion is begun at 9 AM. At 1 PM on the same day, a blood sample is taken; the drug concentration is found to be 3 mg/L. What is the probable steady-state drug concentration, for example, after 12 or more hours of infusion?
(A) 3 mg/L
(B) 4 mg/L
(C) 6 mg/L
(D) 9.9 mg/L
(E) 15 mg/L

9. A 30-year-old man is brought to the emergency department in a deep coma. Respiration is severely depressed and he has pinpoint pupils. His friends state that he self-administered a large dose of morphine 6 h earlier. An immediate blood analysis shows a morphine blood level of 0.25 mg/L. Assuming that the V_d of morphine in this patient is 200 L, and the half-life is 3 h, how much morphine did the patient inject 6 h earlier?
(A) 25 mg
(B) 50 mg
(C) 100 mg
(D) 200 mg
(E) Not enough data to predict

10. Gentamicin, an aminoglycoside antibiotic, is sometimes given in intermittent intravenous bolus doses of 100 mg 3 times a day to achieve target peak plasma concentrations of about 5 mg/L. Gentamicin's clearance (normally 5.4 L/h/70 kg) is almost entirely by glomerular filtration. Your patient, however, is found to have a creatinine clearance one third of normal. What should your modified dosage regimen for this patient be?
(A) 20 mg 3 times a day
(B) 33 mg 3 times a day
(C) 72 mg 3 times a day
(D) 100 mg 2 times a day
(E) 150 mg 2 times a day

ANSWERS

1. Maintenance dosage is a function of the target steady-state plasma level, bioavailability, and clearance only:

$$\text{Rate in} = \text{Rate out at steady state}$$

$$\text{Dosage} = \frac{\text{Plasma level}_{ss} \times \text{Clearance}}{\text{Bioavailability}}$$

$$= \frac{4 \text{ mg/L} \times 0.08 \text{ L/min}}{1.0}$$

$$= 0.32 \text{ mg/min}$$

The arithmetic is correct to this point, so you might put down "A" as the answer. Do not fall into this trap! Note that the drug is to be given at **6-h intervals**:

$$= 0.32 \text{ mg/min} \times 60 \text{ min/h} \times 6 \text{ h}$$

$$= 115.2 \text{ mg/dose every 6 h}$$

The answer is **C**.

2. Loading dose is a function of V_d and target plasma concentration:

$$\text{Loading dose} = \frac{V_d \times \text{Target concentration}}{\text{Bioavailability}}$$

$$\text{Loading dose} = \frac{40 \text{ L} \times 4 \text{ mg/L}}{1.0} = 160 \text{ mg}$$

The answer is **D**.

3. Verapamil is metabolized so readily that only the rate of delivery to the liver regulates its disappearance; that is, its elimination is blood flow-limited, not metabolism-limited. Therefore, further increases in liver enzymes could not increase its elimination. However, the rate of elimination of phenytoin is limited by its rate of metabolism since clearance is much less than hepatic blood flow. Therefore, the clearance of phenytoin can rise if some other agent causes an increase in liver enzymes. The answer is **C**.

4. By inspection of the data in the table, it is clear that the steady-state plasma concentration is approximately 4 mg/L. According to the table, 50% of this concentration was reached after 4 h of infusion. According to the constant infusion principle (Figure 3–3), 1 half-life is required to reach one-half of the final concentration; therefore, the half-life of the drug is 4 h. Rearranging the equation for maintenance dosing (dosing rate = CL × Cp), it can be determined that the clearance (CL) = dosing rate/plasma concentration (Cp), or 2 L/h. The volume of distribution (V_d) can be calculated from the half-life equation ($t_{1/2} = 0.693 \times V_d/\text{CL}$) and is equal to 11.5 L. This drug follows first-order kinetics, as indicated by the progressive approach to the steady-state plasma concentration. The answer is **B**.

5. The approach of the drug plasma concentration to steady-state concentration during continuous infusion follows a stereotypical curve (Figure 3–3) that rises rapidly at first and gradually reaches a plateau. It reaches 50% of steady state at 1 half-life, 75% at 2 half-lives, 87.5% at 3, 93.75% at 4, and progressively halves the difference between its current level and 100% of steady state with each half-life. The answer is **E**, 32 h, or 4 half-lives.

6. The drug is being administered continuously and the steady-state concentration (Cp_{ss}) for a continuously administered drug is given by the equation in question 1. Thus,

$$\text{Dosage} = \text{Plasma level}_{ss} \times \text{Clearance}$$

$$1.92 \text{ mg/min} = Cp_{ss} \times \text{CL}$$

Rearranging:

$$Cp_{ss} = \frac{1.92 \text{ mg/min}}{\text{CL}}$$

$$Cp_{ss} = \frac{1.92 \text{ mg/min}}{640 \text{ mL/min}}$$

$$Cp_{ss} = 0.003 \text{ mg/mL or 3 mg/L}$$

The answer is **B**.

7. If the half-life is 1.4 h, the plasma concentration should approach steady state after 8 h (more than 4 half-lives). As indicated in question 9, the steady-state concentration is a function of dosage and clearance, not V_d. If the plasma level is twice that predicted, the clearance in this patient must be half the average value. To reduce the risk of toxicity, the infusion should be halted until the concentration diminishes (1 half-life) and then restarted at half of the previous rate. The answer is **C**.

8. According to the curve that relates plasma concentration to infusion time (Figure 3–3), a drug reaches 50% of its final steady-state concentration in 1 half-life, 75% in 2 half-lives, etc. From 9 AM to 1 PM is 4 h, or 2 half-lives. Therefore, the measured concentration at 1 PM is 75% of the steady-state value ($0.75 \times Cp_{ss}$). The steady-state concentration is 3 mg/L divided by 0.75, or 4 mg/L. The answer is **B**.

9. According to the curve that relates the decline of plasma concentration to time as the drug is eliminated (Figure 3–3), the plasma concentration of morphine was 4 times higher immediately after administration than at the time of the measurement, which occurred 6 h, or 2 half-lives, later. Therefore, the initial plasma concentration was 1 mg/L. Since the amount in the body at any time is equal to $V_d \times$ plasma concentration (text Equation 1), the amount injected was 200 L × 1 mg/L, or 200 mg. The answer is **D**.

10. If the drug is cleared almost entirely by the kidney and creatinine clearance is reduced to one third of normal, the total daily dose should also be reduced to one third. The answer is **B**.

SKILL KEEPER 1 ANSWER: ZERO-ORDER ELIMINATION (SEE CHAPTER 1)

The 3 important drugs that follow zero-order rather than first-order kinetics are ethanol, aspirin, and phenytoin.

SKILL KEEPER 2 ANSWER: FIRST-PASS EFFECT (SEE CHAPTER 1)

The oral route of administration entails passage of the drug through the gastric and intestinal contents, the epithelium and other tissues of the intestinal wall, the portal blood, and the liver before it enters the systemic circulation for distribution to the body. Metabolism by enzymes in any of these tissues, expulsion by drug transporters, and excretion into the bile all may contribute to the first-pass effect of oral administration.

CHECKLIST

When you complete this chapter, you should be able to:

❑ Estimate clearance and volume of distribution from a table or graph of plasma concentrations of a drug over time following a single known dose.

❑ Estimate the half-life of a drug based on its clearance and volume of distribution or from a graph of its plasma concentration over time.

❑ Calculate loading and maintenance dosage regimens for oral or intravenous administration of a drug when given the following information: minimum therapeutic concentration, oral bioavailability, clearance, and volume of distribution.

❑ Calculate the dosage adjustment required for a patient with impaired renal function.

CHAPTER 3 Summary Table

Major Concept	Description
Loading dose	The dose required to achieve a specific plasma drug concentration level (Cp) with a single administration. Because this requires filling the volume of distribution (V_d), the calculation uses the volume of distribution (V_d) equation as: $$\text{Loading dose} = C_p(\text{target}) \times V_d;\ \text{has units of mg}$$
Maintenance dose	The dose required for regular administration to maintain a target plasma level. Because this requires restoring the amount of drug lost to elimination (clearance, CL), the calculation uses the clearance equation as: $$\text{Maintenance dose} = C_p(\text{target}) \times CL;\ \text{has units of mg per time}$$
Half-life	The half-life concept is useful in predicting the time course of falling drug levels after administration is stopped, and in predicting the time course of increase in drug level when repeated administration is begun—see Figure 3–3
Therapeutic window	The therapeutic window is much more useful as a clinical measure of drug safety and as a guide to dosage than the older therapeutic index. The classic therapeutic index, TI, determined from animal measures of therapeutically effective dosage and lethal dosage, is inapplicable to human therapeutics, whereas the minimum therapeutic dosage and the minimum toxic dosage is readily determined in clinical trials

Drug Metabolism

All organisms are exposed to foreign chemical compounds (**xenobiotics**) in the air, water, and food. To ensure elimination of pharmacologically active xenobiotics as well as to terminate the action of many endogenous substances, evolution has provided metabolic pathways that alter their activity and their susceptibility to excretion.

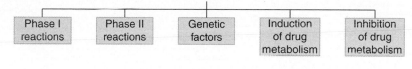

Drug Metabolism

| Phase I reactions | Phase II reactions | Genetic factors | Induction of drug metabolism | Inhibition of drug metabolism |

THE NEED FOR DRUG METABOLISM

Many cells that act as portals for entry of external molecules into the body (eg, pulmonary epithelium, intestinal epithelium) contain transporter molecules (MDR family [P-glycoproteins], MRP family, others) that expel unwanted molecules immediately after absorption. However, some foreign molecules evade these gatekeepers and are absorbed. Therefore, all higher organisms, especially terrestrial animals, require mechanisms for ridding themselves of toxic foreign molecules after they are absorbed, as well as mechanisms for excreting undesirable substances produced within the body. Biotransformation of drugs is one such process. It is an important mechanism by which the body terminates the action of many drugs. In some cases, it serves to *activate* prodrugs. Most drugs are relatively lipid soluble as given, a characteristic needed for absorption across membranes. The same property would result in very slow removal from the body because the unchanged molecule would also be readily reabsorbed from the urine in the renal tubule. The body hastens excretion by transforming many drugs to less lipid-soluble, less readily reabsorbed forms.

High-Yield Terms to Learn

Phase I reactions	Reactions that convert the parent drug to a more polar (water-soluble) or more reactive product by unmasking or inserting a polar functional group such as —OH, —SH, or —NH_2
Phase II reactions	Reactions that increase water solubility by conjugation of the drug molecule with a polar moiety such as glucuronate, acetate, or sulfate
CYP isozymes	Cytochrome P450 enzyme species (eg, CYP2D and CYP3A4) that are responsible for much of drug metabolism. Many isoforms of CYP have been recognized
Enzyme induction	Stimulation of drug-metabolizing capacity; usually manifested in the liver by increased synthesis of smooth endoplasmic reticulum (which contains high concentrations of phase I enzymes)
P-glycoprotein, MDR-1	An ATP-dependent transport molecule found in many epithelial and cancer cells. The transporter expels drug molecules from the cytoplasm into the extracellular space. In epithelial cells, expulsion is via the external or luminal face

TABLE 4–1 Examples of phase I drug-metabolizing reactions.

Reaction Type	Typical Drug Substrates
Oxidations, P450 dependent	
Hydroxylation	Amphetamines, barbiturates, phenytoin, warfarin
N-dealkylation	Caffeine, morphine, theophylline
O-dealkylation	Codeine
N-oxidation	Acetaminophen, nicotine
S-oxidation	Chlorpromazine, cimetidine, thioridazine
Deamination	Amphetamine, diazepam
Oxidations, P450 independent	
Amine oxidation	Epinephrine
Dehydrogenation	Chloral hydrate, ethanol
Reductions	Chloramphenicol, clonazepam, dantrolene, naloxone
Hydrolyses	
Esters	Aspirin, clofibrate, procaine, succinylcholine
Amides	Indomethacin, lidocaine, procainamide

TYPES OF METABOLIC REACTIONS

A. Phase I Reactions

Phase I reactions include oxidation (especially by the **cytochrome P450** group of enzymes, also called **mixed-function oxidases**), reduction, deamination, and hydrolysis. Examples are listed in Table 4–1. These enzymes are found in high concentrations in the smooth endoplasmic reticulum of the liver. They are not highly selective in their substrates, so a relatively small number of P450 isoforms are able to metabolize thousands of drugs. Of the drugs metabolized by phase I cytochrome P450s, approximately 75% are metabolized by just two: CYP3A4 or CYP2D6. Nevertheless, some selectivity can be detected, and optical enantiomers, in particular, are often metabolized at different rates.

B. Phase II Reactions

Phase II reactions are synthetic reactions that involve addition (conjugation) of subgroups to —OH, —NH$_2$, and —SH functions on the drug molecule. The subgroups that are added include glucuronate, acetate, glutathione, glycine, sulfate, and methyl groups. Most of these groups are relatively polar and make the product less lipid-soluble than the original drug molecule. Examples of phase II reactions are listed in Table 4–2. Like phase I enzymes, phase II enzymes are not very selective. Drugs that are metabolized by both routes may undergo phase II metabolism before or after phase I.

TABLE 4–2 Examples of phase II drug-metabolizing reactions.

Reaction Type	Typical Drug Substrates
Glucuronidation	Acetaminophen, diazepam, digoxin, morphine, sulfamethiazole
Acetylation	Clonazepam, dapsone, isoniazid, mescaline, sulfonamides
Glutathione conjugation	Ethacrynic acid, reactive phase I metabolite of acetaminophen
Glycine conjugation	Deoxycholic acid, nicotinic acid (niacin), salicylic acid
Sulfation	Acetaminophen, methyldopa
Methylation	Dopamine, epinephrine, histamine, norepinephrine, thiouracil

Adapted, with permission, from Katzung BG, editor: *Basic & Clinical Pharmacology*, 12th ed. McGraw-Hill, 2012.

SITES OF DRUG METABOLISM

The most important organ for drug metabolism is the liver. The kidneys play an important role in the metabolism of some drugs. A few drugs (eg, esters) are metabolized in many tissues (eg, liver, blood, intestinal wall) because of the wide distribution of their enzymes.

DETERMINANTS OF BIOTRANSFORMATION RATE

The rate of biotransformation of a drug may vary markedly among different individuals. This variation is most often due to genetic or drug-induced differences. For a few drugs, age or disease-related differences in drug metabolism are significant. In humans, gender is important for only a few drugs. (First-pass metabolism of ethanol is greater in men than in women.) On the other hand, a variety of drugs may induce or inhibit drug-metabolizing enzymes to a very significant extent. Smoking is a common cause of enzyme induction in the liver and lung and may increase the metabolism of some drugs. Because the rate of biotransformation is often the primary determinant of clearance, variations in drug metabolism must be considered carefully when designing or modifying a dosage regimen.

A. Genetic Factors

Because recent advances in genomic techniques are making it possible to screen for a huge variety of polymorphisms, it is expected that **pharmacogenomics** will become an important part of patient evaluation in the future, influencing both drug choice and drug dosing. Several drug-metabolizing systems have already been shown to differ among families or populations in genetically determined ways. However, screening for these variants has not yet become common.

1. Hydrolysis of esters—Succinylcholine is an ester that is metabolized in a phase I reaction by plasma cholinesterase ("pseudocholinesterase" or butyrylcholinesterase). In most persons, this process occurs very rapidly, and a single dose of this neuromuscular-blocking drug has a duration of action of about 5 min. Approximately 1 person in 2500 has an abnormal form of this enzyme that metabolizes succinylcholine and similar esters much more slowly. In such persons, the neuromuscular paralysis produced by a single dose of succinylcholine may last many hours.

2. Acetylation of amines—Isoniazid and some other amines such as hydralazine and procainamide are metabolized in a phase II reaction by *N*-acetylation. People who are deficient in acetylation capacity, termed *slow acetylators*, may have prolonged or toxic responses to normal doses of these drugs. Slow acetylators constitute about 50% of white and African American persons in the United States and a much smaller percentage of Asian and Inuit (Eskimo) populations. The slow acetylation trait is inherited as an autosomal recessive gene.

3. Oxidation—The rate of phase I oxidation of debrisoquin, sparteine, phenformin, dextromethorphan, certain beta blockers, and some tricyclic antidepressants by certain P450 isozymes has been shown to be genetically determined.

B. Effects of Other Drugs

Coadministration of certain agents may alter the disposition of many drugs. Mechanisms include the following:

1. Enzyme induction—Induction (increased rate and extent of metabolism) usually results from increased synthesis of cytochrome P450-dependent drug-oxidizing enzymes in the liver as well as the cofactor, heme. Several cytoplasmic drug receptors have been identified that result in activation of the genes for P450 isoforms. Many isozymes of the P450 family exist, and inducers selectively increase subgroups of isozymes. Common inducers of a few of these isozymes and the drugs whose metabolism is increased are listed in Table 4–3. Several days are usually required to reach

TABLE 4–3 A partial list of drugs that significantly induce P450-mediated drug metabolism in humans.

CYP Family Induced	Important Inducers	Drugs Whose Metabolism Is Induced
1A2	Benzo[*a*]pyrene (from tobacco smoke), carbamazepine, phenobarbital, rifampin, omeprazole	Acetaminophen, clozapine, haloperidol, theophylline, tricyclic antidepressants, (*R*)-warfarin
2C9	Barbiturates, especially phenobarbital, phenytoin, primidone, rifampin	Barbiturates, celecoxib, chloramphenicol, doxorubicin, ibuprofen, phenytoin, chlorpromazine, steroids, tolbutamide, (*S*)-warfarin
2C19	Carbamazepine, phenobarbital, phenytoin, rifampin	Diazepam, phenytoin, topiramate, tricyclic antidepressants, (*R*)-warfarin
2E1	Ethanol, isoniazid	Acetaminophen, enflurane, ethanol (minor), halothane
3A4	Barbiturates, carbamazepine, corticosteroids, efavirenz, phenytoin, rifampin, pioglitazone, St. John's wort	Antiarrhythmics, antidepressants, azole antifungals, benzodiazepines, calcium channel blockers, cyclosporine, delavirdine, doxorubicin, efavirenz, erythromycin, estrogens, HIV protease inhibitors, nefazodone, paclitaxel, proton pump inhibitors, HMG-CoA reductase inhibitors, rifabutin, rifampin, sildenafil, SSRIs, tamoxifen, trazodone, vinca alkaloids

SSRIs, selective serotonin reuptake inhibitors.

TABLE 4-4 A partial list of drugs that significantly inhibit P450-mediated drug metabolism in humans.

CYP Family Inhibited	Inhibitors	Drugs Whose Metabolism Is Inhibited
1A2	Cimetidine, fluoroquinolones, grapefruit juice, macrolides, isoniazid, zileuton	Acetaminophen, clozapine, haloperidol, theophylline, tricyclic antidepressants, (R)-warfarin
2C9	Amiodarone, chloramphenicol, cimetidine, isoniazid, metronidazole, SSRIs, zafirlukast	Barbiturates, celecoxib, chloramphenicol, doxorubicin, ibuprofen, phenytoin, chlorpromazine, steroids, tolbutamide, (S)-warfarin
2C19	Fluconazole, omeprazole, SSRIs	Diazepam, phenytoin, topiramate, (R)-warfarin
2D6	Amiodarone, cimetidine, quinidine, SSRIs	Antiarrhythmics, antidepressants, beta-blockers, clozapine, flecainide, lidocaine, mexiletine, opioids
3A4	Amiodarone, azole antifungals, cimetidine, clarithromycin, cyclosporine, diltiazem, erythromycin, fluoroquinolones, grapefruit juice, HIV protease inhibitors, metronidazole, quinine, SSRIs, tacrolimus	Antiarrhythmics, antidepressants, azole antifungals, benzodiazepines, calcium channel blockers, cyclosporine, delavirdine, doxorubicin, efavirenz, erythromycin, estrogens, HIV protease inhibitors, nefazodone, paclitaxel, proton pump inhibitors, HMG-CoA reductase inhibitors, rifabutin, rifampin, sildenafil, SSRIs, tamoxifen, trazodone, vinca alkaloids

SSRIs, selective serotonin reuptake inhibitors.

maximum induction; a similar amount of time is required to regress after withdrawal of the inducer. The most common strong inducers of drug metabolism are carbamazepine, phenobarbital, phenytoin, and rifampin.

2. Enzyme inhibition—A few common inhibitors and the drugs whose metabolism is diminished are listed in Table 4–4. The inhibitors of drug metabolism most likely to be involved in serious drug interactions are amiodarone, cimetidine, furanocoumarins present in grapefruit juice, azole antifungals, and the HIV protease inhibitor ritonavir. **Suicide inhibitors** are drugs that are metabolized to products that irreversibly inhibit the metabolizing enzyme. Such agents include ethinyl estradiol, norethindrone, spironolactone, secobarbital, allopurinol, fluroxene, and propylthiouracil. Metabolism may also be decreased by pharmacodynamic factors such as a reduction in blood flow to the metabolizing organ (eg, propranolol reduces hepatic blood flow).

3. Inhibitors of intestinal P-glycoprotein—MDR-1, also known as P-glycoprotein (P-gp), is an important modulator of intestinal drug transport and usually functions to expel drugs from the intestinal mucosa into the lumen, thus contributing to presystemic elimination. (P-gp and other members of the MDR family are also found in the blood-brain barrier and in drug-resistant cancer cells.) Drugs that inhibit intestinal P-gp mimic drug metabolism inhibitors by increasing bioavailability; coadministration of P-gp inhibitors may result in toxic plasma concentrations of drugs given at normally nontoxic dosage. P-gp inhibitors include verapamil, mibefradil (a calcium channel blocker no longer on the market), and furanocoumarin components of grapefruit juice. Important drugs that are normally expelled by P-gp (and are therefore potentially more toxic when given with a P-gp inhibitor) include digoxin, cyclosporine, and saquinavir.

TOXIC METABOLISM

Drug metabolism is not synonymous with drug inactivation. Some drugs are converted to active products by metabolism. If these products are toxic, severe injury may result under some circumstances. An important example is acetaminophen when taken in large overdoses (Figure 4–1). Acetaminophen is conjugated to harmless glucuronide and sulfate metabolites when it is taken in recommended doses by patients with normal liver function. If a large

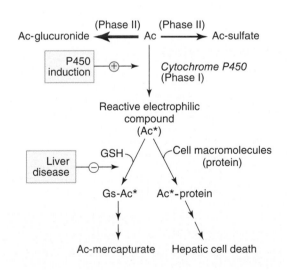

FIGURE 4–1 Metabolism of acetaminophen (Ac) to harmless conjugates or to toxic metabolites. Acetaminophen glucuronide, acetaminophen sulfate, and the mercapturate conjugate of acetaminophen all are nontoxic phase II conjugates. Ac* is the toxic, reactive phase I metabolite. Transformation to the reactive metabolite occurs when hepatic stores of sulfate, glucuronide, and glutathione (GSH, Gs) are depleted or overwhelmed or when phase I enzymes have been induced.

overdose is taken, however, the phase II metabolic pathways are overwhelmed, and a P450-dependent system converts some of the drug to a reactive intermediate (*N*-acetyl-*p*-benzoquinoneimine). This intermediate is conjugated with glutathione to a third harmless product if glutathione stores are adequate. If glutathione stores are exhausted, however, the reactive intermediate combines with sulfhydryl groups on essential hepatic cell proteins, resulting in cell death. Prompt administration of other sulfhydryl donors (eg, acetylcysteine) may be life-saving after an overdose. In severe liver disease, stores of glucuronide, sulfate, and glutathione may be depleted, making the patient more susceptible to hepatic toxicity with near-normal doses of acetaminophen. Enzyme inducers (eg, ethanol) may increase acetaminophen toxicity because they increase phase I metabolism more than phase II metabolism, thus resulting in increased production of the reactive metabolite.

QUESTIONS

1–2. You are planning to treat asthma in a 19-year-old patient with recurrent, episodic attacks of bronchospasm with wheezing. You are concerned about drug interactions caused by changes in drug metabolism in this patient.

1. Drug metabolism in humans usually results in a product that is
   (A) Less lipid soluble than the original drug
   (B) More likely to distribute intracellularly
   (C) More likely to be reabsorbed by kidney tubules
   (D) More lipid soluble than the original drug
   (E) Less water soluble than the original drug

2. If therapy with multiple drugs causes induction of drug metabolism in your asthma patient, it will
   (A) Be associated with increased smooth endoplasmic reticulum
   (B) Be associated with increased rough endoplasmic reticulum
   (C) Be associated with decreased enzymes in the soluble cytoplasmic fraction
   (D) Require 3–4 months to reach completion
   (E) Be irreversible

3. Which of the following factors is likely to increase the duration of action of a drug that is metabolized by CYP3A4 in the liver?
   (A) Chronic administration of phenobarbital before and during therapy with the drug in question
   (B) Chronic therapy with cimetidine
   (C) Displacement from tissue-binding sites by another drug
   (D) Increased cardiac output
   (E) Chronic administration of rifampin

4. Reports of cardiac arrhythmias caused by unusually high blood levels of 2 antihistamines, terfenadine and astemizole, led to their removal from the market. Which of the following best explains these effects?
   (A) Concomitant treatment with phenobarbital
   (B) Use of these drugs by smokers
   (C) A genetic predisposition to metabolize succinylcholine slowly
   (D) Treatment of these patients with ketoconazole, an azole antifungal agent

5. Which of the following drugs is genetically associated with slower metabolism in European Americans and African Americans than in most Asians?
   (A) Cimetidine
   (B) Hydralazine
   (C) Propranolol
   (D) Rifampin
   (E) Succinylcholine

6. Which of the following drugs may inhibit the hepatic microsomal P450 responsible for warfarin metabolism?
   (A) Amiodarone
   (B) Ethanol
   (C) Phenobarbital
   (D) Procainamide
   (E) Rifampin

7. Which of the following drugs, if used chronically, is most likely to increase the toxicity of acetaminophen?
   (A) Cimetidine
   (B) Ethanol
   (C) Ketoconazole
   (D) Procainamide
   (E) Quinidine
   (F) Ritonavir
   (G) Succinylcholine
   (H) Verapamil

8. Which of the following drugs has higher first-pass metabolism in men than in women?
   (A) Cimetidine
   (B) Ethanol
   (C) Ketoconazole
   (D) Procainamide
   (E) Quinidine
   (F) Ritonavir
   (G) Succinylcholine
   (H) Verapamil

9. Which of the following drugs is an established inhibitor of P-glycoprotein (P-gp) drug transporters?
   (A) Cimetidine
   (B) Ethanol
   (C) Ketoconazole
   (D) Procainamide
   (E) Quinidine
   (F) Ritonavir
   (G) Succinylcholine
   (H) Verapamil

10. Which of the following agents, when used in combination with other anti-HIV drugs, permits dose reductions?
   (A) Cimetidine
   (B) Efavirenz
   (C) Ketoconazole
   (D) Procainamide
   (E) Quinidine
   (F) Ritonavir
   (G) Succinylcholine
   (H) Verapamil

ANSWERS

1. Biotransformation usually results in a product that is *less* lipid-soluble. This facilitates elimination of drugs that would otherwise be reabsorbed from the renal tubule. The answer is **A.**

2. The smooth endoplasmic reticulum, which contains the mixed-function oxidase drug-metabolizing enzymes, is selectively increased by inducers. The answer is **A.**

3. Phenobarbital and rifampin can induce drug-metabolizing enzymes and thereby may *reduce* the duration of drug action. Displacement of drug from tissue may transiently increase the intensity of the effect but decreases the volume of distribution. Cimetidine is recognized as an inhibitor of P450 and may also decrease hepatic blood flow under some circumstances. The answer is **B.**

4. Treatment with phenobarbital and smoking are associated with increased drug metabolism and lower, not higher, blood levels. Ketoconazole, itraconazole, erythromycin, and some substances in grapefruit juice slow the metabolism of certain older nonsedating antihistamines (Chapter 16). The answer is **D.**

5. Hydralazine, like procainamide and isoniazid, is metabolized by *N*-acetylation, an enzymatic process that is slow in about 20% of Asians and in about 50% of European Americans and African Americans. The answer is **B.**

6. Amiodarone is an important antiarrhythmic drug and has a well-documented ability to inhibit the hepatic metabolism of many drugs. The answer is **A.**

7. Acetaminophen is normally eliminated by phase II conjugation reactions. The drug's toxicity is caused by an oxidized reactive metabolite produced by phase I oxidizing P450 enzymes. Ethanol (and certain other drugs) induces P450 enzymes and thus reduces the hepatotoxic dose. Alcoholic cirrhosis reduces the hepatotoxic dose even more. The answer is **B.**

8. Ethanol is subject to metabolism in the stomach as well as in the liver. Independent of body weight and other factors, men have greater gastric ethanol metabolism and thus a lower ethanol bioavailability than women. The answer is **B.**

9. Verapamil is an inhibitor of P-glycoprotein drug transporters and has been used to enhance the cytotoxic actions of methotrexate in cancer chemotherapy. The answer is **H.**

10. Ritonavir inhibits hepatic drug metabolism, and its use at low doses in combination regimens has permitted dose reductions of other HIV protease inhibitors (eg, indinavir). The answer is **F.**

CHECKLIST

When you complete this chapter, you should be able to:

❑ List the major phase I and phase II metabolic reactions.

❑ Describe the mechanism of hepatic enzyme induction and list 3 drugs that are known to cause it.

❑ List 3 drugs that inhibit the metabolism of other drugs.

❑ List 3 drugs for which there are well-defined, genetically determined differences in metabolism.

❑ Describe some of the effects of smoking, liver disease, and kidney disease on drug elimination.

❑ Describe the pathways by which acetaminophen is metabolized (1) to harmless products if normal doses are taken and (2) to hepatotoxic products if an overdose is taken.

CHAPTER 4 Summary Table

Major Concept	Description
Drug metabolism vs drug elimination	Termination of drug action requires either removal of the drug from the body (*excretion*) or modification of the drug molecule (*metabolism*) so that it no longer has an effect. Both methods constitute drug *elimination*, and both are very important in the clinical use of drugs. Almost all drugs (or their metabolites) are eventually excreted, but for many, excretion occurs only some time after they have been metabolized to inactive products
Induction and inhibition of drug metabolism	A large number of drugs alter their own metabolism and the metabolism of other drugs either by inducing the synthesis of larger amounts of the metabolizing enzymes (usually P450 enzymes in the liver) or by inhibiting those enzymes. Some drugs both inhibit (acutely) and induce (with chronic administration) drug metabolism
Pharmacogenomic variation in drug metabolism	Genetic variations in drug metabolism undoubtedly occur for many drugs. Specific differences have been defined for (1) succinylcholine and similar esters, (2) procainamide and similar amines, and (3) a miscellaneous group that includes β blockers, antidepressants, and others
Toxic metabolism	Some substances are metabolized to toxic molecules by drug-metabolizing enzymes. Important examples include methyl alcohol, ethylene glycol, and, at high doses or in the presence of liver disease, acetaminophen. See Figure 4–1 and Chapter 23

Drug Evaluation & Regulation

The sale and use of drugs are regulated in almost all countries by governmental agencies. In the United States, regulation is by the Food and Drug Administration (FDA). New drugs are developed in industrial or academic laboratories. Before a new drug can be approved for regular therapeutic use in humans, a series of animal and experimental human studies must be carried out.

New drugs may emerge from a variety of sources. Some are the result of identification of a new target for a disease.

Rational molecular design or screening is then used to find a molecule that selectively alters the function of the target. New drugs may result from the screening of hundreds of compounds against model diseases in animals. In contrast, many (so-called "me-too" drugs) are the result of simple chemical alteration of the pharmacokinetic properties of the original, prototype agent.

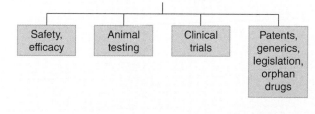

SAFETY & EFFICACY

Because society expects prescription drugs to be safe and effective, governments regulate the development and marketing of new drugs. Current regulations require evidence of relative safety (derived from acute and subacute toxicity testing in animals) and probable therapeutic action (from the pharmacologic profile in animals) before human testing is permitted. Some information about the pharmacokinetics of a compound is also required before clinical evaluation is begun. Chronic toxicity test *results* are generally not required, but testing must be underway before human studies are started. The development of a new drug and its pathway through various levels of testing and regulation are illustrated in Figure 5–1. The cost of development of a new drug, including false starts and discarded molecules, is often several hundred million dollars.

ANIMAL TESTING

The animal testing that is required before human studies can begin is a function of the proposed use and the urgency of the application. Thus, a drug proposed for occasional nonsystemic use requires less extensive testing than one destined for chronic systemic administration.

Because of the urgent need for new agents, anticancer drugs and anti-HIV drugs require less evidence of safety than do drugs used in treatment of less threatening diseases. Urgently needed drugs are often investigated and approved on an accelerated schedule.

A. Acute Toxicity

Acute toxicity studies are required for all new drugs. These studies involve administration of incrementing doses of the agent up to the lethal level in at least 2 species (eg, 1 rodent and 1 nonrodent).

High-Yield Terms to Learn

Mutagenic	An effect on the inheritable characteristics of a cell or organism—a mutation in the DNA; usually tested in microorganisms with the Ames test
Carcinogenic	An effect of inducing malignant characteristics
Teratogenic	An effect on the in utero development of an organism resulting in abnormal structure or function; not generally heritable
Placebo	An inactive "dummy" medication made up to resemble the active investigational formulation as much as possible but lacking therapeutic effect
Single-blind study	A clinical trial in which the investigators—but not the subjects—know which subjects are receiving active drug and which are receiving placebos
Double-blind study	A clinical trial in which neither the subjects nor the investigators know which subjects are receiving placebos; the code is held by a third party
IND	Investigational New Drug Exemption; an application for FDA approval to carry out new drug trials in humans; requires animal data
NDA	New Drug Application; seeks FDA approval to market a new drug for ordinary clinical use. Requires data from clinical trials as well as preclinical (animal) data
Phases 1, 2, and 3 of clinical trials	Three parts of a clinical trial that are usually carried out before submitting an NDA to the FDA
Positive control	A known standard therapy, to be used along with placebo, to evaluate the superiority or inferiority of a new drug in relation to the others available
Orphan drugs	Drugs developed for diseases in which the expected number of patients is small. Some countries bestow certain commercial advantages on companies that develop drugs for uncommon diseases

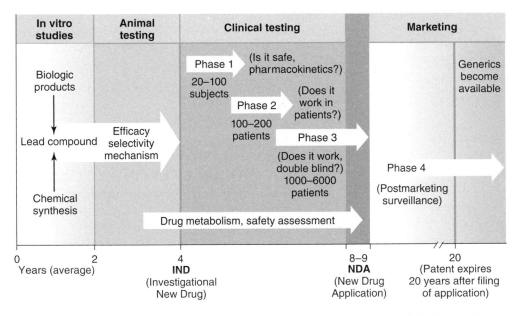

FIGURE 5–1 The development and testing process required to bring a new drug to market in the United States. Some requirements may be different for drugs used in life-threatening diseases. (Reproduced, with permission, from Katzung BG, editor: *Basic & Clinical Pharmacology*, 12th ed. McGraw-Hill, 2012: Fig. 5–1.)

B. Subacute and Chronic Toxicity

Subacute and chronic toxicity testing are required for most agents, especially those intended for chronic use. Tests are usually conducted for 2–4 weeks (subacute) and 6–24 months (chronic), in at least 2 species.

TYPES OF ANIMAL TESTS

Tests done with animals usually include general screening tests for pharmacologic effects, hepatic and renal function monitoring, blood and urine tests, gross and histopathologic examination of tissues, and tests of reproductive effects and carcinogenicity.

A. Pharmacologic Profile

The pharmacologic profile is a description of all the pharmacologic effects of a drug (eg, effects on cardiovascular function, gastrointestinal activity, respiration, renal function, endocrine function, CNS). Both graded and quantal dose-response data are gathered.

B. Reproductive Toxicity

Reproductive toxicity testing involves the study of the fertility effects of the candidate drug and its teratogenic and mutagenic toxicity. The FDA uses a 5-level descriptive scale to summarize information regarding the safety of drugs in pregnancy (Table 5–1). **Teratogenesis** can be defined as the induction of developmental defects in the somatic tissues of the fetus (eg, by exposure of the fetus to a chemical, infection, or radiation). Teratogenesis is studied by treating pregnant female animals of at least 2 species at selected times during early pregnancy when organogenesis is known to take place and by later examining the fetuses or neonates for abnormalities. Examples of drugs known to have teratogenic effects include thalidomide, isotretinoin, valproic acid, ethanol, glucocorticoids, warfarin, lithium, and androgens. **Mutagenesis** is induction of changes in the genetic material of animals of any age and therefore induction of heritable abnormalities. The **Ames test,** the standard in vitro test for mutagenicity, uses a special strain of salmonella bacteria that naturally depends on specific nutrients in the culture medium. Loss of this dependence as a result of exposure to the test drug signals a mutation. Many carcinogens (eg, aflatoxin, cancer chemotherapeutic drugs, and other agents that bind to DNA) have mutagenic effects and test positive in the Ames test. The **dominant lethal test** is an in vivo mutagenicity test carried out in mice. Male animals are exposed to the test substance before mating. Abnormalities in the results of subsequent mating (eg, loss of embryos, deformed fetuses) signal a mutation in the male's germ cells.

C. Carcinogenesis

Carcinogenesis is the induction of malignant characteristics in cells. Carcinogenicity is difficult and expensive to study, and the Ames test is often used to screen chemicals because there is a moderately high degree of correlation between mutagenicity in the Ames test and carcinogenicity in some animal tests, as previously noted. Agents with known carcinogenic effects include coal tar, aflatoxin, dimethylnitrosamine and other nitrosamines, urethane, vinyl chloride, and the polycyclic aromatic hydrocarbons in tobacco smoke (eg, benzo[a]pyrene) and other tobacco products.

CLINICAL TRIALS

Human testing of new drugs in the United States requires approval by institutional committees that monitor the ethical

TABLE 5–1 FDA ratings of drug safety in pregnancy.

Category	Description
A	Controlled studies in women fail to demonstrate a risk to the fetus in the first trimester (and there is no evidence of a risk in later trimesters), and the possibility of fetal harm appears remote
B	Either animal reproduction studies have not demonstrated a fetal risk but there are no controlled studies in pregnant women, or animal reproduction studies have shown an adverse effect (other than a decrease in fertility) that was not confirmed in controlled studies in women in the first trimester (and there is no evidence of a risk in later trimesters)
C	Either studies in animals have revealed adverse effects on the fetus (teratogenic or embryocidal or other) and there are no controlled studies in women, or studies in women and animals are not available. Drugs should be given only when the potential benefit justifies the potential risk to the fetus
D	There is positive evidence of human fetal risk, but the benefits from use in pregnant women may be acceptable despite the risk (eg, if the drug is needed in a life-threatening situation or for a serious disease for which safer drugs cannot be used or are ineffective)
X	Studies in animals or human beings have demonstrated fetal abnormalities or there is evidence of fetal risk based on human experience or both, and the risk of the use of the drug in pregnant women clearly outweighs any possible benefit. The drug is contraindicated in women who are or may become pregnant

(informed consent, patient safety) and scientific aspects (study design, statistical power) of the proposed tests. Such testing also requires the prior approval by the FDA of an **Investigational New Drug Exemption application (IND)**, which is submitted by the manufacturer to the FDA (Figure 5–1). The IND includes all the preclinical data collected up to the time of submission and the detailed proposal for clinical trials. The major clinical testing process is usually divided into 3 phases that are carried out to provide information for a **New Drug Application (NDA)**. The NDA includes all the results of preclinical and clinical testing and constitutes the request for FDA approval of general marketing of the new agent for prescription use. A fourth phase of study (the surveillance phase) follows NDA approval.

A. Phase 1

A phase 1 trial consists of careful evaluation of the dose-response relationship and the pharmacokinetics of the new drug in a small number of normal human volunteers (eg, 20–100). An exception is the phase 1 trials of cancer chemotherapeutic agents and other highly toxic drugs; these are carried out by administering the agents to volunteer patients with the target disease. In phase 1 studies, the acute effects of the agent are studied over a broad range of dosages, starting with one that produces no detectable effect and progressing to one that produces either a significant physiologic response or a very minor toxic effect.

B. Phase 2

A phase 2 trial involves evaluation of a drug in a moderate number of patients (eg, 100–200) with the target disease. A placebo or positive control drug is included in a single-blind or double-blind design. The study is carried out under very carefully controlled conditions, and patients are closely monitored, often in a hospital research ward. The goal is to determine whether the agent has the desired efficacy (ie, produces adequate therapeutic response) at doses that are tolerated by sick patients. Detailed data are collected regarding the pharmacokinetics and pharmacodynamics of the drug in this patient population.

C. Phase 3

A phase 3 trial usually involves many patients (eg, 1000–5000 or more, in many centers) and many clinicians who are using the drug in the manner proposed for its ultimate general use (eg, in outpatients). Such studies usually include placebo and positive controls in a double-blind crossover design. The goals are to explore further, under the conditions of the proposed clinical use, the spectrum of beneficial actions of the new drug, to compare it with older therapies, and to discover toxicities, if any, that occur so infrequently as to be undetectable in phase 2 studies. Very large amounts of data are collected and these studies are usually very expensive.

If the drug successfully completes phase 3, an NDA is submitted to the FDA. If the NDA is approved, the drug can be marketed and phase 4 begins.

D. Phase 4

Phase 4 represents the postmarketing surveillance phase of evaluation, in which it is hoped that toxicities that occur very infrequently will be detected and reported early enough to prevent major therapeutic disasters. Manufacturers are required to inform the FDA at regular intervals of all reported untoward drug reactions. Unlike the first 3 phases, phase 4 has not been rigidly regulated by the FDA in the past. Because so many drugs have been found to be unacceptably toxic only after they have been marketed, there is considerable current interest in making phase 4 surveillance more consistent, effective, and informative.

DRUG PATENTS & GENERIC DRUGS

A patent application is usually submitted around the time that a new drug enters animal testing. In the United States, approval of the patent and completion of the NDA approval process give the originator the right to market the drug without competition from other firms for a period of 20 years from the patent approval date. After expiration of the patent, any company may apply to the FDA for permission to market a generic version of the same drug if they demonstrate that their generic drug molecule is **bioequivalent** (ie, meets certain requirements for content, purity, and bioavailability) to the original product.

> ### SKILL KEEPER: GRADED AND QUANTAL DOSE-RESPONSE CURVES (SEE CHAPTER 2)
>
> *What type of dose-response curve is appropriate for the determination of the therapeutic index of a new drug in mice? What type of dose-response determination is needed for the determination of the minimum effective dose and the maximal efficacy of the drug in humans?*

DRUG LEGISLATION

In the United States, many laws regulating drugs were passed during the 20th century. Refer to Table 5–2 for a partial list of this legislation.

ORPHAN DRUGS

An orphan drug is a drug for a rare disease (one affecting fewer than 200,000 people in the United States). The study of such agents has often been neglected because the sales of an effective agent for an uncommon ailment might not pay the costs of development. In the United States, current legislation provides for tax relief and other incentives designed to encourage the development of orphan drugs.

TABLE 5–2 Selected legislation pertaining to drugs in the United States.

Law	Purpose and Effect
Pure Food and Drug Act of 1906	Prohibited mislabeling and adulteration of foods and drugs (but no requirement for efficacy or safety)
Harrison Narcotics Act of 1914	Established regulations for the use of opium, opioids, and cocaine (marijuana added in 1937)
Food, Drug, and Cosmetics Act of 1938	Required that new drugs be tested for safety as well as purity
Kefauver-Harris Amendment (1962)	Required proof of efficacy as well as safety for new drugs
Dietary Supplement and Health Education Act (1994)	Amended the Food, Drug, and Cosmetics act of 1938 to establish standards for dietary supplements but prohibited the FDA from applying drug efficacy and safety standards to supplements

QUESTIONS

1. Which of the following statements is *most* correct regarding clinical trials of new drugs?
   (A) Phase 1 involves the study of a small number of normal volunteers by highly trained clinical pharmacologists
   (B) Phase 2 involves the use of the new drug in a large number of patients (1000–5000) who have the disease to be treated under conditions of proposed use (eg, outpatients)
   (C) Phase 3 involves the determination of the drug's therapeutic index by the cautious induction of toxicity
   (D) Phase 4 involves the detailed study of toxic effects that have been discovered in phase 3
   (E) Phase 2 requires the use of a positive control (a known effective drug) and a placebo

2. Which of the following statements about animal testing of potential new therapeutic agents is *most* correct?
   (A) Extends at least 3 years to discover late toxicities
   (B) Requires at least 1 primate species (eg, rhesus monkey)
   (C) Requires the submission of histopathologic slides and specimens to the FDA for evaluation by government scientists
   (D) Has good predictability for drug allergy-type reactions
   (E) May be abbreviated in the case of some very toxic agents used in cancer

3. The "dominant lethal" test involves the treatment of a male adult animal with a chemical before mating; the pregnant female is later examined for fetal death and abnormalities. The dominant lethal test therefore is a test of
   (A) Teratogenicity
   (B) Mutagenicity
   (C) Carcinogenicity
   (D) Sperm viability

4. Which of the following would probably *not* be included in an optimal phase 3 clinical trial of a new analgesic drug for mild pain?
   (A) A negative control (placebo)
   (B) A positive control (current standard therapy)
   (C) Double-blind protocol (in which neither the patient nor immediate observers of the patient know which agent is active)
   (D) A group of 1000–5000 subjects with a clinical condition requiring analgesia
   (E) Prior submission of an NDA (new drug application) to the FDA

5. Which of the following statements about the testing of new compounds for potential therapeutic use in the treatment of hypertension is *most* correct?
   (A) Animal tests cannot be used to predict the types of clinical toxicities that may occur because there is no correlation with human toxicity
   (B) Human studies in normal individuals will be done before the drug is used in individuals with hypertension
   (C) The degree of risk must be assessed in at least 3 species of animals, including 1 primate species
   (D) The animal therapeutic index must be known before trial of the agents in humans

6. The Ames test is a method that detects
   (A) Carcinogenesis in primates
   (B) Carcinogenesis in rodents
   (C) Mutagenesis in bacteria
   (D) Teratogenesis in any mammalian species
   (E) Teratogenesis in primates

7. Which of the following statements about new drug development is *most* correct?
   (A) The original manufacturer is protected from generic competition for 20 years after patent approval
   (B) Food supplements and herbal (botanical) remedies are subject to the same FDA regulation as ordinary drugs
   (C) All new drugs must be studied in at least 1 primate species before NDA submission
   (D) Orphan drugs are drugs that are no longer produced by the original manufacturer
   (E) Phase 4 (surveillance) is the most rigidly regulated phase of clinical drug trials

ANSWERS

1. Except for known toxic drugs (eg, cancer chemotherapy drugs), phase 1 is carried out in 25–50 normal volunteers. Phase 2 is carried out in several hundred closely monitored patients with the disease. The therapeutic index is rarely determined in any clinical trial. Phase 4 is the general surveillance phase that follows marketing of the new drug. It is not targeted at specific effects. Positive controls and placebos are not a rigid requirement of any phase of clinical trials, although they are often used in phase 2 and phase 3 studies. The answer is **A**.

2. Drugs proposed for short-term use may not require long-term chronic testing. For some drugs, no primates are used; for other agents, only 1 species is used. The data from the tests, not the evidence itself, must be submitted to the FDA. Prediction of human drug allergy from animal testing is useful but not definitive (see answer 5). The answer is **E.**

3. The description of the test indicates that a chromosomal change (passed from father to fetus) is the toxicity detected. This is a mutation. The answer is **B.**

4. The first 4 items (**A–D**) are correct; they *would* be included. An NDA cannot be acted upon until the first 3 phases of clinical trials have been completed. (The IND must be approved before clinical trials can be conducted.) The answer is **E.**

5. Animal tests in a single species do not always predict human toxicities. However, when these tests are carried out in several species, most acute toxicities that occur in humans also appear in at least 1 animal species. According to current FDA rules, the "degree of risk" must be determined in at least 2 species. Use of primates is not always required. The therapeutic index is not required. Except for cancer chemotherapeutic agents and antivirals used in AIDS, phase 1 clinical trials are carried out in normal subjects. The answer is **B.**

6. The Ames test is carried out in *Salmonella* and detects mutations in the bacterial DNA. Because mutagenic potential is associated with carcinogenic risk for many chemicals, a positive Ames test is often used to claim that a particular agent may be a carcinogen. However, the test itself only detects mutations. The answer is **C.**

7. Food supplements and botanicals are much more loosely regulated than conventional drugs. Primates are not required in any phase of new drug testing, although they are sometimes used. Orphan drugs are those for which the anticipated patient population is smaller than 200,000 patients in the United States. Phase 4 surveillance is the most loosely regulated phase of clinical trials. The answer is **A.**

SKILL KEEPER ANSWER: GRADED AND QUANTAL DOSE-RESPONSE CURVES (CHAPTER 2)

The therapeutic index is the ratio of the median toxic dose, (TD$_{50}$) or median lethal dose (LD$_{50}$) to the effective dose in half the population (ED$_{50}$), determined in a population of subjects. Thus, quantal dose-response experiments are needed to ascertain the therapeutic index. The minimum effective dose and the maximal efficacy of a drug are determined by gradually increasing the dose and noting the responses produced. Graded dose-response experiments are needed for these measurements.

CHECKLIST

When you complete this chapter, you should be able to:

❑ Describe the major animal and clinical studies carried out in drug development.

❑ Describe the purpose of the Investigational New Drug (IND) Exemption and the New Drug Application (NDA).

❑ Define carcinogenesis, mutagenesis, and teratogenesis.

❑ Describe the difference between the FDA regulations for ordinary drugs and those for botanical remedies

CHAPTER 5 Summary Table

Major Concept	Description
Drug safety and efficacy	Standards of safety and efficacy for drugs developed slowly during the 20th century and are still incomplete. Because of heavy lobbying by manufacturers, these standards are still not applied to nutritional supplements and many so-called *alternative medications*. A few of the relevant US laws are listed in Table 5–2.
Preclinical drug testing	All new drugs undergo extensive *preclinical* testing in broken tissue preparations and cell cultures, isolated animal organ preparations, and intact animals. Efforts are made to determine the full range of toxic and therapeutic effects. See Figure 5–1
Clinical drug trials	All new drugs proposed for use in humans must undergo a series of tests in humans. These tests are regulated by the FDA and may be accelerated or retarded depending on the perceived clinical need and possible toxicities. The trials are often divided into 3 phases before marketing is allowed. See Figure 5–1

C H A P T E R

6

Introduction to Autonomic Pharmacology

The autonomic nervous system (ANS) is the major involuntary, unconscious, automatic portion of the nervous system and contrasts in several ways with the somatic (voluntary) nervous system. The anatomy, neurotransmitter chemistry, receptor characteristics, and functional integration of the ANS are discussed in this chapter. Major autonomic drug groups are discussed in Chapters 7 through 10. Drugs in many other groups have significant autonomic effects, many of which are undesirable.

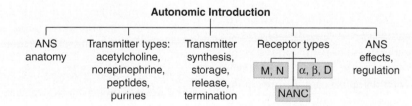

ANATOMIC ASPECTS OF THE ANS

The motor (efferent) portion of the ANS is the major pathway for information transmission from the central nervous system (CNS) to the involuntary effector tissues (smooth muscle, cardiac muscle, and exocrine glands; Figure 6–1). Its 2 major subdivisions are the **parasympathetic** ANS **(PANS)** and the **sympathetic** ANS **(SANS).** The **enteric nervous system (ENS)** is a semiautonomous part of the ANS located in the gastrointestinal tract, with specific functions for the control of this organ system. The ENS consists of the myenteric plexus (plexus of Auerbach) and the submucous plexus (plexus of Meissner); these neurons send sensory input to the parasympathetic and sympathetic nervous systems and receive motor output from them.

There are many sensory (afferent) fibers in autonomic nerves. These are of considerable importance for the physiologic control of the involuntary organs but are directly influenced by only a few drugs.

High-Yield Terms to Learn

Adrenergic	A nerve ending that releases norepinephrine as the primary transmitter; also, a synapse in which norepinephrine is the primary transmitter
Adrenoceptor, adrenergic receptor	A receptor that binds, and is activated by, one of the catecholamine transmitters or hormones (norepinephrine, epinephrine, dopamine) and related drugs
Baroreceptor reflex	The neuronal homeostatic mechanism that maintains a constant arterial blood pressure; the sensory limb originates in the baroreceptors of the carotid sinus and aortic arch; efferent pathways run in parasympathetic and sympathetic nerves
Cholinergic	A nerve ending that releases acetylcholine; also, a synapse in which the primary transmitter is acetylcholine
Cholinoceptor, cholinergic receptor	A receptor that binds, and is activated by, acetylcholine and related drugs
Dopaminergic	A nerve ending that releases dopamine as the primary transmitter; also a synapse in which dopamine is the primary transmitter
Homeostatic reflex	A compensatory mechanism for maintaining a body function at a predetermined level, for example, the baroreceptor reflex for blood pressure
Nonadrenergic, noncholinergic (NANC) system	Nerve fibers associated with autonomic nerves that release purines or peptides, not norepinephrine or acetylcholine
Parasympathetic	The part of the autonomic nervous system that originates in the cranial nerves and sacral part of the spinal cord; the craniosacral autonomic system
Postsynaptic receptor	A receptor located on the distal side of a synapse, for example, on a postganglionic neuron or an autonomic effector cell
Presynaptic receptor	A receptor located on the nerve ending from which the transmitter is released into the synapse; modulates the release of transmitter
Sympathetic	The part of the autonomic nervous system that originates in the thoracic and lumbar parts of the spinal cord

The parasympathetic preganglionic motor fibers originate in cranial nerve nuclei III, VII, IX, and X and in sacral segments (usually S2–S4) of the spinal cord. The sympathetic preganglionic fibers originate in the thoracic (T1–T12) and lumbar (L1–L5) segments of the cord.

Most of the sympathetic ganglia are located in 2 paravertebral chains that lie along the spinal column. A few (the prevertebral ganglia) are located on the anterior aspect of the abdominal aorta. Most of the parasympathetic ganglia are located in the organs innervated and more distant from the spinal cord. Because of the locations of the ganglia, the preganglionic sympathetic fibers are short and the postganglionic fibers are long. The opposite is true for the parasympathetic system: preganglionic fibers are longer and postganglionic fibers are short.

Some receptors that respond to autonomic transmitters and drugs receive no innervation. These include muscarinic receptors on the endothelium of blood vessels, some presynaptic receptors, and, in some species, the adrenoceptors on apocrine sweat glands and α_2 and β adrenoceptors in blood vessels.

NEUROTRANSMITTER ASPECTS OF THE ANS

The synthesis, storage, release, receptor interactions, and termination of action of the neurotransmitters all contribute to the action of autonomic drugs (Figure 6–2).

A. Cholinergic Transmission

Acetylcholine (ACh) is the primary transmitter in all autonomic ganglia and at the synapses between parasympathetic postganglionic neurons and their effector cells. It is the transmitter at postganglionic sympathetic neurons to the thermoregulatory sweat glands. It is also the primary transmitter at the somatic (voluntary) skeletal muscle neuromuscular junction (Figure 6–1).

1. Synthesis and storage—Acetylcholine is synthesized in the nerve terminal by the enzyme choline acetyltransferase (ChAT) from acetyl-CoA (produced in mitochondria) and choline (transported across the cell membrane) (Figure 6–2). The rate-limiting step is probably the transport of choline into the nerve terminal. This transport can be inhibited by the research drug **hemicholinium**. Acetylcholine is actively transported into its vesicles for storage by the vesicle-associated transporter, VAT. This process can be inhibited by another research drug, **vesamicol.**

2. Release of acetylcholine—Release of transmitter stores from vesicles in the nerve ending requires the entry of calcium through calcium channels and triggering of an interaction between **SNARE** (soluble *N*-ethylmaleimide-sensitive-factor attachment protein receptor) proteins. SNARE proteins include v-SNARES associated with the vesicles (**VAMPs, vesicle-associated membrane proteins: synaptobrevin, synaptotagmin**) and t-SNARE proteins associated with the nerve terminal membrane (**SNAPs, synaptosome-associated proteins:**

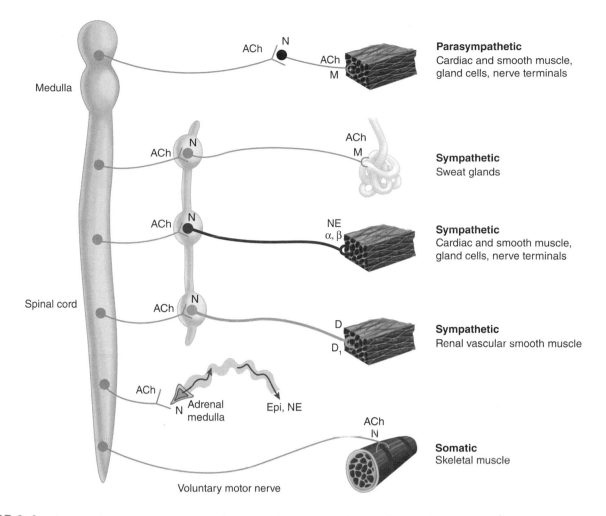

FIGURE 6–1 Schematic diagram comparing some features of the parasympathetic and sympathetic divisions of the autonomic nervous system with the somatic motor system. Parasympathetic ganglia are not shown as discrete structures because most of them are diffusely distributed in the walls of the organs innervated. Only 3 of the more than 20 sympathetic ganglia are shown. α and β, alpha and beta adrenoceptors; ACh, acetylcholine; D, dopamine; D_1, dopamine$_1$ receptors; Epi, epinephrine; M, muscarinic; N, nicotinic; NE, norepinephrine. (Modified and reproduced, with permission, from Katzung BG, editor: *Basic & Clinical Pharmacology,* 12th ed. McGraw-Hill, 2012: Fig. 6–1.)

SNAP25, syntaxin, and others). This interaction results in docking of the vesicle to the terminal membrane and, with influx of calcium, fusion of the membranes of the vesicles with the nerve-ending membranes, the opening of a pore to the extracellular space, and the release of the stored transmitter. The several types of **botulinum toxins** enzymatically alter synaptobrevin or one of the other docking or fusion proteins to prevent the release process.

3. Termination of action of acetylcholine—The action of acetylcholine in the synapse is normally terminated by metabolism to acetate and choline by the enzyme **acetylcholinesterase** in the synaptic cleft. The products are not excreted but are recycled in the body. Inhibition of acetylcholinesterase is an important therapeutic (and potentially toxic) effect of several drugs.

4. Drug effects on synthesis, storage, release, and termination of action of acetylcholine—Drugs that block

the synthesis of acetylcholine (eg, hemicholinium), its storage (eg, vesamicol), or its release (eg, botulinum toxin) are not very useful for systemic therapy because their effects are not sufficiently selective (ie, PANS and SANS ganglia and somatic neuromuscular junctions all may be blocked). However, because botulinum toxin is a very large molecule and diffuses very slowly, it can be used by injection for relatively selective local effects.

SKILL KEEPER: DRUG PERMEATION (SEE CHAPTER 1)

Botulinum toxin is a very large protein molecule and does not diffuse readily when injected into tissue. In spite of this property, it is able to enter cholinergic nerve endings from the extracellular space and block the release of acetylcholine. How might it cross the lipid membrane barrier? The Skill Keeper Answer appears at the end of the chapter.

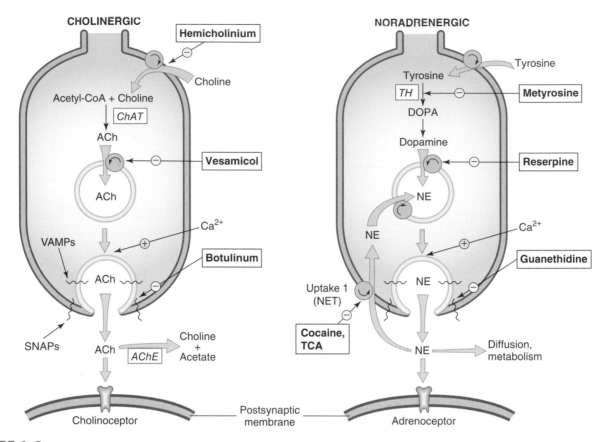

FIGURE 6–2 Characteristics of transmitter synthesis, storage, release, and termination of action at cholinergic and noradrenergic nerve terminals are shown from the top downward. Circles represent transporters; ACh, acetylcholine; AChE, acetylcholinesterase; *ChAT,* choline acetyltransferase; DOPA, dihydroxyphenylalanine; NE, norepinephrine; NET, norepinephrine transporter; TCA, tricyclic antidepressant; *TH,* tyrosine hydroxylase.

B. Adrenergic Transmission

Norepinephrine (NE) is the primary transmitter at the sympathetic postganglionic neuron-effector cell synapses in most tissues. Important exceptions include sympathetic fibers to thermoregulatory (eccrine) sweat glands and probably vasodilator sympathetic fibers in skeletal muscle, which release acetylcholine. Dopamine may be a vasodilator transmitter in renal blood vessels, but norepinephrine is a vasoconstrictor of these vessels.

1. Synthesis and storage—The synthesis of dopamine and norepinephrine requires several steps (Figure 6–2). After transport across the cell membrane, tyrosine is hydroxylated by **tyrosine hydroxylase** (the rate-limiting step) to DOPA (dihydroxyphenylalanine), decarboxylated to dopamine, and (inside the vesicle) hydroxylated to norepinephrine. Tyrosine hydroxylase can be inhibited by **metyrosine.** Norepinephrine and dopamine are transported into vesicles by the vesicular monoamine transporter (VMAT) and are stored there. Monoamine oxidase (MAO) is present on mitochondria in the adrenergic nerve ending and inactivates a portion of the dopamine and norepinephrine in the cytoplasm. Therefore, **MAO inhibitors** may increase the stores of these transmitters and other

amines in the nerve endings (Chapter 30). VMAT can be inhibited by **reserpine**, resulting in depletion of transmitter stores.

2. Release and termination of action—Dopamine and norepinephrine are released from their nerve endings by the same calcium-dependent mechanism responsible for acetylcholine release (see prior discussion). Termination of action, however, is quite different. Metabolism is not responsible for termination of action of the catecholamine transmitters, norepinephrine and dopamine. Rather, **diffusion** and **reuptake** (especially uptake-1, Figure 6–2, by the norepinephrine transporter, **NET,** or the dopamine transporter, **DAT**) reduce their concentration in the synaptic cleft and stop their action. Outside the cleft, these transmitters can be metabolized—by **MAO** and **catechol-O-methyltransferase (COMT)**—and the products of these enzymatic reactions are excreted. Determination of the 24-h excretion of **metanephrine, normetanephrine, 3-methoxy-4-hydroxymandelic acid (VMA),** and other metabolites provides a measure of the total body production of catecholamines, a determination useful in diagnosing conditions such as pheochromocytoma. Inhibition of MAO increases stores of catecholamines and has both therapeutic and toxic potential.

Inhibition of COMT in the brain is useful in Parkinson's disease (Chapter 28).

3. Drug effects on adrenergic transmission—Drugs that block norepinephrine synthesis (eg, metyrosine) or catecholamine storage (eg, reserpine) or release (eg, guanethidine) were used in treatment of several diseases (eg, hypertension) because they block sympathetic but not parasympathetic functions. Other drugs promote catecholamine release (eg, the amphetamine-like agents) and predictably cause sympathomimetic effects.

C. Cotransmitters

Many (probably all) autonomic nerves have transmitter vesicles that contain other transmitter molecules in addition to the primary agents (acetylcholine or norepinephrine) previously described. These cotransmitters may be localized in the same vesicles as the primary transmitter or in a separate population of vesicles. Substances recognized to date as cotransmitters include **ATP (adenosine triphosphate), enkephalins, vasoactive intestinal peptide, neuropeptide Y, substance P, neurotensin, somatostatin,** and others. Their main role in autonomic function appears to involve modulation of synaptic transmission. The same substances function as primary transmitters in other synapses.

RECEPTOR CHARACTERISTICS

The major receptor systems in the ANS include cholinoceptors, adrenoceptors, and dopamine receptors, which have been studied in some detail. The numerous receptors for cotransmitter substances have not been as fully defined.

A. Cholinoceptors

Also referred to as cholinergic receptors, these molecules respond to acetylcholine and its analogs. Cholinoceptors are subdivided as follows (Table 6–1):

1. Muscarinic receptors—As their name suggests, these receptors respond to muscarine (an alkaloid) as well as to acetylcholine. The effects of activation of these receptors resemble those of postganglionic parasympathetic nerve stimulation. Muscarinic receptors are located primarily on autonomic effector cells (including heart, vascular endothelium, smooth muscle, presynaptic nerve terminals, and exocrine glands). Evidence (including their genes) has been found for 5 subtypes, of which 3 appear to be important in peripheral autonomic transmission. All 5 are G-protein-coupled receptors (see Chapter 2).

2. Nicotinic receptors—These receptors are located on Na^+-K^+ ion channels and respond to acetylcholine and nicotine, another acetylcholine mimic (but not to muscarine) by opening the channel. The 2 major nicotinic subtypes are located in ganglia and in skeletal muscle end plates. The nicotinic receptors are the primary receptors for transmission at these sites.

B. Adrenoceptors

Also referred to as adrenergic receptors, adrenoceptors are divided into several subtypes (Table 6–2).

1. Alpha receptors—These are located on vascular smooth muscle, presynaptic nerve terminals, blood platelets, fat cells (lipocytes), and neurons in the brain. Alpha receptors are further divided into 2 major types, α_1 and α_2. These 2 subtypes constitute different families and use different G-coupling proteins.

2. Beta receptors—These receptors are located on most types of smooth muscle, cardiac muscle, some presynaptic nerve terminals, and lipocytes. Beta receptors are divided into 3 major subtypes, β_1, β_2, and β_3. These subtypes are rather similar and use the same G-coupling protein.

C. Dopamine Receptors

Dopamine (D, DA) receptors are a subclass of adrenoceptors but with rather different distribution and function. Dopamine receptors are especially important in the renal and splanchnic vessels and in the brain. Although at least 5 subtypes exist, the D_1 subtype appears to be the most important dopamine receptor on peripheral effector cells. D_2 receptors are found on presynaptic nerve terminals. D_1, D_2, and other types of dopamine receptors also occur in the CNS.

TABLE 6–1 Characteristics of the most important cholinoceptors in the peripheral nervous system.

Receptor	Location	Mechanism	Major Functions
M_1	Nerve endings	G_q-coupled	↑ IP_3, DAG cascade
M_2	Heart, some nerve endings	G_i-coupled	↓ cAMP, activates K^+ channels
M_3	Effector cells: smooth muscle, glands, endothelium	G_q-coupled	↑ IP_3, DAG cascade
N_N	ANS ganglia	Na^+-K^+ ion channel	Depolarizes, evokes action potential
N_M	Neuromuscular end plate	Na^+-K^+ ion channel	Depolarizes, evokes action potential

TABLE 6–2   Characteristics of some important adrenoceptors in the ANS.

Receptor	Location	G Protein	Second Messenger	Major Functions
Alpha$_1$ (α_1)	Effector tissues: smooth muscle, glands	G$_q$	↑ IP$_3$, DAG	↑ Ca^{2+}, causes contraction, secretion
Alpha$_2$ (α_2)	Nerve endings, some smooth muscle	G$_i$	↓ cAMP	↓ Transmitter release (nerves), causes contraction (muscle)
Beta$_1$ (β_1)	Cardiac muscle, juxtaglomerular apparatus	G$_s$	↑ cAMP	↑ Heart rate, ↑ force; ↑ renin release
Beta$_2$ (β_2)	Smooth muscle, liver, heart	G$_s$	↑ cAMP	Relax smooth muscle; ↑ glycogenolysis; ↑ heart rate, force
Beta$_3$ (β_3)	Adipose cells	G$_s$	↑ cAMP	↑ Lipolysis
Dopamine$_1$ (D$_1$)	Smooth muscle	G$_s$	↑ cAMP	Relax renal vascular smooth muscle

ANS, autonomic nervous system.

EFFECTS OF ACTIVATING AUTONOMIC NERVES

Each division of the ANS has specific effects on organ systems. These effects, summarized in Table 6–3, should be memorized.

Dually innervated organs such as the iris of the eye and the sinoatrial node of the heart receive both sympathetic and parasympathetic innervation. The pupil has a natural, intrinsic diameter to which it returns when both divisions of the ANS are blocked. Pharmacologic ganglionic blockade, therefore, causes it to move to its intrinsic size. Similarly, the cardiac sinus node pacemaker rate has an intrinsic value (about 100–110/min) in the absence of both ANS inputs. How will these variables change (increase or decrease) if the ganglia are blocked? The answer is predictable if one knows which system is dominant. For example, both the pupil and, at rest, the sinoatrial node are dominated by the parasympathetic system. Thus, blockade of both systems, with removal of the dominant PANS and nondominant SANS effects, result in mydriasis and tachycardia.

NONADRENERGIC, NONCHOLINERGIC (NANC) TRANSMISSION

Some nerve fibers in autonomic effector tissues do not show the histochemical characteristics of either cholinergic or adrenergic fibers. Some of these are motor fibers that cause the release of ATP and other purines related to it. Purine-evoked responses have been identified in the bronchi, gastrointestinal tract, and urinary tract. Other motor fibers are peptidergic, that is, they release peptides as the primary transmitters (see list in earlier Cotransmitters section). These fibers have been termed "sensory-efferent" or "sensory-local effector" fibers because, when activated by a sensory input, they are capable of releasing transmitter peptides from the sensory ending itself, from local axon branches, and from collaterals that terminate

Other nonadrenergic, noncholinergic fibers have the anatomic characteristics of sensory fibers and contain peptides, such as substance P, that are stored in and released from the fiber terminals. These fibers have been termed "sensory-efferent" or "sensory-local effector" fibers because, when activated by a sensory input, they are capable of releasing transmitter peptides from the sensory ending itself, from local axon branches, and from collaterals that terminate

in the autonomic ganglia. In addition to their neurotransmitter roles, these peptides are potent agonists in many autonomic effector tissues, especially smooth muscle (see Chapter 17).

SITES OF AUTONOMIC DRUG ACTION

Because of the number of steps in the transmission of autonomic commands from the CNS to the effector cells, there are many sites at which autonomic drugs may act. These sites include the CNS centers; the ganglia; the postganglionic nerve terminals; the effector cell receptors; and the mechanisms responsible for transmitter synthesis, storage, release, and termination of action. The most selective effect is achieved by drugs acting at receptors that mediate very selective actions (Table 6–4). Many natural and synthetic toxins have significant effects on autonomic and somatic nerve function.

INTEGRATION OF AUTONOMIC FUNCTION

Functional integration in the ANS is provided mainly through the mechanism of negative feedback and is extremely important in determining the overall response to endogenous and exogenous ANS transmitters and their analogs. This process uses modulatory pre- and postsynaptic receptors at the local level and homeostatic reflexes at the system level.

A. Local Integration

Local feedback control has been found at the level of the nerve endings in all systems investigated. The best documented of these is the negative feedback of norepinephrine upon its own release from adrenergic nerve terminals. This effect is mediated by α_2 receptors located on the presynaptic nerve membrane (Figure 6–3).

Presynaptic receptors that bind the primary transmitter substance and thereby regulate its release are called *autoreceptors*. Transmitter release is also modulated by other presynaptic receptors *(heteroreceptors)*; in the case of adrenergic nerve terminals,

TABLE 6–3 Direct effects of autonomic nerve activity on some organ systems.

| | Effect of | | | |
| | Sympathetic | | Parasympathetic | |
Organ	Action[a]	Receptor[b]	Action[a]	Receptor[b]
Eye				
Iris				
Radial muscle	Contracts	α_1	...	...
Circular muscle	...	...	Contracts	M_3
Ciliary muscle	[Relaxes]	β	Contracts	M_3
Heart				
Sinoatrial node	Accelerates	β_1, β_2	Decelerates	M_2
Ectopic pacemakers	Accelerates	β_1, β_2	...	...
Contractility	Increases	β_1, β_2	Decreases (atria)	[M_2]
Blood vessels				
Skin, splanchnic vessels	Contracts	α	...	...
Skeletal muscle vessels	Relaxes	β_2	...	...
	Contracts	α	...	...
	[Relaxes]	[M^c]	...	...
Bronchiolar smooth muscle	Relaxes	β_2	Contracts	M_3
Gastrointestinal tract				
Smooth muscle				
Walls	Relaxes	α_2,[d] β_2	Contracts	M_3
Sphincters	Contracts	α_1	Relaxes	M_3
Secretion	Inhibits	α_2	Increases	M_3
Myenteric plexus	...	...	Activates	M_1
Genitourinary smooth muscle				
Bladder wall	Relaxes	β_2	Contracts	M_3
Sphincter	Contracts	α_1	Relaxes	M_3
Uterus, pregnant	Relaxes	β_2	...	...
	Contracts	α	Contracts	M_3
Penis, seminal vesicles	Ejaculation	α	Erection	M
Skin				
Pilomotor smooth muscle	Contracts	α	...	...
Sweat glands			...	...
Thermoregulatory	Increases	M	...	...
Apocrine (stress)	Increases	α	...	...
Metabolic functions				
Liver	Gluconeogenesis	β_2, α	...	...
Liver	Glycogenolysis	β_2, α	...	...
Fat cells	Lipolysis	β_3	...	...
Kidney	Renin release	β_1	...	...
Autonomic nerve endings				
Sympathetic	...	...	Decreases NE release	M^e
Parasympathetic	Decreases ACh release	α	...	...

[a]Less important actions are shown in brackets.

[b]Specific receptor type: α, alpha; β, beta; M, muscarinic.

[c]Vascular smooth muscle in skeletal muscle has sympathetic cholinergic dilator fibers.

[d]Probably through presynaptic inhibition of parasympathetic activity.

[e]Probably M_1, but M_2 may participate in some locations.

ACh, acetylcholine; NE, norepinephrine.

Modified and reproduced, with permission, from Katzung BG, editor: *Basic & Clinical Pharmacology*, 12th ed. McGraw-Hill, 2012.

receptors for acetylcholine, histamine, serotonin, prostaglandins, peptides, and other substances have been found. Presynaptic regulation by a variety of endogenous chemicals probably occurs in all nerve fibers.

Postsynaptic modulatory receptors, including M_1 and M_2 muscarinic receptors and at least 1 type of peptidergic receptor, have been found in ganglionic synapses, where nicotinic transmission is primary. These receptors may facilitate or inhibit

TABLE 6–4 **Steps in autonomic transmission: effects of drugs.**

Process	Drug Example	Site	Action
Action potential propagation	Local anesthetics, tetrodotoxin,[a] saxitoxin[b]	Nerve axons	Block sodium channels; block conduction
Transmitter synthesis	Hemicholinium	Cholinergic nerve terminals: membrane	Blocks uptake of choline and slows synthesis of acetylcholine
	Alpha-Methyltyrosine (metyrosine)	Adrenergic nerve terminals and adrenal medulla: cytoplasm	Slows synthesis of norepinephrine
Transmitter storage	Vesamicol	Cholinergic terminals: vesicles	Prevents storage, depletes
	Reserpine	Adrenergic terminals: vesicles	Prevents storage, depletes
Transmitter release	Many[c]	Nerve terminal membrane receptors	Modulate release
	ω-Conotoxin GVIA[d]	Nerve terminal calcium channels	Reduces release
	Botulinum toxin	Cholinergic vesicles	Prevents release
	Alpha-latrotoxin[e]	Cholinergic and adrenergic vesicles	Causes explosive release
	Tyramine, amphetamine	Adrenergic nerve terminals	Promote release
Transmitter uptake after release	Cocaine, tricyclic antidepressants	Adrenergic nerve terminals	Inhibit uptake; increase transmitter effect on postsynaptic receptors
	6-Hydroxydopamine	Adrenergic nerve terminals	Destroys the terminals
Receptor activation or blockade	Norepinephrine	Receptors at adrenergic junctions	Binds α receptors; causes activation
	Phentolamine	Receptors at adrenergic junctions	Binds α receptors; prevents activation
	Isoproterenol	Receptors at adrenergic junctions	Binds β receptors; activates adenylyl cyclase
	Propranolol	Receptors at adrenergic junctions	Binds β receptors; prevents activation
	Nicotine	Receptors at nicotinic cholinergic junctions (autonomic ganglia, neuromuscular end plates)	Binds nicotinic receptors; opens ion channel in post-synaptic membrane
	Hexamethonium	Ganglionic nicotinic receptors	Prevents activation of N_N receptors
	Tubocurarine	Neuromuscular end plates	Prevents activation of N_M receptors
	Bethanechol	Parasympathetic effector cells (smooth muscle, glands)	Binds and activates muscarinic receptors
	Atropine	Parasympathetic effector cells	Binds muscarinic receptors; prevents activation
Enzymatic inactivation of transmitter	Neostigmine	Cholinergic synapses (acetylcholinesterase)	Inhibits enzyme; prolongs and intensifies transmitter action
	Tranylcypromine	Adrenergic nerve terminals (monoamine oxidase)	Inhibits enzyme; increases stored transmitter pool

[a]Toxin of puffer fish, California newt.

[b]Toxin of *Gonyaulax* (red tide organism).

[c]Norepinephrine, dopamine, acetylcholine, angiotensin II, various prostaglandins, etc.

[d]Toxin of marine snails of the genus *Conus*.

[e]Black widow spider venom.

Modified and reproduced, with permission, from Katzung BG, editor: *Basic & Clinical Pharmacology*, 12th ed. McGraw-Hill, 2012.

transmission by evoking slow excitatory or inhibitory postsynaptic potentials (EPSPs or IPSPs).

B. Systemic Reflexes

System reflexes regulate blood pressure, gastrointestinal motility, bladder tone, airway smooth muscle, and other processes.

The control of blood pressure—by the baroreceptor neural reflex and the renin-angiotensin-aldosterone hormonal response—is especially important (Figure 6–4). These homeostatic mechanisms have evolved to maintain mean arterial blood pressure at a level determined by the vasomotor center and renal sensors. Any deviation from this blood pressure "set point" causes a change in ANS activity and renin-angiotensin-aldosterone levels. For example, a

Noradrenergic nerve terminal

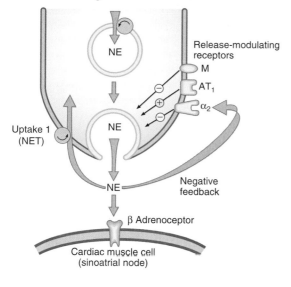

FIGURE 6–3 Local control of autonomic nervous system function via modulation of transmitter release. In the example shown, release of norepinephrine (NE) from a sympathetic nerve ending is modulated by norepinephrine itself, acting on presynaptic α_2 autoreceptors, and by acetylcholine and angiotensin II, acting on heteroreceptors. Many other modulators (see text) influence the release process. AT$_1$, angiotensin II receptor; M, muscarinic receptor; NET, norepinephrine transporter.

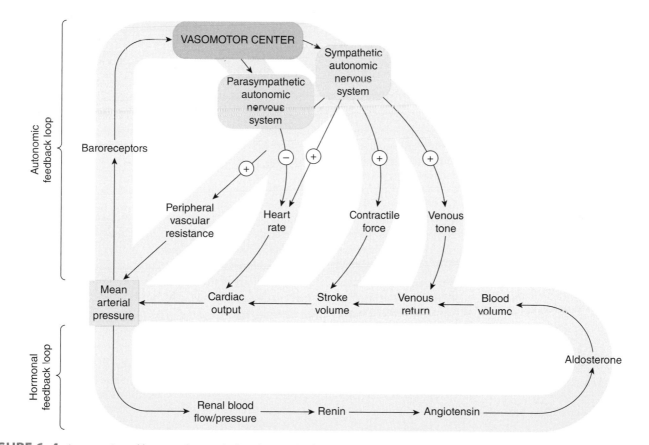

FIGURE 6–4 Autonomic and hormonal control of cardiovascular function. Note that 2 feedback loops are present: the autonomic nervous system loop and the hormonal loop. Each major loop has several components. In the neuronal loop, sensory input to the vasomotor center is via afferent fibers in the ninth and tenth cranial (PANS) nerves. On the efferent side, the sympathetic nervous system directly influences 4 major variables: peripheral vascular resistance, heart rate, contractile force, and venous tone. The parasympathetic nervous system directly influences heart rate. In addition, angiotensin II directly increases peripheral vascular resistance (not shown), and sympathetic nervous system discharge directly increases renin secretion (not shown). Because these control mechanisms have evolved to maintain normal blood pressure, the net feedback effect of each loop is negative; feedback tends to compensate for the change in arterial blood pressure that evoked the response. Thus, decreased blood pressure due to blood loss would be compensated by increased sympathetic outflow and renin release. Conversely, elevated pressure due to the administration of a vasoconstrictor drug would cause reduced sympathetic outflow, decreased renin release, and increased parasympathetic (vagal) outflow. (Modified and reproduced, with permission, from Katzung BG, editor: *Basic & Clinical Pharmacology*, 12th ed. McGraw-Hill, 2012: Fig. 6–7.)

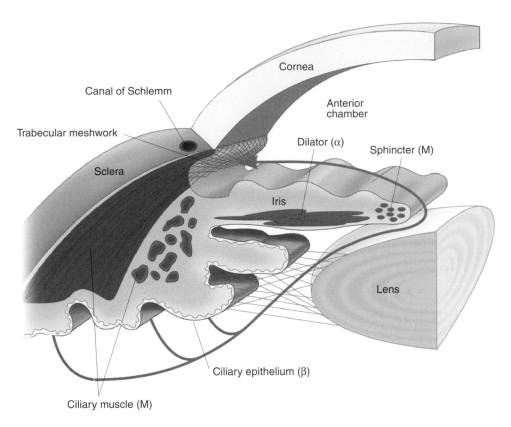

FIGURE 6–5 Some pharmacologic targets in the eye. The diagram illustrates clinically important structures and their receptors. The heavy arrow (blue) illustrates the flow of aqueous humor from its secretion by the ciliary epithelium to its drainage through the canal of Schlemm. M, muscarinic receptor; α, alpha receptor; β, beta receptor. (Modified and reproduced, with permission, from Katzung BG, editor: *Basic & Clinical Pharmacology,* 12th ed. McGraw-Hill, 2012: Fig. 6–9.)

decrease in blood pressure caused by hemorrhage causes increased SANS discharge and renin release. As a result, peripheral vascular resistance, venous tone, heart rate, and cardiac force are increased by norepinephrine released from sympathetic nerves. This ANS response can be blocked with ganglion-blocking drugs such as hexamethonium. Blood volume is replenished by retention of salt and water in the kidney under the influence of increased levels of aldosterone. These compensatory responses may be large enough to overcome some of the actions of drugs. For example, the chronic treatment of hypertension with a vasodilator such as hydralazine will be unsuccessful when the compensatory tachycardia (via the baroreceptor reflex) and the salt and water retention (via the renin system response) are not prevented through the use of additional drugs.

C. Complex Organ Control: The Eye

The eye contains multiple tissues, several of them under autonomic control (Figure 6–5). The pupil, discussed previously, is under reciprocal control by the SANS (via α receptors on the pupillary dilator muscle) and the PANS (via muscarinic receptors on the pupillary constrictor). The ciliary muscle, which controls

accommodation, is under primary control of muscarinic receptors innervated by the PANS, with insignificant contributions from the SANS. The ciliary *epithelium,* on the other hand, has important β receptors that have a permissive effect on aqueous humor secretion. Each of these receptors is an important target of drugs that are discussed in the following chapters.

QUESTIONS

1. A 3-year-old child has swallowed the contents of 2 bottles of a nasal decongestant whose primary ingredient is a potent, selective α-adrenoceptor agonist drug. Which of the following is a sign of α-receptor activation that may occur in this patient?
   (A) Bronchodilation
   (B) Cardiac acceleration (tachycardia)
   (C) Pupillary dilation (mydriasis)
   (D) Renin release from the kidneys
   (E) Vasodilation of the splanchnic vessels

2. Ms Green is a 60-year-old woman with poorly controlled hypertension of 170/110 mm Hg. She is to receive minoxidil. The active metabolite of minoxidil is a powerful arteriolar vasodilator that does not act on autonomic receptors. Which of the following effects will be observed if no other drugs are used?
   (A) Tachycardia and increased cardiac contractility
   (B) Tachycardia and decreased cardiac output
   (C) Decreased mean arterial pressure and decreased cardiac contractility
   (D) Decreased mean arterial pressure and increased salt and water excretion by the kidney
   (E) No change in mean arterial pressure and decreased cardiac contractility

3. Full activation of the sympathetic nervous system, as in the fight-or-flight reaction, may occur during maximal exercise. Which of the following effects is likely to occur?
   (A) Bronchoconstriction
   (B) Increased intestinal motility
   (C) Decreased renal blood flow
   (D) Miosis
   (E) Decreased heart rate (bradycardia)

Questions 4–5. For these questions, use the accompanying diagram. Assume that the diagram can represent either the sympathetic or the parasympathetic system.

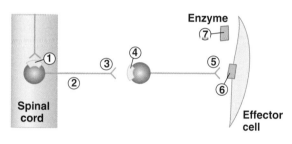

4. Norepinephrine acts at which of the following sites in the diagram?
   (A) Sites 1 and 2
   (B) Sites 3 and 4
   (C) Sites 5 and 6

5. If the effector cell in the diagram is a thermoregulatory sweat gland, which of the following transmitters is released from structure 5?
   (A) Acetylcholine
   (B) Dopamine
   (C) Epinephrine
   (D) Norepinephrine

6. Nicotinic receptor sites do *not* include which one of the following sites?
   (A) Bronchial smooth muscle
   (B) Adrenal medullary cells
   (C) Parasympathetic ganglia
   (D) Skeletal muscle end plates
   (E) Sympathetic ganglia

7. Several children at a summer camp were hospitalized with symptoms thought to be due to ingestion of food containing botulinum toxin. Which one of the following signs or symptoms is consistent with the diagnosis of botulinum poisoning?
   (A) Bronchospasm
   (B) Cycloplegia
   (C) Diarrhea
   (D) Skeletal muscle spasms
   (E) Hyperventilation

8. Which one of the following is the neurotransmitter agent normally released in the sinoatrial node of the heart in response to a blood pressure increase?
   (A) Acetylcholine
   (B) Dopamine
   (C) Epinephrine
   (D) Glutamate
   (E) Norepinephrine

Questions 9-10. Assume that the diagram below represents a sympathetic postganglionic nerve ending.

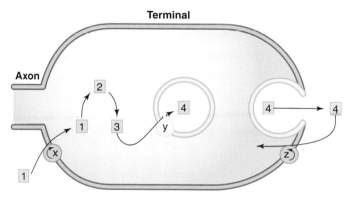

9. Which of the following blocks the carrier represented by "y" in the diagram?
   (A) Amphetamine
   (B) Botulinum toxin
   (C) Cocaine
   (D) Hemicholinium
   (E) Reserpine

10. Which of the following inhibits the carrier denoted "z" in the diagram?
    (A) Cocaine
    (B) Dopamine
    (C) Hemicholinium
    (D) Reserpine
    (E) Vesamicol

ANSWERS

1. Mydriasis can be caused by contraction of the radial fibers of the iris; these smooth muscle cells have α receptors. All the other responses are mediated by β adrenoceptors (Table 6–4). The answer is **C.**

2. Because of the compensatory responses, a drug that directly decreases blood pressure through a decrease in peripheral vascular resistance will cause a reflex increase in sympathetic outflow, an increase in renin release, and a decrease in parasympathetic outflow. As a result, heart rate and cardiac force will increase. In addition, salt and water retention will occur. The answer is **A.**

3. Sympathetic discharge causes constriction of the renal resistance vessels and a fall in renal blood flow. This is the typical response in severe exercise or hypotension. The other effects are parasympathomimetic actions. The answer is **C**.

4. Norepinephrine acts at presynaptic α_2 regulatory receptors (site 5) and postsynaptic α_1 adrenoceptors (site 6). It may be metabolized by enzymes outside the synapse or transported back into the nerve terminal. The answer is **C**.

5. The nerves innervating the thermoregulatory (eccrine) sweat glands are sympathetic *cholinergic* nerves. The answer is **A**.

6. Both types of ganglia and the skeletal muscle neuromuscular junction have nicotinic cholinoceptors, as does the adrenal medulla (a modified form of sympathetic postganglionic neuron tissue). Bronchial smooth muscle contains muscarinic cholinoceptors and noncholinergic receptors. The answer is **A**.

7. Botulinum toxin impairs all types of cholinergic transmission, including transmission at ganglionic synapses and somatic motor nerve endings. Botulinum toxin prevents discharge of vesicular transmitter content from cholinergic nerve endings. All of the signs listed except cycloplegia indicate increased muscle contraction; cycloplegia (paralysis of accommodation) results in blurred near vision. The answer is **B**.

8. Acetylcholine is the transmitter at parasympathetic nerve endings innervating the sinus node (nerve endings of the vagus nerve). When blood pressure increases, the parasympathetic system is activated and heart rate slows. The answer is **A**.

9. The vesicular carrier in the diagram transports dopamine and norepinephrine into the vesicles for storage. It can be blocked by reserpine. The answer is **E**.

10. The reuptake carrier in sympathetic postganglionic nerve endings can be blocked by cocaine or tricyclic antidepressants. Hemicholiniums and vesamicol block transporters in cholinergic nerves. The answer is **A**.

SKILL KEEPER ANSWER: DRUG PERMEATION (SEE CHAPTER 1)

Botulinum toxin is too large to cross membranes by means of lipid or aqueous diffusion. It must bind to membrane receptors and enter by endocytosis. Botulinum-binding receptors for endocytosis are present on cholinergic neurons but not adrenergic neurons.

CHECKLIST

When you complete this chapter, you should be able to:

❏ Describe the steps in the synthesis, storage, release, and termination of action of the major autonomic transmitters.

❏ Name 2 cotransmitter substances.

❏ Name the major types of autonomic receptors and the tissues in which they are found.

❏ Describe the organ system effects of stimulation of the parasympathetic and sympathetic systems.

❏ Name examples of inhibitors of acetylcholine and norepinephrine synthesis, storage, and release. Predict the effects of these inhibitors on the function of the major organ systems.

❏ List the determinants of blood pressure and describe the baroreceptor reflex response for the following perturbations: (1) blood loss, (2) administration of a vasodilator, (3) a vasoconstrictor, (4) a cardiac stimulant, (5) a cardiac depressant.

❏ Describe the results of transplantation of the heart (with interruption of its autonomic nerves) on cardiac function.

❏ Describe the actions of several toxins that affect nerve function: tetrodotoxin, saxitoxin, botulinum toxins, and latrotoxin.

SUMMARY TABLE: Introductory Autonomic Drugs

Drug	Comment
Acetylcholine	Primary transmitter at cholinergic nerve endings (preganglionic ANS, postganglionic parasympathetic, postganglionic sympathetic to thermoregulatory sweat glands, and somatic neuromuscular end plates)
Amphetamine	Sympathomimetic drug that facilitates the release of catecholamines from adrenergic nerve endings
Botulinum toxin	Bacterial toxin that enzymatically disables release of acetylcholine from cholinergic nerve endings
Cocaine	Sympathomimetic drug that impairs reuptake of catecholamine transmitters (norepinephrine, dopamine) by adrenergic nerve endings; also local anesthetic
Dopamine	Important central nervous system (CNS) transmitter with some peripheral effects (renal vasodilation, cardiac stimulation)
Epinephrine	Hormone released from adrenal medulla, neurotransmitter in CNS
Hemicholiniums	Drugs that inhibit transport of choline into cholinergic nerve endings
Hexamethonium	Research drug that blocks all ANS ganglia and prevents autonomic compensatory reflexes
Metanephrine	Product of epinephrine and norepinephrine metabolism
Metyrosine	Inhibitor of tyrosine hydroxylase, the rate-limiting enzyme in norepinephrine synthesis
Norepinephrine	Primary transmitter at most sympathetic postganglionic nerve endings; important CNS transmitter
Reserpine	Drug that inhibits VMAT, transporter of dopamine and norepinephrine into transmitter vesicles of adrenergic nerves
Tetrodotoxin, saxitoxin	Toxins that block sodium channels and thereby limit transmission in all nerve fibers
Vesamicol	Drug that inhibits VAT, transporter of acetylcholine into its transmitter vesicles

7

Cholinoceptor-Activating & Cholinesterase-Inhibiting Drugs

Drugs with acetylcholine-like effects (**cholinomimetics**) consist of 2 major subgroups on the basis of their mode of action (ie, whether they act directly at the acetylcholine receptor or indirectly through inhibition of cholinesterase). Drugs in the direct-acting subgroup are further subdivided on the basis of

their spectrum of action (ie, whether they act on muscarinic or nicotinic cholinoceptors).

Acetylcholine may be considered the prototype that acts directly at both muscarinic and nicotinic receptors. **Neostigmine** is a prototype for the indirect-acting cholinesterase inhibitors.

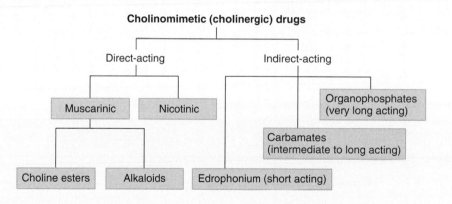

DIRECT-ACTING CHOLINOMIMETIC AGONISTS

This class comprises a group of choline esters (**acetylcholine, methacholine, carbachol**, and **bethanechol**) and a second group of naturally occurring alkaloids (**muscarine, pilocarpine, nicotine, lobeline**). Newer drugs are occasionally introduced for special applications. The members differ in their spectrum of action (amount of muscarinic versus nicotinic stimulation) and in their pharmacokinetics (Table 7–1). Both factors influence their clinical use.

A. Classification

Muscarinic agonists are parasympathomimetic; that is, they mimic the actions of parasympathetic nerve stimulation in addition to other effects. Five subgroups of muscarinic receptors have been identified (Table 7–2), but the muscarinic agonists available for clinical use activate them nonselectively. Nicotinic agonists are rarely classified on the basis of whether ganglionic or neuromuscular stimulation predominates; agonist selectivity is limited. On the other hand, relatively selective *antagonists* are available for the two nicotinic receptor types (Chapter 8).

High-Yield Terms to Learn

Choline ester	A cholinomimetic drug consisting of choline (an alcohol) esterified with an acidic substance, (eg, acetic or carbamic acid); usually poorly lipid-soluble
Cholinergic crisis	The clinical condition of excessive activation of cholinoceptors; it may include skeletal muscle weakness as well as parasympathetic signs
Cholinomimetic alkaloid	A drug with weakly basic properties (usually of plant origin) whose effects resemble those of acetylcholine; usually lipid-soluble
Cyclospasm	Marked contraction of the ciliary muscle; maximum accommodation for close vision
Direct-acting cholinomimetic	A drug that binds and activates cholinoceptors; the effects mimic those of acetylcholine
Endothelium-derived relaxing factor (EDRF)	A potent vasodilator substance, largely nitric oxide (NO), that is released from vascular endothelial cells
Indirect-acting cholinomimetic	A drug that amplifies the effects of endogenous acetylcholine by inhibiting acetylcholinesterase
Muscarinic agonist	A cholinomimetic drug that binds muscarinic receptors and has primarily muscarine-like actions
Myasthenic crisis	In patients with myasthenia, an acute worsening of symptoms; usually relieved by increasing cholinomimetic treatment
Nicotinic agonist	A cholinomimetic drug that binds nicotinic receptors and has primarily nicotine-like actions
Organophosphate	An ester of phosphoric acid and an alcohol that inhibits cholinesterase
Organophosphate aging	A process whereby the organophosphate, after binding to cholinesterase, is chemically modified and becomes more firmly bound to the enzyme
Parasympathomimetic	A drug whose effects resemble those of stimulating the parasympathetic nerves

TABLE 7–1 Some cholinomimetics: spectrum of action and pharmacokinetics.

Drug	Spectrum of Action[a]	Pharmacokinetic Features
Direct-acting		
Acetylcholine	B	Rapidly hydrolyzed by cholinesterase (ChE); duration of action 5–30 s; poor lipid solubility
Bethanechol	M	Resistant to ChE; orally active, poor lipid solubility; duration of action 30 min to 2 h
Carbachol	B	Like bethanechol
Pilocarpine	M	Not an ester, good lipid solubility; duration of action 30 min to 2 h
Nicotine	N	Like pilocarpine; duration of action 1–6 h; high lipid solubility
Varenicline	N	Partial agonist at N receptors, high lipid solubility; duration 12–24 h
Indirect-acting		
Edrophonium	B	Alcohol, quaternary amine, poor lipid solubility, not orally active; duration of action 5–15 min
Neostigmine	B	Carbamate, quaternary amine, poor lipid solubility, orally active; duration of action 30 min to 2 h or more
Physostigmine	B	Carbamate, tertiary amine, good lipid solubility, orally active; duration of action 30 min to 2 h
Pyridostigmine	B	Carbamate, like neostigmine, but longer duration of action (4–8 h)
Echothiophate	B	Organophosphate, moderate lipid solubility; duration of action 2–7 days
Parathion	B	Organophosphate, high lipid solubility; duration of action 7–30 days

[a]B, both M and N; M, muscarinic; N, nicotinic.

TABLE 7–2 Cholinoceptor types and their postreceptor mechanisms.

Receptor Type	G Protein	Postreceptor Mechanisms
M_1	G_q	↑ IP_3, DAG cascade
M_2	G_i	↓ cAMP synthesis
M_3	G_q	↑ IP_3, DAG cascade
M_4	G_i	↓ cAMP synthesis
M_5	G_q	↑ IP_3, DAG cascade
N_M	None	Na^+/K^+ depolarizing current
N_N	None	Na^+/K^+ depolarizing current

cAMP, cyclic adenosine monophosphate; DAG, diacylglycerol; IP_3 inositol-1,4,5-trisphosphate.

> ### SKILL KEEPER: DRUG METABOLISM (SEE CHAPTER 4)
>
> *Acetylcholine is metabolized in the body by hydrolysis of the ester bond. Is this a phase I or phase II metabolic reaction?* The Skill Keeper Answer appears at the end of the chapter.

B. Molecular Mechanisms of Action

1. Muscarinic mechanism—Muscarinic receptors are G protein-coupled receptors (GPCRs) (Table 7–2). G_q protein coupling of M_1 and M_3 muscarinic receptors to phospholipase C, a membrane-bound enzyme, leads to the release of the second messengers, **diacylglycerol (DAG)** and **inositol-1,4,5-trisphosphate (IP_3)**. DAG modulates the action of protein kinase C, an enzyme important in secretion, whereas IP_3 evokes the release of calcium from intracellular storage sites, which results in contraction in smooth muscle. M_2 muscarinic receptors couple to adenylyl cyclase through the inhibitory G_i-coupling protein. A third mechanism couples the same M_2 receptors via the βγ subunit of the G protein to potassium channels in the heart and elsewhere; muscarinic agonists facilitate opening of these channels. M_4 and M_5 receptors may be important in the central nervous system (CNS) but have not been shown to play major roles in peripheral organs.

2. Nicotinic mechanism—The mechanism of nicotinic action has been clearly defined. The nicotinic acetylcholine ACh receptor is located on a channel protein that is selective for sodium and potassium. When the receptor is activated, the channel opens and depolarization of the cell occurs as a direct result of the influx of sodium, causing an excitatory postsynaptic potential (EPSP). If large enough, the EPSP evokes a propagated action potential in the surrounding membrane. The nicotinic

receptors on sympathetic and parasympathetic ganglion cells (N_N, also denoted N_G) differ slightly from those on neuromuscular end plates (N_M).

C. Tissue and Organ Effects

The tissue and organ system effects of cholinomimetics are summarized in Table 7–3. Note that vasodilation (and decreased blood pressure) is not a parasympathomimetic response (ie, it is not evoked by parasympathetic nerve discharge, even though directly acting cholinomimetics cause vasodilation). This vasodilation results from the release of endothelium-derived relaxing factor (EDRF; nitric oxide and possibly other substances) in the vessels, mediated by *uninnervated* muscarinic receptors on the endothelial cells. Note also that decreased blood pressure evokes the baroreceptor reflex, resulting in strong compensatory sympathetic discharge to the heart. As a result, injections of small to moderate amounts of direct-acting muscarinic cholinomimetics often cause *tachycardia*, whereas parasympathetic (vagal) nerve discharge to the heart causes *bradycardia*. Another effect seen with cholinomimetic drugs but not with parasympathetic nerve stimulation is thermoregulatory sweating; this is a *sympathetic* cholinergic effect (see Chapter 6).

The tissue and organ level effects of nicotinic ganglionic stimulation depend on the autonomic innervation of the organ involved. The blood vessels are dominated by sympathetic innervation; therefore, nicotinic receptor activation results in vasoconstriction mediated by sympathetic postganglionic nerve discharge. The gut is dominated by parasympathetic control; nicotinic drugs increase motility and secretion because of increased parasympathetic postganglionic neuron discharge. Nicotinic neuromuscular end plate activation by direct-acting drugs results in fasciculations and spasm of the muscles involved. Prolonged activation results in paralysis (see Chapter 27), which is an important hazard of exposure to nicotine-containing and organophosphate insecticides.

D. Clinical Use

Several clinical conditions benefit from an increase in cholinergic activity, including glaucoma, Sjogren's syndrome, and loss of normal PANS activity in the bowel and bladder. Direct-acting nicotinic agonists are used in smoking cessation and to produce skeletal muscle paralysis (**succinylcholine**, Chapter 27). Indirect-acting agents are used when increased nicotinic activation is needed at the neuromuscular junction (see discussion of myasthenia gravis). Nicotine is still used as an insecticide. **Varenicline** is a newer nicotinic agonist with partial agonist properties. It appears to reduce craving in persons addicted to nicotine.

E. Toxicity

The signs and symptoms of overdosage are readily predicted from the general pharmacology of acetylcholine.

1. Muscarinic toxicity—These effects include CNS stimulation (uncommon with choline esters and pilocarpine), miosis, spasm

TABLE 7–3 **Effects of cholinomimetics on major organ systems.**

Organ	Response[a]
CNS	Complex stimulatory effects. Nicotine: elevation of mood, alerting, addiction; physostigmine: convulsions; excessive concentrations may cause coma
Eye	
Sphincter muscle of iris	Contraction (miosis)
Ciliary muscle	Contraction (accommodation for near vision), cyclospasm
Heart	
Sinoatrial node	Decrease in rate (negative chronotropy), but note important reflex response in intact subject (see text)
Atria	Decrease in contractile force (negative inotropy); decrease in refractory period
Atrioventricular node	Decrease in conduction velocity (negative dromotropy), increase in refractory period
Ventricles	Small decrease in contractile force
Blood vessels	Dilation via release of EDRF from endothelium
Bronchi	Contraction (bronchoconstriction)
Gastrointestinal tract	
Motility	Increase in smooth muscle contraction, peristalsis
Sphincters	Decrease in tone, relaxation. (Exception: gastroesophageal sphincter contracts)
Urinary bladder	
Detrusor	Increase in contraction
Trigone and sphincter	Relaxation; voiding
Skeletal muscle	Activation of neuromuscular end plates, contraction
Glands (exocrine)	Increased secretion (thermoregulatory sweating, lacrimation, salivation, bronchial secretion, gastrointestinal glands)

[a]Only the direct effects are indicated; homeostatic responses to these direct actions may be important (see text).

EDRF, endothelium-derived relaxing factor (primarily nitric oxide).

of accommodation, bronchoconstriction, excessive gastrointestinal and genitourinary smooth muscle activity, increased secretory activity (sweat glands, airway, gastrointestinal tract, lacrimal glands), and vasodilation. Transient bradycardia occurs, followed by reflex tachycardia if the drug is administered as an intravenous bolus; reflex tachycardia occurs otherwise. Muscarine and similar alkaloids are found in certain mushrooms (*Inocybe* species and *Amanita muscaria*) and are responsible for the short-acting form of mushroom poisoning, which is characterized by nausea, vomiting, and diarrhea. (The much more dangerous and potentially lethal form of mushroom poisoning from *Amanita phalloides* and related species involves initial vomiting and diarrhea but is followed by hepatic and renal necrosis. It is not caused by muscarinic agonists but by amanitin and phalloidin, RNA polymerase inhibitors.)

2. Nicotinic toxicity—Toxic effects include ganglionic stimulation and block and neuromuscular end plate depolarization leading to fasciculations and then paralysis. CNS toxicity includes stimulation (including convulsions) followed by depression. Nicotine in small doses is strongly addicting.

INDIRECT-ACTING AGONISTS

A. Classification and Prototypes

Hundreds of indirect-acting cholinomimetic drugs have been synthesized in 2 major chemical classes: carbamic acid esters (**carbamates**) and phosphoric acid esters (**organophosphates**). **Neostigmine** is a prototypic carbamate, whereas **parathion,** an important insecticide, is a prototypic organophosphate. A third class has only one clinically useful member: **edrophonium** is an alcohol (not an ester) with a very short duration of action.

B. Mechanism of Action

Both carbamate and organophosphate inhibitors bind to cholinesterase and undergo prompt hydrolysis. The alcohol portion of the molecule is then released. The acidic portion (carbamate ion or phosphate ion) is released much more slowly, preventing the binding and hydrolysis of endogenous acetylcholine. As a result, these drugs **amplify** acetylcholine effects wherever the transmitter is released. Edrophonium, though not an ester, has sufficient affinity for the enzyme active site to similarly prevent access of acetylcholine for 5–15 min. After hydrolysis, carbamates are released by cholinesterase over a period of 2–8 h. Organophosphates are long-acting drugs; they form an extremely stable phosphate complex with the enzyme. After initial hydrolysis, the phosphoric acid residue is released over periods of days to weeks. Recovery is due in part to synthesis of new enzyme.

C. Effects

By inhibiting cholinesterase, these agents cause an increase in the concentration, half-life, and actions of acetylcholine in synapses where acetylcholine is released physiologically. Therefore, the indirect agents have muscarinic or nicotinic effects depending on which organ system is under consideration. Cholinesterase inhibitors do not have significant actions at uninnervated sites where acetylcholine is not normally released (eg, vascular endothelial cells).

D. Clinical Use

The clinical applications of the indirect-acting cholinomimetics are predictable from a consideration of the organs and the diseases that benefit from an amplification of cholinergic activity. These applications are summarized in the Drug Summary Table. Carbamates, which include **neostigmine, physostigmine, pyridostigmine**, and **ambenonium**, are used far more commonly in therapeutics than are organophosphates. The treatment of myasthenia is especially important. (Because myasthenia is an autoimmune disorder, treatment may also include thymectomy and immunosuppressant drugs.) **Rivastigmine**, a carbamate, and several other cholinesterase inhibitors are used exclusively in Alzheimer's disease. A portion of their action may be due to other, unknown mechanisms. Although their effects are modest and temporary, these drugs are frequently used in this devastating condition. Some carbamates (eg, **carbaryl**) are used in agriculture as insecticides. Two organophosphates used in medicine are **malathion** (a scabicide) and **metrifonate** (an antihelminthic agent).

Edrophonium is used for the rapid reversal of nondepolarizing neuromuscular blockade (Chapter 27), in the diagnosis of myasthenia, and in differentiating myasthenic crisis from cholinergic crisis in patients with this disease. Because cholinergic crisis can result in muscle weakness like that of myasthenic crisis, distinguishing the 2 conditions may be difficult. Administration of a short-acting cholinomimetic, such as edrophonium, will improve muscle strength in myasthenic crisis but weaken it in cholinergic crisis.

E. Toxicity

In addition to their therapeutic uses, some indirect-acting agents (especially organophosphates) have clinical importance because of accidental exposures to toxic amounts of pesticides. The most toxic of these drugs (eg, parathion) can be rapidly fatal if exposure is not immediately recognized and treated. After standard protection of vital signs (see Chapter 58), the antidote of first choice is the antimuscarinic agent **atropine**, but this drug has no effect on the nicotinic signs of toxicity. Nicotinic toxicity is treated by regenerating active cholinesterase. Immediately after binding to cholinesterase, most organophosphate inhibitors can be removed from the enzyme by the use of regenerator compounds such as **pralidoxime** (see Chapter 8), and this may reverse both nicotinic and muscarinic signs. If the enzyme-phosphate binding is allowed to persist, however, aging (a further chemical change) occurs and regenerator drugs can no longer remove the inhibitor. Treatment is described in more detail in Chapter 8.

Because of their toxicity and short persistence in the environment, organophosphates are used extensively in agriculture as insecticides and antihelminthic agents; examples are malathion and parathion. Some of these agents (eg, malathion, dichlorvos) are relatively safe in humans because they are metabolized rapidly to inactive products in mammals (and birds) but not in insects. Some are prodrugs (eg, malathion, parathion) and must be metabolized to the active product (malaoxon from malathion, paraoxon from parathion). The signs and symptoms of poisoning are the same as those described for the direct-acting agents, with the following exceptions: vasodilation is a late and uncommon effect; bradycardia is more common than tachycardia; CNS stimulation is common with organophosphate and physostigmine overdosage and includes convulsions, followed by respiratory and cardiovascular depression. The spectrum of toxicity can be remembered with the aid of the mnemonic DUMBBELSS (diarrhea, urination, miosis, bronchoconstriction, bradycardia, excitation [of skeletal muscle and CNS], lacrimation, and salivation and sweating).

QUESTIONS

1. A 30-year-old woman undergoes abdominal surgery. In spite of minimal tissue damage, complete ileus (absence of bowel motility) follows, and she complains of severe bloating. She also finds it difficult to urinate. Mild cholinomimetic stimulation with bethanechol or neostigmine is often effective in relieving these complications of surgery. Neostigmine and bethanechol in moderate doses have significantly *different* effects on which one of the following?
   (A) Gastric secretion
   (B) Neuromuscular end plate
   (C) Salivary glands
   (D) Sweat glands
   (E) Ureteral tone

2. Parathion has which one of the following characteristics?
   (A) It is inactivated by conversion to paraoxon
   (B) It is less toxic to humans than malathion
   (C) It is more persistent in the environment than DDT
   (D) It is poorly absorbed through skin and lungs
   (E) If treated early, its toxicity may be partly reversed by pralidoxime

3. Ms Brown has been treated for myasthenia gravis for several years. She reports to the emergency department complaining of recent onset of weakness of her hands, diplopia, and difficulty swallowing. She may be suffering from a change in response to her myasthenia therapy, that is, a cholinergic or a myasthenic crisis. Which of the following is the best drug for distinguishing between myasthenic crisis (insufficient therapy) and cholinergic crisis (excessive therapy)?
(A) Atropine
(B) Edrophonium
(C) Physostigmine
(D) Pralidoxime
(E) Pyridostigmine

4. A crop duster pilot has been accidentally exposed to a high concentration of a highly toxic agricultural organophosphate insecticide. If untreated, the cause of death from such exposure would probably be
(A) Cardiac arrhythmia
(B) Gastrointestinal bleeding
(C) Heart failure
(D) Hypotension
(E) Respiratory failure

5. Mr Green has just been diagnosed with dysautonomia (chronic idiopathic autonomic insufficiency). You are considering different therapies for his disease. Pyridostigmine and neostigmine may cause which one of the following?
(A) Bronchodilation
(B) Cycloplegia
(C) Diarrhea
(D) Irreversible inhibition of acetylcholinesterase
(E) Reduced gastric acid secretion

6. Parasympathetic nerve stimulation and a slow infusion of bethanechol will each:
(A) Cause ganglion cell depolarization
(B) Cause skeletal muscle end plate depolarization
(C) Cause vasodilation
(D) Increase bladder tone
(E) Increase heart rate

7. Actions and clinical uses of muscarinic cholinoceptor agonists include which one of the following?
(A) Bronchodilation (asthma)
(B) Improved aqueous humor drainage (glaucoma)
(C) Decreased gastrointestinal motility (diarrhea)
(D) Decreased neuromuscular transmission and relaxation of skeletal muscle (during surgical anesthesia)
(E) Increased sweating (fever)

8. Which of the following is a direct-acting cholinomimetic that is lipid-soluble and is used to facilitate smoking cessation?
(A) Acetylcholine
(B) Bethanechol
(C) Neostigmine
(D) Physostigmine
(E) Varenicline

9. A 3-year-old child is admitted after taking a drug from her parents' medicine cabinet. The signs suggest that the drug is an indirect-acting cholinomimetic with little or no CNS effect and a duration of action of about 2–4 h. Which of the following is the most likely cause of these effects?
(A) Acetylcholine
(B) Bethanechol
(C) Neostigmine
(D) Physostigmine
(E) Pilocarpine

10. Which of the following is the primary second-messenger process in the contraction of the ciliary muscle when focusing on near objects?
(A) cAMP (cyclic adenosine monophosphate)
(B) DAG (diacylglycerol)
(C) Depolarizing influx of sodium ions via a channel
(D) IP_3 (inositol 1,4,5-trisphosphate)
(E) NO (nitric oxide)

ANSWERS

1. Because neostigmine acts on the enzyme cholinesterase, which is present at all cholinergic synapses, this drug increases acetylcholine effects at nicotinic junctions as well as muscarinic ones. Bethanechol, on the other hand, is a direct-acting agent that is selective for muscarinic receptors and has no effect on nicotinic junctions such as the skeletal muscle end plate. The answer is **B**.

2. The "-thion" organophosphates (those containing the P=S bond) are activated, not inactivated, by conversion to "-oxon" (P=O) derivatives. They are less stable than halogenated hydrocarbon insecticides of the DDT type; therefore, they are less persistent in the environment. Parathion is more toxic than malathion. It is very lipid-soluble and rapidly absorbed through the lungs and skin. Pralidoxime has very high affinity for the phosphorus atom and is a chemical antagonist of organophosphates. The answer is **E**.

3. Any of the cholinesterase inhibitors (choices B, C, or E) would effectively correct myasthenic crisis. However, because cholinergic crisis (if that is what is causing the symptoms) would be worsened by a cholinomimetic, we choose the shortest-acting cholinesterase inhibitor, edrophonium. The answer is **B**.

4. Respiratory failure, from neuromuscular paralysis or CNS depression, is the most important cause of acute deaths in cholinesterase inhibitor toxicity. The answer is **E**.

5. Cholinesterase inhibition is typically associated with increased (never decreased) bowel activity. (Fortunately, many patients become tolerant to this effect.) The answer is **C**.

6. Choice **(E)** is not correct because the vagus slows the heart. Parasympathetic nerve stimulation does not cause vasodilation (most vessels do not receive parasympathetic innervation), so choice **(C)** is incorrect. Ganglion cells and the end plate contain nicotinic receptors, which are not affected by bethanechol, a direct-acting muscarinic agonist. The answer is **D**.

7. Muscarinic agonists cause accommodation and cyclospasm, the opposite of paralysis of accommodation (cycloplegia). In open-angle glaucoma, this results in increased outflow of aqueous and decreased intraocular pressure. These agents may cause broncho*spasm* but have no effect on neuromuscular transmission. They may *cause* diarrhea and are not used in its treatment. Muscarinic agonists may also cause sweating, but drug-induced sweating is of no value in the treatment of fever. The answer is **B**.

8. Varenicline is a lipid-soluble partial agonist at nicotinic receptors and is used to reduce craving for tobacco in smokers. The answer is **E**.

9. Neostigmine is the prototypical indirect-acting cholinomimetic; it is a quaternary (charged) substance with poor lipid solubility; its duration of action is about 2–4 h. Physostigmine is similar but has good lipid solubility and significant CNS effects. The answer is **C**.

10. Cholinomimetics cause smooth muscle contraction mainly through the release of intracellular calcium. This release is triggered by an increase in IP_3 acting on receptors in the endoplasmic reticulum. The answer is **D**.

SKILL KEEPER ANSWER: DRUG METABOLISM (SEE CHAPTER 4)

The esters acetylcholine and methacholine are hydrolyzed by acetylcholinesterase. Hydrolytic drug metabolism reactions are classified as phase I.

CHECKLIST

When you complete this chapter, you should be able to:

❑ List the locations and types of acetylcholine receptors in the major organ systems (CNS, autonomic ganglia, eye, heart, vessels, bronchi, gut, genitourinary tract, skeletal muscle, exocrine glands).

❑ Describe the second messengers involved and the effects of acetylcholine on the major organs

❑ List the major clinical uses of cholinomimetic agonists.

❑ Describe the pharmacodynamic differences between direct-acting and indirect-acting cholinomimetic agents.

❑ List the major pharmacokinetic differences of the direct- and indirect-acting cholinomimetics.

❑ List the major signs and symptoms of (1) organophosphate insecticide poisoning and (2) acute nicotine toxicity.

DRUG SUMMARY TABLE: Cholinoceptor-Activating & Cholinesterase-Inhibiting Drugs

Subclass	Mechanism of Action	Clinical and Other Applications	Pharmacokinetics	Toxicities, Interactions
Direct-acting, muscarinic agonists				
Bethanechol	Activates muscarinic (M) receptors • increases IP_3 and DAG	Bladder and bowel atony, for example, after surgery or spinal cord injury	Oral, IM activity Poor lipid solubility: does not enter CNS • Duration: 0.3–2 h	All parasympathomimetic effects: cyclospasm, diarrhea, urinary urgency, plus vasodilation, reflex tachycardia, and sweating
Pilocarpine	Same as bethanechol • may also activate EPSP via M receptors in ganglia	Sjögren's syndrome (increases salivation) • was used in glaucoma (causes miosis, cyclospasm)	Oral, IM activity Good lipid solubility, topical activity in eye	Similar to bethanechol but may cause vasoconstriction via ganglionic effect
Muscarine	Same as bethanechol	Alkaloid found in mushrooms	Low lipid solubility but readily absorbed from gut	Mushroom poisoning of fast-onset type
Direct-acting, nicotinic agonists				
Nicotine	Activates all nicotinic (N) receptors • opens Na^+-K^+ channels in ganglia and neuromuscular end plates	Smoking cessation (also used as insecticide)	High lipid solubility, absorbed by all routes • For smoking cessation, usually used as gum or transdermal patch • Duration: 4–6 h	Generalized ganglionic stimulation: hypertension, tachycardia, nausea, vomiting, diarrhea Major overdose: convulsions, paralysis, coma
Varenicline	A partial agonist at N receptors	Smoking cessation	High lipid solubility, oral activity • Duration: ~12 h	Hypertension, sweating, sensory disturbance, diarrhea, polyuria, menstrual disturbance
Succinylcholine	N-receptor agonist, moderately selective for neuromuscular end plate (N_M receptors)	Muscle relaxation (see Chapter 27)	Highly polar, used IV • Duration: 5–10 min	Initial muscle spasms and postoperative pain • Prolonged action in persons with abnormal butyrylcholinesterase
Indirect-acting, alcohol				
Edrophonium	Inhibitor of cholinesterase • amplifier of endogenously released ACh	Reversal of N_M block by nondepolarizing drugs • diagnosis of myasthenia gravis	Highly polar • used IV • Duration: 5–10 min	Increased parasympathetic effects, especially nausea, vomiting, diarrhea, urinary urgency
Indirect-acting, carbamates				
Neostigmine	Like edrophonium plus small direct nicotinic agonist action	Reversal of N_M block, treatment of myasthenia	Moderately polar but orally active • Duration: 2–4 h	Like edrophonium but longer duration
Pyridostigmine	Like edrophonium	Treatment of myasthenia	Moderately polar but orally active • Duration: 4–8 h	Like edrophonium but longer duration
Physostigmine	Like edrophonium	Reversal of severe atropine poisoning (IV) • occasionally used in acute glaucoma (topical)	Lipid soluble • can be used topically in the eye • Duration: 2–4 h	Like edrophonium but longer duration plus CNS effects: seizures

Indirect-acting, organophosphates				
Parathion	Like edrophonium	Insecticide only · Duration: days to weeks	Highly lipid-soluble	Highly dangerous insecticide · causes all parasympathetic effects plus muscle paralysis and coma
Malathion	Like edrophonium	Insecticide and scabicide (topical) · Duration: days	Highly lipid-soluble but metabolized to inactive products in mammals and birds	Much safer insecticide than parathion
Sarin, tabun, others	Like parathion	Nerve gases · terrorist threat	Like parathion but more rapid action	Rapidly lethal
Indirect-acting, for Alzheimer's disease				
Rivastigmine, galantamine, donepezil; tacrine is obsolete	Cholinesterase inhibition plus variable other poorly understood effects	Alzheimer's disease	Lipid soluble, enter CNS · Half-lives: 1.5–70 h	Nausea, vomiting

ACh, acetylcholine; DAG, diacylglycerol; EPSP, excitatory postsynaptic potential; IP_3, inositol-1,4,5-trisphosphate.

Cholinoceptor Blockers & Cholinesterase Regenerators

C H A P T E R

8

The cholinoceptor antagonists are readily grouped into subclasses on the basis of their spectrum of action (ie, block of muscarinic versus nicotinic receptors). These drugs are pharmacologic antagonists or inverse agonists (eg, atropine). A special subgroup, the cholinesterase regenerators, are not receptor blockers but rather are chemical antagonists of organophosphate cholinesterase inhibitors.

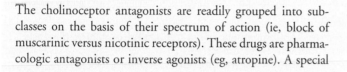

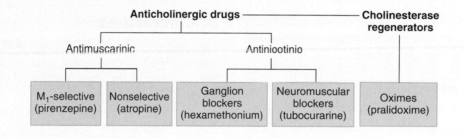

MUSCARINIC ANTAGONISTS

A. Classification and Pharmacokinetics

1. Classification of the muscarinic antagonists—Muscarinic antagonists can be subdivided according to their selectivity for specific M receptors or their lack of such selectivity. Although the division of muscarinic receptors into subgroups is well documented (Chapters 6 and 7), only 2 distinctly receptor-selective M_1 antagonists have reached clinical trials (eg, pirenzepine, telenzepine). However, as noted later, several agents in use in the United States are somewhat selective for the M_3 subtype. Most of the drugs in general use in the United States are relatively nonspecific. The muscarinic blockers can also be subdivided on the basis of their primary clinical target organs (central nervous system [CNS], eye, bronchi, or gastrointestinal and genitourinary tracts). Drugs used for their effects on the CNS or the eye must be sufficiently lipid-soluble to cross lipid barriers. A major determinant of this property is the presence or absence

of a permanently charged (quaternary) amine group in the drug molecule because charged molecules are less lipid-soluble.

2. Pharmacokinetics—**Atropine** is the prototypical nonselective muscarinic blocker. This alkaloid is found in *Atropa belladonna* and many other plants. Because it is a tertiary amine, atropine is relatively lipid-soluble and readily crosses membrane barriers. The drug is well distributed into the CNS, the eye, and other organs. It is eliminated partially by metabolism in the liver and partially unchanged in the urine; half-life is approximately 2 h; duration of action of normal doses is 4–8 h except in the eye (see Drug Summary Table).

In ophthalmology, topical activity (the ability to enter the eye after conjunctival administration) and duration of action are important in determining the usefulness of several antimuscarinic drugs (see Clinical Uses). Similar ability to cross lipid barriers is essential for the agents used in parkinsonism. In contrast, the drugs used for their antisecretory or antispastic actions in the gut,

High-Yield Terms to Learn

Anticholinergic	A drug that blocks muscarinic or nicotinic receptors, but commonly used to mean antimuscarinic
Antimuscarinic	A drug that blocks muscarinic but not nicotinic receptors
Atropine fever	Hyperthermia induced by antimuscarinic drugs; caused mainly by inhibition of sweating
Atropine flush	Marked cutaneous vasodilation of the arms and upper torso and head by antimuscarinic drugs; mechanism unknown
Cholinesterase regenerator	A chemical antagonist that binds the phosphorus of organophosphates and displaces acetylcholinesterase
Cycloplegia	Paralysis of accommodation; inability to focus on close objects
Depolarizing blockade	Flaccid skeletal muscle paralysis caused by persistent depolarization of the neuromuscular end plate
Miotic	A drug that constricts the pupil
Mydriatic	A drug that dilates the pupil
Nondepolarizing blockade	Flaccid skeletal muscle paralysis caused by blockade of the nicotinic receptor and prevention of end plate depolarization
Parasympatholytic, parasympathoplegic	A drug that reduces the effects of parasympathetic nerve stimulation, usually by blockade of the muscarinic receptors of autonomic effector tissues

bladder, and bronchi are often selected for minimum CNS activity; these drugs may incorporate quaternary amine groups to limit penetration through the blood–brain barrier.

B. Mechanism of Action

Although several are inverse agonists, muscarinic blocking agents act like competitive (surmountable) pharmacologic antagonists; their blocking effects can be overcome by increased concentrations of muscarinic agonists.

C. Effects

The peripheral actions of muscarinic blockers are mostly predictable effects derived from cholinoceptor blockade (Table 8–1). These include the ocular, gastrointestinal, genitourinary, and secretory effects. The CNS effects are less predictable. CNS effects seen at therapeutic concentrations include sedation, reduction of motion sickness, and, as previously noted, reduction of some of the signs of parkinsonism. Cardiovascular effects at therapeutic doses include an initial slowing of heart rate caused by central or presynaptic vagal effects followed by the tachycardia and decreased atrioventricular conduction time that would be predicted from peripheral vagal blockade. M_1-selective agents (not currently available in the United States) may be somewhat selective for the gastrointestinal tract.

SKILL KEEPER: DRUG IONIZATION (SEE CHAPTER 1)

The pK$_a$ of atropine, a weak base, is 9.7. What fraction of atropine (an amine) is in the lipid-soluble form in urine of pH 7.7? The Skill Keeper Answer appears at the end of the chapter.

D. Clinical Uses

The muscarinic blockers have several useful therapeutic applications in the CNS, eye, bronchi, gut, and urinary bladder. These uses are listed in the Drug Summary Table at the end of this chapter.

1. CNS—Scopolamine is standard therapy for motion sickness; it is one of the most effective agents available for this condition. A transdermal patch formulation is available. Benztropine, biperiden, and trihexyphenidyl are representative of several antimuscarinic agents used in parkinsonism. Although not as effective as levodopa (see Chapter 28), these agents may be useful as adjuncts or when patients become unresponsive to levodopa. Benztropine is sometimes used parenterally to treat acute dystonias caused by antipsychotic medications.

2. Eye—Antimuscarinic drugs are used to cause mydriasis, as indicated by the origin of the name belladonna ("beautiful lady") from the ancient cosmetic use of extracts of the *Atropa belladonna* plant to dilate the pupils. They also cause cycloplegia and paralyze accommodation. In descending order of duration of action, these drugs are **atropine** (>72 h), **homatropine** (24 h), **cyclopentolate** (2–12 h), and **tropicamide** (0.5–4 h). These agents are all well absorbed from the conjunctival sac into the eye.

3. Bronchi—Parenteral atropine has long been used to reduce airway secretions during general anesthesia. **Ipratropium** is a quaternary antimuscarinic agent used by inhalation to promote bronchodilation in asthma and chronic obstructive pulmonary disease (COPD). Although not as efficacious as β agonists, ipratropium is less likely to cause tachycardia and cardiac arrhythmias in sensitive patients. It has very few antimuscarinic

TABLE 8–1 Effects of muscarinic blocking drugs.

Organ	Effect	Mechanism
CNS	Sedation, anti-motion sickness action, antiparkinson action, amnesia, delirium	Block of muscarinic receptors, several subtypes
Eye	Cycloplegia, mydriasis	Block of M_3 receptors
Bronchi	Bronchodilation, especially if constricted	Block of M_3 receptors
Gastrointestinal tract	Relaxation, slowed peristalsis, reduced salivation	Block of M_1, M_3 receptors
Genitourinary tract	Relaxation of bladder wall, urinary retention	Block of M_3 and possibly M_1 receptors
Heart	Initial bradycardia, especially at low doses, then tachycardia	Tachycardia from block of M_2 receptors in the sinoatrial node
Blood vessels	Block of muscarinic vasodilation; not manifest unless a muscarinic agonist is present	Block of M_3 receptors on endothelium of vessels
Glands	Marked reduction of salivation, moderate reduction of lacrimation, sweating; less reduction of gastric secretion	Block of M_1, M_3 receptors
Skeletal muscle	None	

effects outside the lungs because it is poorly absorbed and rapidly metabolized. **Tiotropium** is a newer analog with a longer duration of action.

4. Gut—Atropine, **methscopolamine,** and **propantheline** were used in the past to reduce acid secretion in acid-peptic disease, but are now obsolete for this indication because they are not as effective as H_2 blockers (Chapter 16) and proton pump inhibitors (Chapter 59), and they cause far more frequent and severe adverse effects. The M_1-selective inhibitor pirenzepine is available in Europe for the treatment of peptic ulcer. Muscarinic blockers can also be used to reduce cramping and hypermotility in transient diarrheas, but drugs such as diphenoxylate and loperamide (Chapter 31) are more effective.

5. Bladder—Oxybutynin, **tolterodine,** or similar agents may be used to reduce urgency in mild cystitis and to reduce bladder spasms after urologic surgery. **Tolterodine, darifenacin, solifenacin,** and **fesoterodine** are promoted for the treatment of stress incontinence.

E. Toxicity

A traditional mnemonic for atropine toxicity is "Dry as a bone, red as a beet, mad as a hatter." This description reflects both predictable antimuscarinic effects and some unpredictable actions.

1. Predictable toxicities—Antimuscarinic actions lead to several important and potentially dangerous effects. Blockade of thermoregulatory sweating may result in hyperthermia or "atropine fever." This is the most dangerous effect of the antimuscarinic drugs in children and is potentially lethal in infants. Sweating, salivation, and lacrimation are all significantly

reduced or stopped ("dry as a bone"). Moderate tachycardia is common, and severe tachycardia or arrhythmias are common with large overdoses. In the elderly, important toxicities include acute angle-closure glaucoma and urinary retention, especially in men with prostatic hyperplasia. Constipation and blurred vision are common adverse effects in all age groups.

2. Other toxicities—Toxicities not predictable from peripheral autonomic actions include CNS and cardiovascular effects. CNS toxicity includes sedation, amnesia, and delirium or hallucinations ("mad as a hatter"); convulsions may also occur. Central muscarinic receptors are probably involved. Other drug groups with antimuscarinic effects, for example, tricyclic antidepressants, may cause hallucinations or delirium in the elderly, who are especially susceptible to antimuscarinic toxicity. At very high doses, intraventricular conduction may be blocked; this action is probably not mediated by muscarinic blockade and is difficult to treat. Dilation of the cutaneous vessels of the arms, head, neck, and trunk also occurs at these doses; the resulting "atropine flush" ("red as a beet") may be diagnostic of overdose with these drugs. The mechanism is unknown.

3. Treatment of toxicity—Treatment of toxicity is usually symptomatic. Severe tachycardia may require cautious administration of small doses of physostigmine. Hyperthermia can usually be managed with cooling blankets or evaporative cooling.

F. Contraindications

The antimuscarinic agents should be used cautiously in infants because of the danger of hyperthermia. The drugs are relatively contraindicated in persons with glaucoma, especially the closed-angle form, and in men with prostatic hyperplasia.

NICOTINIC ANTAGONISTS

A. Ganglion-Blocking Drugs

Blockers of ganglionic nicotinic receptors act like competitive pharmacologic antagonists, although there is evidence that some also block the pore of the nicotinic channel itself. These drugs were the first successful agents for the treatment of hypertension. **Hexamethonium** (C6, a prototype), **mecamylamine**, and several other ganglion blockers were extensively used for this disease. Unfortunately, the adverse effects of ganglion blockade in hypertension are so severe (both sympathetic and parasympathetic divisions are blocked) that patients were unable to tolerate them for long periods (Table 8–2). **Trimethaphan** was the ganglion blocker most recently used in clinical practice, but it too has been almost abandoned. It is poorly lipid-soluble, inactive orally, and has a short half-life. It was used intravenously to treat severe accelerated hypertension (malignant hypertension) and to produce controlled hypotension.

Recent interest has focused on nicotinic receptors in the CNS and their relation to nicotine addiction and to Tourette's syndrome. Paradoxically, nicotine (in the form of nicotine gum or patches), **varenicline** (a partial agonist given by mouth), and mecamylamine, a nicotinic ganglion blocker that enters the CNS, have all been shown to have some benefit in smoking cessation.

Because ganglion blockers interrupt sympathetic control of venous tone, they cause marked venous pooling; postural hypotension is a major manifestation of this effect. Other toxicities of ganglion-blocking drugs include dry mouth, blurred vision, constipation, and severe sexual dysfunction (Table 8–2). As a result, ganglion blockers are rarely used.

B. Neuromuscular-Blocking Drugs

Neuromuscular-blocking drugs are important for producing complete skeletal muscle relaxation in surgery; new ones are introduced regularly. They are discussed in greater detail in Chapter 27.

CHOLINESTERASE REGENERATORS

Pralidoxime is the prototype cholinesterase regenerator. These *chemical* antagonists contain an oxime group, which has an extremely high affinity for the phosphorus atom in organophosphate insecticides. Because the affinity of the oxime group for phosphorus exceeds the affinity of the enzyme-active site for phosphorus, these agents are able to bind the inhibitor and displace the enzyme (if aging has not occurred). The active enzyme is thus regenerated. Pralidoxime, the oxime currently available in the United States, may be used to treat patients exposed to insecticides, such as parathion, or to nerve gases.

QUESTIONS

Questions 1–2. A 2-year-old child has been admitted to the emergency department. Antimuscarinic drug overdose is suspected.

1. Probable signs of atropine overdose include which one of the following?
   (A) Gastrointestinal smooth muscle cramping
   (B) Increased heart rate
   (C) Increased gastric secretion
   (D) Pupillary constriction
   (E) Urinary frequency

2. Which of the following is the most dangerous effect of belladonna alkaloids in infants and toddlers?
   (A) Dehydration
   (B) Hallucinations
   (C) Hypertension
   (D) Hyperthermia
   (E) Intraventricular heart block

3. Which one of the following can be blocked by atropine?
   (A) Decreased blood pressure caused by hexamethonium
   (B) Increased blood pressure caused by nicotine
   (C) Increased skeletal muscle strength caused by neostigmine
   (D) Tachycardia caused by exercise
   (E) Tachycardia caused by infusion of acetylcholine

TABLE 8–2 Effects of ganglion-blocking drugs.

Organ	Effects
CNS	Antinicotinic action may include reduction of nicotine craving and amelioration of Tourette's syndrome (mecamylamine only)
Eye	Moderate mydriasis and cycloplegia
Bronchi	Little effect; asthmatics may note some bronchodilation
Gastrointestinal tract	Marked reduction of motility, constipation may be severe
Genitourinary tract	Reduced contractility of the bladder; impairment of erection (parasympathetic block) and ejaculation (sympathetic block)
Heart	Moderate tachycardia and reduction in force and cardiac output at rest; block of exercise-induced changes
Vessels	Reduction in arteriolar and venous tone, dose-dependent reduction in blood pressure; orthostatic hypotension usually marked
Glands	Reductions in salivation, lacrimation, sweating, and gastric secretion
Skeletal muscle	No significant effect

Questions 4–5. Two new synthetic drugs (X and Y) are to be studied for their cardiovascular effects. The drugs are given to three anesthetized animals while the blood pressure is recorded. The first animal has received no pretreatment (control), the second has received an effective dose of a long-acting ganglion blocker, and the third has received an effective dose of a long-acting muscarinic antagonist.

4. Drug X caused a 50 mm Hg rise in mean blood pressure in the control animal, no blood pressure change in the ganglion-blocked animal, and a 75 mm mean blood pressure rise in the atropine-pretreated animal. Drug X is probably a drug similar to
   (A) Acetylcholine
   (B) Atropine
   (C) Epinephrine
   (D) Hexamethonium
   (E) Nicotine

5. The net changes induced by drug Y in these experiments are shown in the following graph.

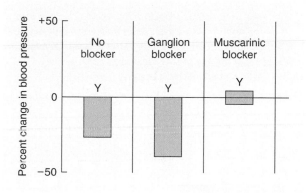

Drug Y is probably a drug similar to
   (A) Acetylcholine
   (B) Edrophonium
   (C) Hexamethonium
   (D) Nicotine
   (E) Pralidoxime

6. A 30-year-old man has been treated with several autonomic drugs for 4 weeks. He is now admitted to the emergency department showing signs of drug toxicity. Which of the following signs would distinguish between an overdose of a ganglion blocker versus a muscarinic blocker?
   (A) Blurred vision
   (B) Dry mouth, constipation
   (C) Mydriasis
   (D) Postural hypotension
   (E) Tachycardia

7. Accepted therapeutic indications for the use of antimuscarinic drugs include all of the following *except*
   (A) Atrial fibrillation
   (B) Motion sickness
   (C) Parkinson's disease
   (D) Postoperative bladder spasm
   (E) To antidote parathion poisoning

8. Which of the following is an expected effect of a therapeutic dose of an antimuscarinic drug?
   (A) Decreased cAMP (cyclic adenosine monophosphate) in cardiac muscle
   (B) Decreased DAG (diacylglycerol) in salivary gland tissue
   (C) Increased IP_3 (inositol trisphosphate) in intestinal smooth muscle
   (D) Increased potassium efflux from smooth muscle
   (E) Increased sodium influx into the skeletal muscle end plate

9. Which one of the following drugs causes vasodilation that can be blocked by atropine?
   (A) Benztropine
   (B) Bethanechol
   (C) Botulinum
   (D) Cyclopentolate
   (E) Edrophonium
   (F) Neostigmine
   (G) Pralidoxime

10. Which one of the following drugs has a very high affinity for the phosphorus atom in parathion and is often used to treat life-threatening insecticide toxicity?
    (A) Atropine
    (B) Benztropine
    (C) Bethanechol
    (D) Botulinum
    (E) Cyclopentolate
    (F) Neostigmine
    (G) Pralidoxime

ANSWERS

1. Tachycardia is a characteristic atropine overdose effect. Bradycardia is sometimes observed after small doses. The answer is **B.**

2. Choices **B, D,** and **E** are all possible effects of the atropine group. In infants, however, the most dangerous effect is hyperthermia. Deaths with body temperatures in excess of 42°C have occurred after the use of atropine-containing eye drops in children. The answer is **D.**

3. Atropine blocks muscarinic receptors and inhibits parasympathomimetic effects. Nicotine can induce both parasympathomimetic and sympathomimetic effects by virtue of its ganglion-stimulating action. Hypertension and exercise-induced tachycardia reflect sympathetic discharge and therefore would not be blocked by atropine. The answer is **E.**

4. Drug X causes an increase in blood pressure that is blocked by a ganglion blocker but not by a muscarinic blocker. The pressor response is actually increased by pretreatment with atropine, a muscarinic blocker, suggesting that compensatory vagal discharge might have blunted the full response. This description fits a ganglion stimulant like nicotine but not epinephrine, since epinephrine's pressor effects are produced at α receptors, not in the ganglia. The answer is **E.**

5. Drug Y causes a decrease in blood pressure that is blocked by a muscarinic blocker but not by a ganglion blocker. Therefore, the depressor effect must be evoked at a site distal

to the ganglia. In fact, the drop in blood pressure is actually greater in the presence of ganglion blockade, suggesting that compensatory sympathetic discharge might have blunted the full depressor action of drug Y in the control animal. The description fits a direct-acting muscarinic stimulant such as acetylcholine (given in high dosage). Indirect-acting cholinomimetics (cholinesterase inhibitors) would not produce this pattern because the vascular muscarinic receptors involved in the depressor response are not innervated and are unresponsive to indirectly acting agents. The answer is **A.**

6. Both ganglion blockers and muscarinic blockers can cause mydriasis, increase resting heart rate, blur vision, and cause dry mouth and constipation, because these are determined largely by parasympathetic tone. Postural hypotension, on the other hand, is a sign of sympathetic blockade, which would occur with ganglion blockers but not muscarinic blockers (Chapter 6). The answer is **D.**

7. Atrial fibrillation and other arrhythmias are not responsive to antimuscarinic agents. The answer is **A.**

8. Muscarinic M_1 and M_3 receptors mediate increases in IP_3 and DAG in target tissues (intestine, salivary glands). M_2 receptors (heart) mediate a decrease in cAMP and an increase in potassium permeability. Antimuscarinic agents block these effects. The answer is **B.**

9. Bethanechol (Chapter 7) causes vasodilation by activating muscarinic receptors on the endothelium of blood vessels. This effect can be blocked by atropine. The answer is **B.**

10. Pralidoxime has a very high affinity for the phosphorus atom in organophosphate insecticides. The answer is **G.**

SKILL KEEPER ANSWER: DRUG IONIZATION (SEE CHAPTER 1)

The pK_a of atropine is 9.7. According to the Henderson-Hasselbalch equation,

$$Log\ (protonated/unprotonated) = pK_a - pH$$
$$Log\ (P/U) = 9.7 - 7.7$$
$$Log\ (P/U) = 2$$
$$P/U = antilog\ (2)$$
$$= 100/1$$

Therefore, about 99% of the drug is in the protonated form, 1% in the unprotonated form. Since atropine is a weak base, it is the unprotonated form that is lipid soluble. Therefore, about 1% of the atropine in the urine is lipid soluble.

CHECKLIST

When you complete this chapter, you should be able to:

❑ Describe the effects of atropine on the major organ systems (CNS, eye, heart, vessels, bronchi, gut, genitourinary tract, exocrine glands, skeletal muscle).

❑ List the signs, symptoms, and treatment of atropine overdose.

❑ List the major clinical indications and contraindications for the use of muscarinic antagonists.

❑ Describe the effects of the ganglion-blocking nicotinic antagonists.

❑ List one antimuscarinic agent promoted for each of the following uses: to produce mydriasis and cycloplegia; to treat parkinsonism, asthma, bladder spasm, and the muscarinic toxicity of insecticides.

❑ Describe the mechanism of action and clinical use of pralidoxime.

DRUG SUMMARY TABLE: Cholinoceptor Blockers & Cholinesterase Regenerators

Subclass	Mechanism of Action	Clinical Applications	Pharmacokinetics	Toxicities, Interactions
Antimuscarinic, nonselective				
Atropine	Competitive pharmacologic antagonist at all M receptors	Mydriatic, cycloplegic • antidote for cholinesterase inhibitor toxicity	Lipid-soluble Duration: 2–4 h except in eye: ≥72 h	All parasympatholytic effects plus sedation, delirium, hyperthermia, flushing

Benztropine, others: antiparkinsonism; oral and parenteral
Dicyclomine, glycopyrrolate: oral, parenteral for gastrointestinal applications
Homatropine, cyclopentolate, tropicamide: topical ophthalmic use to produce mydriasis, cycloplegia
Ipratropium, tiotropium: inhaled for asthma, chronic obstructive pulmonary disease
Oxybutynin: oral, transdermal, promoted for urinary urgency, incontinence
Scopolamine: anti-motion sickness via transdermal patch
Trospium: oral, for urinary urgency

Subclass	Mechanism of Action	Clinical Applications	Pharmacokinetics	Toxicities, Interactions
Antimuscarinic, selective				
Darifenacin, fesoterodine, solifenacin, tolterodine	Like atropine, but modest selectivity for M_3 receptors	Urinary urgency, incontinence	Oral Duration: 12–24 h	Excessive parasympatholytic effects
Pirenzepine, telenzepine	Significant M_1 selectivity	Peptic disease (not available in USA)	Oral	Excessive parasympatholytic effects
Antinicotinic ganglion blockers				
Hexamethonium	Selective block of N_N receptors	Obsolete; was used for hypertension	Oral, parenteral	Block of all autonomic effects

Trimethaphan: IV only, short-acting; was used for hypertensive emergencies and controlled hypotension
Mecamylamine: oral, enters CNS; investigational use for smoking cessation

Antinicotinic neuromuscular blockers
See Chapter 27

Subclass	Mechanism of Action	Clinical Applications	Pharmacokinetics	Toxicities, Interactions
Regenerator				
Pralidoxime	Chemical antagonist of organophosphates	Organophosphate poisoning	Parenteral	Muscle weakness

Sympathomimetics

The sympathomimetics constitute a very important group of drugs used for cardiovascular, respiratory, and other conditions. They are readily divided into subgroups on the basis of their spectrum of action (α-, β-, or dopamine-receptor affinity) or mode of action (direct or indirect).

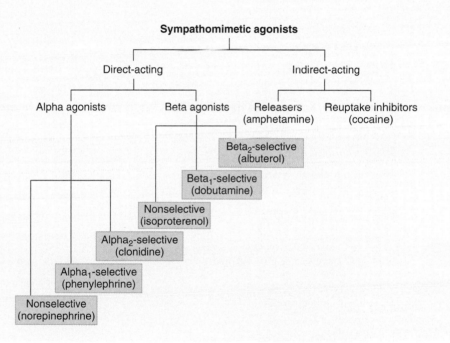

CLASSIFICATION

A. Spectrum of Action

Adrenoceptors are classified as α, β, or dopamine receptors; these groups are further subdivided into subgroups. The distribution of these receptors is set forth in Table 9–1. **Epinephrine** may be considered a single prototype agonist with effects at all α- and β-receptor types. Alternatively, separate prototypes, **phenylephrine** (an α agonist) and **isoproterenol** (β) may be defined. The just-mentioned drugs have relatively little effect on dopamine receptors, but **dopamine** itself is a potent dopamine receptor agonist and, when given as a drug, can also activate β receptors (intermediate doses) and α receptors (larger doses).

B. Mode of Action

Sympathomimetic agonists may directly activate their adrenoceptors, or they may act indirectly to increase the concentration of endogenous catecholamine transmitter in the synapse. **Amphetamine** derivatives and **tyramine** cause the release of stored catecholamines; they are therefore mainly indirect in their mode of action. **Cocaine** and the **tricyclic antidepressants** exhibit another form of indirect action; these drugs inhibit reuptake of

High-Yield Terms to Learn

Anorexiant	A drug that decreases appetite (causes anorexia)
Catecholamine	A dihydroxyphenylethylamine derivative (eg, norepinephrine, epinephrine), a relatively polar molecule that is readily metabolized by catechol-*O*-methyltransferase
Decongestant	An α-agonist drug that reduces conjunctival, nasal, or oropharyngeal mucosal vasodilation by constricting blood vessels in the submucosal tissue
Mydriatic	A drug that causes dilation of the pupil; opposite of miotic
Phenylisopropylamine	A derivative of phenylisopropylamine (eg, amphetamine, ephedrine). Unlike catecholamines, phenylisopropylamines usually have oral activity, a long half-life, CNS activity, and cause release of stored catecholamines
Selective α agonist, β agonist	Drugs that have relatively greater effects on α or β adrenoceptors; none are *absolutely* selective or specific
Sympathomimetic	A drug that mimics stimulation of the sympathetic autonomic nervous system
Reuptake inhibitor	An indirect-acting drug that increases the activity of transmitters in the synapse by inhibiting their reuptake into the presynaptic nerve ending. May act selectively on noradrenergic, serotonergic, or both types of nerve endings

TABLE 9–1 Types of adrenoceptors, some of the peripheral tissues in which they are found, and their major effects.

Type	Tissue	Actions
α_1	Most vascular smooth muscle	Contracts ($\uparrow$ vascular resistance)
	Pupillary dilator muscle	Contracts (mydriasis)
	Pilomotor smooth muscle	Contracts (erects hair)
	Liver (in some species, eg, rat)	Stimulates glycogenolysis
α_2	Adrenergic and cholinergic nerve terminals	Inhibits transmitter release
	Platelets	Stimulates aggregation
	Some vascular smooth muscle	Contracts
	Fat cells	Inhibits lipolysis
	Pancreatic β (B) cells	Inhibits insulin release
β_1	Heart	Stimulates rate and force
	Juxtaglomerular cells of kidney	Stimulates renin release
β_2	Airways, uterine, and vascular smooth muscle	Relaxes
	Liver (human)	Stimulates glycogenolysis
	Pancreatic β (B) cells	Stimulates insulin release
	Somatic motor neuron terminals (voluntary muscle)	Causes tremor
	Heart	Stimulates rate and force
β_3	Fat cells	Stimulates lipolysis
Dopamine$_1$ (D$_1$)	Renal and other splanchnic blood vessels	Dilates ($\downarrow$ resistance)
Dopamine$_2$ (D$_2$)	Nerve terminals	Inhibits adenylyl cyclase

catecholamines by the norepinephrine transporter (NET) and the dopamine transporter (DAT) in nerve terminals (see Figure 6–2) and thus increase the synaptic activity of released transmitter.

Blockade of metabolism (ie, block of catechol-*O*-methyltransferase [COMT] and monoamine oxidase [MAO]) has little direct effect on autonomic activity, but MAO inhibition increases the stores of catecholamines and related molecules in adrenergic synaptic vesicles and thus may potentiate the action of indirect-acting sympathomimetics that cause the release of stored transmitter.

CHEMISTRY & PHARMACOKINETICS

The endogenous adrenoceptor agonists (**epinephrine, norepinephrine,** and **dopamine**) are **catecholamines** and are rapidly metabolized by COMT and MAO. If used as drugs, these adrenoceptor agonists are inactive by the oral route and must be given parenterally. When released from nerve endings, they are subsequently taken up (by NET or DAT) into nerve endings and into perisynaptic cells; this uptake may also occur with norepinephrine, epinephrine, and dopamine given as drugs. These agonists have a short duration of action. When given parenterally, they do not enter the central nervous system (CNS) in significant amounts. Isoproterenol, a synthetic catecholamine, is similar to the endogenous transmitters but is not readily taken up into nerve endings. **Phenylisopropylamines,** for example, **amphetamines,** are resistant to MAO; most of them are not catecholamines and are therefore also resistant to COMT. Phenylisopropylamines are orally active; they enter the CNS, and their effects last much longer than do those of catecholamines. **Tyramine,** which is not a phenylisopropylamine, is rapidly metabolized by MAO except in patients who are taking an MAO inhibitor drug. MAO inhibitors are sometimes used in the treatment of depression (see Chapter 30).

MECHANISMS OF ACTION

A. Alpha Receptor Effects

Alpha$_1$ receptor effects are mediated primarily by the trimeric coupling protein G$_q$. When G$_q$ is activated, the alpha moiety of this protein activates the enzyme phospholipase C, resulting in the release of inositol-1,4,5-trisphosphate (IP$_3$) and diacylglycerol (DAG) from membrane lipids. Calcium is subsequently released from stores in smooth muscle cells by IP$_3$, and enzymes are activated by DAG. Direct gating of calcium channels may also play a role in increasing intracellular calcium concentration. Alpha$_2$ receptor activation results in inhibition of adenylyl cyclase via the coupling protein G$_i$.

B. Beta Receptor Effects

Beta receptors (β_1, β_2, and β_3) stimulate adenylyl cyclase via the coupling protein G$_s$, which leads to an increase in cyclic adenosine monophosphate (cAMP) concentration in the cell.

C. Dopamine Receptor Effects

Dopamine D$_1$ receptors activate adenylyl cyclase via G$_s$ and increase cAMP in neurons and vascular smooth muscle. Dopamine D$_2$ receptors are more important in the brain but probably also play a significant role as presynaptic receptors on peripheral nerves. These receptors reduce the synthesis of cAMP via G$_i$.

ORGAN SYSTEM EFFECTS

A. Central Nervous System

Catecholamines do not enter the CNS effectively. Sympathomimetics that do enter the CNS (eg, amphetamines) have a spectrum of stimulant effects, beginning with mild alerting or reduction of fatigue and progressing to anorexia, euphoria, and insomnia. Some of these central effects probably reflect the release of dopamine in certain dopaminergic tracts. Repeated dosing of amphetamines results in the rapid development of tolerance and dependence. These CNS effects reflect the amplification of dopamine's action in the ventral tegmental area and other CNS nuclei (see Chapter 32). Very high doses of amphetamines lead to marked anxiety or aggressiveness, paranoia, and, less commonly, seizures. Overdoses of cocaine very commonly result in seizures.

B. Eye

The smooth muscle of the pupillary dilator responds to topical **phenylephrine** and similar α agonists with contraction and mydriasis. Accommodation is not significantly affected. Outflow of aqueous humor may be facilitated by nonselective α agonists, with a subsequent reduction of intraocular pressure. This probably occurs via the uveoscleral drainage system. Alpha$_2$-selective agonists also reduce intraocular pressure, apparently by reducing synthesis of aqueous humor.

C. Bronchi

The smooth muscle of the bronchi relaxes markedly in response to β_2 agonists. These agents are the most efficacious and reliable drugs for reversing bronchospasm.

D. Gastrointestinal Tract

The gastrointestinal tract is well endowed with both α and β receptors, located both on smooth muscle and on neurons of the enteric nervous system. Activation of either α or β receptors leads to relaxation of the smooth muscle. Alpha$_2$ agonists may also decrease salt and water secretion into the intestine.

E. Genitourinary Tract

The genitourinary tract contains α receptors in the bladder trigone and sphincter area; these receptors mediate contraction of the sphincter. In men, α_1 receptors mediate prostatic smooth muscle contraction. Sympathomimetics are sometimes used to increase sphincter tone. Beta$_2$ agonists may cause significant

TABLE 9–2 Effects of prototypical sympathomimetics on vascular resistance, blood pressure, and heart rate.

Drug	Skin, Splanchnic Vascular Resistance	Skeletal Muscle Vascular Resistance	Renal Vascular Resistance	Mean Blood Pressure	Heart Rate
Phenylephrine	↑↑↑	↑	↑	↑↑	↓[1]
Isoproterenol	—	↓↓	—	↓↓	↑↑
Norepinephrine	↑↑↑↑	↑↑	↑	↑↑↑	↓[1]

[1]Compensatory reflex response.

uterine relaxation in pregnant women near term, but the doses required also cause significant tachycardia.

F. Vascular System

Different vascular beds respond differently, depending on their dominant receptor type (Tables 9–1 and 9–2).

1. Alpha₁ agonists—Alpha$_1$ agonists (eg, **phenylephrine**) contract vascular smooth muscle, especially in skin and splanchnic blood vessels, and increase peripheral vascular resistance and venous pressure. Because these drugs increase blood pressure, they often evoke a compensatory reflex bradycardia.

2. Alpha₂ agonists—Alpha$_2$ agonists (eg, **clonidine**) cause vasoconstriction when administered intravenously or topically (eg, as a nasal spray), but when given orally they accumulate in the CNS and *reduce* sympathetic outflow and blood pressure as described in Chapter 11.

3. Beta agonists—Beta$_2$ agonists (eg, **albuterol, metaproterenol, terbutaline**) cause significant reduction in arteriolar tone in the skeletal muscle vascular bed and can reduce peripheral vascular resistance and arterial blood pressure. Beta$_1$ agonists have relatively little effect on vessels.

4. Dopamine—Dopamine causes vasodilation in the splanchnic and renal vascular beds by activating D$_1$ receptors. This effect can be very useful in the treatment of renal failure associated with shock. At higher doses, dopamine activates β receptors in the heart and elsewhere; at still higher doses, α receptors are activated.

G. Heart

The heart is well supplied with β$_1$ and β$_2$ receptors. The β$_1$ receptors predominate in some parts of the heart; both β receptors mediate increased rate of cardiac pacemakers (normal and abnormal), increased atrioventricular node conduction velocity, and increased cardiac force.

H. Net Cardiovascular Actions

Sympathomimetics with both α and β$_1$ effects (eg, **norepinephrine**) may cause a reflex increase in vagal outflow because they increase blood pressure and evoke the baroreceptor reflex. This reflex vagal effect may dominate any direct beta effects on the heart rate, so that a slow infusion of norepinephrine typically causes increased blood pressure and *bradycardia* (Figure 9–1; Table 9–2). If the reflex is blocked (eg, by a ganglion blocker or antimuscarinic drug), norepinephrine will cause a direct β$_1$-mediated *tachycardia*. A pure α agonist (eg, phenylephrine) routinely slows heart rate via the baroreceptor reflex, whereas a pure β agonist (eg, isoproterenol) almost always increases the rate.

The diastolic blood pressure is affected mainly by peripheral vascular resistance and the heart rate. (The heart rate is important because the diastolic interval determines the outflow of blood from the arterial compartment.) The adrenoceptors with the greatest effects on vascular resistance are α and β$_2$ receptors. The pulse pressure (the systolic minus the diastolic pressure) is determined mainly by the stroke volume (a function of force of cardiac contraction), which is influenced by β$_1$ receptors. The systolic pressure is the sum of the diastolic and the pulse pressures and is therefore a function of both α and β effects.

I. Metabolic and Hormonal Effects

Beta$_1$ agonists increase renin secretion. Beta$_2$ agonists increase insulin secretion. They also increase glycogenolysis in the liver. The resulting hyperglycemia is countered by the increased insulin levels. Transport of glucose out of the liver is associated initially with hyperkalemia; transport into peripheral organs (especially skeletal muscle) is accompanied by movement of potassium into these cells, resulting in a later hypokalemia. All β agonists appear to stimulate lipolysis via the β$_3$ receptor.

> ### SKILL KEEPER: BLOOD PRESSURE CONTROL MECHANISMS IN PHEOCHROMOCYTOMA (SEE CHAPTER 6)
>
> *Patients with pheochromocytoma may have this tumor for several months or even years before symptoms or signs lead to a diagnosis. Predict the probable compensatory responses to a chronic increase in blood pressure caused by a tumor releasing large amounts of norepinephrine. The Skill Keeper Answer appears at the end of the chapter.*

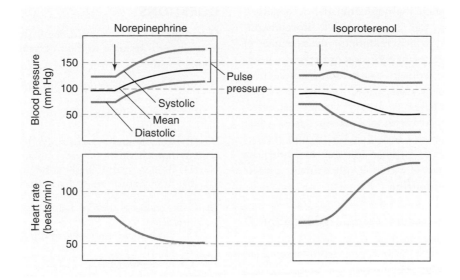

FIGURE 9–1 Typical effects of norepinephrine and isoproterenol on blood pressure and heart rate. Note that the pulse pressure is only slightly increased by norepinephrine but is markedly increased by isoproterenol (see text). The reduction in heart rate caused by norepinephrine is the result of baroreceptor reflex activation of vagal outflow to the heart.

CLINICAL USES

Pharmacokinetic characteristics and clinical applications of selected sympathomimetics are shown in the Drug Summary Table.

A. Anaphylaxis

Epinephrine is the **drug of choice** for the immediate treatment of anaphylactic shock because it is an effective physiologic antagonist of many of the mediators of anaphylaxis. Antihistamines and corticosteroids may also be used, but these agents are neither as efficacious as epinephrine nor as rapid acting.

B. Central Nervous System

The phenylisopropylamines such as **amphetamine** are widely used and abused for their CNS effects. Legitimate indications include narcolepsy and, with appropriate adjuncts, weight reduction. The anorexiant effect may be helpful in initiating weight loss but is insufficient to maintain the loss unless patients also receive intensive dietary and psychological counseling and support. **Methylphenidate** and other amphetamine analogs have been heavily used in attention deficit disorder. The drugs are abused or misused for the purpose of deferring sleep and for their mood-elevating, euphoria-producing action. They have a high addiction liability (see Chapter 32).

C. Eye

The α agonists, especially **phenylephrine** and **tetrahydrozoline,** are often used to reduce the conjunctival itching and congestion caused by irritation or allergy. Phenylephrine is also an effective mydriatic. These drugs do not cause cycloplegia. Newer α₂ agonists are in current use for glaucoma and include **apraclonidine** and **brimonidine.** As noted, the α₂-selective agonists appear to reduce aqueous synthesis. See Table 10–3 for a summary of drugs used in glaucoma.

D. Bronchi

The β agonists, especially the β₂-selective agonists, are **drugs of choice** in the treatment of acute asthmatic bronchoconstriction. The short-acting β₂-selective agonists (eg, **albuterol, metaproterenol, terbutaline**) are not recommended for prophylaxis, but they are safe and effective and may be lifesaving in the treatment of bronchospasm. Much longer-acting β₂-selective agonists, **salmeterol, formoterol,** and **indacaterol** are used in combination with corticosteroids for prophylaxis; they are not indicated for the treatment of acute symptoms, see Chapter 20.

E. Cardiovascular Applications

1. Conditions in which an *increase* in blood flow is desired—In acute heart failure and some types of shock, an increase in cardiac output and blood flow to the tissues is needed. Beta₁ agonists may be useful in this situation because they increase cardiac contractility and reduce (to some degree) afterload by decreasing the impedance to ventricular ejection through a small β₂ effect. **Norepinephrine**, in contrast to earlier impressions, is an effective agent in septic and cardiogenic shock. **Dobutamine** and **dopamine** are also used. Unfortunately, the arrhythmogenic effects of these drugs may be dose-limiting.

2. Conditions in which a *decrease* in blood flow or increase in blood pressure is desired—Alpha₁ agonists are useful in situations in which vasoconstriction is appropriate.

These include local hemostatic (**epinephrine**) and decongestant effects (**phenylephrine**) as well as spinal shock (**norepinephrine, phenylephrine**), in which temporary maintenance of blood pressure may help maintain perfusion of the brain, heart, and kidneys. Shock due to septicemia or myocardial infarction, on the other hand, is usually made worse by vasoconstrictors, because sympathetic discharge is usually already increased. Alpha agonists are often mixed with local anesthetics to reduce the loss of anesthetic from the area of injection into the circulation. Chronic orthostatic hypotension due to inadequate sympathetic tone can be treated with oral **ephedrine** or a newer orally active α_1 agonist, **midodrine**.

3. Conditions in which acute cardiac stimulation is desired—**Epinephrine** has been used in cardiac arrest by intravenous and direct intracardiac injection. **Isoproterenol** has been used for atrioventricular (AV) block.

F. Genitourinary Tract

Beta$_2$ agonists (**ritodrine, terbutaline**) are sometimes used to suppress premature labor, but the cardiac stimulant effect may be hazardous to both mother and fetus. Nonsteroidal anti-inflammatory drugs, calcium channel blockers, and magnesium are also used for this indication.

Long-acting oral sympathomimetics such as ephedrine are sometimes used to improve urinary continence in the elderly and in children with enuresis. This action is mediated by α receptors in the trigone of the bladder and, in men, the smooth muscle of the prostate.

TOXICITY

Because of their limited penetration into the brain, **catecholamines** have little CNS toxicity when given systemically. In the periphery, their adverse effects are extensions of their pharmacologic alpha or beta actions: excessive vasoconstriction, cardiac arrhythmias, myocardial infarction, hemorrhagic stroke, and pulmonary edema or hemorrhage.

The **phenylisopropylamines** may produce mild to severe CNS toxicity, depending on dosage. In small doses, they induce nervousness, anorexia, and insomnia; in higher doses, they may cause anxiety, aggressiveness, or paranoid behavior. Convulsions may occur. Peripherally acting agents have toxicities that are predictable on the basis of the receptors they activate. Thus, α_1 agonists cause hypertension, and β_1 agonists cause sinus tachycardia and serious arrhythmias. Beta$_2$ agonists cause skeletal muscle tremor. It is important to note that none of these drugs is perfectly selective; at high doses, β_1-selective agents have β_2 actions and vice versa. Cocaine is of special importance as a drug of abuse: its major toxicities include cardiac arrhythmias or infarction and convulsions. A fatal outcome is more common with acute cocaine overdose than with any other sympathomimetic.

QUESTIONS

Questions 1–2. A 7-year-old boy with a previous history of bee sting allergy is brought to the emergency department after being stung by 3 bees.

1. Which of the following are probable signs of the anaphylactic reaction to bee stings?
   - (A) Bronchodilation, tachycardia, hypertension, vomiting, diarrhea
   - (B) Bronchospasm, tachycardia, hypotension
   - (C) Bronchodilation, bradycardia, vomiting, diarrhea
   - (D) Bronchospasm, bradycardia, hypotension, diarrhea
   - (E) Bronchodilation, tachycardia, vomiting, diarrhea

2. If this child has signs of anaphylaxis, what is the treatment of choice?
   - (A) Diphenhydramine (an antihistamine)
   - (B) Ephedrine
   - (C) Epinephrine
   - (D) Methylprednisolone (a corticosteroid)
   - (E) Phenylephrine

3. A 65-year-old woman with long-standing diabetes mellitus is admitted to the ward from the emergency department, and you wish to examine her retinas for possible changes. Which of the following drugs is a good choice when pupillary dilation—but not cycloplegia—is desired?
   - (A) Isoproterenol
   - (B) Norepinephrine
   - (C) Phenylephrine
   - (D) Pilocarpine
   - (E) Tropicamide

4. A 30-year-old man is admitted to the emergency department after taking a suicidal overdose of reserpine. His blood pressure is 50/0 mm Hg and heart rate is 40 bpm. Which of the following would be the most effective cardiovascular stimulant?
   - (A) Amphetamine
   - (B) Clonidine
   - (C) Cocaine
   - (D) Norepinephrine
   - (E) Tyramine

5. An anesthetized dog is prepared for recording blood pressure and heart rate in a study of a new blocking drug. Results show that the new drug prevents the tachycardia evoked by isoproterenol? Which of the following standard agents does the new drug most resemble?
   - (A) Atropine
   - (B) Hexamethonium
   - (C) Phentolamine (an α blocker)
   - (D) Physostigmine
   - (E) Propranolol (a β blocker)

6. Your new 10-year-old patient has asthma, and you decide to treat her with a β_2 agonist. In considering the possible drug effects in this patient, you would note that β_2 stimulants frequently cause
   - (A) Direct stimulation of renin release
   - (B) Hypoglycemia
   - (C) Increased cGMP (cyclic guanine monophosphate) in mast cells
   - (D) Skeletal muscle tremor
   - (E) Vasodilation in the skin

7. Mr Green, a 54-year-old man, had a cardiac transplant 6 months ago. His current blood pressure is 120/70 mm Hg and heart rate is 100 bpm. Which of the following drugs would have the *least* effect on Mr Green's heart rate?
(A) Albuterol
(B) Epinephrine
(C) Isoproterenol
(D) Norepinephrine
(E) Phenylephrine

Questions 8–9. Several new drugs with autonomic actions are being studied in phase 1 clinical trials. Autonomic drugs X and Y were given in moderate doses as intravenous boluses to normal volunteers. The systolic and diastolic blood pressures changed as shown in the diagram below.

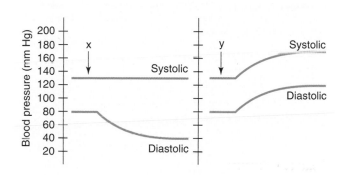

8. Which of the following drugs most resembles drug X?
(A) Atropine
(B) Bethanechol
(C) Epinephrine
(D) Isoproterenol
(E) Norepinephrine

9. Which of the following most resembles drug Y?
(A) Atropine
(B) Bethanechol
(C) Epinephrine
(D) Isoproterenol
(E) Norepinephrine

10. A new drug was given by subcutaneous injection to 25 normal subjects in a phase 1 clinical trial. The cardiovascular effects are summarized in the table below.

Variable	Control	Peak Drug Effect
Systolic BP (mm Hg)	116	144
Diastolic BP (mm Hg)	76	96
Cardiac output (L/min)	5.4	4.7
Heart rate (beats/min)	71.2	54.3

Which of the following drugs does the new experimental agent most resemble?
(A) Atropine
(B) Epinephrine
(C) Isoproterenol
(D) Phenylephrine
(E) Physostigmine

ANSWERS

1. Anaphylaxis is caused by the release of several mediators. Leukotrienes and certain proteins are the most important of these. They cause bronchospasm and laryngeal edema and marked vasodilation with severe hypotension. Tachycardia is a common reflex response to the hypotension. Gastrointestinal disturbance is not as common nor as dangerous. The answer is **B.**

2. The treatment of anaphylaxis requires a powerful physiologic antagonist with the ability to cause bronchodilation (β_2 effect), and vasoconstriction (α effect). Epinephrine is the most effective agent with these properties. Antihistamines and corticosteroids are sometimes used as supplementary agents, but the use of epinephrine is mandatory. The answer is **C.**

3. Antimuscarinics (tropicamide) are mydriatic and cycloplegic; α-sympathomimetic agonists are only mydriatic. Isoproterenol has negligible effects on the eye. Norepinephrine penetrates the conjunctiva poorly and would produce intense vasoconstriction. Pilocarpine causes *miosis*. The answer is **C.**

4. A large overdose of reserpine causes marked depletion of stored catecholamine transmitter. The indirect-acting agents (amphetamines, cocaine, and tyramine) act through catecholamines in (or released from) the nerve terminal and would therefore be ineffective in this patient. Clonidine acts primarily on presynaptic nerve endings although it can activate α_2 receptors located elsewhere. Norepinephrine has the necessary combination of direct action and a spectrum that includes α_1, α_2, and β_1 effects. The answer is **D.**

5. When considering questions that may involve reflex homeostatic responses, it helps to recall the pathway and receptors involved in the baroceptor reflex. In the case of isoproterenol-induced tachycardia, a reflex is evoked by the β_2-mediated decrease in blood pressure. This reflex will be processed by the vasomotor center and result in increased sympathetic autonomic nervous system outflow to the sinus node to increase heart rate. This reflex would be blocked by a ganglion blocker such as hexamethonium. However, isoproterenol also causes tachycardia *directly* by activating the β receptors in the sinus node, an effect not blocked by ganglion blockers. Only a β blocker (propranolol) will prevent both the reflex tachycardia and the direct tachycardia induced by isoproterenol. The answer is **F.**

6. Tremor is a common β_2 effect. Blood vessels in the skin have almost exclusively α (vasoconstrictor) receptors. Stimulation of renin release is a β_1 effect. Beta$_2$ agonists cause *hyper*glycemia. The answer is **D.**

7. Heart transplantation involves the cutting of autonomic nerves to the heart. As a result, autonomic nerve endings degenerate, and cardiac transmitter stores are absent for 2 years or longer after surgery. Therefore, indirect-acting sympathomimetics are ineffective in changing heart rate. All the drugs listed are direct-acting, and all but phenylephrine have significant effects on β receptors. Phenylephrine usually causes reflex bradycardia, which requires intact vagal innervation. The answer is **E.** (Note that denervation may result in upregulation of both β_1 and β_2 receptors so that direct-acting β agonists have a *greater* than normal effect.)

8. The drug X dose caused a decrease in diastolic blood pressure and little change in systolic pressure. Thus, there was a large increase in pulse pressure. The decrease in diastolic pressure

suggests that the drug decreased vascular resistance, that is, it must have significant muscarinic or β-agonist effects. The fact that it also markedly increased pulse pressure suggests that it strongly increased stroke volume, a β-agonist effect. The drug with these beta effects is isoproterenol (Figure 9–1). The answer is **D.**

9. Drug Y caused a marked increase in diastolic pressure, suggesting strong α vasoconstrictor effects. It also caused a small increase in pulse pressure, suggesting some β-agonist action. An increase in stroke volume may also result from increased venous return (an α-agonist effect) and stroke volume. The drug that best matches this description is norepinephrine. The answer is **E.**

10. The investigational agent caused a marked increase in diastolic pressure but a small increase in pulse pressure (from 40 to 48 mm Hg). These changes suggest a strong alpha effect on vessels but an increase in venous return and stroke volume or a small β-agonist action in the heart. The heart rate decreased markedly, reflecting a baroreceptor reflex compensatory response. Note that the stroke volume increased slightly (cardiac output divided by heart rate—from 75.8 to 86.6 mL). This is to be expected even in the absence of beta effects if bradycardia causes increased diastolic filling time. The drug behaves most like a pure α agonist. The answer is **D.**

SKILL KEEPER ANSWER: BLOOD PRESSURE CONTROL MECHANISMS IN PHEOCHROMOCYTOMA (SEE CHAPTER 6)

Because the control mechanisms that attempt to maintain blood pressure constant are intact in patients with pheochromocytoma (they are reset in patients with ordinary "essential" hypertension), a number of compensatory changes are observed in pheochromocytoma patients (see Figure 6–4). These include reduced renin, angiotensin, and aldosterone levels in the blood. Reduced aldosterone causes more salt and water to be excreted by the kidney, reducing blood volume. Since the red cell mass is not affected, hematocrit is often increased. If the tumor releases only norepinephrine, a compensatory bradycardia may also be present, but most patients release enough epinephrine to maintain heart rate at a normal or even increased level.

CHECKLIST

When you complete this chapter, you should be able to:

❑ Name a typical nonselective α agonist, a selective α_2 agonist, a nonselective β agonist, a selective β_1 agonist, selective β_2 agonists, an α_1, α_2, β_1 agonist, and an α_1, α_2, β_1, β_2 agonist.

❑ List tissues that contain significant numbers of α_1 or α_2 receptors.

❑ List tissues that contain significant numbers of β_1 or β_2 receptors.

❑ Describe the major organ system effects of a pure α agonist, a pure β agonist, and a mixed α and β agonist.

❑ Describe a clinical situation in which the effects of an indirect sympathomimetic would differ from those of a direct agonist.

❑ List the major clinical applications of the adrenoceptor agonists.

DRUG SUMMARY TABLE: Sympathomimetics

Subclass	Mechanism of Action	Clinical Applications	Pharmacokinetics	Toxicities, Interactions
Direct-acting catecholamines				
Epinephrine	α_1, α_2, β_1, β_2, β_3 agonist	Anaphylaxis • hemostatic • cardiac arrest	Parenteral and topical only • does not enter CNS • Duration: short	Hypertension, arrhythmia, stroke, myocardial infarction, pulmonary edema
Norepinephrine	α_1, α_2, β_1 agonist	Shock	Like epinephrine • IV only	Vasospasm, tissue necrosis, excessive blood pressure increase, arrhythmias, infarction
Dopamine	D_1, α_1, α_2, β_1, β_2, β_3 agonist	Shock, especially with renal shutdown • sometimes used in heart failure	Like epinephrine • IV only	Cardiovascular disturbance, arrhythmias

Isoproterenol: β_1, β_2, β_3 agonist; primary use is by nebulizer in acute asthma and IV, in AV block
Dobutamine: β_1 agonist; primary use is in acute heart failure to increase cardiac output

Subclass	Mechanism of Action	Clinical Applications	Pharmacokinetics	Toxicities, Interactions
Noncatecholamines				
Phenylephrine	α_1, α_2 agonist	Decongestant, mydriatic, neurogenic hypotension	Oral, inhalant, topical, and parenteral • Duration: 15–60 min	Hypertension, stroke, myocardial infarction

Subclass	Mechanism of Action	Clinical Applications	Pharmacokinetics	Toxicities, Interactions
Noncatecholamine β-selective				
Albuterol, metaproterenol, terbutaline	β_2 agonist	Prompt onset for acute bronchospasm	Inhalant via aerosol canister • Duration: 2–6 h	Tachycardia, tremor

Salmeterol, formoterol, indacaterol: β_2 agonists; slow onset, long action. Not useful in acute bronchospasm, used only with corticosteroids for prophylaxis of asthma

Subclass	Mechanism of Action	Clinical Applications	Pharmacokinetics	Toxicities, Interactions
Indirect-acting phenylisopropylamines				
Amphetamine, methamphetamine	Displaces stored catecholamines from nerve endings	Anorexiant, ADHD, narcolepsy	Oral and parenteral • Duration: $\geq$4–6 h	High addiction liability. Paranoia, aggression; insomnia; hypertension

Ephedrine: displacer like amphetamine; oral activity; duration 4–6 h. Sometimes used for narcolepsy, idiopathic postural hypotension, enuresis. Lower addiction liability than amphetamines

Subclass	Mechanism of Action	Clinical Applications	Pharmacokinetics	Toxicities, Interactions
Cocaine				
Cocaine	Blocks norepinephrine reuptake (NET) and dopamine reuptake (DAT)	Local anesthetic with intrinsic hemostatic action	Parenteral only Duration: 2 h	Very high addiction liability. Hypertension, arrhythmias, seizures
Tyramine				
Tyramine	Displaces stored catecholamines	No clinical use but found in fermented foods	Normally high first-pass effect, but in patients taking MAO inhibitors it is absorbed	Hypertension, arrhythmias, stroke, myocardial infarction

ADHD, attention-deficit hyperactivity disorder; CNS, central nervous system; DAT, dopamine transporter; MAO, monoamine oxidase.

Adrenoceptor Blockers

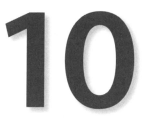

C H A P T E R

10

Alpha- and beta-adrenoceptor-blocking agents are divided into primary subgroups on the basis of their receptor selectivity. All of these agents are pharmacologic antagonists or partial agonists.

Because α and β blockers differ markedly in their effects and clinical applications, these drugs are considered separately in the following discussion.

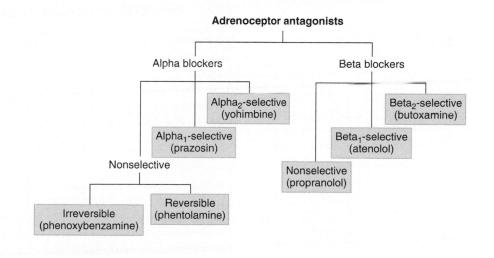

ALPHA-BLOCKING DRUGS

A. Classification

Subdivisions of the α blockers are based on selective affinity for α_1 versus α_2 receptors or a lack thereof. Other features used to classify the α-blocking drugs are their reversibility and duration of action.

Irreversible, long-acting—Phenoxybenzamine is the prototypical long-acting, irreversible α blocker. It is only slightly α_1-selective. **Reversible, shorter-acting—Phentolamine** is a competitive, reversible blocking agent that does not distinguish between α_1 and α_2 receptors. **Alpha$_1$-selective—Prazosin** is a highly selective, reversible pharmacologic α_1 blocker. Doxazosin, terazosin, and tamsulosin are similar drugs. The advantage of α_1 selectivity is discussed in the following text. **Alpha$_2$-selective—Yohimbine** and **rauwolscine** are α_2-selective competitive pharmacologic antagonists. They are used primarily in research applications.

B. Pharmacokinetics

Alpha-blocking drugs are all active by the oral as well as the parenteral route, although phentolamine is rarely given orally. Phenoxybenzamine has a short elimination half-life but a long duration of action—about 48 h—because it binds covalently to its receptor. Phentolamine has a duration of action of 2–4 h when used orally and 20–40 min when given parenterally. Prazosin and the other α_1-selective blockers act for 8–24 h.

High-Yield Terms to Learn

Competitive blocker	A surmountable antagonist (eg, phentolamine); one that can be overcome by increasing the dose of agonist
Epinephrine reversal	Conversion of the pressor response to epinephrine (typical of large doses) to a blood pressure–lowering effect; caused by α blockers, which unmask the β_2 effects of epinephrine
Intrinsic sympathomimetic activity (ISA)	Partial agonist action by adrenoceptor blockers; typical of several β blockers (eg, pindolol, acebutolol)
Irreversible blocker	A nonsurmountable inhibitor, usually because of covalent bond formation (eg, phenoxybenzamine)
Membrane-stabilizing activity (MSA)	Local anesthetic action; typical of several β blockers (eg, propranolol)
Orthostatic hypotension	Hypotension that is most marked in the upright position; caused by venous pooling (typical of α blockade) or inadequate blood volume (caused by blood loss or excessive diuresis)
Partial agonist	A drug (eg, pindolol) that produces a smaller maximal effect than a full agonist and therefore can inhibit the effect of a full agonist
Pheochromocytoma	A tumor consisting of cells that release varying amounts of norepinephrine and epinephrine into the circulation

C. Mechanism of Action

Phenoxybenzamine binds covalently to the α receptor, thereby producing an irreversible (insurmountable) blockade. The other agents are competitive antagonists, and their effects can be surmounted by increased concentrations of agonist. This difference may be important in the treatment of pheochromocytoma because a massive release of catecholamines from the tumor may overcome a reversible blockade.

D. Effects

1. Nonselective blockers—These agents cause a predictable blockade of α-mediated responses to sympathetic nervous system discharge and exogenous sympathomimetics (ie, the α responses listed in Table 9–1). The most important effects of nonselective α blockers are those on the cardiovascular system: a reduction in vascular tone with a reduction of both arterial and venous pressures. There are no significant direct cardiac effects. However, the nonselective α blockers do cause baroreceptor reflex-mediated tachycardia as a result of the drop in mean arterial pressure (see Figure 6–4). This tachycardia may be exaggerated because the α_2 receptors on adrenergic nerve terminals in the heart, which normally reduce the net release of norepinephrine, are also blocked (see Figure 6–3).

Epinephrine reversal (Figure 10–1) is a predictable effect in a patient who has received an α blocker. The term refers to a reversal of the blood pressure effect of large doses of epinephrine, from a pressor response (mediated by α receptors) to a depressor response (mediated by β_2 receptors). The effect is not observed with phenylephrine or norepinephrine because these drugs lack sufficient β_2 effects. Epinephrine reversal is occasionally seen as an unexpected (but predictable) effect of drugs for which α blockade is an adverse effect (eg, some phenothiazine tranquilizers, antihistamines).

2. Selective α blockers—Because prazosin and its analogs block vascular α_1 receptors much more effectively than the α_2-modulatory receptors associated with cardiac sympathetic nerve endings, these drugs cause much less reflex tachycardia than the nonselective α blockers when reducing blood pressure. These drugs also have useful effects on smooth muscle in the prostate.

E. Clinical Uses

1. Nonselective α blockers—Nonselective α blockers have limited clinical applications. The best-documented application is in the presurgical management of pheochromocytoma. Such patients may have severe hypertension and reduced blood volume, which should be corrected before subjecting the patient to the stress of surgery. Phenoxybenzamine is usually used during this preparatory phase; phentolamine is sometimes used during surgery. Phenoxybenzamine also has serotonin receptor-blocking effects, which justify its occasional use in carcinoid tumor, as well as H$_1$ antihistaminic effects, which lead to its use in mastocytosis.

Accidental local infiltration of potent α agonists such as norepinephrine may lead to tissue ischemia and necrosis if not promptly reversed; infiltration of the ischemic area with phentolamine is sometimes used to prevent tissue damage. Overdose with drugs of abuse such as amphetamine, cocaine, or phenylpropanolamine may lead to severe hypertension because of their indirect sympathomimetic actions. This hypertension usually responds well to α blockers. Sudden cessation of clonidine therapy leads to rebound hypertension (Chapter 11); this phenomenon is often treated with phentolamine.

Raynaud's phenomenon sometimes responds to α blockers, but their efficacy in this condition is not well documented. Phentolamine or yohimbine has been used by direct injection to cause penile erection in men with erectile dysfunction, but phosphodiesterase inhibitors are more popular (see Chapter 12).

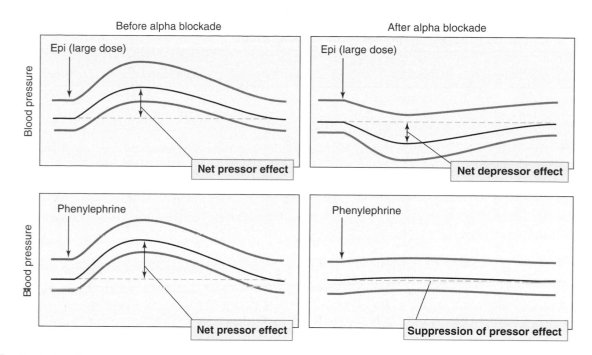

FIGURE 10–1 The effects of an α blocker, for example, phentolamine, on the blood pressure responses to epinephrine (epi) and phenylephrine. The epinephrine response exhibits reversal of the mean blood pressure change from a net increase (the α response) to a net decrease (the β_2 response). The response to phenylephrine is suppressed but not reversed, because phenylephrine lacks β action.

2. Selective α blockers—Prazosin, doxazosin, and terazosin are used in hypertension (Chapter 11). These α_1 blockers, tamsulosin, and silodosin are also used to reduce urinary hesitancy and prevent urinary retention in men with benign prostatic hyperplasia.

F. Toxicity

The most important toxicities of the α blockers are simple extensions of their α-blocking effects. The main manifestations are orthostatic hypotension and, in the case of the nonselective agents, marked reflex tachycardia. Tachycardia is less common and less severe with α_1-selective blockers. Phentolamine also has some non-alpha-mediated vasodilating effects. In patients with coronary disease, angina may be precipitated by the tachycardia. Oral administration of some of these drugs can cause nausea and vomiting. The α_1-selective agents are associated with an exaggerated orthostatic hypotensive response to the first dose in some patients. Therefore, the first dose is usually small and taken just before going to bed.

BETA-BLOCKING DRUGS

A. Classification, Subgroups, and Mechanisms

All of the β blockers used clinically are competitive pharmacologic antagonists. **Propranolol** is the prototype. Drugs in this group are usually classified into subgroups on the basis of β_1 selectivity, partial agonist activity, local anesthetic action, and lipid-solubility (Table 10–1).

1. Receptor selectivity—Beta$_1$-receptor selectivity (β_1 block > β_2 block) is a property of **acebutolol, atenolol, esmolol, metoprolol,** and several other β blockers. This property may be an advantage when treating patients with asthma. **Nadolol, propranolol**, and **timolol** are typical nonselective β blockers.

　　Labetalol and **carvedilol** have combined α- and β-blocking actions. These drugs are optically active, and different isomers have α- or β-blocking action. **Nebivolol** has vasodilating action in addition to β_1-selective antagonism.

2. Partial agonist activity—Partial agonist activity ("intrinsic sympathomimetic activity") may be an advantage in treating patients with asthma because these drugs (eg, **pindolol, acebutolol**)—at least in theory—are less likely to cause bronchospasm. In contrast, full antagonists such as propranolol are more likely to cause severe bronchospasm in patients with airway disease.

3. Local anesthetic activity—Local anesthetic activity ("membrane-stabilizing activity") is a disadvantage when β blockers are used topically in the eye because it decreases protective reflexes and increases the risk of corneal ulceration. Local anesthetic effects are absent from **timolol** and several other β blockers that are useful in glaucoma.

4. Pharmacokinetics—Most of the systemic agents have been developed for chronic oral use, but bioavailability and duration

TABLE 10–1 Properties of several β-adrenoceptor-blocking drugs.

Drug	Selectivity	Partial Agonist Activity	Local Anesthetic Activity	Lipid Solubility	Elimination Half-Life
Acebutolol	β_1	Yes	Yes	Low	3–4 h
Atenolol	β_1	No	No	Low	6–9 h
Carvedilol[a]	None	No	No	Moderate	7–10 h
Esmolol	β_1	No	No	Low	10 min
Labetalol[a]	None	Yes[b]	Yes	Low	5 h
Metoprolol	β_1	No	Yes	Moderate	3–4 h
Nadolol	None	No	No	Low	14–24 h
Pindolol	None	Yes	Yes	Moderate	3–4 h
Propranolol	None	No	Yes	High	3.5–6 h
Timolol	None	No	No	Moderate	4–5 h

[a]Also causes α-receptor blockade.

[b]Partial agonist effect at β_2 receptors.

Modified, with permission, from Katzung BG, editor: *Basic & Clinical Pharmacology*, 12th ed., McGraw-Hill, 2012: p. 159.

of action vary widely (Table 10–1). Esmolol is a short-acting ester β blocker that is used only parenterally. Nadolol is the longest-acting β blocker. Acebutolol, atenolol, and nadolol are less lipid-soluble than other β blockers and probably enter the central nervous system (CNS) to a lesser extent.

> ### SKILL KEEPER: PARTIAL AGONIST ACTION (SEE CHAPTER 2)
>
> *Draw a concentration-response graph showing the effect of increasing concentrations of albuterol on airway diameter (as a percentage of maximum) in the presence of a large concentration of pindolol. On the same graph, draw the curves for the percentage of receptors bound to albuterol and to pindolol at each concentration. The Skill Keeper Answer appears at the end of the chapter.*

B. Effects and Clinical Uses

Most of the organ-level effects of β blockers are predictable from blockade of the β-receptor–mediated effects of sympathetic discharge. The clinical applications of β blockade are remarkably broad (see the Drug Summary Table). The treatment of open-angle glaucoma involves the use of several groups of autonomic drugs as well as other agents (Table 10–2). The cardiovascular applications of β blockers—especially in hypertension, angina, and arrhythmias—are extremely important. Treatment

of chronic (not acute) heart failure has become an important application of β blockers. Several large clinical trials have shown that some, but not all, β blockers can reduce morbidity and mortality when used properly in heart failure (see Chapter 13). Labetalol, carvedilol, and metoprolol appear to be beneficial in this application. Pheochromocytoma is sometimes treated with combined α- and β-blocking agents (eg, labetalol), especially if the tumor is producing large amounts of epinephrine as well as norepinephrine.

C. Toxicity

Cardiovascular adverse effects, which are extensions of the β blockade induced by these agents, include bradycardia, atrioventricular blockade, and heart failure. Patients with airway disease may suffer severe asthma attacks. Beta blockers have been shown experimentally to reduce insulin secretion, but this does not appear to be a clinically important effect. However, premonitory symptoms of hypoglycemia from insulin overdosage (tachycardia, tremor, and anxiety) may be masked by β blockers, and mobilization of glucose from the liver and sequestration of K^+ in skeletal muscle may be impaired. CNS adverse effects include sedation, fatigue, and sleep alterations. Atenolol, nadolol, and several other less lipid-soluble β blockers are claimed to have less marked CNS action because they do not enter the CNS as readily as other members of this group. Sexual dysfunction has been reported for most of the β blockers in some patients.

TABLE 10–2 Drugs used in glaucoma.

Group, Drugs	Mechanism	Method of Administration
Beta blockers		
Timolol, others	Decreased secretion of aqueous humor from the ciliary epithelium	Topical drops
Prostaglandins		
Latanoprost, others	Increased aqueous outflow	Topical drops
Cholinomimetics		
Pilocarpine, physostigmine	Ciliary muscle contraction, opening of trabecular meshwork, increased outflow	Topical drops or gel, plastic film slow-release insert
Alpha agonists		
Nonselective: epinephrine	Increased outflow via uveoscleral veins	Topical drops (obsolete)
Alpha$_2$-selective agonists		
Apraclonidine, brimonidine	Decreased aqueous secretion	Topical drops
Carbonic anhydrase inhibitors		
Acetazolamide, dorzolamide	Decreased aqueous secretion due to lack of HCO_3^-	Oral (acetazolamide) or topical (others)
Osmotic agents		
Mannitol	Removal of water from eye	IV (for acute closed-angle glaucoma)

Modified and reproduced, with permission, from Katzung BG, editor: *Basic & Clinical Pharmacology*, 12th ed. McGraw-Hill, 2012, p. 161.

QUESTIONS

1. A patient is to receive epinephrine. She has previously received an adrenoceptor-blocking agent. Which of the following effects of epinephrine would be blocked by phentolamine but not by metoprolol?
   (A) Cardiac stimulation
   (B) Increase of cAMP (cyclic adenosine monophosphate) in fat
   (C) Mydriasis
   (D) Relaxation of bronchial smooth muscle
   (E) Relaxation of the uterus

2. Clinical studies have shown that adrenoceptor blockers have many useful effects in patients. However, a number of drug toxicities have been documented. Adverse effects that limit the use of adrenoceptor blockers include which one of the following?
   (A) Bronchoconstriction from α-blocking agents
   (B) Acute heart failure exacerbation from β blockers
   (C) Impaired blood sugar response with α blockers
   (D) Increased intraocular pressure with β blockers
   (E) Sleep disturbances from α-blocking drugs

Questions 3–6. Four new synthetic drugs (designated W, X, Y, and Z) are to be studied for their cardiovascular effects. They are given to 4 anesthetized animals while the heart rate is recorded. The first animal has received no pretreatment (control); the second has received an effective dose of hexamethonium; the third has received an effective dose of atropine; and the fourth has received an effective dose of phenoxybenzamine. The net changes induced by the new drugs (not by the blocking drugs) are described in the following questions.

3. Drug W increased heart rate in the control animal, the atropine-pretreated animal, and the phenoxybenzamine-pretreated animal. However, drug W had no effect on heart rate in the hexamethonium-pretreated animal. Drug W is probably a drug similar to
   (A) Acetylcholine
   (B) Edrophonium
   (C) Isoproterenol
   (D) Nicotine
   (E) Norepinephrine

4. Drug X had the effects shown in the table below.

In the Animal Receiving	Heart Rate Response to Drug X Was
No pretreatment	↓
Hexamethonium	↑
Atropine	↑
Phenoxybenzamine	↑

Drug X is probably a drug similar to
(A) Acetylcholine
(B) Albuterol
(C) Edrophonium
(D) Isoproterenol
(E) Norepinephrine

5. Drug Y had the effects shown in the table below.

In the Animal Receiving	Heart Rate Response to Drug Y Was
No pretreatment	↑
Hexamethonium	↑
Atropine	↑
Phenoxybenzamine	↑

Drug Y is probably a drug similar to
(A) Acetylcholine
(B) Edrophonium
(C) Isoproterenol
(D) Norepinephrine
(E) Prazosin

6. The results of the test of drug Z are shown in the graph.

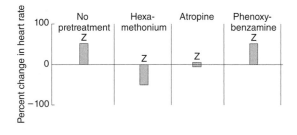

Drug Z is probably a drug similar to
(A) Acetylcholine
(B) Edrophonium
(C) Isoproterenol
(D) Norepinephrine
(E) Pralidoxime

7. When given to a patient, phentolamine blocks which one of the following?
(A) Bradycardia induced by phenylephrine
(B) Bronchodilation induced by epinephrine
(C) Increased cardiac contractile force induced by norepinephrine
(D) Miosis induced by acetylcholine
(E) Vasodilation induced by isoproterenol

8. Your 75-year-old patient with angina and glaucoma is to receive a β-blocking drug. Which of the following statements is most correct regarding β-blocking drugs?
(A) Esmolol's pharmacokinetics are compatible with chronic topical use
(B) Metoprolol blocks β_2 receptors selectively
(C) Nadolol lacks β_2-blocking action
(D) Pindolol is a β antagonist with high membrane-stabilizing (local anesthetic) activity
(E) Timolol lacks the local anesthetic effects of propranolol

9. A 56-year-old man has hypertension and an enlarged prostate, which biopsy shows to be benign prostatic hyperplasia. He complains of urinary retention. Which of the following drugs would be the most appropriate initial therapy?
(A) Albuterol
(B) Atenolol
(C) Metoprolol
(D) Prazosin
(E) Timolol

10. A new drug was administered to an anesthetized animal with the results shown here. A large dose of epinephrine (epi) was administered before and after the new agent for comparison.

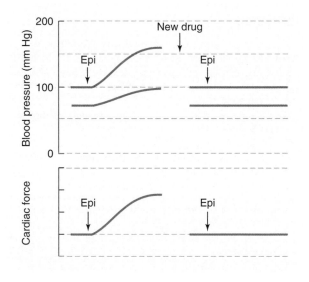

Which of the following agents does the new drug most closely resemble?
(A) Atenolol
(B) Atropine
(C) Labetalol
(D) Phenoxybenzamine
(E) Propranolol

ANSWERS

1. Mydriasis caused by contraction of the pupillary dilator radial smooth muscle is mediated by α receptors. All the other effects listed are mediated by β receptors. The answer is **C.**

2. Although *chronic* heart failure is often treated with β blockers, acute heart failure can be precipitated by these drugs. Choices **A, C,** and **E** reverse the correct pairing of receptor subtype (α versus β) with effect. Choice **D** reverses the direction of change of intraocular pressure. The answer is **B.**

3. In developing a strategy for this type of question, consider first the actions of the known blocking drugs. Hexamethonium blocks reflexes as well as the direct action of nicotine. Atropine would block direct muscarinic effects of an unknown drug (if it had any) or reflex slowing of the heart mediated by the vagus. Phenoxybenzamine blocks only α-receptor-mediated processes. If the response produced in the nonpretreated animal is blocked or reversed by hexamethonium, it is probably a direct nicotinic effect or a reflex response to hypotension. In that case, consider all the receptors involved in mediating the reflex. Drug W causes tachycardia that is prevented by ganglion blockade. The only drug in the list of choices that causes hypotension and tachycardia that is not blocked by atropine is isoproterenol, and the tachycardia caused by isoproterenol is not blocked by ganglionic blockade. Thus, drug W must be nicotine. The answer is **D.**

4. Drug X causes slowing of the heart rate, but this is converted into tachycardia by hexamethonium and atropine, demonstrating that the bradycardia is caused by reflex vagal discharge. Phenoxybenzamine also reverses the bradycardia to tachycardia, suggesting that α receptors are needed to induce the reflex bradycardia and that X also has direct β-agonist actions. The choices that evoke a vagal reflex bradycardia (vasoconstrictors) but can also cause direct tachycardia (beta agonists) are limited; the answer is **E.**

5. Drug Y causes tachycardia that is not significantly influenced by any of the blockers; therefore, drug Y must have a direct β-agonist effect on the heart. The answer is **C.**

6. Drug Z causes tachycardia that is converted to bradycardia by hexamethonium and blocked completely by atropine. This indicates that the tachycardia is a reflex evoked by vasodilation. Drug Z causes bradycardia when the ganglia are blocked, indicating that it also has a direct muscarinic action on the heart. This is confirmed by the ability of atropine to block both the tachycardia and the bradycardia. The answer is **A.**

7. Phenylephrine, an α agonist, induces bradycardia through the baroreceptor reflex. Blockade of this drug's α-mediated vasoconstrictor effect prevents the bradycardia. The answer is **A.**

8. Esmolol is a short-acting β blocker for parenteral use only. Nadolol is a nonselective β blocker, and metoprolol is a β₁-selective blocker. Timolol is useful in glaucoma because it does not anesthetize the cornea. The answer is **E.**

9. An α blocker is appropriate therapy in a man with both hypertension and benign prostatic hyperplasia because both conditions involve contraction of smooth muscle containing α receptors. The answer is **D.**

10. The new drug blocks both the α-mediated effects (increased diastolic and mean arterial blood pressure) and β-mediated action (increased cardiac force). In addition, it does not cause epinephrine reversal. Therefore, the drug must have both α- and β-blocking effects. The answer is **C.**

SKILL KEEPER ANSWER: PARTIAL AGONIST ACTION (SEE CHAPTER 2)

Because pindolol is a partial agonist at β receptors, the concentration–response curve will show a bronchodilating effect at zero albuterol concentration. As albuterol concentration increases, the airway diameter also increases. The binding curves will show pindolol binding starting at 100% of receptors and going to zero as albuterol concentration increases, with albuterol binding starting at zero and going to 100%.

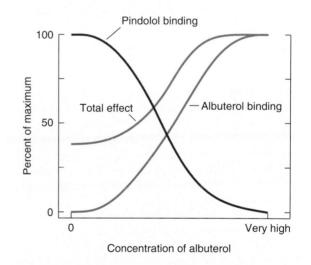

CHECKLIST

When you complete this chapter, you should be able to:

❑ Describe and compare the effects of an α blocker on the blood pressure and heart rate responses to epinephrine, norepinephrine, and phenylephrine.

❑ Compare the pharmacodynamics of propranolol, labetalol, metoprolol, and pindolol.

❑ Compare the pharmacokinetics of propranolol, atenolol, esmolol, and nadolol.

❑ Describe the clinical indications and toxicities of typical α and β blockers.

DRUG SUMMARY TABLE: Adrenoceptor Blockers

Subclass	Mechanism of Action	Clinical Applications	Pharmacokinetics	Toxicities, Interactions
Nonselective α blockers				
Phentolamine	Competitive pharmacologic antagonism at α receptors	Pheochromocytoma, antidote to overdose of α agonists	Oral, IV • short half-life Duration: 2–4 h	Orthostatic hypotension • reflex tachycardia
Phenoxybenzamine	Irreversible (covalent) binding to α receptors	Pheochromocytoma, carcinoid, mastocytosis, Raynaud's phenomenon	Oral, short half-life but long duration of action (24–48 h)	Orthostatic hypotension, reflex tachycardia • gastrointestinal irritation
α₁-Selective blockers				
Prazosin	Competitive antagonism at α₁ receptors	Hypertension, benign prostatic hyperplasia	Oral Duration: 8 h	Orthostatic hypotension (especially first dose), but little reflex tachycardia
Doxazosin, terazosin: like prazosin; longer duration of action (12–24 h) *Tamsulosin, silodosin:* like prazosin, approved only for benign prostatic hyperplasia				
α₂-Selective blockers				
Yohimbine	Competitive antagonism at α₂ receptors	Obsolete use for erectile dysfunction • research use	Oral, parenteral	Tachycardia • gastrointestinal upset
Nonselective β blockers				
Propranolol	Competitive block of β receptors, local anesthetic effect	Angina, arrhythmias (treatment and prophylaxis), hypertension, thyrotoxicosis, tremor, stage fright, migraine	Oral and IV Duration: 4–6 h. Ready entry into CNS	Excessive β blockade: bronchospasm (can be fatal in asthmatics), atrioventricular block, heart failure • CNS sedation, lethargy, sleep disturbances
Timolol, betaxolol: lack local anesthetic action; useful in glaucoma *Pindolol:* partial agonist action; possibly safer in asthma *Nadolol:* like propranolol but longer action (up to 24 h) and less CNS effect				
β₁-Selective blockers				
Atenolol	Competitive block of β₁ receptors	Hypertension, angina, arrhythmias	Oral Duration: 6–9 h	Like propranolol with somewhat less danger of bronchospasm
Esmolol: IV agent for perioperative and thyroid storm arrhythmias, hypertensive emergency *Metoprolol:* like atenolol, oral, shown to reduce mortality in heart failure *Nebivolol:* new oral β₁-selective blocker with additional vasodilating action				
β₂-Selective blockers				
Butoxamine	Competitive block of β₂ receptors	None • research use only	—	Bronchospasm
α + β blockers				
Labetalol	Four isomers; 2 bind and block both α and β receptors	Hypertension, hypertensive emergencies (IV)	Oral and IV Duration: 5 h	Like atenolol
Carvedilol: like labetalol, 2 isomers; shown to reduce mortality in heart failure				

Drugs Used in Hypertension

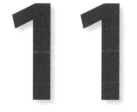

C H A P T E R

11

Antihypertensive drugs are organized around a clinical indication—the need to treat a disease—rather than a receptor type. The drugs covered in this unit have a variety of mechanisms of action including diuresis, sympathoplegia, vasodilation, and antagonism of angiotensin, and many agents are available in most categories. A single renin inhibitor has recently been added to the drugs used in this condition.

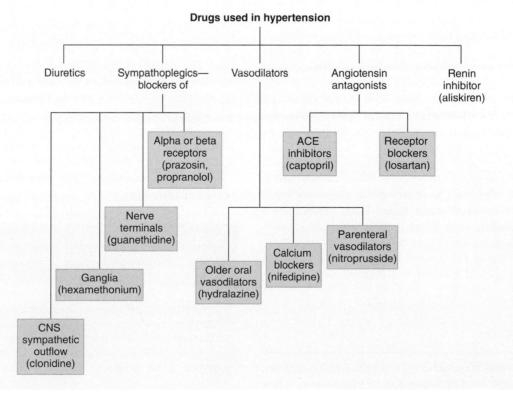

Drugs used in hypertension

Diuretics

Sympathoplegics— blockers of

Vasodilators

Angiotensin antagonists

Renin inhibitor (aliskiren)

Alpha or beta receptors (prazosin, propranolol)

Nerve terminals (guanethidine)

Ganglia (hexamethonium)

CNS sympathetic outflow (clonidine)

ACE inhibitors (captopril)

Receptor blockers (losartan)

Parenteral vasodilators (nitroprusside)

Calcium blockers (nifedipine)

Older oral vasodilators (hydralazine)

High-Yield Terms to Learn

Baroreceptor reflex	Primary autonomic mechanism for blood pressure homeostasis; involves sensory input from carotid sinus and aorta to the vasomotor center and output via the parasympathetic and sympathetic motor nerves
Catecholamine reuptake pump (norepinephrine transporter [NET])	Nerve terminal transporter responsible for recycling norepinephrine after release into the synapse
Catecholamine vesicle pump	Storage vesicle transporter that pumps amine from cytoplasm into vesicle; also called vesicle monoamine transporter (VMAT)
End-organ damage	Vascular damage in heart, kidney, retina, or brain
Essential hypertension	Hypertension of unknown etiology; also called primary hypertension
False transmitter	Substance, for example, octopamine, stored in vesicles and released into synaptic cleft but lacking the effect of the true transmitter, for example, norepinephrine
Hypertensive emergency ("malignant hypertension")	An accelerated form of severe hypertension associated with rising blood pressure and rapidly progressing damage to vessels and end organs. Often signaled by renal damage, encephalopathy, and retinal hemorrhages or by angina, stroke, or myocardial infarction
Orthostatic hypotension	Hypotension on assuming upright posture; postural hypotension
Postganglionic neuron blocker	Drug that blocks transmission by an action in the terminals of the postganglionic nerves
Rebound hypertension	Elevated blood pressure (usually above pretreatment levels) resulting from loss of antihypertensive drug effect
Reflex tachycardia	Tachycardia resulting from lowering of blood pressure; mediated by the baroreceptor reflex
Stepped care	Progressive addition of drugs to a regimen, starting with one (usually a diuretic) and adding in stepwise fashion a sympatholytic, an ACE inhibitor, and (sometimes) a vasodilator
Sympatholytic, sympathoplegic	Drug that reduces effects of the sympathetic nervous system

Less than 20% of cases of hypertension are due to ("secondary" to) factors that can be clearly defined and corrected. This type of hypertension is associated with pheochromocytoma, coarctation of the aorta, renal vascular disease, adrenal cortical tumors, and a few other rare conditions. Most cases of hypertension are idiopathic, also called "primary" or "essential" hypertension. The strategies for treating idiopathic hypertension are based on the determinants of arterial pressure (see Figure 6–4). These strategies include reductions of blood volume, sympathetic effects, vascular smooth muscle tension, and angiotensin effects. Unfortunately, the baroreceptor reflex and the renin response in primary hypertension are reset to maintain the higher blood pressure. As a result, they respond to lower blood pressure with compensatory homeostatic responses, which may be significant (Table 11–1). As indicated in Figure 11–1, these compensatory responses can be counteracted with β blockers and diuretics or angiotensin antagonists.

DIURETICS

Diuretics are covered in greater detail in Chapter 15 but are mentioned here because of their importance in hypertension. These drugs lower blood pressure by reduction of blood volume and probably also by a direct vascular effect that is not fully understood. The diuretics most important for treating hypertension are the **thiazides** (eg, hydrochlorothiazide) and the **loop diuretics** (eg, furosemide). Thiazides may be adequate in mild hypertension, but the loop agents are used in moderate and severe hypertension and in hypertensive emergencies. Compensatory responses to blood pressure lowering by diuretics are minimal (Table 11–1). When thiazides are given, the maximal antihypertensive effect is often achieved with doses lower than those required for the maximal diuretic effect.

SKILL KEEPER 1: DEVELOPMENT OF NEW ANTIHYPERTENSIVE DRUGS (SEE CHAPTER 5)

A new drug is under development for the treatment of hypertension. What types of data will the producer of this drug have to provide to carry out clinical trials? What data will be needed to market the drug? The Skill Keeper Answer appears at the end of the chapter.

TABLE 11–1 Compensatory responses to antihypertensive drugs.

Class and Drug	Compensatory Responses
Diuretics (thiazides, loop agents)	Minimal
Sympathoplegics	
Centrally acting (clonidine, methyldopa)	Salt and water retention
Ganglion blockers (obsolete)	Salt and water retention
Alpha$_1$-selective blockers	Salt and water retention, slight tachycardia
Beta blockers	Minimal
Vasodilators	
Hydralazine	Salt and water retention, moderate tachycardia
Minoxidil	Marked salt and water retention, marked tachycardia
Nifedipine, other calcium channel blockers	Minor salt and water retention
Nitroprusside	Salt and water retention
Angiotensin antagonists (ACE inhibitors, ARBs)	Minimal

SYMPATHOPLEGICS

Sympathoplegic drugs interfere with sympathetic (SANS) control of cardiovascular function. The result is a reduction of one or more of the following: venous tone, heart rate, contractile force of the heart, cardiac output, and total peripheral resistance (see Figure 6–4). Compensatory responses are marked for some of these agents (Table 11–1). Sympathoplegics are subdivided by anatomic site of action (Figure 11–2).

A. Baroreceptor-Sensitizing Agents

A few natural products, such as veratrum alkaloids, appear to increase sensitivity of baroreceptor sensory nerves and reduce SANS outflow while increasing vagal tone to the heart. These agents are toxic and no clinically available drugs act at this site.

B. Central Nervous System-Active Agents

Alpha$_2$-selective agonists (eg, **clonidine, methyldopa**) cause a decrease in sympathetic outflow by activation of α_2 receptors in the CNS. These drugs readily enter the CNS when given orally. Methyldopa is a prodrug; it is converted to **methylnorepinephrine** in the brain. Clonidine and methyldopa reduce blood pressure by reducing cardiac output, vascular resistance, or both. The major compensatory response is salt retention. Sudden discontinuation of clonidine causes rebound hypertension, which

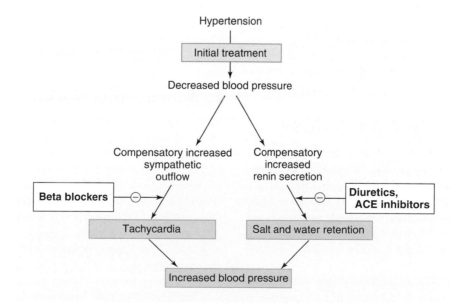

FIGURE 11–1 Compensatory responses (*orange boxes*) to decreased blood pressure when treating hypertension. The initial treatment that causes the compensatory responses might be a vasodilator. Arrows with minus signs indicate drugs used (*white boxes*) to minimize the compensatory responses. ACE, angiotensin-converting enzyme.

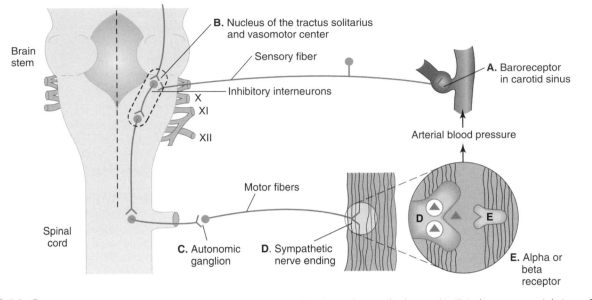

FIGURE 11–2 Baroreceptor reflex arc and sites of action of sympathoplegic drugs. The letters (A–E) indicate potential sites of action of subgroups of sympathoplegics. No clinically useful drugs act at the baroreceptor (site A), but drugs are available for each of the other sites.

may be severe. This rebound increase in blood pressure can be controlled by reinstitution of clonidine therapy or administration of α blockers such as phentolamine. Methyldopa occasionally causes hematologic immunotoxicity, detected initially by test tube agglutination of red blood cells (positive Coombs' test), and in some patients progressing to hemolytic anemia. Both drugs may cause sedation—methyldopa more so at therapeutic dosage.

C. Ganglion-Blocking Drugs

Nicotinic blockers that act in the ganglia are very efficacious, but because their adverse effects are severe, they are now considered obsolete. **Hexamethonium** and **trimethaphan** are extremely powerful blood pressure-lowering drugs.

D. Postganglionic Sympathetic Nerve Terminal Blockers

Drugs that deplete the adrenergic nerve terminal of its norepinephrine stores (eg, **reserpine**) or that deplete and block release of the stores (eg, **guanethidine, guanadrel**) can lower blood pressure. The major compensatory response is salt and water retention. In high dosages, these drugs are very efficacious but produce severe adverse effects and are now considered obsolete for hypertension.

Monoamine oxidase (MAO) inhibitors were once used in hypertension because they cause the formation of a false transmitter (octopamine) in sympathetic postganglionic neuron terminals and lower blood pressure. This octopamine is stored, along with increased amounts of norepinephrine, in the transmitter vesicles. SANS nerve impulses then release a mixture of octopamine

(which has very low efficacy) and norepinephrine, resulting in a smaller than normal increase in vascular resistance. Large doses of indirect-acting sympathomimetics, on the other hand (eg, the tyramine in a meal of fermented foods), may cause release of very large amounts of stored norepinephrine (along with the octopamine) and result in a hypertensive crisis. (Recall that tyramine normally has very low bioavailability because of metabolism by MAO. In the presence of MAO inhibitors, it has much higher bioavailability.) Because of this risk and the availability of better drugs, MAO inhibitors are no longer used in hypertension. However, they are still occasionally used for treatment of severe depressive disorder (Chapter 30).

E. Adrenoceptor Blockers

Alpha$_1$-selective agents (eg, **prazosin, doxazosin, terazosin**) are moderately effective antihypertensive drugs. Alpha blockers reduce vascular resistance and venous return. The nonselective α blockers (phentolamine, phenoxybenzamine) are of no value in chronic hypertension because of excessive tachycardia. Alpha$_1$-selective adrenoceptor blockers are relatively free of the severe adverse effects of the nonselective α blockers and postganglionic nerve terminal sympathoplegic agents. They do, however, cause orthostatic hypotension, especially with the first few doses. On the other hand, they relax smooth muscle in the prostate, which is useful in benign prostatic hyperplasia.

Beta blockers are used very heavily in the treatment of hypertension. **Propranolol** is the prototype, and **atenolol, metoprolol,** and **carvedilol** are among the most popular. They initially reduce cardiac output, but after a few days their action may include a decrease in vascular resistance as a contributing effect.

The latter effect may result from reduced angiotensin levels (β blockers reduce renin release from the kidney). **Nebivolol** is a newer β blocker with some direct vasodilator action. Potential adverse effects are listed in the Drug Summary Table. As noted in Chapter 10, $β_1$-selective blockers with fewer CNS effects may have some advantages over the nonselective and more lipid-soluble agents.

VASODILATORS

Drugs that dilate blood vessels by acting directly on smooth muscle cells through nonautonomic mechanisms are useful in treating some hypertensive patients. Vasodilators act by four major mechanisms: release of nitric oxide, opening of potassium channels (which leads to hyperpolarization), blockade of calcium channels, and activation of D_1 dopamine receptors (Table 11–2). Compensatory responses are listed in Table 11–1.

A. Hydralazine and Minoxidil

These older vasodilators have more effect on arterioles than on veins. They are orally active and suitable for chronic therapy. Hydralazine apparently acts through the release of nitric oxide from endothelial cells. However, it is rarely used at high dosage because of its toxicity (Drug Summary Table). Hydralazine-induced lupus erythematosus is reversible upon stopping the drug, and lupus is uncommon at dosages below 200 mg/d.

Minoxidil is extremely efficacious, and systemic administration is reserved for severe hypertension. Minoxidil is a prodrug; its metabolite, minoxidil sulfate, is a potassium channel opener that hyperpolarizes and relaxes vascular smooth muscle. The compensatory responses to minoxidil (Figure 11–1) require the concomitant use of diuretics and β blockers. Because it can cause hirsutism, minoxidil is also available as a topical agent for the treatment of baldness.

B. Calcium Channel-Blocking Agents

Calcium channel blockers (eg, **nifedipine, verapamil, diltiazem**) are effective vasodilators; because they are moderately efficacious and orally active, these drugs are suitable for chronic use in hypertension of any severity. Verapamil and diltiazem also reduce cardiac output in most patients. Nifedipine is the prototype **dihydropyridine** calcium channel blocker, and many other dihydropyridines are available (eg, **amlodipine, felodipine, isradipine**). Because they produce fewer compensatory responses, the calcium channel blockers are much more commonly used than hydralazine or minoxidil. They are discussed in greater detail in Chapter 12.

C. Nitroprusside, Diazoxide, and Fenoldopam

These parenteral vasodilators are used in hypertensive emergencies. Nitroprusside is a light-sensitive, short-acting agent (duration of action is a few minutes) that must be infused continuously. The release of nitric oxide (from the drug molecule itself) stimulates guanylyl cyclase and increases cyclic guanine monophosphate (cGMP) concentration in smooth muscle.

Diazoxide is a thiazide derivative but lacks diuretic properties. It is given as intravenous boluses or as an infusion and has duration of action of several hours. Diazoxide opens potassium channels, thus hyperpolarizing and relaxing smooth muscle cells. This drug also reduces insulin release and can be used to treat hypoglycemia caused by insulin-producing tumors.

Dopamine D_1 receptor activation by fenoldopam causes prompt, marked arteriolar vasodilation. This drug is given by intravenous infusion. It has a short duration of action (10 min) and is used for hypertensive emergencies.

ANGIOTENSIN ANTAGONISTS & A RENIN INHIBITOR

The two primary groups of angiotensin antagonists are the **angiotensin-converting enzyme (ACE) inhibitors** and the **angiotensin II receptor blockers (ARBs)**. ACE inhibitors (eg, **captopril**), which inhibit the enzyme variously known as angiotensin-converting enzyme, kininase II, and peptidyl dipeptidase, cause a *reduction* in blood levels of angiotensin II and aldosterone and an *increase* in endogenous vasodilators of the kinin family (bradykinin; Figure 11–3). ACE inhibitors have a low incidence of serious adverse effects when given in normal dosage (except in pregnancy) and produce minimal compensatory responses (Table 11–1). The ACE inhibitors are useful in heart failure and diabetes as well as in hypertension. The toxicities of ACE inhibitors include cough (up to 30% of patients) and renal damage in occasional patients with preexisting renal vascular disease and in the fetus (although they *protect* the diabetic kidney). These drugs are absolutely contraindicated in pregnancy. The second group of angiotensin antagonists, the receptor blockers, is represented by the orally active agents **losartan,** valsartan, irbesartan, candesartan, and other ARBs, which competitively inhibit angiotensin II at its AT_1 receptor site. ARBs appear to be as effective in lowering blood pressure as the ACE inhibitors and have the advantage of a lower incidence of cough. However, like the ACE inhibitors, they do cause fetal renal toxicity and are thus contraindicated in pregnancy.

TABLE 11–2 Mechanisms of action of vasodilators.

Mechanism of Smooth Muscle Relaxation	Examples
Release of nitric oxide from drug or endothelium	Nitroprusside, hydralazine
Hyperpolarization of vascular smooth muscle through opening of potassium channels	Minoxidil sulfate, diazoxide
Reduction of calcium influx via L-type channels	Verapamil, diltiazem, nifedipine
Activation of dopamine D_1 receptors	Fenoldopam

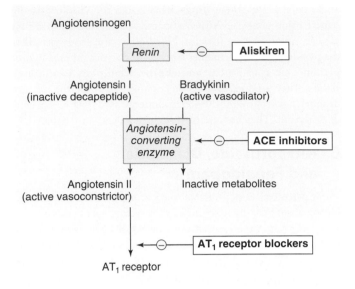

FIGURE 11–3 Actions of aliskiren, angiotensin-converting enzyme inhibitors, and AT$_1$ receptor blockers. Renin converts angiotensinogen to angiotensin I. Block by aliskiren blocks the sequence at its start. ACE is responsible for activating angiotensin I to angiotensin II and for inactivating bradykinin, a vasodilator normally present in very low concentrations. Block of this enzyme thus decreases the concentration of a vasoconstrictor and increases the concentration of a vasodilator. The AT$_1$ receptor antagonists lack the effect on bradykinin levels, which may explain the lower incidence of cough observed with these agents.

The newest drug in the antihypertensive group is **aliskiren**, an inhibitor of renin's action on its substrate, angiotensinogen. It thus reduces the formation of angiotensin I and, in consequence, angiotensin II. Toxicities include headache and diarrhea. It does not appear to cause cough, but it is not yet known whether it has the other toxicities of the angiotensin antagonists. It does not show reproductive toxicity in animals but is considered to be contraindicated in pregnancy because of the toxicity of ACE inhibitors and ARBs.

Angiotensin antagonists and renin inhibitors reduce aldosterone levels (angiotensin II is a major stimulant of aldosterone release) and cause potassium retention. If the patient has renal impairment, is consuming a high-potassium diet, or is taking other drugs that tend to conserve potassium, potassium concentrations may reach toxic levels.

CLINICAL USES OF ANTIHYPERTENSIVE DRUGS

A. Stepped Care (Polypharmacy)

Therapy of hypertension is complex because the disease is symptomless until far advanced and because the drugs may cause major compensatory responses and significant toxicities.

However, overall toxicity can be reduced and compensatory responses minimized by the use of multiple drugs at lower dosages in patients with moderate or severe hypertension. Typically, drugs are added to a patient's regimen in stepwise fashion; each additional agent is chosen from a different subgroup until adequate blood pressure control has been achieved. The usual steps include (1) lifestyle measures such as salt restriction and weight reduction, (2) diuretics (a thiazide), (3) sympathoplegics (a β blocker), (4) ACE inhibitors, and (5) vasodilators. The vasodilator chosen first is usually a calcium channel blocker. The ability of drugs in steps 2 and 3 to control the compensatory responses induced by the others should be noted (eg, propranolol reduces the tachycardia induced by hydralazine). Thus, rational polypharmacy minimizes toxicities while producing additive or supra-additive therapeutic effects.

> ### SKILL KEEPER 2: COMPENSATORY RESPONSES TO ANTIHYPERTENSIVE DRUGS (SEE CHAPTER 6)
>
> *If hydralazine is administered in moderate dosage for several weeks, compensatory cardiac and renal responses will be observed. Specify the exact mechanisms and structures involved in these responses.* The Skill Keeper Answer appears at the end of the chapter.

B. Monotherapy

It has been found in large clinical studies that many patients do well on a single drug (eg, an ACE inhibitor, calcium channel blocker, or combined α and β blocker). This approach to the treatment of mild and moderate hypertension has become more popular than stepped care because of its simplicity, better patient compliance, and—with modern drugs—a relatively low incidence of toxicity.

C. Age and Ethnicity

Older patients of most races respond better to diuretics and β blockers than to ACE inhibitors. African Americans of all ages respond better to diuretics and calcium channel blockers, and they respond less well to ACE inhibitors. There is considerable interindividual variability in metabolism of β blockers.

D. Hypertensive Emergency

Hypertensive emergency (formerly called malignant hypertension) is an accelerated form of severe hypertension associated with rising blood pressure and rapidly progressing damage to vessels and end organs. Management of hypertensive emergency must be carried out on an urgent basis in the hospital. Powerful vasodilators (nitroprusside, fenoldopam, or diazoxide) are combined with diuretics (furosemide) and β blockers to lower blood pressure to the 140–160/90–110 mm Hg range promptly (within a few hours). Further reduction is then pursued more slowly.

QUESTIONS

1. A 32-year-old woman with hypertension wishes to become pregnant. Her physician informs her that she will have to switch to another antihypertensive drug. Which of the following drugs is absolutely contraindicated in pregnancy?
   (A) Atenolol
   (B) Captopril
   (C) Methyldopa
   (D) Prazosin
   (E) Propranolol

2. A patient is admitted to the emergency department with severe tachycardia after a drug overdose. His family reports that he has been depressed about his hypertension. Which one of the following drugs increases the heart rate in a dose-dependent manner?
   (A) Captopril
   (B) Hydrochlorothiazide
   (C) Minoxidil
   (D) Prazosin
   (E) Verapamil

3. Which one of the following is characteristic of captopril treatment in patients with essential hypertension?
   (A) Competitively blocks angiotensin II at its receptor
   (B) Decreases angiotensin II concentration in the blood
   (C) Decreases renin concentration in the blood
   (D) Increases sodium and decreases potassium in the blood
   (E) Decreases sodium and increases potassium in the urine

4. A 73-year-old man with a history of falling at home is found to have moderately severe hypertension. Which of the following drug groups is most likely to cause postural hypotension and thus an increased risk of falls?
   (A) ACE inhibitors
   (B) Alpha-receptor blockers
   (C) Arteriolar dilators
   (D) Beta$_1$-selective receptor blockers
   (E) Nonselective β blockers

5. A significant number of patients started on ACE inhibitor therapy for hypertension are intolerant and must be switched to a different class of drug. What is the most common manifestation of this intolerance?
   (A) Diarrhea
   (B) Glaucoma
   (C) Incessant cough
   (D) Lupus-like syndrome
   (E) Vomiting

6. Which one of the following is a significant unwanted effect of the drug named?
   (A) Heart failure with hydralazine
   (B) Hemolytic anemia with atenolol
   (C) Fetal damage with losartan
   (D) Lupus-like syndrome with hydrochlorothiazide
   (E) Tachycardia with verapamil

7. Comparison of prazosin with atenolol shows that
   (A) Both decrease heart rate
   (B) Both increase cardiac output
   (C) Both increase renin secretion
   (D) Both increase sympathetic outflow from the CNS
   (E) Both produce orthostatic hypotension

8. A patient with hypertension is to receive a calcium channel blocker. Verapamil is associated with which one of the following?
   (A) Diarrhea
   (B) Hypoglycemia
   (C) Increased PR interval
   (D) Tachycardia
   (E) Thyrotoxicosis

9. A 45-year-old man is brought to the emergency department with mental obtundation. He is found to have a blood pressure of 220/160 and retinal hemorrhages. Which one of the following is used in severe hypertensive emergencies, is short-acting, acts on a G protein-coupled receptor, and must be given by intravenous infusion?
   (A) Aliskiren
   (B) Captopril
   (C) Fenoldopam
   (D) Hydralazine
   (E) Losartan
   (F) Metoprolol
   (G) Nifedipine
   (H) Prazosin
   (I) Propranolol

10. Which of the following is very short-acting and acts by releasing nitric oxide?
    (A) Atenolol
    (B) Captopril
    (C) Diltiazem
    (D) Fenoldopam
    (E) Hydrochlorothiazide
    (F) Losartan
    (G) Minoxidil
    (H) Nitroprusside
    (I) Prazosin

ANSWERS

1. Methyldopa is often recommended in pregnant patients because it has a good safety record. Alpha (choice D) and β blockers (choices A and E) are not contraindicated. In contrast, ACE inhibitors (choice B) and ARBs have been shown to be teratogenic. The answer is **B**.

2. Neither ACE inhibitors (choice A) nor diuretics (choice B) significantly increase heart rate. Although dihydropyridine calcium channel blockers do not usually reduce rate markedly (and may increase it), verapamil and diltiazem do inhibit the sinoatrial node and predictably decrease rate. Direct vasodilators (choice C) and α blockers (choice D) regularly *increase* heart rate but minoxidil, a very efficacious vasodilator causes severe tachycardia that must be controlled with β blockers. The answer is **C**.

3. Converting enzyme inhibitors act on the enzyme, not on the angiotensin receptor. The plasma renin level may increase as a result of the compensatory response to reduced angiotensin II. ACE inhibitors increase blood potassium and urine sodium. The answer is **B**.

4. Postural (orthostatic) hypotension is usually due to venous pooling. Venous pooling is normally prevented by α-receptor activation. The answer is **B**. (Postural hypotension may also occur in patients with hypovolemia owing to excessive diuretic treatment.)

5. Chronic, intolerable cough is an important adverse effect of captopril and other ACE inhibitors. It may be relieved by prior administration of aspirin. These drugs are very commonly used in hypertensive diabetic patients because of their proven benefits in *reducing* diabetic renal damage. The ACE inhibitors do not cause glaucoma or gastrointestinal disturbances. The answer is **C.**

6. Hydralazine (choice A) is sometimes used in heart failure. Beta blockers (choice B) are not associated with hematologic abnormalities, but methyldopa is. The thiazide diuretics (choice D) often cause mild hyperglycemia, hyperuricemia, and hyperlipidemia but not lupus; hydralazine is associated with a lupus-like syndrome. Verapamil (choice E) often causes bradycardia, not tachycardia. ARBs (choice C) may cause damage to the fetal kidney, and they are contraindicated in pregnancy. The answer is **C.**

7. Atenolol, but not prazosin, may decrease heart rate (choice A). Prazosin—but not atenolol—may increase cardiac output, a compensatory effect (choice B). Prazosin may increase renin output (a compensatory response), but β blockers inhibit its release by the kidney (choice C). By reducing blood pressure, both may increase central sympathetic outflow (a compensatory response). Beta blockers do not cause orthostatic hypotension. The answer is **D.**

8. Calcium channel blockers do not cause diarrhea and are sometimes associated with constipation, probably through inhibition of calcium influx in intestinal smooth muscle. Hypoglycemia is not a common effect of any of the antihypertensive drugs. Thyroid disorders are not associated with calcium blockers. However, calcium blockers, especially verapamil and diltiazem, are associated with depression of calcium-dependent processes in the heart, for example, contractility, heart rate, and atrioventricular conduction. Therefore, *bradycardia* and increased PR interval may be expected. The dihydropyridines do not often cause cardiac depression, probably because they evoke increased sympathetic outflow as a result of their dominant vascular effects. The answer is **C.**

9. Fenoldopam, nitroprusside, and propranolol are the drugs in the list that have been used in hypertensive emergencies. Fenoldopam and nitroprusside are used by infusion only, but nitroprusside releases nitric oxide, which acts on intracellular guanylyl cyclase. The answer is **C.**

10. The two agents in this list that act via a nitric oxide mechanism are hydralazine and nitroprusside (see Table 11–2). However, hydralazine has a duration of action of hours, whereas nitroprusside acts for seconds to minutes and must be given by intravenous infusion. The answer is **H.**

SKILL KEEPER 1 ANSWER: DEVELOPMENT OF NEW ANTIHYPERTENSIVE DRUGS (SEE CHAPTER 5)

The FDA requires a broad range of animal data, provided by the developer in an investigational new drug (IND) application, before clinical trials can be started. These data must show that the drug has the expected effects on blood pressure in animals and has low and well-defined toxicity in at least two species. A new drug application (NDA) must be submitted and approved before marketing can begin. This application usually requires data on pharmacokinetics in volunteers (phase 1), efficacy and safety in a small group of closely observed patients (phase 2), and efficacy and safety in a much larger group of patients under conditions of actual use (phase 3).

SKILL KEEPER 2 ANSWER: COMPENSATORY RESPONSES TO ANTIHYPERTENSIVE DRUGS (SEE CHAPTER 6)

The compensatory responses to hydralazine are tachycardia and salt and water retention. These responses are generated by the baroreceptor and renin-angiotensin-aldosterone mechanisms summarized in Figures 6–4 and 11–1. The motor limb of the sympathetic response consists of outflow from the vasomotor center to the heart and vessels, as shown in Figure 11–2. You should be able to reproduce these diagrams from memory.

CHECKLIST

When you complete this chapter, you should be able to:

❑ List the 4 major groups of antihypertensive drugs, and give examples of drugs in each group. (Renin inhibitors are not considered an independent major group; can you name the drug that acts by this mechanism?)

❑ Describe the compensatory responses, if any, to each of the 4 major types of antihypertensive drugs.

❑ List the major sites of action of sympathoplegic drugs in clinical use, and give examples of drugs that act at each site.

❑ List the 4 mechanisms of action of vasodilator drugs.

❑ List the major antihypertensive vasodilator drugs and describe their effects.

❑ Describe the differences between the 2 types of angiotensin antagonists.

❑ List the major toxicities of the prototype antihypertensive agents.

DRUG SUMMARY TABLE: Drugs Used in Hypertension

Subclass	Mechanism of Action	Clinical Applications	Pharmacokinetics	Toxicities, Interactions
Diuretics (see also Chapter 15)				
Hydrochlorothiazide, chlorthalidone	Block Na/Cl transporter in distal convoluted tubule	Hypertension, mild edema	Oral Duration: 8–12 h	Hypokalemia, hyperglycemia, hyperuricemia, hyperlipidemia
Furosemide	Block Na/K/2Cl transporter in thick ascending limb	Hypertension, heart failure, edema, hypercalcemia	Oral, parenteral Duration: 2–3 h	Hypokalemia, hypovolemia, ototoxicity
Sympathoplegics				
Centrally acting				
Clonidine	Agonist at α_2 receptors • in CNS this results in decreased SANS outflow	Hypertension	Oral and transdermal Oral duration: 2–3 days • transdermal 1 wk	Sedation, danger of severe rebound hypertension if suddenly stopped
Methyldopa	Prodrug converted to methylnorepinephrine in CNS, with result like clonidine	Hypertension	Oral Duration: 12–24 h	Sedation, induces hemolytic antibodies
Ganglion blockers				
Hexamethonium	Obsolete prototype nicotinic acetylcholine (ACh) receptor blocker in ganglia • blocks all ANS transmission	None	Oral, parenteral	Severe orthostatic hypotension, constipation, blurred vision, sexual dysfunction

Trimethaphan: IV, rarely used short-acting ganglion blocker for hypertensive emergencies, controlled hypotension
Mecamylamine: oral ganglion blocker, several hours' duration, experimental use in smoking cessation

Postganglionic neuron blockers				
Reserpine	Blocks vesicular pump (VMAT) in adrenergic neurons	Obsolete in hypertension, Huntington's disease	Oral Duration: 5 days	Sedation • severe psychiatric depression (high doses)

Guanadrel: blocks reuptake of norepinephrine (NET) and depletes stores; oral, long duration; severe orthostatic hypotension (guanethidine, a similar drug, was withdrawn in the United States)

Alpha blockers				
Prazosin	Selective α_1 blocker • reduces peripheral vascular resistance • prostatic smooth muscle tone	Mild hypertension, benign prostatic hyperplasia	Oral Duration: 6–8 h	First dose orthostatic hypotension

Doxazosin, terazosin: similar to prazosin but longer duration of action

Beta blockers				
Propranolol	Prototype nonselective β blocker • reduces cardiac output • possible secondary reduction in renin release	Hypertension • many other applications (see Chapter 10)	Oral, parenteral Duration: 6–8 h (extended release forms available)	Bronchospasm in asthmatics • excessive cardiac depression, sexual dysfunction, sedation, sleep disturbances

Atenolol, metoprolol: like propranolol but β_1-selective; fewer adverse effects
Labetalol, carvedilol: combined α and β blockade; oral and parenteral

(Continued)

DRUG SUMMARY TABLE: Drugs Used in Hypertension (*Continued*)

Subclass	Mechanism of Action	Clinical Applications	Pharmacokinetics	Toxicities, Interactions
Vasodilators, oral				
Calcium channel blockers				
Verapamil, diltiazem	Prototype L-type calcium channel blockers • combine moderate vascular effect with strong cardiac effect	Hypertension, angina, arrhythmias	Oral, parenteral Duration: 6–8 h	Excessive cardiac depression • constipation
Nifedipine, other dihydropyridines: oral and parenteral; greater vasodilator than cardiodepressant effects				
Older oral vasodilators				
Hydralazine	Probably causes release of nitric acid (NO) by endothelial cells • causes arteriolar dilation	Hypertension (also used in heart failure in combination with isosorbide dinitrate)	Oral Duration: 6–8 h	Tachycardia, salt and water retention, lupus-like syndrome
Minoxidil	Prodrug, sulfate metabolite opens K^+ channels, causes arteriolar smooth muscle hyperpolarization and vasodilation	Severe hypertension • male-pattern baldness	Oral, topical Duration: 6–8 h	Marked tachycardia, salt and water retention • hirsutism
Vasodilators, parenteral				
Nitroprusside	Releases NO from drug molecule	Hypertensive emergencies • cardiac decompensation	Parenteral only Duration: minutes • requires constant infusion	Excessive hypotension • prolonged infusion may cause thiocyanate and cyanide toxicity
Diazoxide	K^+ channel opener in smooth muscle, secretory cells	Hypertensive emergencies • hypoglycemia due to insulin-secreting tumors	Parenteral for hypertension, oral for insulinoma	Hyperglycemia • edema, excessive hypotension
Fenoldopam	D_1 agonist • causes arteriolar dilation	Hypertensive emergencies	Parenteral only, very short duration	Excessive hypotension
Renin antagonist				
Aliskiren	Renin inhibitor • reduces angiotensin I synthesis	Hypertension	Oral Duration: 12 h	Angioedema, renal impairment
Angiotensin antagonists				
ACE inhibitors				
Captopril	ACE inhibitor • reduces angiotensin II synthesis	Hypertension, diabetic renal disease, heart failure	Oral Half-life: 2.2 h but large doses provide duration of 12 h	Hyperkalemia • teratogen • cough
Benazepril, enalapril, lisinopril, others: like captopril but longer half-lives				
Angiotensin II receptor blockers (ARBs)				
Losartan	Blocks AT_1 receptors	Hypertension	Oral Duration: 6–8 h	Hyperkalemia • teratogen
Candesartan, irbesartan, others: like losartan				

ACE, angiotensin-converting enzyme; ANS, autonomic nervous system; CNS, central nervous system; SANS, sympathetic autonomic nervous system.

Drugs Used in the Treatment of Angina Pectoris

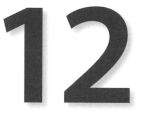

Angina pectoris refers to a strangling or pressure-like pain caused by cardiac ischemia. The pain is usually located substernally but is sometimes perceived in the neck, shoulder and arm, or epigastrium. Women develop angina at a later age than men and are less likely to have classic substernal pain. Drugs used in angina exploit two main strategies: reduction of oxygen demand and increase of oxygen delivery to the myocardium.

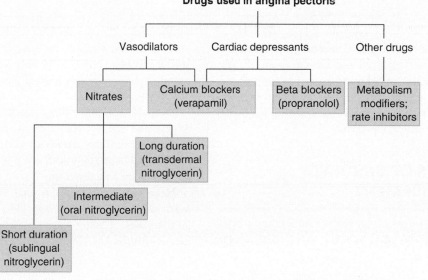

PATHOPHYSIOLOGY OF ANGINA

A. Types of Angina

1. Atherosclerotic angina—Atherosclerotic angina is also known as angina of effort or classic angina. It is associated with atheromatous plaques that partially occlude one or more coronary arteries. When cardiac work increases (eg, in exercise), the obstruction of flow and inadequate oxygen delivery results in the accumulation of acidic metabolites and ischemic changes that stimulate myocardial pain endings. Rest usually leads to complete relief of the pain within 15 min. Atherosclerotic angina constitutes about 90% of angina cases.

2. Vasospastic angina—Vasospastic angina, also known as rest angina, variant angina, or Prinzmetal's angina, is responsible for less than 10% of cases. It involves reversible spasm of coronaries, usually at the site of an atherosclerotic plaque. Spasm may occur at any time, even during sleep. Vasospastic angina may deteriorate into unstable angina.

High-Yield Terms to Learn

Angina of effort, classic angina, atherosclerotic angina	Angina pectoris (crushing, strangling chest pain) that is precipitated by exertion
Vasospastic angina, variant angina, Prinzmetal's angina	Angina precipitated by reversible spasm of coronary vessels, often at rest
Coronary vasodilator	Older, incorrect name for drugs useful in angina; some potent coronary vasodilators are ineffective in angina
"Monday disease"	Industrial disease caused by chronic exposure to vasodilating concentrations of organic nitrates in the workplace; characterized by headache, dizziness, and tachycardia on return to work after 2 days absence
Nitrate tolerance, tachyphylaxis	Loss of effect of a nitrate vasodilator when exposure is prolonged beyond 10–12 h
Unstable angina	Rapidly progressing increase in frequency and severity of anginal attacks; an acute coronary syndrome that often heralds imminent myocardial infarction
Preload	Filling pressure of the heart, dependent on venous tone and blood volume; determines end-diastolic fiber length and tension
Afterload	Impedance to ejection of stroke volume; determined by arterial blood pressure and arterial stiffness; determines systolic fiber tension
Intramyocardial fiber tension	Force exerted by myocardial fibers, especially ventricular fibers at any given time; a primary determinant of O_2 requirement
Double product	The product of heart rate and systolic blood pressure; an estimate of cardiac work
Myocardial revascularization	Mechanical intervention to improve O_2 delivery to the myocardium by angioplasty or bypass grafting

3. Unstable angina—A third type of angina—unstable or crescendo angina, also known as **acute coronary syndrome**—is characterized by increased frequency and severity of attacks that result from a combination of atherosclerotic plaques, platelet aggregation at fractured plaques, and vasospasm. Unstable angina is thought to be the immediate precursor of a myocardial infarction and is treated as a medical emergency.

DETERMINANTS OF CARDIAC OXYGEN REQUIREMENT

The pharmacologic treatment of coronary insufficiency is based on the physiologic factors that control myocardial oxygen requirement. A major determinant is **myocardial fiber tension** (the higher the tension, the greater the oxygen requirement). Several variables contribute to fiber tension (Figure 12–1), as discussed next. Note that several of these variables are increased by sympathetic discharge.

Preload (diastolic filling pressure) is a function of blood volume and venous tone. Venous tone is mainly controlled by sympathetic outflow. **Afterload** is determined by arterial blood pressure and large artery stiffness. It is one of the systolic determinants of oxygen requirement.

Heart rate contributes to total fiber tension because at fast heart rates, fibers spend more time at systolic tension levels. Furthermore, at faster rates, diastole is abbreviated, and diastole constitutes the time available for coronary flow (coronary

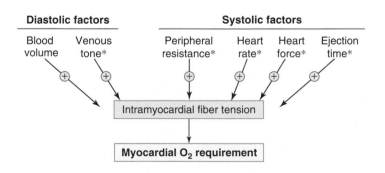

FIGURE 12–1 Determinants of the volume of oxygen required by the heart. Both diastolic and systolic factors contribute to the oxygen requirement; most of these factors are directly influenced by sympathetic discharge (venous tone, peripheral resistance, heart rate, and heart force) as noted by the asterisks.

blood flow is low or nil during systole). Heart rate and systolic blood pressure may be multiplied to yield the **double product,** a measure of cardiac work and therefore of oxygen requirement. As intensity of exercise (eg, running on a treadmill) increases, demand for cardiac output increases, so the double product also increases. However, the double product is sensitive to sympathetic tone, as is cardiac oxygen demand (Figure 12–1). In patients with atherosclerotic angina, effective drugs reduce the double product by reducing cardiac work without reducing exercise capacity.

Force of cardiac contraction is another systolic factor controlled mainly by sympathetic outflow to the heart. **Ejection time** for ventricular contraction is inversely related to force of contraction but is also influenced by impedance to outflow. Increased ejection time (prolonged systole) increases oxygen requirement.

THERAPEUTIC STRATEGIES

The defect that causes anginal pain is inadequate coronary oxygen delivery relative to the myocardial oxygen requirement. This defect can be corrected—at present—in 2 ways: by **increasing oxygen delivery** and by **reducing oxygen requirement** (Figure 12–2). Traditional pharmacologic therapies include the **nitrates**, the **calcium channel blockers**, and the **β blockers**.

A newer strategy attempts to increase the **efficiency of oxygen utilization** by shifting the energy substrate preference of the heart from fatty acids to glucose. Drugs that may act by this mechanism are termed partial fatty acid oxidation inhibitors (**pFOX inhibitors**) and include **ranolazine** and trimetazidine. However, more

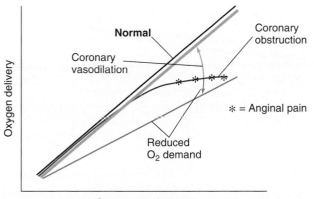

FIGURE 12–2 Strategies for the treatment of effort angina. When coronary flow is adequate, O_2 delivery increases as O_2 requirement increases with exercise (*black line*). Angina is characterized by reduced coronary oxygen delivery versus oxygen requirement (*curve in red line*), and anginal pain occurs as the oxygen debt increases. In some cases, this can be corrected by increasing oxygen delivery (revascularization or, in the case of reversible vasospasm, nitrates and calcium channel blockers, *brown line*). More often, drugs are used to reduce oxygen requirement (nitrates, β blockers, and calcium channel blockers) and cause a shift to the *green line.*

recent evidence suggests that the major mechanism of action of ranolazine is inhibition of late sodium current (see below). Another new group of antianginal drugs selectively reduces heart rate with no other detectable hemodynamic effects. These investigational drugs (**ivabradine** is the prototype) act by inhibition of the sinoatrial pacemaker current, I_f.

The nitrates, calcium blockers, and β blockers all reduce the oxygen requirement in atherosclerotic angina. Nitrates and calcium channel blockers (but not β blockers) can also increase oxygen delivery by reducing spasm in vasospastic angina. **Myocardial revascularization** corrects coronary obstruction either by bypass grafting or by angioplasty (enlargement of the lumen by means of a special catheter). Therapy of unstable angina differs from that of stable angina in that urgent angioplasty is the treatment of choice in most patients and platelet clotting is the major target of drug therapy. A variety of platelet inhibitors are used in this condition (see Chapter 34). Intravenous nitroglycerin is sometimes of value.

NITRATES

A. Classification and Pharmacokinetics

Nitroglycerin (the active ingredient in dynamite) is the most important of the therapeutic nitrates and is available in forms that provide a range of durations of action from 10–20 min (sublingual for relief of acute attacks) to 8–10 h (transdermal for prophylaxis) (see the Drug Summary Table at the end of the chapter). Nitroglycerin (glyceryl trinitrate) is rapidly denitrated in the liver and in smooth muscle—first to the dinitrate (glyceryl dinitrate), which retains a significant vasodilating effect; and more slowly to the mononitrate, which is much less active. Because of the high enzyme activity in the liver, the first-pass effect for nitroglycerin is about 90%. The efficacy of oral (swallowed) nitroglycerin probably results from the high levels of glyceryl dinitrate in the blood. The effects of sublingual nitroglycerin are mainly the result of the unchanged drug because this route avoids the first-pass effect (see Chapters 1 and 3).

Other nitrates are similar to nitroglycerin in their pharmacokinetics and pharmacodynamics. Isosorbide dinitrate is another commonly used nitrate; it is available in sublingual and oral forms. Isosorbide dinitrate is rapidly denitrated in the liver and smooth muscle to isosorbide mononitrate, which is also active. Isosorbide mononitrate is available as a separate drug for oral use. Several other nitrates are available for oral use and, like the oral nitroglycerin preparation, have an intermediate duration of action (4–6 h). Amyl nitrite is a volatile and rapid-acting vasodilator that was used for angina by the inhalational route but is now rarely prescribed.

B. Mechanism of Action

Nitrates release nitric oxide (NO) within smooth muscle cells, probably through the action of the mitochondrial enzyme aldehyde dehydrogenase-2 (ALD2). NO stimulates guanylyl cyclase and causes an increase of the second messenger cGMP (cyclic guanosine monophosphate); the latter results in smooth muscle

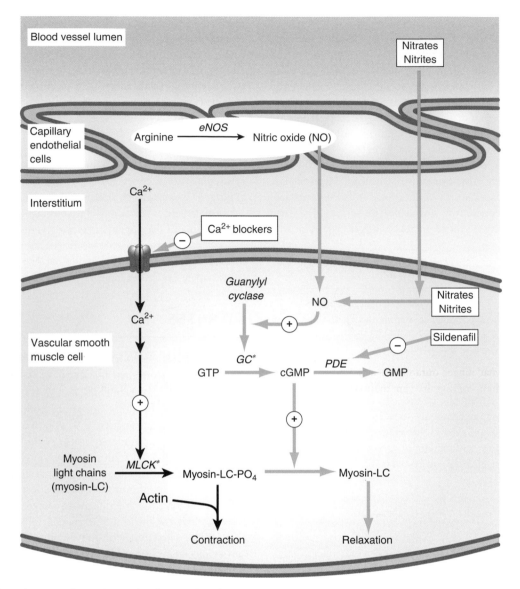

FIGURE 12–3 Mechanisms of smooth muscle relaxation by calcium channel blockers and nitrates. Contraction results from phosphorylation of myosin light chains (MLC) by myosin light-chain kinase (MLCK). MLCK is activated by Ca^{2+}, so calcium channel blockers reduce this step. Relaxation follows when the phosphorylated light chains are dephosphorylated, a process facilitated by cyclic guanosine monophosphate (cGMP). Nitrates and other sources of nitric oxide (NO) increase cGMP synthesis, and phosphodiesterase (PDE) inhibitors reduce cGMP metabolism. eNOS, endothelial nitric oxide synthase; GC, activated guanylyl cyclase; GTP, guanosine triphosphate. (Modified and reproduced, with permission, from Katzung BG, editor: *Basic & Clinical Pharmacology,* 12th ed. McGraw-Hill, 2012: Fig. 12–2.)

relaxation by dephosphorylation of myosin light-chain phosphate (Figure 12–3). Note that this mechanism is identical to that of nitroprusside (see Chapter 11).

C. Organ System Effects

1. Cardiovascular—Smooth muscle relaxation by nitrates leads to an important degree of venodilation, which results in reduced cardiac size and cardiac output through reduced preload. Relaxation of arterial smooth muscle may increase flow through partially occluded epicardial coronary vessels. Reduced afterload, from arteriolar dilation of resistance vessels, may contribute to an

increase in ejection and a further decrease in cardiac size. Some studies suggest that of the vascular beds, the veins are the most sensitive, arteries less so, and arterioles least sensitive. Venodilation leads to decreased diastolic heart size and fiber tension. Arteriolar dilation leads to reduced peripheral resistance and blood pressure. These changes contribute to an overall reduction in myocardial fiber tension, oxygen consumption, and the double product. Thus, the primary mechanism of therapeutic benefit in atherosclerotic angina is reduction of the oxygen requirement. A secondary mechanism—namely, an increase in coronary flow via collateral vessels in ischemic areas—has also been proposed. In vasospastic angina, a reversal of coronary spasm and increased flow can be demonstrated.

Nitrates have no direct effects on cardiac muscle, but significant reflex tachycardia and increased force of contraction are common results when nitroglycerin reduces the blood pressure. These compensatory effects result from the baroreceptor mechanism shown in Figure 6–4.

2. Other organs—Nitrates relax the smooth muscle of the bronchi, gastrointestinal tract, and genitourinary tract, but these effects are too small to be clinically useful. Intravenous nitroglycerin (sometimes used in unstable angina) reduces platelet aggregation. There are no clinically useful effects on other tissues.

D. Clinical Uses

As previously noted, nitroglycerin is available in several formulations (see Drug Summary Table). The standard form for treatment of acute anginal pain is the sublingual tablet or spray, which has a duration of action of 10–20 min. Sublingual isosorbide dinitrate is similar with a duration of 30 min. Oral (swallowed) normal-release formulations of nitroglycerin and isosorbide dinitrate have durations of action of 4–6 h. Sustained-release oral forms have a somewhat longer duration of action. Transdermal formulations (ointment or patch) can maintain blood levels for up to 24 h. Tolerance develops after 8–10 h, however, with rapidly diminishing effectiveness thereafter. It is therefore recommended that nitroglycerin patches be removed after 10–12 h to allow recovery of sensitivity to the drug.

E. Toxicity of Nitrates and Nitrites

The most common toxic effects of nitrates are the responses evoked by vasodilation. These include tachycardia (from the baroreceptor reflex), orthostatic hypotension (a direct extension of the venodilator effect), and throbbing headache from meningeal artery vasodilation.

Nitrates interact with sildenafil and similar drugs promoted for erectile dysfunction. These agents inhibit a phosphodiesterase isoform (PDE5) that metabolizes cGMP in smooth muscle (Figure 12–4). The increased cGMP in erectile smooth muscle relaxes it, allowing for greater inflow of blood and more effective and prolonged erection. This effect also occurs in vascular smooth muscle. As a result, the combination of nitrates (through increased production of cGMP) and a PDE5 inhibitor (through decreased breakdown of cGMP) causes a synergistic relaxation of vascular smooth muscle with potentially dangerous hypotension and inadequate perfusion of critical organs.

Nitrites are of significant toxicologic importance because they cause methemoglobinemia at high blood concentrations. This same effect has a potential antidotal action in cyanide poisoning (see later discussion). The nitrates do not cause methemoglobinemia. In the past, the nitrates were responsible for several occupational diseases in munitions factories in which workplace contamination by these volatile chemicals was severe. The most common of these diseases was "Monday disease," that is, the alternating development of tolerance (during the work week) and

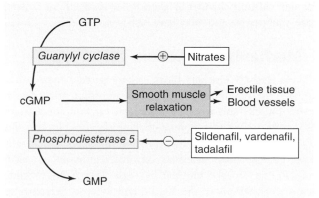

FIGURE 12–4 Mechanism of the interaction between nitrates and drugs used in erectile dysfunction. Because these drug groups increase cyclic guanosine monophosphate (cGMP) by complementary mechanisms, they can have a synergistic effect on blood pressure resulting in dangerous hypotension. GTP, guanosine triphosphate.

loss of tolerance (over the weekend) for the vasodilating action and its associated tachycardia and resulting in headache (from cranial vasodilation), tachycardia, and dizziness (from orthostatic hypotension) every Monday.

F. Nitrites in the Treatment of Cyanide Poisoning

Cyanide ion rapidly complexes with the iron in cytochrome oxidase, resulting in a block of oxidative metabolism and cell death. Fortunately, the iron in methemoglobin has a higher affinity for cyanide than does the iron in cytochrome oxidase. Nitrites convert the ferrous iron in hemoglobin to the ferric form, yielding methemoglobin. Therefore, cyanide poisoning can be treated by a 3-step procedure: (1) immediate exposure to amyl nitrite, followed by (2) intravenous administration of sodium nitrite, which rapidly increases the methemoglobin level to the degree necessary to remove a significant amount of cyanide from cytochrome oxidase. This is followed by (3) intravenous sodium thiosulfate, which converts cyanomethemoglobin resulting from step 2 to thiocyanate and methemoglobin. Thiocyanate is much less toxic than cyanide and is excreted by the kidney. (It should be noted that excessive methemoglobinemia is fatal because methemoglobin is a very poor oxygen carrier.) Recently, hydroxocobalamin, a form of vitamin B_{12}, has become the preferred method of treating cyanide poisoning (see Chapter 58).

CALCIUM CHANNEL-BLOCKING DRUGS

A. Classification and Pharmacokinetics

Several types of calcium channel blockers are approved for use in angina; these drugs are typified by **nifedipine**, a **dihydropyridine**, and several other dihydropyridines; **diltiazem**; and **verapamil**.

Although calcium channel blockers differ markedly in structure, all are orally active and most have half-lives of 3–6 h.

B. Mechanism of Action

Calcium channel blockers block voltage-gated L-type calcium channels, the calcium channels most important in cardiac and smooth muscle, and reduce intracellular calcium concentration and muscle contractility. None of these channel blockers interferes with calcium-dependent neurotransmission or hormone release because these processes use different types of calcium channels that are not blocked by these agents. Nerve ending calcium channels are of the N-, P-, and R-types. Secretory cells use L-type channels, but these channels are less sensitive to the calcium blockers than are cardiac and smooth muscle L-type channels.

C. Effects and Clinical Use

Calcium blockers relax blood vessels and, to a lesser extent, the uterus, bronchi, and gut. The rate and contractility of the heart are reduced by diltiazem and verapamil. Because they block calcium-dependent conduction in the atrioventricular (AV) node, verapamil and diltiazem may be used to treat AV nodal arrhythmias (see Chapter 14). Nifedipine and other dihydropyridines evoke greater vasodilation, and the resulting sympathetic reflex prevents bradycardia and may actually increase heart rate. All the calcium channel blockers reduce blood pressure and reduce the double product in patients with angina.

Calcium blockers are effective as prophylactic therapy in both effort and vasospastic angina; nifedipine has also been used to abort acute anginal attacks but use of the prompt-release form is discouraged (see Skill Keeper). In severe atherosclerotic angina, these drugs are particularly valuable when combined with nitrates (Table 12–1). In addition to well-established uses in angina, hypertension, and supraventricular tachycardia, some of these agents are used in migraine, preterm labor, stroke, and Raynaud's phenomenon.

D. Toxicity

The calcium channel blockers cause constipation, pretibial edema, nausea, flushing, and dizziness. More serious adverse effects include heart failure, AV blockade, and sinus node depression; these are most common with verapamil and least common with the dihydropyridines.

BETA-BLOCKING DRUGS

A. Classification and Mechanism of Action

These drugs are described in detail in Chapter 10. Because they reduce cardiac work (and oxygen demand), all β blockers are effective in the prophylaxis of atherosclerotic angina attacks.

B. Effects and Clinical Use

Actions include both beneficial antianginal effects (decreased heart rate, cardiac force, blood pressure) and detrimental effects (increased heart size, longer ejection period; Table 12–1). Like nitrates and calcium channel blockers, β blockers reduce cardiac work, the double product, and oxygen demand.

Beta blockers are used only for prophylactic therapy of angina; they are of no value in an acute attack. They are effective in preventing exercise-induced angina but are ineffective against the vasospastic form. The combination of β blockers and nitrates is useful because the adverse undesirable compensatory effects

TABLE 12–1 Effects of nitrates alone or with beta blockers or calcium channel blockers in angina pectoris.[a]

	Nitrates Alone	Beta Blockers or Calcium Channel Blockers Alone	Combined Nitrates and Beta Blockers or Calcium Channel Blockers
Heart rate	*Reflex increase*	**Decrease**	**Decrease**
Arterial pressure	**Decrease**	**Decrease**	**Decrease**
End-diastolic pressure	**Decrease**	*Increase*	**Decrease**
Contractility	*Reflex increase*	**Decrease**	No effect or decrease
Ejection time	Reflex decrease	*Increase*	No effect
Net myocardial oxygen requirement	**Decrease**	**Decrease**	**Decrease**

[a]Undesirable effects (effects that increase oxygen requirement) are shown in *italics;* major beneficial effects are shown in **bold**.

evoked by the nitrates (tachycardia and increased cardiac force) are prevented or reduced by β blockade (Table 12–1).

C. Toxicity

See Chapter 10.

NEWER DRUGS

Ranolazine appears to act mainly by reducing a late, prolonged sodium current in myocardial cells. The decrease in intracellular sodium causes an increase in calcium expulsion via the Na/Ca transporter (see Chapter 13) and a reduction in cardiac force and work. As noted previously, it may also alter cardiac metabolism. Ranolazine is moderately effective in angina prophylaxis. **Ivabradine**, an investigational drug, inhibits the I_f sodium current in the sinoatrial node. The reduction in this hyperpolarization-induced inward pacemaker current results in decreased heart rate and consequently decreased cardiac work.

NONPHARMACOLOGIC THERAPY

Myocardial revascularization by coronary artery bypass grafting (CABG) and percutaneous transluminal coronary angioplasty (PTCA) are extremely important in the treatment of severe angina. These are the only methods capable of consistently increasing coronary flow in atherosclerotic angina and increasing the double product.

QUESTIONS

Questions 1–4. A 60-year-old man presents to his primary care physician with a complaint of severe chest pain when he walks uphill to his home in cold weather. The pain disappears when he rests. After evaluation and discussion of treatment options, a decision is made to treat him with nitroglycerin.

1. Which of the following is a common direct or reflex effect of nitroglycerin?
   (A) Decreased heart rate
   (B) Decreased venous capacitance
   (C) Increased afterload
   (D) Increased cardiac force
   (E) Increased diastolic myocardial fiber tension

2. In advising the patient about the adverse effects he may notice, you point out that nitroglycerin in moderate doses often produces certain symptoms. Which of the following effects might occur due to the mechanism listed?
   (A) Apnea due to cranial vasodilation
   (B) Dizziness due to reduced cardiac force of contraction
   (C) Diuresis due to sympathetic discharge
   (D) Headache due to meningeal vasodilation
   (E) Hypertension due to reflex tachycardia

3. One year later, the patient returns complaining that his nitroglycerin works well when he takes it for an acute attack but that he is now having more frequent attacks and would like something to *prevent* them. Useful drugs for the prophylaxis of angina of effort include
   (A) Amyl nitrite
   (B) Diltiazem
   (C) Esmolol
   (D) Sublingual isosorbide dinitrate
   (E) Sublingual nitroglycerin

4. If a β blocker were to be used for prophylaxis in this patient, what is the most probable mechanism of action in angina?
   (A) Block of exercise-induced tachycardia
   (B) Decreased end-diastolic ventricular volume
   (C) Increased double product
   (D) Increased cardiac force
   (E) Decreased ventricular ejection time

5. A new 60-year-old patient presents to the medical clinic with hypertension and angina. In considering adverse effects of possible drugs for these conditions, you note that an adverse effect that nitroglycerin and prazosin have in common is
   (A) Bradycardia
   (B) Impaired sexual function
   (C) Lupus erythematosus syndrome
   (D) Orthostatic hypotension
   (E) Throbbing headache

6. A man is admitted to the emergency department with a brownish cyanotic appearance, marked shortness of breath, and hypotension. Which of the following is most likely to cause methemoglobinemia?
   (A) Amyl nitrite
   (B) Isosorbide dinitrate
   (C) Isosorbide mononitrate
   (D) Nitroglycerin
   (E) Sodium cyanide

7. Another patient is admitted to the emergency department after a drug overdose. He is noted to have hypotension and severe tachycardia. He has been receiving therapy for hypertension and angina. Which of the following drugs often causes tachycardia?
   (A) Clonidine
   (B) Diltiazem
   (C) Isosorbide dinitrate
   (D) Propranolol
   (E) Verapamil

8. A 45-year-old woman with hyperlipidemia and frequent migraine headaches develops angina of effort. Which of the following is relatively contraindicated because of her migraines?
   (A) Amlodipine
   (B) Diltiazem
   (C) Metoprolol
   (D) Nitroglycerin
   (E) Verapamil

9. When nitrates are used in combination with other drugs for the treatment of angina, which one of the following combinations results in additive effects on the variable specified?
   (A) Beta blockers and nitrates on end-diastolic cardiac size
   (B) Beta blockers and nitrates on heart rate
   (C) Calcium channel blockers and β blockers on cardiac force
   (D) Beta blockers and nitrates on venous tone
   (E) Calcium channel blockers and nitrates on heart rate

10. Certain drugs can cause severe hypotension when combined with nitrates. Which of the following interacts with nitroglycerin by inhibiting the metabolism of cGMP?
    (A) Atenolol
    (B) Hydralazine
    (C) Isosorbide mononitrate
    (D) Nifedipine
    (E) Ranolazine
    (F) Sildenafil
    (G) Terbutaline

ANSWERS

1. Nitroglycerin *increases* heart rate and venous capacitance and *decreases* afterload and diastolic fiber tension. It increases cardiac contractile force because the decrease in blood pressure evokes a compensatory increase in sympathetic discharge. The answer is **D.**

2. Nitroglycerin causes hypotension as a result of arterial and venous dilation. Dilation of arteries in the head has no effect on central nervous system function but does cause headache. The answer is **D.**

3. The calcium channel blockers and the β blockers are generally effective in reducing the number of attacks of angina of effort, and most have durations of 4–8 h. Oral and transdermal nitrates have similar or longer durations. Amyl nitrite, the sublingual nitrates, and esmolol (an intravenous β blocker) have short durations of action and are of no value in prophylaxis. The answer is **B.**

4. Propranolol blocks tachycardia but has none of the other effects listed. Only revascularization increases double product; drugs that decrease cardiac work increase exercise time by decreasing double product. The answer is **A.**

5. Both drugs cause venodilation and reduce venous return sufficiently to cause some degree of postural hypotension. Throbbing headache is a problem only with the nitrates, and bradycardia and lupus with neither of them. The answer is **D.**

6. Read carefully! Nitrites, not nitrates, cause methemoglobinemia in adults. Methemoglobinemia is deliberately induced in one of the treatments of cyanide poisoning. The answer is **A.**

7. Isosorbide dinitrate (like all the nitrates) can cause reflex tachycardia, but all the other drugs listed here slow heart rate. The answer is **C.**

8. Acute migraine headache is associated with vasodilation of meningeal arteries. Of the drugs listed, only nitroglycerin is commonly associated with headache. In fact, calcium channel blockers and β blockers have been used with some success as prophylaxis for migraine. The answer is **D.**

9. The effects of β blockers (or calcium channel blockers) and nitrates on heart size, force, venous tone, and heart rate are *opposite*. The effects of β blockers and calcium channel blockers are the same. The answer is **C.**

10. Sildenafil inhibits phosphodiesterase 5, an enzyme that inactivates cGMP. The nitrates (via nitric oxide) increase the synthesis of cGMP. This combination is synergistic. The answer is **F.**

SKILL KEEPER ANSWER: NIFEDIPINE CARDIOTOXICITY (SEE CHAPTER 6)

Several studies have suggested that patients receiving prompt-release nifedipine may have an increased risk of myocardial infarction. Slow-release formulations do not seem to impose this risk. These observations have been explained as follows: Rapid-acting vasodilators—such as nifedipine in its prompt-release formulation—cause significant and sudden reduction in blood pressure. The drop in blood pressure evokes increased sympathetic outflow to the cardiovascular system and increases heart rate and force of contraction as shown in Figure 6–4. These changes can markedly increase cardiac oxygen requirement. If coronary blood flow does not increase sufficiently to match the increased requirement, ischemia and necrosis can result.

CHECKLIST

When you complete this chapter, you should be able to:

❑ Describe the pathophysiology of effort angina and vasospastic angina and the major determinants of cardiac oxygen consumption.

❑ List the strategies and drug targets for relief of anginal pain.

❑ Contrast the therapeutic and adverse effects of nitrates, β blockers, and calcium channel blockers when used for angina.

❑ Explain why the combination of a nitrate with a β blocker or a calcium channel blocker may be more effective than either alone.

❑ Explain why the combination of a nitrate and sildenafil is potentially dangerous.

❑ Contrast the effects of medical therapy and surgical therapy of angina.

DRUG SUMMARY TABLE: Drugs Used in Angina

Subclass	Mechanism of Action	Clinical Applications	Pharmacokinetics	Toxicities, Interactions
Short-acting nitrate				
Nitroglycerin, sublingual (SL)	Releases nitric oxide (NO), increases cGMP (cyclic guanosine monophosphate), and relaxes vascular smooth muscle	Acute angina pectoris • acute coronary syndrome	Rapid onset (1 min) • short duration (15 min)	Tachycardia, orthostatic hypotension, headache
Isosorbide dinitrate (SL): like nitroglycerin SL but slightly longer acting (20–30 min)				
Intermediate-acting nitrate				
Nitroglycerin, oral	Like nitroglycerin SL • active metabolite dinitroglycerin	Prophylaxis of angina	Slow onset • Duration: 2–4 h	Same as nitroglycerin SL
Isosorbide dinitrate and mononitrate, oral: like nitroglycerin oral				
Other oral nitrates: like nitroglycerin oral				
Long-acting nitrate				
Transdermal nitroglycerin	Like nitroglycerin oral	Prophylaxis of angina	Slow onset • long duration of absorption: 24 h • duration of effect: 10 h (tachyphylaxis)	Same as nitroglycerin SL • loss of response is common after 10–12 h exposure to drug
Ultrashort-acting nitrite				
Amyl nitrite	Same as nitroglycerin SL	Obsolete for angina • some recreational use	Vapors are inhaled • onset seconds Duration: 1–5 min	Same as nitroglycerine SL
Calcium channel blockers				
Verapamil	Blocks L-type Ca^{2+} channels in smooth muscle and heart • decreases intracellular Ca^{2+}	Angina (both atherosclerotic and vasospastic), hypertension • AV-nodal arrhythmias; migraine	Oral, parenteral Duration: 6–8 h	Constipation, pretibial edema, flushing, dizziness Higher doses: cardiac depression, hypotension
Diltiazem: like verapamil; shorter half-life				
Nifedipine	Dihydropyridine Ca^{2+} channel blocker; vascular > cardiac effect	Angina, hypertension	Oral • slow-release form Duration: 6–8 h	Like verapamil • less constipation, cardiac effect
Amlodipine, felodipine, nicardipine, nisoldipine: like nifedipine				
Beta blockers				
Propranolol	Blocks sympathetic effects on heart and blood pressure • reduces renin release	Angina, hypertension, arrhythmias, migraine, performance anxiety	Oral, parenteral Duration: 6 h	See Chapter 10
Atenolol, metoprolol, other β blockers: like propranolol; most have longer duration of action				
Other antianginal drugs				
Ranolazine	Blocks late Na^+ current in myocardium, reduces cardiac work	Angina	Oral Duration: 10–12 h	QT prolongation on ECG • inhibits CYP3A and 2D6
Ivabradine	Blocks pacemaker Na^+ current (I_f) in sinoatrial node, reduces heart rate	Investigational: angina, heart failure	Oral, administered twice daily	Unknown

Drugs Used in Heart Failure

Heart failure results when cardiac output is inadequate for the needs of the body. A defect in cardiac contractility is complicated by multiple compensatory processes that further weaken the failing heart. The drugs used in heart failure fall into 3 major groups with varying targets and actions.

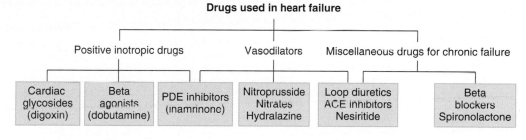

Drugs used in heart failure

Positive inotropic drugs — Vasodilators — Miscellaneous drugs for chronic failure

| Cardiac glycosides (digoxin) | Beta agonists (dobutamine) | PDE inhibitors (inamrinone) | Nitroprusside Nitrates Hydralazine | Loop diuretics ACE inhibitors Nesiritide | Beta blockers Spironolactone |

PATHOPHYSIOLOGY

Heart failure is an extremely serious cardiac condition associated with a high mortality rate. The fundamental physiologic defect in heart failure is a **decrease in cardiac output** relative to the needs of the body, and the major manifestations are dyspnea and fatigue. The causes of heart failure are still not completely understood. In some cases, it can be ascribed to simple loss of functional myocardium, as in myocardial infarction. It is frequently associated with chronic hypertension, valvular disease, coronary artery disease, and a variety of cardiomyopathies. About one third of cases are due to a reduction of cardiac contractile force and ejection fraction (systolic failure). Another third is caused by stiffening or other changes of the ventricles that prevent adequate filling during diastole; ejection fraction may be normal (diastolic failure). The remainder of cases can be attributed to a combination of systolic and diastolic dysfunction. The natural history of heart failure is characterized by a slow deterioration of cardiac function, punctuated by episodes of acute cardiac decompensation that are often associated with pulmonary or peripheral edema or both (congestion).

The reduction in cardiac output is best shown by the ventricular function curve (Frank-Starling curve; Figure 13–1). The changes in the ventricular function curve reflect some compensatory responses of the body and may also be used to demonstrate the response to drugs. As ventricular ejection decreases, the end-diastolic fiber length increases, as shown by the shift from point A to point B in Figure 13–1. Operation at point B is intrinsically less efficient than operation at shorter fiber lengths because of the increase in myocardial oxygen requirement associated with increased fiber tension and length (see Figure 12–1).

The homeostatic responses of the body to depressed cardiac output are extremely important and are mediated mainly by the sympathetic nervous system and the renin-angiotensin-aldosterone system. They are summarized in Figure 13–2. Increased blood volume results in edema and pulmonary congestion and contributes to the increased end-diastolic fiber length. Cardiomegaly (enlargement of the heart)—a slower compensatory response, mediated at least in part by sympathetic discharge and angiotensin II, is common. Although these compensatory responses can temporarily improve cardiac output (point C in Figure 13–1), they also increase the load on the heart, and the increased load contributes to further long-term decline in cardiac function. Apoptosis is a later response, and results in a reduction in the number of functioning myocytes. Evidence suggests that catecholamines, angiotensin II, and aldosterone play a direct role in these changes.

High-Yield Terms to Learn

End-diastolic fiber length	The length of the ventricular fibers at the end of diastole; a determinant of the force of the following contraction
Heart failure	A condition in which the cardiac output is insufficient for the needs of the body. Low-output failure may be due to decreased stroke volume (systolic failure) or decreased filling (diastolic failure)
PDE inhibitor	Phosphodiesterase inhibitor; a drug that inhibits one or more enzymes that degrade cAMP (and other cyclic nucleotides). Examples: high concentrations of theophylline, inamrinone
Premature ventricular beat	An abnormal beat arising from a cell below the AV node—often from a Purkinje fiber, sometimes from a ventricular fiber
Sodium pump (Na⁺/K⁺ ATPase)	A transport molecule in the membranes of all vertebrate cells; responsible for the maintenance of normal low intracellular sodium and high intracellular potassium concentrations; it uses ATP to pump these ions against their concentration gradients
Sodium-calcium exchanger	A transport molecule in the membrane of many cells that pumps one calcium atom outward against its concentration gradient in exchange for three sodium ions moving inward down their concentration gradient
Ventricular function curve	The graph that relates cardiac output, stroke volume, etc, to filling pressure or end-diastolic fiber length; also known as the Frank-Starling curve
Ventricular tachycardia	An arrhythmia consisting entirely or largely of beats originating below the AV node

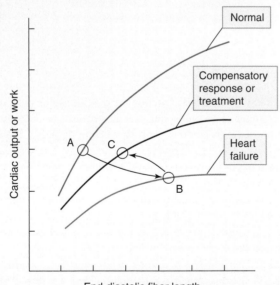

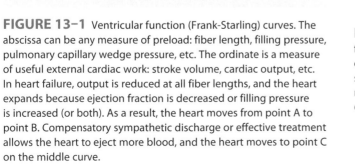

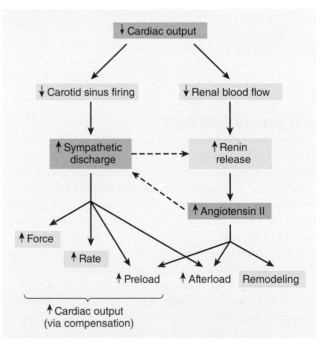

FIGURE 13–1 Ventricular function (Frank-Starling) curves. The abscissa can be any measure of preload: fiber length, filling pressure, pulmonary capillary wedge pressure, etc. The ordinate is a measure of useful external cardiac work: stroke volume, cardiac output, etc. In heart failure, output is reduced at all fiber lengths, and the heart expands because ejection fraction is decreased or filling pressure is increased (or both). As a result, the heart moves from point A to point B. Compensatory sympathetic discharge or effective treatment allows the heart to eject more blood, and the heart moves to point C on the middle curve.

FIGURE 13–2 Compensatory responses that occur in heart failure. These responses play an important role in the progression of the disease. Dashed arrows indicate interactions between the sympathetic and the renin-angiotensin systems. (Modified and reproduced, with permission, from Katzung BG, editor: *Basic & Clinical Pharmacology*, 12th ed. McGraw-Hill, 2012: Fig. 13–2.)

THERAPEUTIC STRATEGIES

Pharmacologic therapies for heart failure include the removal of retained salt and water with diuretics; reduction of afterload and salt and water retention by means of angiotensin-converting enzyme (ACE) inhibitors; reduction of excessive sympathetic stimulation by means of β blockers; reduction of preload or afterload with vasodilators; and in systolic failure, direct augmentation of depressed cardiac contractility with positive inotropic drugs such as digitalis glycosides. Considerable evidence indicates that angiotensin antagonists, certain β-adrenoceptor blockers, and the aldosterone antagonists spironolactone and eplerenone also have long-term beneficial effects. The use of diuretics is discussed in Chapter 15.

Current clinical evidence suggests that acute heart failure should be treated with a **loop diuretic**; if very severe, a prompt-acting positive inotropic agent such as a **β agonist** or **phosphodiesterase inhibitor,** and **vasodilators** should be used as required to optimize filling pressures and blood pressure. Chronic failure is best treated with diuretics (often a loop agent plus spironolactone) plus an **ACE inhibitor** and, if tolerated, a **β blocker**. Digitalis may be helpful if systolic dysfunction is prominent. Nesiritide, a recombinant form of brain natriuretic peptide, has vasodilating and diuretic properties and has been heavily promoted for use in acute failure.

CARDIAC GLYCOSIDES

Digitalis glycosides are no longer considered first-line drugs in the treatment of heart failure. However, because they are not discussed elsewhere in this book, we begin our discussion with this group.

A. Prototypes and Pharmacokinetics

All cardiac glycosides include a steroid nucleus and a lactone ring; most also have one or more sugar residues. The cardiac glycosides are often called "digitalis" because several come from the digitalis (foxglove) plant. **Digoxin** is the prototype agent and the only one commonly used in the United States. A very similar molecule, digitoxin, which also comes from the foxglove, is no longer available in the United States. Digoxin has an oral bioavailability of 60–75%, and a half-life of 36–40 h. Elimination is by renal excretion (about 60%) and hepatic metabolism (40%).

B. Mechanism of Action

Inhibition of Na^+/K^+ ATPase of the cell membrane by digitalis is well documented and is considered to be the primary biochemical mechanism of action (Figure 13–3). Inhibition of Na^+/K^+ ATPase results in a small increase in intracellular sodium. The increased sodium alters the driving force for sodium-calcium exchange by the exchanger, NCX, so that less calcium is removed from the cell. The increased intracellular calcium is stored in the sarcoplasmic reticulum and upon release increases contractile force. Other mechanisms of action for digitalis have been proposed, but they

are probably not as important as inhibition of the ATPase. The consequences of Na^+/K^+ ATPase inhibition are seen in both the mechanical and the electrical function of the heart. Digitalis also modifies autonomic outflow, and this action has effects on the electrical properties of the heart.

C. Cardiac Effects

1. Mechanical effects—The increase in contractility evoked by digitalis results in increased ventricular ejection, decreased end-systolic and end-diastolic size, increased cardiac output, and increased renal perfusion. These beneficial effects permit a decrease in the compensatory sympathetic and renal responses previously described. The decrease in sympathetic tone is especially beneficial: reduced heart rate, preload, and afterload permit the heart to function more efficiently (point C in Figure 13–1 may approach point A as the function curve approaches normal).

2. Electrical effects—Electrical effects include early cardiac parasympathomimetic responses and later arrhythmogenic actions. They are summarized in Table 13–1.

a. Early responses—Increased PR interval, caused by the decrease in atrioventricular (AV) conduction velocity, and flattening of the T wave are common electrocardiogram (ECG) effects. The effects on the atria and AV node are largely parasympathetic (mediated by the vagus nerve) and can be partially blocked by atropine. The increase in the AV nodal refractory period is particularly important when atrial flutter or fibrillation is present because the refractoriness of the AV node determines the ventricular rate in these arrhythmias. The effect of digitalis is to slow ventricular rate. Shortened QT, inversion of the T, and ST depression may occur later.

b. Toxic responses—Increased automaticity, caused by intracellular calcium overload, is the most important manifestation of digitalis toxicity. Intracellular calcium overload results in delayed afterdepolarizations, which may evoke extrasystoles, tachycardia, or fibrillation in any part of the heart. In the ventricles, the extrasystoles are recognized as premature ventricular beats (PVBs). When PVBs are coupled to normal beats in a 1:1 fashion, the rhythm is called bigeminy (Figure 13–4).

D. Clinical Uses

1. Congestive heart failure—Digitalis is the traditional positive inotropic agent used in the treatment of chronic heart failure. However, careful clinical studies indicate that while digitalis may improve functional status (reducing symptoms), it does not prolong life. Other agents (diuretics, ACE inhibitors, vasodilators) may be equally effective and less toxic, and some of these alternative therapies do prolong life (see later discussion). Because the half-lives of cardiac glycosides are long, the drugs accumulate significantly in the body, and dosing regimens must be carefully designed and monitored.

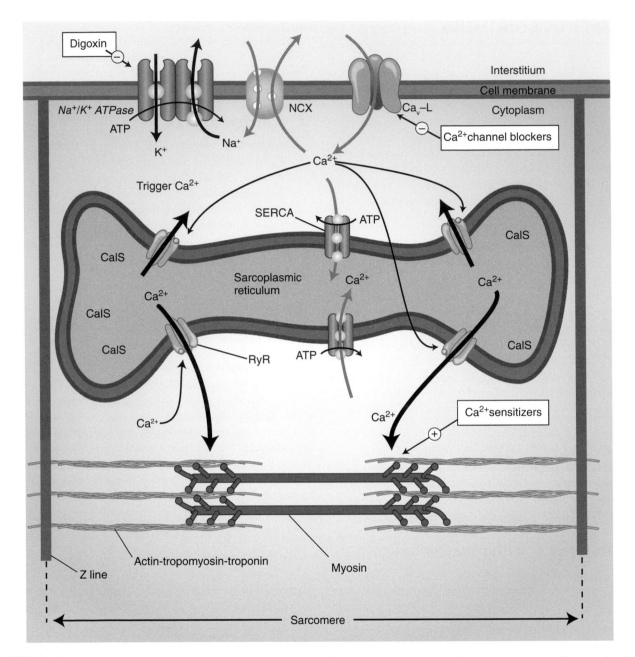

FIGURE 13–3 Schematic diagram of a cardiac sarcomere with the cellular components involved in excitation-contraction coupling and the sites of action of several drugs. Factors involved in excitation-contraction coupling include Na^+/K^+ ATPase; Na^+/Ca^{2+} exchanger, NCX; voltage-gated calcium channel (Ca_V-L); calcium transporter (SERCA) in the wall of the sarcoplasmic reticulum (SR); calcium release channel in the SR, RyR (ryanodine receptor); and the site of calcium interaction with the troponin-tropomyosin system. CalS, calsequestrin, a calcium-binding protein in the SR. (Modified and reproduced, with permission, from Katzung BG, editor: *Basic & Clinical Pharmacology*, 11th ed. McGraw-Hill, 2009: Fig. 13–1.)

2. Atrial fibrillation—In atrial flutter and fibrillation, it is desirable to reduce the conduction velocity or increase the refractory period of the AV node so that ventricular rate is controlled within a range compatible with efficient filling and ejection. The parasympathomimetic action of digitalis often accomplishes this therapeutic objective, although high doses may be required. Alternative drugs for rate control include β blockers and calcium channel blockers, but these drugs have negative inotropic effects.

E. Interactions

Quinidine causes a well-documented reduction in digoxin clearance and can increase the serum digoxin level if digoxin dosage is not adjusted. Several other drugs have the same effect (amiodarone, verapamil, others), but the interactions with these drugs are not clinically significant. Digitalis toxicity, especially arrhythmogenesis, is increased by hypokalemia, hypomagnesemia, and hypercalcemia.

TABLE 13–1 Major actions of cardiac glycosides on cardiac electrical function.

Variable	Tissue		
	Atrial Muscle	AV Node	Purkinje System, Ventricles
Effective refractory period	↓ (PANS)	↑ (PANS)	↓ (Direct)
Conduction velocity	↑ (PANS)	↓ (PANS)	Negligible
Automaticity	↑ (Direct)	↑ (Direct)	↑ (Direct)
Electrocardiogram before arrhythmias	Negligible	↑ PR interval	↓ QT interval; T-wave inversion; ST-segment depression
Arrhythmias	Atrial tachycardia, fibrillation	AV nodal tachycardia, AV blockade	Premature ventricular beats, bigeminy, ventricular tachycardia, ventricular fibrillation

AV, atrioventricular; PANS, parasympathomimetic actions; direct, direct membrane actions.

Loop diuretics and thiazides, which are always included in the treatment of heart failure, may significantly reduce serum potassium and thus precipitate digitalis toxicity. Digitalis-induced vomiting may deplete serum magnesium and similarly facilitate toxicity. These ion interactions are important in treating digitalis toxicity.

F. Digitalis Toxicity

The major signs of digitalis toxicity are arrhythmias, nausea, vomiting, and diarrhea. Rarely, confusion or hallucinations and visual or endocrine aberrations may occur. Arrhythmias are common and dangerous. Chronic intoxication is an extension of the therapeutic effect of the drug and is caused by excessive calcium accumulation in cardiac cells (calcium overload). This overload triggers abnormal automaticity and the arrhythmias noted in Table 13–1.

Severe, acute intoxication caused by suicidal or accidental extreme overdose results in cardiac depression leading to cardiac arrest rather than tachycardia or fibrillation.

Treatment of digitalis toxicity includes several steps, as follows.

1. Correction of potassium or magnesium deficiency—
Correction of potassium deficiency (caused, eg, by diuretic use) is useful in chronic digitalis intoxication. Mild toxicity may often be managed by omitting 1 or 2 doses of digitalis and giving oral or parenteral K^+ supplements. Severe acute intoxication (as in suicidal

overdoses) usually causes marked hyperkalemia and should not be treated with supplemental potassium.

2. Antiarrhythmic drugs—
Antiarrhythmic drugs may be useful if increased automaticity is prominent and does not respond to normalization of serum potassium. Agents that do not severely impair cardiac contractility (eg, lidocaine or phenytoin) are favored, but drugs such as propranolol have also been used successfully. Severe acute digitalis overdose usually causes marked *inhibition* of all cardiac pacemakers, and an electronic pacemaker may be required. Antiarrhythmic drugs are dangerous in such patients.

3. Digoxin antibodies—
Digoxin antibodies (Fab fragments; Digibind) are extremely effective and should always be used if other therapies appear to be failing. They are effective for poisoning with many cardiac glycosides in addition to digoxin and may save patients who would otherwise die.

> ### SKILL KEEPER: MAINTENANCE DOSE CALCULATIONS (SEE CHAPTER 3)
>
> *Digoxin has a narrow therapeutic window, and its dosing must be carefully managed. The drug's minimum effective concentration is about 1 ng/mL. About 60% is excreted in the urine; the rest is metabolized in the liver. The normal clearance of digoxin is 7 L/h/70 kg; volume of distribution is 500 L/70 kg; and bioavailability is 70%. If your 70-kg patient's renal function is only 30% of normal, what daily oral maintenance dosage should be used to achieve a safe plasma concentration of 1 ng/mL? The Skill Keeper Answer appears at the end of the chapter.*

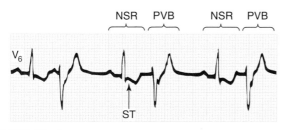

FIGURE 13–4 Electrocardiographic record showing digitalis-induced bigeminy. The complexes marked NSR are normal sinus rhythm beats; an inverted T wave and depressed ST segment are present. The complexes marked PVB are premature ventricular beats.

OTHER DRUGS USED IN CONGESTIVE HEART FAILURE

The other major agents used in heart failure include diuretics, ACE inhibitors, β_1-selective sympathomimetics, β blockers, phosphodiesterase inhibitors, and vasodilators.

A. Diuretics

Diuretics are the first-line therapy for both systolic and diastolic failure and are used in heart failure before digitalis and other drugs are considered. **Furosemide** is a very useful agent for immediate reduction of the pulmonary congestion and severe edema associated with acute heart failure and for moderate or severe chronic failure. Thiazides such as **hydrochlorothiazide** are sometimes sufficient for mild chronic failure. Clinical studies suggest that **spironolactone** and **eplerenone** (aldosterone antagonist diuretics) have significant long-term benefits and can reduce mortality in chronic failure. Diuretics are discussed in Chapter 15.

B. Angiotensin Antagonists

These agents have been shown to reduce morbidity and mortality in chronic heart failure. Although they have no direct positive inotropic action, angiotensin antagonists reduce aldosterone secretion, salt and water retention, and vascular resistance (see Chapter 11). They are now considered, along with diuretics, to be first-line drugs for chronic heart failure. The angiotensin receptor blockers (ARBs, eg, **losartan**) appear to have the same benefits as ACE inhibitors (eg, **captopril**), although experience with ARBs is not as extensive.

C. Beta₁-Adrenoceptor Agonists

Dobutamine and **dopamine** are often useful in acute failure in which systolic function is markedly depressed (see Chapter 9). However, they are not appropriate for chronic failure because of tolerance, lack of oral efficacy, and significant arrhythmogenic effects.

D. Beta-Adrenoceptor Antagonists

Several β blockers (**carvedilol, labetalol, metoprolol,** Chapter 10) have been shown in long-term studies to reduce progression of *chronic* heart failure. This benefit of β blockers had long been recognized in patients with hypertrophic cardiomyopathy but has also been shown to occur in patients without cardiomyopathy. **Nebivolol,** a newer β blocker with vasodilator effects, is investigational in heart failure. Beta blockers are not of value in acute failure and may be detrimental if systolic dysfunction is marked.

E. Phosphodiesterase Inhibitors

Inamrinone and **milrinone** are the major representatives of this infrequently used group. Theophylline (in the form of its salt, **aminophylline**) was commonly used for acute failure in the past. These drugs increase cyclic adenosine monophosphate (cAMP) by inhibiting its breakdown by phosphodiesterase and cause an increase in cardiac intracellular calcium similar to that produced by β-adrenoceptor agonists. Phosphodiesterase inhibitors also cause vasodilation, which may be responsible for a major part of their beneficial effect. At sufficiently high concentrations, these agents may increase the sensitivity of the contractile protein system to calcium. These agents should not be used in chronic failure because they have been shown to increase morbidity and mortality.

F. Vasodilators

Vasodilator therapy with **nitroprusside** or **nitroglycerin** is often used for acute severe failure with congestion. The use of these vasodilator drugs is based on the reduction in cardiac size and improved efficiency that can be achieved with proper adjustment of venous return (preload) and reduction of impedance to ventricular ejection (afterload). Vasodilator therapy can be dramatically effective, especially in cases in which increased afterload is a major factor in causing the failure (eg, continuing hypertension in an individual who has just had an infarct). The natriuretic peptide **nesiritide** acts chiefly by causing vasodilation, although it does have natriuretic effects as well. It is given by IV infusion for acute failure only. Nesiritide has significant renal toxicity and renal function must be monitored. Chronic heart failure sometimes responds favorably to oral vasodilators such as **hydralazine** or **isosorbide dinitrate** (or both), and this combination has been shown to reduce mortality in African Americans. Calcium channel blockers (eg, verapamil) are of no value in heart failure.

G. Nonpharmacologic Therapy

A variety of surgical procedures to remove nonfunctional regions of damaged myocardium have been attempted with mixed results. Resynchronization of right and left ventricular contraction by means of a pacemaker has been beneficial in patients with long QRS (indicating conduction abnormalities). Patients with coronary artery disease and heart failure may have improved systolic function after coronary revascularization.

QUESTIONS

Questions 1–2. A 73-year-old man with an inadequate response to other drugs is to receive digoxin for heart failure.

1. Which of the following is the best-documented mechanism of beneficial action of cardiac glycosides?
   (A) A decrease in calcium uptake by the sarcoplasmic reticulum
   (B) An increase in ATP synthesis
   (C) A modification of the actin molecule
   (D) An increase in systolic cytoplasmic calcium levels
   (E) A block of cardiac β adrenoceptors

2. After your patient has been receiving digoxin for 3 wk, he presents to the emergency department with an arrhythmia. Which one of the following is most likely to contribute to the arrhythmogenic effect of digoxin?
   (A) Increased parasympathetic discharge
   (B) Increased intracellular calcium
   (C) Decreased sympathetic discharge
   (D) Decreased intracellular ATP
   (E) Increased extracellular potassium

3. A patient who has been taking digoxin for several years for atrial fibrillation and chronic heart failure is about to receive atropine for another condition. A common effect of digoxin (at therapeutic blood levels) that can be almost entirely blocked by atropine is
   (A) Decreased appetite
   (B) Headaches
   (C) Increased atrial contractility
   (D) Increased PR interval on ECG
   (E) Tachycardia

4. A 65-year-old woman has been admitted to the coronary care unit with a left ventricular myocardial infarction. She develops acute severe heart failure with marked pulmonary edema, but no evidence of peripheral edema or weight gain. Which one of the following drugs would be most useful?
   (A) Digoxin
   (B) Furosemide
   (C) Minoxidil
   (D) Propranolol
   (E) Spironolactone

5. An 82-year-old woman has long-standing heart failure. Which one of the following drugs has been shown to reduce mortality in chronic heart failure?
   (A) Atenolol
   (B) Digoxin
   (C) Dobutamine
   (D) Furosemide
   (E) Spironolactone

6. Which row in the following table correctly shows the major effects of full therapeutic doses of digoxin on the AV node and the ECG?

Row	AV Refractory Period	QT Interval	T Wave
(A)	Increased	Increased	Upright
(B)	Increased	Decreased	Inverted
(C)	Decreased	Increased	Upright
(D)	Decreased	Decreased	Upright
(E)	Decreased	Increased	Inverted

7. Which one of the following drugs is associated with clinically useful or physiologically important positive inotropic effect?
   (A) Captopril
   (B) Dobutamine
   (C) Enalapril
   (D) Losartan
   (E) Nesiritide

8. A 38-year-old man who has been running a marathon collapses and is brought to the emergency department. He is found to have a left ventricular myocardial infarction and heart failure with significant pulmonary edema. The first-line drug of choice in most cases of heart failure is
   (A) Atenolol
   (B) Captopril
   (C) Carvedilol
   (D) Digoxin
   (E) Diltiazem
   (F) Dobutamine
   (G) Enalapril
   (H) Furosemide
   (I) Metoprolol
   (J) Spironolactone

9. Which of the following has been shown to prolong life in patients with chronic congestive failure in spite of having a negative inotropic effect on cardiac contractility?
   (A) Carvedilol
   (B) Digoxin
   (C) Dobutamine
   (D) Enalapril
   (E) Furosemide

10. A 5-year-old child is brought to the emergency department with sinus arrest and a ventricular rate of 35 bpm. An empty bottle of his uncle's digoxin was found where he was playing. Which of the following is the drug of choice in treating a severe overdose of digoxin?
    (A) Digoxin antibodies
    (B) Lidocaine infusion
    (C) Magnesium infusion
    (D) Phenytoin by mouth
    (E) Potassium by mouth

ANSWERS

1. Digitalis does not decrease calcium uptake by the sarcoplasmic reticulum or increase ATP synthesis; it does not modify actin. Cardiac adrenoceptors are not blocked. The most accurate description of digitalis's mechanism in this list is that it increases systolic cytoplasmic calcium indirectly by inhibiting Na^+/K^+ ATPase and altering Na/Ca exchange. The answer is **D**.

2. The effects of digitalis include increased vagal action on the heart (not arrhythmogenic) and increased intracellular calcium, including calcium overload, the most important cause of toxicity. Decreased sympathetic discharge and increased extracellular potassium and magnesium *reduce* digitalis arrhythmogenesis. The answer is **B**.

3. The parasympathomimetic effects of digitalis can be blocked by muscarinic blockers such as atropine. The only parasympathomimetic effect in the list provided is increased PR interval, representing slowing of AV conduction. The answer is **D**.

4. Acute severe congestive failure with pulmonary edema often requires a vasodilator that reduces intravascular pressures in the lungs. Furosemide has such vasodilating actions in the context of acute failure. Pulmonary edema also involves a shift of fluid from the intravascular compartment to the lungs. Minoxidil would decrease arterial pressure and increase the heart rate excessively. Digoxin has a slow onset of action and lacks vasodilating effects. Spironolactone is useful in chronic

failure but not in acute pulmonary edema. Pulmonary vaso-dilation and removal of edema fluid by diuresis are accomplished by furosemide. The answer is **B.**

5. Of the drugs listed, only spironolactone has been shown to reduce mortality in this highly lethal disease. Digoxin, dobutamine, and furosemide are used in the management of symptoms. The answer is **E.**

6. Digitalis increases the AV node refractory period—a parasympathomimetic action. Its effects on the ventricles include shortened action potential and QT interval, and a change in repolarization with flattening or inversion of the T wave. The answer is **B.**

7. Although they are extremely useful in heart failure, ACE inhibitors (eg, captopril, enalapril), and angiotensin receptor blockers (ARBs, eg, losartan) have no positive inotropic effect on the heart. Nesiritide is a vasodilator with diuretic effects and renal toxicity. The answer is **B.**

8. In both systolic and diastolic heart failure, the initial treatment of choice is usually furosemide. The answer is **H.**

9. Several β blockers, including carvedilol, have been shown to prolong life in heart failure patients even though these drugs have a negative inotropic action on the heart. Their benefits presumably result from some other effect, and at least one β blocker has failed to show a mortality benefit. The answer is **A.**

10. The drug of choice in severe, massive overdose with any cardiac glycoside is digoxin antibody, Digibind. The other drugs listed are used in moderate overdosage associated with increased automaticity. The answer is **A.**

SKILL KEEPER ANSWER: MAINTENANCE DOSE CALCULATIONS (SEE CHAPTER 3)

Maintenance dosage is equal to $CL \times Cp \div F$, so

Maintenance dosage for a patient with normal renal function

$= 7 \text{ L/h} \times 1 \text{ ng/mL} \div 0.7 = 7 \text{ L/h} \times 1 \text{ mcg/L} \div 0.7$

$= 10 \text{ mcg/h} \times 24 \text{ h/d} = 240 \text{ mcg/d} = 0.24 \text{ mg/d}$

But this patient has only 30% of normal renal function, so

CL (total) $= 0.3 \times$ CL (renal [60% of total])

$\qquad\qquad\quad + $ CL (liver [40% of total])

CL (total) $= 0.3 \times 0.6 \times 7 \text{ L/h} + 0.4 \times 7 \text{ L/h}$, and

CL (total) $= 1.26 \text{ L/h} + 2.8 \text{ L/h} = 4.06 \text{ L/h}$, and

Maintenance dosage $= 4.06 \text{ L/h} \times 1 \text{ mcg/L} \div 0.7$

$\qquad\qquad\qquad\quad = 5.8 \text{ mcg/h} = 139 \text{ mcg/d} = 0.14 \text{ mg/d}$

CHECKLIST

When you complete this chapter, you should be able to:

❑ Describe the strategies and list the major drug groups used in the treatment of acute heart failure and chronic failure.

❑ Describe the mechanism of action of digitalis and its major effects. Indicate why digitalis is no longer considered a first-line therapy for chronic heart failure.

❑ Describe the nature and mechanism of digitalis's toxic effects on the heart.

❑ List some positive inotropic drugs other than digitalis that have been used in heart failure.

❑ Explain the beneficial effects of diuretics, vasodilators, ACE inhibitors, and other drugs that lack positive inotropic effects in heart failure.

DRUG SUMMARY TABLE: Drugs Used in Heart Failure

Subclass	Mechanism of Action	Clinical Applications	Pharmacokinetics	Toxicities, Interactions
Diuretics				
Furosemide	Reduces preload, edema by powerful diuretic action on thick ascending limb in nephron • vasodilating effect on pulmonary vessels	Acute and chronic heart failure, especially acute pulmonary edema • other edematous conditions, hypercalcemia (see Chapter 15)	Oral, parenteral Duration: 2–4 h	Ototoxicity • hypovolemia, hypokalemia
Spironolactone	Antagonist of aldosterone in kidney plus poorly understood reduction in mortality	Chronic heart failure, aldosteronism	Oral Duration: 24–48 h	Hyperkalemia • gynecomastia
Eplerenone: similar to spironolactone but lacks gynecomastia effect				
Angiotensin-converting enzyme (ACE) inhibitors				
Captopril	Blocks angiotensin-converting enzyme, reduces AII levels, decreases vascular tone and aldosterone secretion	Heart failure, hypertension, diabetes	Oral; short half-life but large doses used Duration: 12–24 h	Cough, renal damage, hyperkalemia
Benazepril, enalapril, others: like captopril *Losartan, candesartan, others:* angiotensin receptor blockers (see Chapter 11)				
Positive inotropic drugs				
Cardiac glycosides: digoxin	Inhibits Na^+/K^+ ATPase sodium pump and increases intracellular Na^+, decreasing Ca^{2+} expulsion and increasing cardiac contractility	Heart failure, nodal arrhythmias	Oral, parenteral Duration: 40 h	Arrhythmogenic! Nausea, vomiting, diarrhea, visual changes (rare)
Sympathomimetics: dobutamine	β_1-Selective sympathomimetic, increases cAMP and force of contraction	Acute heart failure	Parenteral Duration: a few minutes	Arrhythmias
Beta blockers				
Carvedilol, metoprolol, bisoprolol	Poorly understood reduction of mortality, possibly by decreasing remodeling	Chronic heart failure	Oral Duration varies (see Chapter 10)	Cardiac depression (see Chapter 10)
Vasodilators				
Nitroprusside	Rapid, powerful vasodilation reduces preload and afterload	Acute severe decompensated failure	IV only Duration: a few minutes	Excessive hypotension • thiocyanate and cyanide toxicity
Hydralazine + isosorbide dinitrate	Poorly understood reduction in mortality	Chronic failure in African Americans	Oral	Headache, tachycardia
Nesiritide	Atrial peptide vasodilator, diuretic	Acute severe decompensated failure	Parenteral Duration: a few minutes	Renal damage, hypotension

cAMP, cyclic adenosine monophosphate.

Antiarrhythmic Drugs

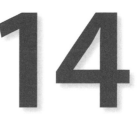

Cardiac arrhythmias are the most common cause of death in patients with a myocardial infarction or terminal heart failure. They are also the most serious manifestation of digitalis toxicity and are often associated with anesthesia, hyperthyroidism, and electrolyte disorders. The drugs used for arrhythmias fall into five major groups or classes, but most have very low therapeutic indices and when feasible, nondrug therapies (cardioversion, pacemakers, ablation, implanted defibrillators) are used.

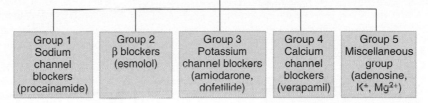

Drugs used in cardiac arrhythmias

| Group 1 Sodium channel blockers (procainamide) | Group 2 β blockers (esmolol) | Group 3 Potassium channel blockers (amiodarone, dofetilide) | Group 4 Calcium channel blockers (verapamil) | Group 5 Miscellaneous group (adenosine, K+, Mg2+) |

PATHOPHYSIOLOGY

A. Nature of Arrhythmias

Normal electrical cardiac function (**normal sinus rhythm, NSR**) is dependent on generation of an impulse in the normal sinoatrial (SA) node pacemaker and its conduction through the atrial muscle, through the atrioventricular (AV) node, through the Purkinje conduction system, to the ventricular muscle (Figure 14–1). Normal pacemaking and conduction require normal action potentials (dependent on sodium, calcium, and potassium channel activity) under appropriate autonomic control. Arrhythmias (also called dysrhythmias) are therefore defined by exclusion, that is, any rhythm that is not normal sinus rhythm is an arrhythmia.

Abnormal **automaticity** and abnormal (reentrant) **conduction** are the 2 major mechanisms for arrhythmias. A few of the clinically important arrhythmias are **atrial flutter, atrial fibrillation (AFib), atrioventricular nodal reentry** (a common type of supraventricular tachycardia [SVT]), **premature ventricular beats (PVBs), ventricular tachycardia (VT),** and **ventricular fibrillation** (VF). Examples of electrocardiographic (ECG) recordings of normal sinus rhythm and some of these common arrhythmias are shown in Figure 14–2. **Torsades de pointes** is a ventricular arrhythmia of great pharmacologic importance because it is often *induced* by antiarrhythmic and other drugs that change the shape of the action potential and prolong the QT interval. It has the ECG morphology of a polymorphic ventricular tachycardia, often displaying waxing and waning QRS amplitude. Torsades is also associated with **long QT syndrome,** a heritable abnormal prolongation of the QT interval caused by mutations in the I_K or I_{Na} channel proteins.

B. Normal Electrical Activity in the Cardiac Cell

The cellular action potentials shown in Figure 14–1 are the result of ion fluxes through voltage-gated channels and carrier mechanisms. These processes are diagrammed in Figure 14–3. In most parts of the heart, sodium channel (I_{Na}) dominates the upstroke (phase 0) of the action potential (AP) and is the most important determinant of its conduction velocity. After a very brief activation, the sodium current enters a more prolonged period of inactivation. In the calcium-dependent AV node, calcium current (I_{Ca}) dominates the upstroke and the AP conduction velocity. The plateau of the AP (phase 2) is dominated by calcium current (I_{Ca}) and one or more potassium-repolarizing currents (referred to as a

High-Yield Terms to Learn

Abnormal automaticity	Pacemaker activity that originates anywhere other than in the sinoatrial node
Abnormal conduction	Conduction of an impulse that does not follow the path defined in Figure 14–1 or reenters tissue previously excited
Atrial, ventricular fibrillation (AFib, VF)	Arrhythmias involving rapid reentry and chaotic movement of impulses through the tissue of the atria or ventricles. Ventricular, but not atrial, fibrillation is fatal if not terminated within a few minutes
Group (class) 1, 2, 3, and 4 drugs	A method for classifying antiarrhythmic drugs, sometimes called the Singh-Vaughan Williams classification; based loosely on the channel or receptor affected
Reentrant arrhythmias	Arrhythmias of abnormal conduction; they involve the repetitive movement of an impulse through tissue previously excited by the same impulse
Effective refractory period	The time that must pass after the upstroke of a conducted impulse in a part of the heart before a new action potential can be propagated in that cell or tissue
Selective depression	The ability of certain drugs to selectively depress areas of excitable membrane that are most susceptible, leaving other areas relatively unaffected
Supraventricular tachycardia (SVT)	A reentrant arrhythmia that travels through the AV node; it may also be conducted through atrial tissue as part of the reentrant circuit
Ventricular tachycardia (VT)	A very common arrhythmia, often associated with myocardial infarction; ventricular tachycardia may involve abnormal automaticity or abnormal conduction, usually impairs cardiac output, and may deteriorate into ventricular fibrillation; for these reasons it requires prompt management

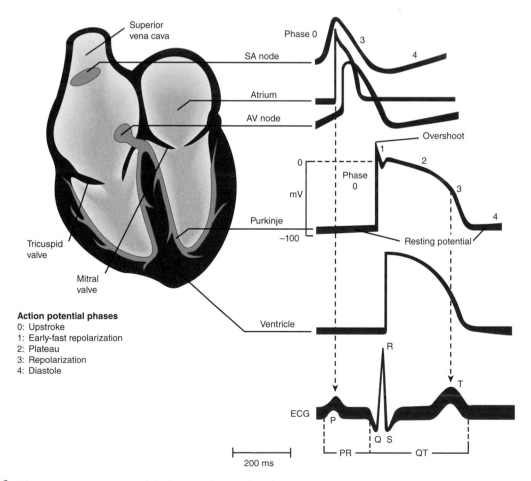

FIGURE 14–1 Schematic representation of the heart and normal cardiac electrical activity (intracellular recordings from areas indicated and ECG). The ECG is the body surface manifestation of the depolarization and repolarization waves of the heart. The P wave is generated by atrial depolarization, the QRS by ventricular muscle depolarization, and the T wave by ventricular repolarization. The PR interval is a measure of conduction time from atrium to ventricle through the atrioventricular (AV) node, and the QRS duration indicates the time required for all of the ventricular cells to be activated (ie, the intraventricular conduction time). The QT interval reflects the duration of the ventricular action potential. SA, sinoatrial. (Reproduced, with permission, from Katzung BG, editor: *Basic & Clinical Pharmacology,* 12th ed. McGraw-Hill, 2012: Fig. 14–1.)

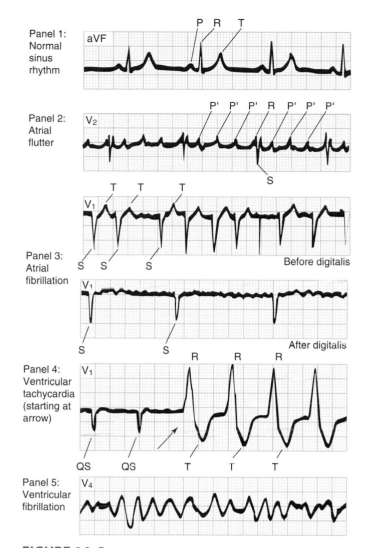

Panel 1: Normal sinus rhythm — aVF

Panel 2: Atrial flutter — V₂

Panel 3: Atrial fibrillation — V₁ Before digitalis / V₁ After digitalis

Panel 4: Ventricular tachycardia (starting at arrow) — V₁

Panel 5: Ventricular fibrillation — V₄

FIGURE 14–2 Typical ECGs of normal sinus rhythm and some common arrhythmias. Major waves (P, Q, R, S, and T) are labeled in each electrocardiographic record except in panel 5, in which electrical activity is completely disorganized and none of these deflections are recognizable. (Modified and reproduced, with permission, from Goldman MJ: *Principles of Clinical Electrocardiography*, 11th ed. McGraw-Hill, 1982.)

class as I_K). At the end of the plateau, I_K causes rapid repolarization (phase 3).

The refractory period of the sodium-dependent cardiac cells is a function of how rapidly sodium channels recover from inactivation. Recovery from inactivation depends on both the membrane potential, which varies with repolarization time and the extracellular potassium concentration, and on the actions of drugs that bind to the sodium channel (ie, sodium channel blockers). Similarly, in the calcium-dependent AV node, the duration of refractoriness is dependent on the rate of recovery from inactivation of the calcium channels. The carrier processes (sodium pump and sodium–calcium exchanger) contribute little to the shape of the AP, but they are critical for the maintenance of the ion gradients on which the sodium, calcium, and potassium currents depend. Antiarrhythmic

drugs act on 1 or more of the 3 major currents (I_{Na}, I_{Ca}, I_K) or on the β adrenoceptors that modulate these currents.

C. Drug Classification

The antiarrhythmic agents are usually classified using a system loosely based on the channel or receptor involved. As indicated by the overview figure on the first page of this chapter, this system specifies 4 groups or classes, usually denoted by the numerals 1 through 4, plus a miscellaneous group (see also Table 14–1 and Drug Summary Table).

1. Sodium channel blockers
2. Beta-adrenoceptor blockers
3. Potassium channel blockers
4. Calcium channel blockers

The **miscellaneous** group includes adenosine, potassium ion, and magnesium ion.

GROUP 1 ANTIARRHYTHMICS (LOCAL ANESTHETICS)

A. Prototypes and Mechanism of Action

The group 1 drugs are further subdivided on the basis of their effects on AP duration (Figure 14–4). Group 1A agents (prototype **procainamide**) prolong the AP. Group 1B drugs (prototype **lidocaine**) shorten the AP in some cardiac tissues. Group 1C drugs (prototype **flecainide**) have no effect on AP duration.

All group 1 drugs slow conduction in ischemic and depolarized cells and slow or abolish abnormal pacemakers wherever these processes depend on sodium channels. The most selective agents (those in group 1B) have significant effects on sodium channels in ischemic tissue, but negligible effects on channels in normal cells. In contrast, less selective group 1 drugs (groups 1A and 1C) cause some reduction of I_{Na} even in normal cells.

Useful sodium channel-blocking drugs bind to their receptors much more readily when the channel is open or inactivated than when it is fully repolarized and resting. Therefore, these antiarrhythmic drugs block channels in abnormal tissue more effectively than channels in normal tissue. They are **use dependent** or **state dependent** in their action (ie, they selectively depress tissue that is frequently depolarizing, eg, during a fast tachycardia; or tissue that is relatively depolarized during rest, eg, by hypoxia). The effects of the major group 1 drugs are summarized in Table 14–1 and in Figure 14–4.

1. Drugs with group 1A action—Procainamide is a group 1A prototype. Other drugs with group 1A actions include quinidine and disopyramide. **Amiodarone,** often classified in group 3, also has typical group 1A actions. These drugs affect both atrial and ventricular arrhythmias. They block I_{Na} and therefore slow conduction velocity in the atria, Purkinje fibers, and ventricular cells. At high doses they may slow AV conduction. These effects are summarized in Table 14–1. Amiodarone has similar effects on sodium current (I_{Na} block) and has the greatest AP-prolonging effect (I_K block).

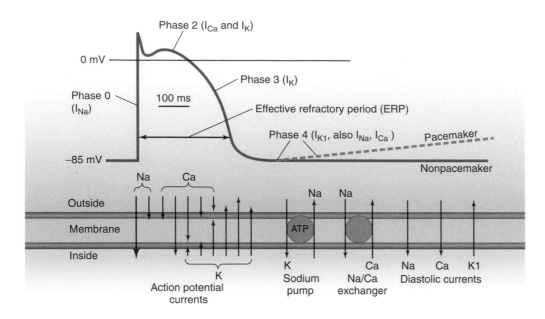

FIGURE 14–3 Components of the membrane action potential (AP) in a typical Purkinje or ventricular cardiac cell. The deflections of the AP, designated as phases 0–3, are generated by several ionic currents. The actions of the sodium pump and sodium–calcium exchanger are mainly involved in maintaining ionic steady state during repetitive activity. Note that small but significant currents occur during diastole (phase 4) in addition to the pump and exchanger activity. In non-pacemaker cells, the outward potassium current during phase 4 is sufficient to maintain a stable negative resting potential as shown by the solid line at the right end of the tracing. In pacemaker cells, however, the potassium current is smaller and the depolarizing currents (sodium, calcium, or both) during phase 4 are large enough to gradually depolarize the cell during diastole (*dashed line*). ATP, adenosine triphosphate.

2. Drugs with group 1B actions—Lidocaine is the prototype 1B drug and is used exclusively by the IV or IM routes. **Mexiletine** is an orally active 1B agent. These drugs selectively affect ischemic or depolarized Purkinje and ventricular tissue and have little effect on atrial tissue; the drugs reduce AP duration in some cells, but because they slow recovery of sodium channels from inactivation, they do not shorten (and may even prolong) the effective refractory period. Because these agents have little effect on normal cardiac cells, they have little effect on the ECG (Table 14–1). **Phenytoin,** an anticonvulsant and not a true local anesthetic, is sometimes classified with the group 1B antiarrhythmic agents because it can be used to reverse digitalis-induced

TABLE 14–1 Properties of the prototype antiarrhythmic drugs.

Drug	Group	PR Interval	QRS Duration	QT Interval
Procainamide, disopyramide, quinidine	1A	↑ or ↓[a]	↑↑	↑↑
Lidocaine, mexiletine	1B	—	—[b]	—, ↓[c]
Flecainide	1C	↑ (slight)	↑↑	—
Propranolol, esmolol	2	↑↑	—	—
Amiodarone	3, 1A, 2, 4	↑	↑↑	↑↑↑↑
Ibutilide, dofetilide	3	—	—	↑↑↑
Sotalol	3, 2	↑↑	—	↑↑↑
Verapamil	4	↑↑	—	—
Adenosine	Misc	↑↑↑	—	—

[a]PR interval may decrease owing to antimuscarinic action or increase owing to channel-blocking action.

[b]Lidocaine, mexiletine, and some other group 1B drugs slow conduction through ischemic, depolarized ventricular cells but not in normal tissue.

[c]Decreased QT in Purkinje cells.

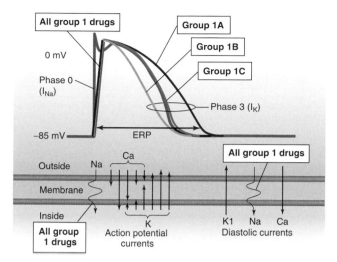

FIGURE 14–4 Schematic diagram of the effects of group 1 agents. Note that all group 1 drugs reduce both phase 0 and phase 4 sodium currents (*wavy lines*) in susceptible cells. Group 1A drugs also reduce phase 3 potassium current (I_K) and prolong the action potential (AP) duration. This results in significant prolongation of the effective refractory period (ERP). Group 1B and group 1C drugs have different (or no) effects on potassium current and thus shorten or have no effect on the AP duration. However, all group 1 drugs prolong the ERP by slowing recovery of sodium channels from inactivation.

arrhythmias. It resembles lidocaine in lacking significant effects on the normal ECG.

3. Drugs with group 1C action—Flecainide is the prototype drug with group 1C actions. Other members of this group are used outside the United States and may be available in this country in special circumstances. These drugs have no effect on ventricular AP duration or the QT interval. They are powerful depressants of sodium current, however, and can markedly slow conduction velocity in atrial and ventricular cells. They increase the QRS duration of the ECG.

B. Pharmacokinetics, Clinical Uses, and Toxicities

Pharmacokinetics of the major drugs are listed in the Drug Summary Table at the end of the chapter.

1. Group 1A drugs—Procainamide can be used in all types of arrhythmias: atrial and ventricular arrhythmias are most responsive. **Quinidine** and **disopyramide** have similar effects but are used much less frequently. Procainamide is also commonly used in arrhythmias during the acute phase of myocardial infarction.

Procainamide may cause hypotension and a reversible syndrome similar to lupus erythematosus. Quinidine causes cinchonism (headache, vertigo, tinnitus); cardiac depression; gastrointestinal upset; and autoimmune reactions (eg, thrombocytopenic

purpura). As noted in Chapter 13, quinidine reduces the clearance of digoxin and may increase the serum concentration of the glycoside significantly. Disopyramide has marked antimuscarinic effects and may precipitate heart failure. All group 1A drugs may precipitate new arrhythmias. Torsades de pointes is particularly associated with quinidine and other drugs that prolong AP duration (except **amiodarone**). The toxicities of amiodarone are discussed in the following text.

Hyperkalemia usually exacerbates the cardiac toxicity of group 1 drugs. Treatment of overdose with these agents is often carried out with sodium lactate (to reverse drug-induced arrhythmias) and pressor sympathomimetics (to reverse drug-induced hypotension) if indicated.

2. Group 1B drugs—Lidocaine is useful in acute ischemic ventricular arrhythmias, for example, after myocardial infarction. Atrial arrhythmias are not responsive unless caused by digitalis. **Mexiletine** has similar actions and is given orally for chronic arrhythmias and for certain types of neuropathic pain. Lidocaine is usually given intravenously, but intramuscular administration is also possible. It is never given orally because it has a very high first-pass effect and its metabolites are potentially cardiotoxic.

Lidocaine and mexiletine occasionally cause typical local anesthetic toxicity (ie, central nervous system [CNS] stimulation, including convulsions); cardiovascular depression (usually minor); and allergy (usually rashes but may extend to anaphylaxis). These drugs may also precipitate arrhythmias, but this is much less common than with group 1A drugs. Hyperkalemia increases cardiac toxicity.

3. Group 1C drugs—Flecainide is effective in both atrial and ventricular arrhythmias but is approved only for refractory ventricular tachycardias and for certain intractable supraventricular arrhythmias. Flecainide and its congeners are more likely than other antiarrhythmic drugs to exacerbate or precipitate arrhythmias (*proarrhythmic* effect). This toxicity was dramatically demonstrated by the Cardiac Arrhythmia Suppression Trial (CAST), a large clinical trial of the prophylactic use of group 1C drugs in myocardial infarction survivors. The trial results showed that group 1C drugs caused greater mortality than placebo. For this reason, the group 1C drugs are now restricted to use in persistent arrhythmias that fail to respond to other drugs. Group 1C drugs also cause local anesthetic-like CNS toxicity. Hyperkalemia increases the cardiac toxicity of these agents.

GROUP 2 ANTIARRHYTHMICS (BETA BLOCKERS)

A. Prototypes, Mechanisms, and Effects

Beta blockers are discussed in more detail in Chapter 10. **Propranolol** and **esmolol** are prototypic antiarrhythmic β blockers. Their mechanism in arrhythmias is primarily cardiac β-adrenoceptor blockade and reduction in cAMP, which results in the reduction of both sodium and calcium currents and the suppression of abnormal pacemakers. The AV node is particularly sensitive to β blockers and the PR interval is usually prolonged by group 2 drugs (Table 14–1). Under some conditions, these drugs may have some direct local anesthetic (sodium channel-blocking) effect in the heart, but this is probably rare at the concentrations achieved clinically. **Sotalol** and **amiodarone**, generally classified as group 3 drugs, also have group 2 β-blocking effects.

B. Clinical Uses and Toxicities

Esmolol, a very short-acting β blocker for intravenous administration, is used exclusively in acute arrhythmias. Propranolol, metoprolol, and timolol are commonly used as prophylactic drugs in patients who have had a myocardial infarction.

The toxicities of β blockers are the same in patients with arrhythmias as in patients with other conditions (Chapter 10 and Drug Summary Table). While patients with arrhythmias are often more prone to β-blocker-induced depression of cardiac output than are patients with normal hearts, it should be noted that judicious use of these drugs reduces progression of chronic heart failure (Chapter 13) and reduces the incidence of potentially fatal arrhythmias in this condition.

> ### SKILL KEEPER: CHARACTERISTICS OF β BLOCKERS (SEE CHAPTER 10)
>
> *Describe the important subgroups of β blockers and their major pharmacokinetic and pharmacodynamic features.* The Skill Keeper Answer appears at the end of the chapter.

GROUP 3 ANTIARRHYTHMICS (POTASSIUM I_K CHANNEL BLOCKERS)

A. Prototypes, Mechanisms, and Effects

Dofetilide and **ibutilide** are typical group 3 drugs. **Sotalol** is a chiral compound (ie, it has 2 optical isomers). One isomer is an effective β blocker, and both isomers contribute to the antiarrhythmic action. The clinical preparation contains both isomers. **Amiodarone** is usually classified as a group 3 drug because it blocks the same K channels and markedly prolongs AP duration as well as blocking sodium channels. **Dronedarone** is a new drug, similar to amiodarone but less efficacious and less toxic.

The hallmark of group 3 drugs is prolongation of the AP duration. This AP prolongation is caused by blockade of I_K potassium channels, chiefly I_{Kr}, that are responsible for the repolarization of the AP (Figure 14–5). AP prolongation results in an increase in effective refractory period and reduces the ability of the heart to respond to rapid tachycardias. Sotalol, ibutilide, dofetilide, and amiodarone (and group 1A drugs; see prior discussion) produce this effect on most cardiac cells; the action of these drugs is, therefore, apparent in the ECG as an increase in QT interval (Table 14–1).

B. Clinical Uses and Toxicities

See the Drug Summary Table.

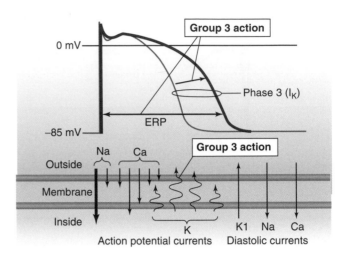

FIGURE 14–5 Schematic diagram of the effects of group 3 agents. All group 3 drugs prolong the AP duration in susceptible cardiac cells by reducing the outward (repolarizing) phase 3 potassium current (I_K, *wavy lines*). The main effect is to prolong the effective refractory period (ERP). Note that the phase 4 diastolic potassium current (I_{K1}) is not affected by these drugs.

C. Amiodarone: A Special Case

Amiodarone is useful in most types of arrhythmias and is considered the most efficacious of all antiarrhythmic drugs. This may be because it has a broad spectrum: It blocks sodium, calcium, and potassium channels and β adrenoceptors. Because of its toxicities, however, amiodarone is approved for use mainly in arrhythmias that are resistant to other drugs. Nevertheless, it is used very extensively, off label, in a wide variety of arrhythmias because of its superior efficacy.

Amiodarone causes microcrystalline deposits in the cornea and skin, thyroid dysfunction (hyper- or hypothyroidism), paresthesias, tremor, and pulmonary fibrosis. Amiodarone rarely causes new arrhythmias, perhaps because it blocks calcium channels and β receptors as well as sodium and potassium channels. **Dronedarone**, an amiodarone analog that may be less toxic, is also approved. Like amiodarone, it acts on sodium, potassium, and calcium channels, but at present it is approved only for the treatment of atrial fibrillation or flutter.

GROUP 4 ANTIARRHYTHMICS (CALCIUM L-TYPE CHANNEL BLOCKERS)

A. Prototypes, Mechanisms, and Effects

Verapamil is the prototype. **Diltiazem** is also an effective antiarrhythmic drug. Nifedipine and the other dihydropyridines are *not* useful as antiarrhythmics, probably because they decrease arterial pressure enough to evoke a compensatory sympathetic discharge to the heart. The latter effect facilitates rather than suppresses arrhythmias.

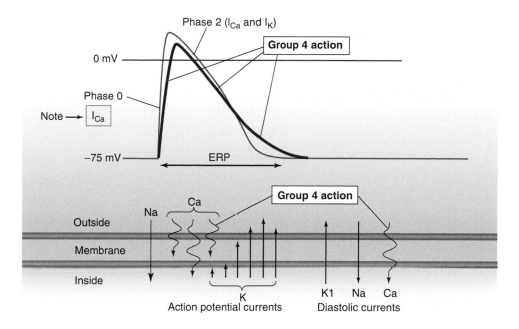

FIGURE 14–6 Schematic diagram of the effects of group 4 drugs in a calcium-dependent cardiac cell in the AV node (note that the AP upstroke in this figure is due mainly to calcium current). Group 4 drugs reduce inward calcium current during the AP and during phase 4 (*wavy lines*). As a result, conduction velocity is slowed in the AV node and refractoriness is prolonged. Pacemaker depolarization during phase 4 is slowed as well if caused by excessive calcium current. ERP, effective refractory period.

Verapamil and diltiazem are effective in arrhythmias that must traverse calcium-dependent cardiac tissue such as the AV node. These agents cause a state- and use-dependent selective depression of calcium current (Figure 14–6). AV conduction velocity is decreased, and effective refractory period and PR interval are increased by these drugs (Table 14–1).

B. Clinical Use and Toxicities

Calcium channel blockers are effective for converting AV nodal reentry (also known as nodal tachycardia) to normal sinus rhythm. Their major use is in the prevention of these nodal arrhythmias in patients prone to recurrence. These drugs are orally active; and also available for parenteral use (see Drug Summary Table). The most important toxicity of these drugs is excessive depression of cardiac contractility, AV conduction, and blood pressure. These agents should be avoided in ventricular tachycardias. See Chapter 12 for additional discussion of toxicity. Amiodarone has moderate calcium channel-blocking activity.

MISCELLANEOUS ANTIARRHYTHMIC DRUGS

A. Adenosine

Adenosine is a normal component of the body, but when given in high doses (6–12 mg) as an intravenous bolus, the drug markedly slows or completely blocks conduction in the atrioventricular node (Table 14–1), probably by hyperpolarizing this tissue (through increased I_{K1}) and by reducing calcium current.

Adenosine is extremely effective in abolishing AV nodal arrhythmia, and because of its very low toxicity it has become the drug of choice for this arrhythmia. Adenosine has an extremely short duration of action (about 15 s). Toxicity includes flushing and hypotension, but because of their short duration these effects do not limit the use of the drug. Transient chest pain and dyspnea (probably due to bronchoconstriction) may also occur.

B. Potassium Ion

Potassium depresses ectopic pacemakers, including those caused by digitalis toxicity. Hypokalemia is associated with an increased incidence of arrhythmias, especially in patients receiving digitalis. Conversely, excessive potassium levels depress conduction and can cause reentry arrhythmias. Therefore, when treating arrhythmias, serum potassium should be measured and normalized if abnormal.

C. Magnesium Ion

Magnesium appears to have similar depressant effects as potassium on digitalis-induced arrhythmias. Magnesium also appears to be effective in some cases of torsades de pointes arrhythmia.

NONPHARMACOLOGIC TREATMENT OF ARRHYTHMIAS

It should be noted that electrical methods of treatment of arrhythmias have become very important. These methods include (1) external defibrillation, (2) implanted defibrillators, (3) implanted pacemakers, and (4) radiofrequency ablation of arrhythmogenic foci via a catheter.

QUESTIONS

Questions 1–2. A 76-year-old patient with rheumatoid arthritis and chronic heart disease is being considered for treatment with procainamide. She is already receiving digoxin, hydrochlorothiazide, and potassium supplements for her cardiac condition.

1. In deciding on a treatment regimen with procainamide for this patient, which of the following statements is *most* correct?
   (A) A possible drug interaction with digoxin suggests that digoxin blood levels should be obtained before and after starting procainamide
   (B) Hyperkalemia should be avoided to reduce the likelihood of procainamide toxicity
   (C) Procainamide cannot be used if the patient has asthma because it has a β-blocking effect
   (D) Procainamide has a duration of action of 36–40 h
   (E) Procainamide is not active by the oral route

2. If this patient should take an overdose and manifest severe acute procainamide toxicity with markedly prolonged QRS, which of the following should be given immediately?
   (A) A calcium chelator such as EDTA
   (B) Digitalis
   (C) Nitroprusside
   (D) Potassium chloride
   (E) Sodium lactate

3. A 57-year-old man is admitted to the emergency department with an irregular heart rate. The ECG shows an inferior myocardial infarction and ventricular tachycardia. Lidocaine is ordered. When used as an antiarrhythmic drug, lidocaine typically
   (A) Increases action potential duration
   (B) Increases contractility
   (C) Increases PR interval
   (D) Reduces abnormal automaticity
   (E) Reduces resting potential

4. A 36-year-old woman with a history of poorly controlled thyrotoxicosis has recurrent episodes of tachycardia with severe shortness of breath. When she is admitted to the emergency department with one of these episodes, which of the following drugs would be *most* suitable?
   (A) Amiodarone
   (B) Disopyramide
   (C) Esmolol
   (D) Quinidine
   (E) Verapamil

5. A 16-year-old girl has paroxysmal attacks of rapid heart rate with palpitations and shortness of breath. These episodes occasionally terminate spontaneously but often require a visit to the emergency department of the local hospital. Her ECG during these episodes reveals an AV nodal tachycardia. The antiarrhythmic of choice in most cases of acute AV nodal tachycardia is
   (A) Adenosine
   (B) Amiodarone
   (C) Flecainide
   (D) Propranolol
   (E) Verapamil

6. A 55-year-old man is admitted to the emergency department and is found to have an abnormal ECG. Overdose of an antiarrhythmic drug is considered. Which of the following drugs is correctly paired with its ECG effects?
   (A) Quinidine: Increased PR and decreased QT intervals
   (B) Flecainide: Increased PR, QRS, and QT intervals
   (C) Verapamil: Increased PR interval
   (D) Lidocaine: Decreased QRS and PR interval
   (E) Metoprolol: Increased QRS duration

7. A 60-year-old man comes to the emergency department with severe chest pain. ECG reveals ventricular tachycardia with occasional normal sinus beats, and ST-segment changes suggestive of ischemia. A diagnosis of myocardial infarction is made, and the man is admitted to the cardiac intensive care unit. His arrhythmia should be treated immediately with
   (A) Adenosine
   (B) Digoxin
   (C) Lidocaine
   (D) Quinidine
   (E) Verapamil

8. Which of the following drugs slows conduction through the AV node and has its primary action directly on L-type calcium channels?
   (A) Adenosine
   (B) Amiodarone
   (C) Diltiazem
   (D) Esmolol
   (E) Flecainide
   (F) Lidocaine
   (G) Mexiletine
   (H) Procainamide
   (I) Quinidine

9. When working in outlying fields, this 62-year-old farmer is away from his house for 12–14 h at a time. He has an arrhythmia that requires chronic therapy. Which of the following has the longest half-life of all antiarrhythmic drugs?
   (A) Adenosine
   (B) Amiodarone
   (C) Disopyramide
   (D) Esmolol
   (E) Flecainide
   (F) Lidocaine
   (G) Mexiletine
   (H) Procainamide
   (I) Quinidine
   (J) Verapamil

10. A drug was tested in the electrophysiology laboratory to determine its effects on the cardiac action potential in ventricular cells. The results are shown in the diagram.

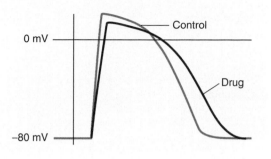

Which of the following drugs does this agent most resemble?
(A) Adenosine
(B) Flecainide
(C) Mexiletine
(D) Procainamide
(E) Verapamil

ANSWERS

1. Hyperkalemia facilitates procainamide toxicity. Procainamide is active by the oral route and has a duration of action of 2–4 h (in the prompt-release form). Procainamide has no significant documented interaction with digoxin and little or no β-blocking action. The answer is **B.**

2. The most effective therapy for procainamide toxicity appears to be concentrated sodium lactate. This drug may (1) increase sodium current by increasing the ionic gradient and (2) reduce drug-receptor binding by alkalinizing the tissue. The answer is **E.**

3. Lidocaine reduces automaticity in the ventricles; the drug does not alter resting potential or AP duration and does not increase contractility. The answer is **D.**

4. Beta blockers are the most effective agents in acute thyrotoxic arrhythmias. Esmolol is a parenteral, rapid-acting β blocker. The answer is **C.**

5. Calcium channel blockers are effective in supraventricular AV nodal tachycardias. However, adenosine is just as effective in most acute nodal tachycardias and is less toxic because of its extremely short duration of action. The answer is **A.**

6. All the associations listed are incorrect except verapamil (see Table 14–1). This group 4 drug increases PR interval and has little effect on the other ECG variables. The answer is **C.**

7. Lidocaine has limited applications as an antiarrhythmic drug, but emergency treatment of myocardial infarction arrhythmias is one of the most important. Lidocaine is also useful in digoxin-induced arrhythmias. After recovery from the acute phase of a myocardial infarction, β blockers are used for 2 yrs or more to prevent sudden death arrhythmias. The answer is **C.**

8. Diltiazem is the calcium channel blocker in this list. (Beta blockers also slow AV conduction but have much smaller effects on calcium channels.) The answer is **C.**

9. Amiodarone has the longest half-life of all the antiarrhythmics (weeks). The answer is **B.**

10. The drug effect shown in the diagram includes slowing of the upstroke of the AP and prolongation of repolarization or AP duration. This is most typical of group 1A drugs. The answer is **D,** procainamide.

CHECKLIST

When you complete this chapter, you should be able to:

❏ Describe the distinguishing electrophysiologic and ECG effects of the 4 major groups of antiarrhythmic drugs and adenosine.

❏ List 2 or 3 of the most important drugs in each of the 4 groups.

❏ List the major toxicities of those drugs.

❏ Describe the mechanism of selective depression by local anesthetic antiarrhythmic agents.

❏ Explain how hyperkalemia, hypokalemia, or an antiarrhythmic drug can cause an arrhythmia.

DRUG SUMMARY TABLE: Antiarrhythmic Drugs

Subclass	Mechanism of Action	Clinical Applications	Pharmacokinetics	Toxicities, Interactions
Group 1A				
Procainamide	Use- and state-dependent block of I_{Na} channels • some block of I_K channels. Slowed conduction velocity and pacemaker activity • prolonged action potential duration and refractory period	Atrial and ventricular arrhythmias, especially after myocardial infarction	Oral and parenteral • oral slow-release forms available Duration: 2-3 h	Increased arrhythmias, hypotension, lupus-like syndrome
Disopyramide: similar to procainamide but longer duration of action; toxicity includes antimuscarinic effects and heart failure				
Quinidine: similar to procainamide but toxicity includes cinchonism (tinnitus, headache, gastrointestinal disturbance) and thrombocytopenia				
Group 1B				
Lidocaine	Highly selective use- and state-dependent I_{Na} block; minimal effect in normal tissue; no effect on I_K	Ventricular arrhythmias post-myocardial infarction and digitalis-induced arrhythmias	IV and IM Duration: 1-2 h	Central nervous system (CNS) sedation or excitation
Mexiletine: similar to lidocaine but oral activity and longer duration of action				
Group 1C				
Flecainide	Selective use- and state-dependent block of I_{Na} • slowed conduction velocity and pacemaker activity	Refractory arrhythmias	Oral Duration: 20 h	Increased arrhythmias • CNS excitation
Group 2				
Propranolol	Block of β receptors; slowed pacemaker activity	Postmyocardial infarction as prophylaxis against sudden death ventricular fibrillation; thyrotoxicosis	Oral, parenteral Duration: 4-6 h	Bronchospasm • cardiac depression, atrioventricular (AV) block, hypotension (see Chapter 10)
Metoprolol: similar to propranolol but β₁-selective				
Esmolol: selective β₁-receptor blockade; IV only, 10-min duration. Used in perioperative and thyrotoxicosis arrhythmias				

(Continued)

DRUG SUMMARY TABLE: Antiarrhythmic Drugs (*Continued*)

Subclass	Mechanism of Action	Clinical Applications	Pharmacokinetics	Toxicities, Interactions
Group 3				
Amiodarone	Strong I_K block produces marked prolongation of action potential and refractory period. Group 1 activity slows conduction velocity • groups 2 and 4 activity confer additional antiarrhythmic activity	Refractory arrhythmias • used off-label in many arrhythmias (broad spectrum of therapeutic action)	Oral, parenteral Half-life and duration of action: 1–10 wk	Thyroid abnormalities, deposits in skin and cornea, pulmonary fibrosis, optic neuritis • torsades is rare with amiodarone
Sotalol	I_K block and β-adrenoceptor block	Ventricular arrhythmias and atrial fibrillation	Oral Duration: 7 h	Dose-related torsades de pointes • cardiac depression
Ibutilide	Selective I_K block • prolonged action potential and QT interval	Treatment of acute atrial fibrillation	Ibutilide is IV only Duration: 6 h	Torsades de pointes
Dofetilide	Like ibutilide	Treatment and prophylaxis of atrial fibrillation	Oral Duration: 7 h	Torsades de pointes
Group 4				
Verapamil	State- and use-dependent I_{Ca} block slows conduction in AV node and pacemaker activity • PR interval prolongation	AV nodal arrhythmias, especially in prophylaxis	Oral, parenteral Duration: 7 h	Cardiac depression • constipation, hypotension
Diltiazem	Like verapamil	Rate control in atrial fibrillation	Oral, parenteral Duration: 6 h	Like verapamil
Dihydropyridines: calcium channel blockers but not useful in arrhythmias; sometimes precipitate them				
Miscellaneous				
Adenosine	Increase in diastolic I_K of AV node that causes marked hyperpolarization and conduction block • reduced I_{Ca}	Acute nodal tachycardias	IV only Duration: 10–15 s	Flushing, bronchospasm, chest pain, headache
Potassium ion	Increase in all K currents, decreased automaticity, decreased digitalis toxicity	Digitalis toxicity and other arrhythmias if serum K is low	Oral or IV	Both hypokalemia and hyperkalemia are associated with arrhythmogenesis. Severe hyperkalemia causes cardiac arrest
Magnesium ion	Poorly understood, possible increase in Na^+/K^+ ATPase activity	Digitalis arrhythmias and other arrhythmias if serum Mg is low	IV	Muscle weakness • severe hypermagnesemia can cause respiratory paralysis

Diuretic Agents

Each segment of the nephron—proximal convoluted tubule (PCT), thick ascending limb of the loop of Henle (TAL), distal convoluted tubule (DCT), and cortical collecting tubule (CCT)—has a different mechanism for reabsorbing sodium and other ions. The subgroups of the sodium-excreting diuretics are based on these sites and processes in the nephron. Several other drugs alter water excretion predominantly. The effects of the diuretic agents are predictable from knowledge of the function of the segment of the nephron in which they act.

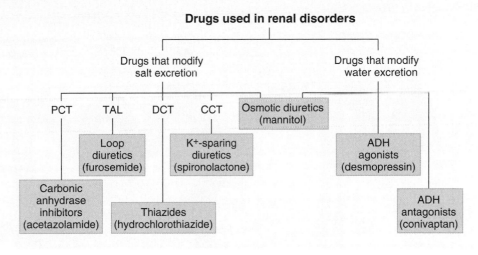

RENAL TRANSPORT MECHANISMS & DIURETIC DRUG GROUPS

The kidney filters plasma water and solutes at the glomerulus at a very high rate (180 L/day) and must recover a significant percentage of most of these substances before excretion in the urine. The major transport mechanisms for the recovery of ions and water in the various segments of the nephron are shown in Figure 15–1. Because the mechanisms for reabsorption of salt and water differ in each of the 4 major tubular segments, the diuretics acting in these segments have differing mechanisms of action. Most diuretics act from the luminal side of the membrane. An exception is the aldosterone receptor antagonist group (eg, spironolactone and eplerenone); these drugs enter the collecting tubule cell from the basolateral side and bind to the cytoplasmic aldosterone receptor.

PROXIMAL CONVOLUTED TUBULE (PCT)

This segment carries out isosmotic reabsorption of amino acids, glucose, and numerous cations. It is also the major site for sodium chloride and sodium bicarbonate reabsorption. The proximal tubule is responsible for 60–70% of the total reabsorption of sodium. No currently available drug directly acts on NaCl reabsorption in the PCT. The mechanism for bicarbonate reabsorption is shown in Figure 15–2. Bicarbonate itself is poorly reabsorbed through the luminal membrane, but conversion of bicarbonate to carbon dioxide via carbonic acid permits rapid reabsorption of the carbon dioxide. Bicarbonate can then be regenerated from carbon dioxide within the tubular cell and transported into the interstitium. Sodium is separately reabsorbed from the lumen in exchange for hydrogen ions (NHE3 transporter) and transported

High-Yield Terms to Learn

Bicarbonate diuretic	A diuretic that selectively increases sodium bicarbonate excretion. Example: a carbonic anhydrase inhibitor
Diluting segment	A segment of the nephron that removes solute without water; the thick ascending limb and the distal convoluted tubule are active salt-absorbing segments that are not permeable by water
Hyperchloremic metabolic acidosis	A shift in body electrolyte and pH balance involving elevated chloride, diminished bicarbonate concentration, and a decrease in pH in the blood. Typical result of bicarbonate diuresis
Hypokalemic metabolic alkalosis	A shift in body electrolyte balance and pH involving a decrease in serum potassium and an increase in blood pH. Typical result of loop and thiazide diuretic actions
Nephrogenic diabetes insipidus	Loss of urine-concentrating ability in the kidney caused by lack of responsiveness to antidiuretic hormone (ADH is normal or high)
Pituitary diabetes insipidus	Loss of urine-concentrating ability in the kidney caused by lack of antidiuretic hormone (ADH is low or absent)
Potassium-sparing diuretic	A diuretic that reduces the exchange of potassium for sodium in the collecting tubule; a drug that increases sodium and reduces potassium excretion. Example: aldosterone antagonists
Uricosuric diuretic	A diuretic that increases uric acid excretion, usually by inhibiting uric acid reabsorption in the proximal tubule. Example: ethacrynic acid

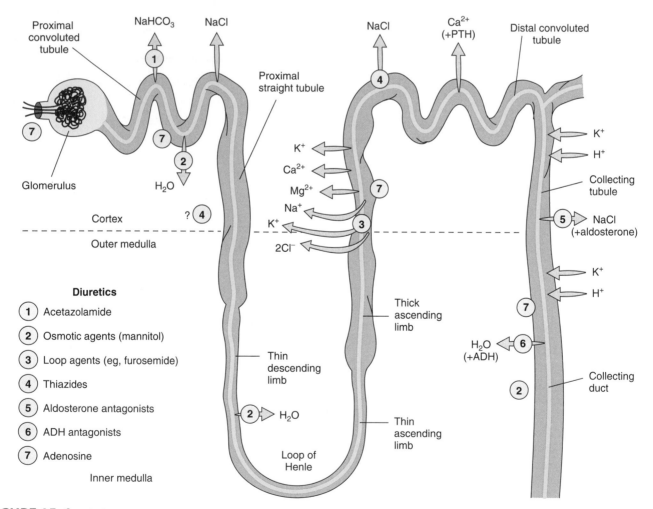

FIGURE 15–1 Tubule transport systems in the kidney and sites of action of diuretics. Circles with arrows denote known ion cotransporters that are targets of the diuretics indicated by the numerals. Question marks denote preliminary or incompletely documented suggestions for the location of certain drug effects. (Modified and reproduced, with permission, from Katzung BG, editor: *Basic & Clinical Pharmacology,* 12th ed. McGraw-Hill, 2012: Fig. 15–1.)

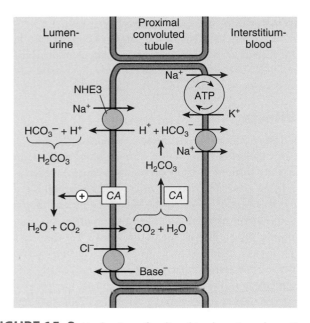

FIGURE 15–2 Mechanism of sodium bicarbonate reabsorption in the proximal tubule cell. NHE3, Na^+/H^+ exchanger 3; CA, carbonic anhydrase. (Reproduced, with permission, from Katzung BG, editor: *Basic & Clinical Pharmacology*, 12th ed. McGraw-Hill, 2012: Fig. 15–2.)

into the interstitial space by the sodium-potassium pump (Na^+/K^+ ATPase). Carbonic anhydrase, the enzyme required for the bicarbonate reabsorption process on the brush border and in the cytoplasm, is the target of carbonic anhydrase inhibitor drugs. Active secretion and reabsorption of weak acids and bases also occurs in the proximal tubule. Most weak acid transport occurs in the straight S_2 segment, distal to the convoluted part. Uric acid transport is especially important and is targeted by some of the drugs used in treating gout (Chapter 36). Weak bases are transported in the S_1 and S_2 segments.

CARBONIC ANHYDRASE INHIBITORS

A. Prototypes and Mechanism of Action

Acetazolamide is the prototypic agent. These diuretics are sulfonamide derivatives. The mechanism of action is inhibition of carbonic anhydrase in the brush border and cytoplasm (Figure 15–2). Carbonic anhydrase is also found in other tissues and plays an important role in the secretion of cerebrospinal fluid and aqueous humor. Acetazolamide inhibits carbonic anhydrase in all tissues of the body.

B. Effects

The major renal effect is bicarbonate diuresis (ie, sodium bicarbonate is excreted); body bicarbonate is depleted, and metabolic acidosis results. As increased sodium is presented to the cortical collecting tubule, some of the excess sodium is reabsorbed and potassium is secreted, resulting in significant potassium wasting (Table 15–1). As a result of bicarbonate depletion, sodium bicarbonate excretion slows—even with continued diuretic administration—and the diuresis is self-limiting within 2–3 days. Secretion of bicarbonate into aqueous humor by the ciliary epithelium in the eye and into the cerebrospinal fluid by the choroid plexus is reduced. In the eye, a useful reduction in intraocular pressure can be achieved. In the central nervous system (CNS), acidosis of the cerebrospinal fluid results in hyperventilation, which can protect against high-altitude sickness. The ocular and cerebrospinal fluid effects are not self-limiting.

C. Clinical Uses and Toxicity

Acetazolamide is used parenterally in the treatment of severe acute glaucoma (see Table 10–3). Acetazolamide can also be administered orally, but topical analogs are available (**dorzolamide**, **brinzolamide**) for chronic use in the eye. Acetazolamide is also used to prevent acute mountain (high-altitude) sickness. It is used for the diuretic effect only if edema is accompanied by significant metabolic alkalosis.

Drowsiness and paresthesia toxicities are commonly reported after oral therapy. Cross-allergenicity between these and all other sulfonamide derivatives (other sulfonamide diuretics, hypoglycemic agents, antibacterial sulfonamides) is uncommon but can occur. Alkalinization of the urine by these drugs may cause precipitation of calcium salts and formation of renal stones. Renal potassium wasting may be marked. Patients with hepatic impairment often excrete large amounts of ammonia in the urine in the form of ammonium ion. If they are given acetazolamide, alkalinization

TABLE 15–1 Electrolyte changes produced by diuretic drugs.

Group	Amount in Urine			Body pH
	NaCl	NaHCO₃	K⁺	
Carbonic anhydrase inhibitors	↑[a]	↑↑↑[a]	↑[a]	Acidosis[b]
Loop diuretics	↑↑↑↑	—	↑	Alkalosis
Thiazides	↑↑	↑,—	↑	Alkalosis
K⁺-sparing diuretics	↑	—	↓	Acidosis

[a]Self-limited (2–3 days).
[b]Not self-limited.

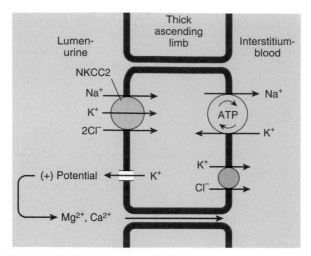

FIGURE 15–3 Mechanism of sodium, potassium, and chloride reabsorption by the transporter NKCC2 in the thick ascending limb of the loop of Henle. Note that pumping of potassium into the cell from both the lumen and the interstitium would result in unphysiologically high intracellular K⁺ concentration. This is avoided by movement of K⁺ down its concentration gradient back into the lumen, carrying with it excess positive charge. This positive charge drives the reabsorption of calcium and magnesium. (Reproduced, with permission, from Katzung BG, editor: *Basic & Clinical Pharmacology*, 12th ed. McGraw-Hill, 2012: Fig. 15–3.)

of the urine prevents conversion of ammonia to ammonium ion. As a result, they may develop hepatic encephalopathy because of increased ammonia reabsorption and hyperammonemia.

THICK ASCENDING LIMB OF THE LOOP OF HENLE (TAL)

This segment pumps sodium, potassium, and chloride out of the lumen into the interstitium of the kidney. It is also a major site of calcium and magnesium reabsorption, as shown in Figure 15–3. Reabsorption of sodium, potassium, and chloride are all accomplished by a Na⁺/K⁺/2Cl⁻ carrier (NKCC2), which is the target of the **loop diuretics.** This cotransporter provides part of the concentration gradient for the countercurrent concentrating mechanism in the kidney and is responsible for the reabsorption of 20–30% of the sodium filtered at the glomerulus. Because potassium is pumped into the cell from both the luminal and basal sides, an escape route must be provided; this occurs into the lumen via a potassium-selective channel. Because the potassium diffusing through these channels is not accompanied by an anion, a net positive charge is set up in the lumen. This positive potential drives the reabsorption of calcium and magnesium.

LOOP DIURETICS

A. Prototypes and Mechanism of Action

Furosemide is the prototypical loop agent. Furosemide, **bumetanide,** and **torsemide** are sulfonamide derivatives.

Ethacrynic acid is a phenoxyacetic acid derivative; it is not a sulfonamide but acts by the same mechanism. Loop diuretics inhibit the cotransport of sodium, potassium, and chloride (NKCC2, Figure 15–3). The loop diuretics are relatively short-acting (diuresis usually occurs over a 4-h period following a dose).

B. Effects

A full dose of a loop diuretic produces a massive sodium chloride diuresis if glomerular filtration is normal; blood volume may be significantly reduced. If tissue perfusion is adequate, edema fluid is rapidly excreted. The diluting ability of the nephron is reduced because the loop of Henle is the site of significant dilution of urine. Inhibition of the Na⁺/K⁺/2Cl⁻ transporter also results in loss of the lumen-positive potential, which reduces reabsorption of divalent cations as well. As a result, calcium excretion is significantly increased. Ethacrynic acid is a moderately effective uricosuric drug if blood volume is maintained. The presentation of large amounts of sodium to the collecting tubule may result in significant potassium wasting and excretion of protons; hypokalemic alkalosis may result (Table 15–1). Loop diuretics also reduce pulmonary vascular pressures; the mechanism is not known.

Prostaglandins are important in maintaining glomerular filtration. When synthesis of prostaglandins is inhibited, for example, by nonsteroidal anti-inflammatory drugs (Chapter 36), the efficacy of most diuretics decreases.

C. Clinical Use and Toxicities

The major application of loop diuretics is in the treatment of edematous states (eg, heart failure, ascites, and acute pulmonary edema). They are sometimes used in hypertension if response to thiazides is inadequate, but the short duration of action of loop diuretics is a disadvantage in this condition. A less common but important application is in the treatment of severe hypercalcemia. This life-threatening condition can often be managed with large doses of furosemide together with parenteral volume and electrolyte (sodium and potassium chloride) replacement. It should be noted that diuresis *without* volume replacement results in hemoconcentration; serum calcium concentration then will not diminish and may even increase further.

Loop diuretics usually induce hypokalemic metabolic alkalosis (Table 15–1). Because large amounts of sodium are presented to the collecting tubules, potassium wasting may be severe. Because they are so efficacious, loop diuretics can cause hypovolemia and cardiovascular complications. Ototoxicity is an important toxic effect of the loop agents. The sulfonamides in this group may rarely cause typical sulfonamide allergy.

DISTAL CONVOLUTED TUBULE (DCT)

This segment actively pumps sodium and chloride out of the lumen of the nephron via the Na⁺/Cl⁻ carrier (NCC) shown in Figure 15–4. This cotransporter is the target of the **thiazide diuretics.** The distal convoluted tubule is responsible for approximately 5–8% of sodium reabsorption. Calcium is also reabsorbed

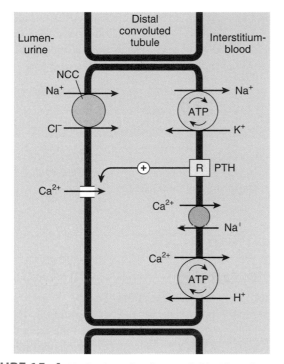

FIGURE 15–4 Mechanism of sodium and chloride reabsorption by the transporter NCC in the distal convoluted tubule. A separate reabsorptive mechanism, modulated by parathyroid hormone (PTH), is present for movement of calcium into the cell from the urine. This calcium must be transported via the sodium-calcium exchanger back into the blood. R, PTH receptor. (Reproduced, with permission, from Katzung BG, editor: *Basic & Clinical Pharmacology*, 12th ed. McGraw-Hill, 2012: Fig. 15–4.)

in this segment under the control of parathyroid hormone (PTH). Removal of the reabsorbed calcium back into the blood requires the sodium-calcium exchange process discussed in Chapter 13.

THIAZIDE DIURETICS

A. Prototypes and Mechanism of Action

Hydrochlorothiazide, the prototypical agent, and all the other members of this group are sulfonamide derivatives. A few derivatives that lack the typical thiazide ring in their structure nevertheless have effects identical with those of thiazides and are therefore considered thiazide-like. The major action of thiazides is to inhibit sodium chloride transport in the early segment of the distal convoluted tubule (NCC, Figure 15–4). Thiazides are active by the oral route and have a duration of action of 6–12 h, considerably longer than most loop diuretics.

B. Effects

In full doses, thiazides produce moderate but sustained sodium and chloride diuresis. Hypokalemic metabolic alkalosis may occur (Table 15–1). Reduction in the transport of sodium from the lumen into the tubular cell reduces intracellular sodium and promotes sodium-calcium exchange at the basolateral membrane.

As a result, reabsorption of calcium from the urine is increased, and urine calcium content is decreased—the *opposite* of the effect of loop diuretics. Because they act in a diluting segment of the nephron, thiazides may reduce the excretion of water and cause dilutional hyponatremia. Thiazides also reduce blood pressure, and the maximal pressure-lowering effect occurs at doses lower than the maximal diuretic doses (see Chapter 11). Inhibition of renal prostaglandin synthesis reduces the efficacy of the thiazides. When a thiazide is used with a loop diuretic, a synergistic effect occurs with marked diuresis.

C. Clinical Use and Toxicities

The major application of thiazides is in hypertension, for which their long duration and moderate intensity of action are particularly useful. Chronic therapy of edematous conditions such as mild heart failure is another application, although loop diuretics are usually preferred. Chronic renal calcium stone formation can sometimes be controlled with thiazides because they reduce urine calcium concentration.

Massive sodium diuresis with hyponatremia is an uncommon but dangerous early toxicity of thiazides. Chronic therapy is often associated with potassium wasting, since an increased sodium load is presented to the collecting tubules; the cortical collecting tubules compensate by reabsorbing sodium and excreting potassium. Diabetic patients may have significant hyperglycemia. Serum uric acid and lipid levels are also increased in some persons. Thiazides are sulfonamides and share potential sulfonamide allergenicity.

CORTICAL COLLECTING TUBULE (CCT)

The final segment of the nephron is the last tubular site of sodium reabsorption and is controlled by aldosterone (Figure 15–5), a steroid hormone secreted by the adrenal cortex. This segment is responsible for reabsorbing 2–5% of the total filtered sodium under normal circumstances; more if aldosterone is increased. The reabsorption of sodium occurs via channels (ENaC, not a transporter) and is accompanied by loss of potassium or hydrogen ions. The collecting tubule is thus the primary site of acidification of the urine and the last site of potassium excretion. The aldosterone receptor and the sodium channels are sites of action of the **potassium-sparing diuretics.** Reabsorption of water occurs in the medullary collecting tubule under the control of antidiuretic hormone (ADH).

POTASSIUM-SPARING DIURETICS

A. Prototypes and Mechanism of Action

Spironolactone and **eplerenone** are steroid derivatives and act as pharmacologic antagonists of aldosterone in the collecting tubules. By combining with and blocking the intracellular aldosterone receptor, these drugs reduce the expression of genes that code for the epithelial sodium ion channel (ENaC) and Na$^+$/K$^+$ ATPase. **Amiloride** and **triamterene** act by blocking the

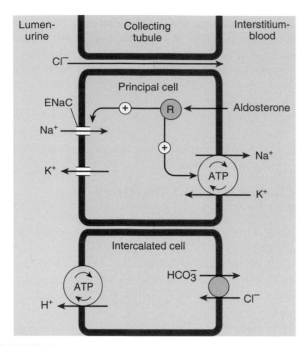

FIGURE 15–5 Mechanism of sodium, potassium, and hydrogen ion movement in the collecting tubule cells. Synthesis of Na⁺/K⁺ ATPase, and the epithelial sodium channels (ENaC) and potassium channels is under the control of aldosterone, which combines with an intracellular receptor, *R*, before entering the nucleus. (Reproduced, with permission, from Katzung BG, editor: *Basic & Clinical Pharmacology*, 12th ed. McGraw-Hill, 2012: Fig. 15–5.)

epithelial sodium channels in the same portion of the nephron (Figure 15–5). (These drugs do *not* block I_{Na} channels in excitable membranes.) Spironolactone and eplerenone have slow onsets and offsets of action (24–72 h). Amiloride and triamterene have durations of action of 12–24 h.

B. Effects

All drugs in this class cause an increase in sodium clearance and a decrease in potassium and hydrogen ion excretion and therefore qualify as potassium-sparing diuretics. They may cause hyperkalemic metabolic acidosis (Table 15–1).

C. Clinical Use and Toxicities

Potassium wasting caused by chronic therapy with loop or thiazide diuretics, if not controlled by dietary potassium supplements, usually responds to these drugs. They are commonly combined with a thiazide in a single pill.

Aldosteronism (eg, the elevated serum aldosterone levels that occur in cirrhosis) is an important indication for spironolactone. Aldosteronism is also a feature of heart failure, and spironolactone and eplerenone have been shown to have significant long-term benefits in this condition (Chapter 13). Some of this effect may occur in the heart, an action that is not yet understood.

The most important toxic effect of potassium-sparing diuretics is hyperkalemia. These drugs should never be given with potassium supplements. Other aldosterone antagonists (eg, angiotensin [ACE]

inhibitors and angiotensin receptor blockers [ARBs]), if used at all, should be used with caution. Spironolactone can cause endocrine abnormalities, including gynecomastia and antiandrogenic effects. Eplerenone has less affinity for gonadal steroid receptors.

> ### SKILL KEEPER: DIURETIC COMBINATIONS AND ELECTROLYTES (SEE CHAPTER 13)
>
> *Describe the possible interactions of cardiac glycosides (digoxin) with the major classes of diuretics.* The Skill Keeper Answer appears at the end of the chapter.

OSMOTIC DIURETICS

A. Prototypes and Mechanism of Action

Mannitol, the prototypical osmotic diuretic, is given intravenously. Other drugs often classified with mannitol (but rarely used) include glycerin, isosorbide (not isosorbide dinitrate), and urea. Because they are freely filtered at the glomerulus but poorly reabsorbed from the tubule, they remain in the lumen and "hold" water by virtue of their osmotic effect. The major location for this action is the proximal convoluted tubule. Reabsorption of water is also reduced in the descending limb of the loop of Henle and the collecting tubule.

B. Effects

The volume of urine is increased. Most filtered solutes are excreted in larger amounts unless they are actively reabsorbed. Sodium excretion is usually increased because the rate of urine flow through the tubule is greatly accelerated and sodium transporters cannot handle the volume rapidly enough. Mannitol can also reduce brain volume and intracranial pressure by osmotically extracting water from the tissue into the blood. A similar effect occurs in the eye.

C. Clinical Use and Toxicities

The osmotic drugs are used to maintain high urine flow (eg, when renal blood flow is reduced and in conditions of solute overload from severe hemolysis, rhabdomyolysis, or tumor lysis syndrome). Mannitol and several other osmotic agents are useful in reducing intraocular pressure in acute glaucoma and intracranial pressure in neurologic conditions.

Removal of water from the intracellular compartment may cause hyponatremia and pulmonary edema. As the water is excreted, hypernatremia may follow. Headache, nausea, and vomiting are common.

ANTIDIURETIC HORMONE AGONISTS & ANTAGONISTS

A. Prototypes and Mechanism of Action

Antidiuretic hormone (ADH) and **desmopressin** are prototypical ADH agonists. They are peptides and must be given

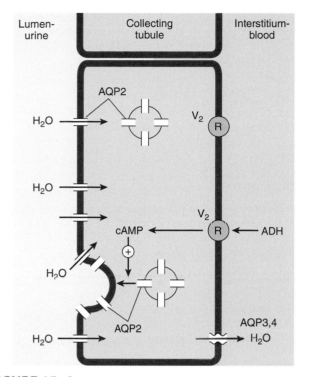

FIGURE 15–6 Mechanism of water transport across the membranes of collecting duct cells. Aquaporins 3 and 4 (AQP3, 4) are normally present in the basolateral membranes, but the luminal water channel, AQP2, is inserted only in the presence of ADH or similar antidiuretic peptides acting on the vasopressin V_2 receptor. (Reproduced, with permission, from Katzung BG, editor: *Basic & Clinical Pharmacology,* 12th ed. McGraw-Hill, 2012: Fig. 15–6.)

parenterally. **Conivaptan** and **tolvaptan** are ADH *antagonists.* Demeclocycline was previously used for this purpose. Lithium also has ADH-antagonist effects but is never used for this purpose.

ADH facilitates water reabsorption from the collecting tubule by activation of V_2 receptors, which stimulate adenylyl cyclase via G_s. The increased cyclic adenosine monophosphate (cAMP) causes the insertion of additional aquaporin AQP2 water channels into the luminal membrane in this part of the tubule (Figure 15–6). Conivaptan is an ADH inhibitor at V_{1a} and V_2 receptors. Tolvaptan is a more selective V_2 blocker with little V_1 affinity. Demeclocycline and lithium inhibit the action of ADH at some point distal to the generation of cAMP and presumably interfere with the insertion of water channels into the membrane.

B. Effects and Clinical Uses

1. Agonists—ADH and desmopressin reduce urine volume and increase its concentration. ADH and desmopressin are useful in pituitary diabetes insipidus. They are of no value in the nephrogenic form of the disease, but salt restriction, water restriction, thiazides, and loop diuretics may be used. These therapies reduce blood volume, a very strong stimulus to proximal tubular reabsorption. The proximal tubule thus substitutes—in part—for the deficient concentrating function of the collecting tubule in nephrogenic diabetes insipidus.

2. Antagonists—ADH antagonists oppose the actions of ADH and other naturally occurring peptides that act on the same V_2 receptor. Such peptides are produced by certain tumors (eg, small cell carcinoma of the lung) and can cause significant water retention and dangerous hyponatremia. This **syndrome of inappropriate ADH secretion (SIADH)** can be treated with demeclocycline and conivaptan. Lithium also works but has greater toxicity.

C. Toxicity

In the presence of ADH or desmopressin, a large water load may cause dangerous hyponatremia. Large doses of either peptide may cause hypertension in some persons.

Conivaptan and tolvaptan may cause demyelination with serious neurologic consequences if hyponatremia is corrected too rapidly. Conivaptan may cause infusion site reactions. In children younger than 8 years, demeclocycline (like other tetracyclines) causes bone and teeth abnormalities. Lithium causes nephrogenic diabetes insipidus as a toxic effect; because of its other toxicities, the drug is never used to treat SIADH.

QUESTIONS

1. A 70-year-old retired businessman is admitted with a history of recurrent heart failure and metabolic derangements. He has marked peripheral edema and metabolic alkalosis. Which of the following drugs is *most* appropriate for the treatment of his edema?
   (A) Acetazolamide
   (B) Digoxin
   (C) Dobutamine
   (D) Hydrochlorothiazide
   (E) Spironolactone

2. A 50-year-old man has a history of frequent episodes of renal colic with calcium-containing renal stones. A careful workup indicates that he has a defect in proximal tubular calcium reabsorption, which results in high concentrations of calcium salts in the tubular urine. The most useful diuretic agent in the treatment of recurrent calcium stones is
   (A) Acetazolamide
   (B) Furosemide
   (C) Hydrochlorothiazide
   (D) Mannitol
   (E) Spironolactone

3. Which of the following is an important effect of chronic therapy with loop diuretics?
   (A) Decreased urinary excretion of calcium
   (B) Elevation of blood pressure
   (C) Elevation of pulmonary vascular pressure
   (D) Metabolic acidosis
   (E) Ototoxicity

4. Which drug is correctly associated with its actions in the following table? (+ indicates increase and − indicates decrease.)

Choice	Drug	Urine Na⁺	Urine K⁺	Metabolic change
A	Acetazolamide	+++	+	Alkalosis
B	Furosemide	++	−	Alkalosis
C	Hydrochlorothiazide	+	++	Acidosis
D	Spironolactone	+	−	Acidosis
E	Mannitol	−	++	Alkalosis

5. Which of the following diuretics would be most useful in the acute treatment of a comatose patient with brain injury and cerebral edema?
   (A) Acetazolamide
   (B) Amiloride
   (C) Ethacrynic acid
   (D) Furosemide
   (E) Mannitol

6. A 62-year-old man with advanced prostate cancer is admitted to the emergency department with mental obtundation. An electrolyte panel shows a serum calcium of 16.5 (normal ~8.5–10.5 mg/dL). Which of the following therapies would be most useful in the management of severe hypercalcemia?
   (A) Acetazolamide plus saline infusion
   (B) Furosemide plus saline infusion
   (C) Hydrochlorothiazide plus saline infusion
   (D) Mannitol plus saline infusion
   (E) Spironolactone plus saline infusion

7. A 60-year-old patient complains of paresthesias and occasional nausea associated with one of her drugs. She is found to have hyperchloremic metabolic acidosis. She is probably taking
   (A) Acetazolamide for glaucoma
   (B) Amiloride for edema associated with aldosteronism
   (C) Furosemide for severe hypertension and heart failure
   (D) Hydrochlorothiazide for hypertension
   (E) Mannitol for cerebral edema

8. A 70-year-old woman is admitted to the emergency department because of a "fainting spell" at home. She appears to have suffered no trauma from her fall, but her blood pressure is 120/60 when lying down and 60/20 when she sits up. Neurologic examination and an ECG are within normal limits when she is lying down. Questioning reveals that she has recently started taking "water pills" (diuretics) for a heart condition. Which of the following drugs is the most likely cause of her fainting spell?
   (A) Acetazolamide
   (B) Amiloride
   (C) Furosemide
   (D) Hydrochlorothiazide
   (E) Spironolactone

9. A 58-year-old woman with lung cancer has abnormally low serum osmolality. A drug that increases the formation of dilute urine and is used to treat SIADH is
   (A) Acetazolamide
   (B) Amiloride
   (C) Conivaptan
   (D) Desmopressin
   (E) Ethacrynic acid
   (F) Furosemide
   (G) Hydrochlorothiazide
   (H) Mannitol
   (I) Spironolactone
   (J) Triamterene

10. A graduate student is planning to make a high-altitude climb in South America while on vacation. He will not have time to acclimate slowly to altitude. A drug that is useful in preventing high-altitude sickness is
   (A) Acetazolamide
   (B) Amiloride
   (C) Demeclocycline
   (D) Desmopressin
   (E) Ethacrynic acid

ANSWERS

1. Although acetazolamide is rarely used in heart failure, carbonic anhydrase inhibitors are quite valuable in patients with edema *and* metabolic alkalosis. The high bicarbonate levels in these patients make them particularly susceptible to the action of carbonic anhydrase inhibitors. Digoxin is useful in chronic systolic failure but is not first-line therapy. Dobutamine is appropriate only when diuresis has already been accomplished in severe acute failure. Hydrochlorothiazide and spironolactone are not adequate for first-line therapy of edema in failure. The answer is **A.**

2. The thiazides are useful in the prevention of calcium stones because these drugs reduce tubular calcium concentration, probably by increasing passive proximal tubular and distal convoluted tubule reabsorption of calcium. In contrast, the loop agents facilitate calcium excretion. The answer is **C.**

3. Loop diuretics increase urinary calcium excretion and decrease blood pressure (in hypertension) and pulmonary vascular pressure. They cause metabolic alkalosis. Loop diuretics also cause ototoxicity. The answer is **E.**

4. Acetazolamide causes metabolic acidosis. Furosemide causes a marked increase in sodium and a moderate increase in potassium excretion. Thiazides cause alkalosis and a greater increase in sodium than potassium excretion. Mannitol causes a small increase in both sodium and potassium excretion and no change in body pH. Spironolactone causes the changes indicated. The answer is **D.**

5. An osmotic agent is needed to remove water from the cells of the edematous brain and reduce intracranial pressure rapidly. The answer is **E.**

6. Diuretic therapy of hypercalcemia requires a reduction in calcium reabsorption in the thick ascending limb, an effect of loop diuretics. However, a loop diuretic alone would reduce blood volume around the remaining calcium so that serum calcium would not decrease appropriately. Therefore, saline infusion should accompany the loop diuretic. The answer is **B.**

7. Paresthesias and gastrointestinal distress are common adverse effects of acetazolamide, especially when it is taken chronically, as in glaucoma. The observation that the patient has metabolic acidosis also suggests the use of acetazolamide. The answer is **A.**

8. The case history suggests that the syncope (fainting) is associated with diuretic use. Complications of diuretics that can result in syncope include both postural hypotension (which this patient exhibits) due to excessive reduction of blood volume and arrhythmias due to excessive potassium loss. Potassium wasting is more common with thiazides (because of their long duration of action), but these drugs rarely cause reduction of blood volume sufficient to result in orthostatic hypotension. The answer is **C,** furosemide.

9. Inability to form dilute urine in the fully hydrated condition is characteristic of SIADH. Antagonists of ADH are needed to treat this condition. The answer is **C,** conivaptan.

10. Carbonic anhydrase inhibitors are useful in the prevention of altitude sickness. The answer is **A.**

SKILL KEEPER ANSWER: DIGITALIS AND DIURETICS (SEE CHAPTER 13)

Digoxin toxicity is facilitated by hypokalemia. Therefore, potassium-wasting diuretics (eg, loop agents, thiazides), which are often needed in heart failure, can increase the risk of a fatal digitalis arrhythmia. Carbonic anhydrase inhibitors, though also potassium-wasting agents, are rarely used for their systemic and diuretic effects and are therefore less likely to be involved in digitalis toxicity. The potassium-sparing diuretics, in contrast to the other groups, can be useful in preventing such interactions.

CHECKLIST

When you complete this chapter, you should be able to:

❑ List 5 major types of diuretics and relate them to their sites of action.

❑ Describe 2 drugs that reduce potassium loss during sodium diuresis.

❑ Describe a therapy that reduces calcium excretion in patients who have recurrent urinary stones.

❑ Describe a treatment for severe acute hypercalcemia in a patient with advanced carcinoma.

❑ Describe a method for reducing urine volume in nephrogenic diabetes insipidus.

❑ List the major applications and the toxicities of acetazolamide, thiazides, loop diuretics, and potassium-sparing diuretics.

DRUG SUMMARY TABLE: Diuretic Agents

Subclass	Mechanism of Action	Clinical Applications	Pharmacokinetics	Toxicities, Interactions
Carbonic anhydrase inhibitors				
Acetazolamide	Inhibits carbonic anhydrase. In proximal tubule, bicarbonate reabsorption is blocked and Na^+ is excreted with HCO_3^-. In glaucoma, secretion of aqueous humor is reduced, and in mountain sickness, metabolic acidosis increases respiration	Glaucoma, mountain sickness • edema with alkalosis	Oral, parenteral Diuresis is self-limiting, but effects in glaucoma and mountain sickness persist	Metabolic acidosis; sedation, paresthesias. Hyperammonemia in cirrhosis
Dorzolamide, brinzolamide: topical carbonic anhydrase inhibitors for glaucoma only				
Loop diuretics				
Furosemide, also bumetanide, torsemide	Inhibit $Na^+/K^+/2Cl^-$ transporter in thick ascending limb of loop of Henle. Cause powerful diuresis and increased Ca^{2+} excretion	Heart failure, pulmonary edema, severe hypertension; other forms of edema	Oral, parenteral	Metabolic hypokalemic alkalosis • ototoxicity • hypovolemia • efficacy is reduced by nonsteroidal anti-inflammatory drugs. Sulfonamide allergy (rare).
Ethacrynic acid: like furosemide but not a sulfonamide and has some uricosuric effect				
Thiazide diuretics				
Hydrochlorothiazide, many other thiazides	Inhibit Na^+/Cl^- transporter in distal convoluted tubule. Cause moderate diuresis and reduced excretion of calcium	Hypertension, mild heart failure, hypercalciuria with stones • syndrome of inappropriate ADH secretion	Oral	Metabolic hypokalemic alkalosis • early hyponatremia • increased serum glucose, lipids, uric acid • efficacy is reduced by nonsteroidal anti-inflammatory drugs. Sulfonamide allergy (rare)
Chlorthalidone: not a thiazide, but effects are indistinguishable from those of thiazides				
K⁺-sparing diuretics				
Spironolactone, eplerenone	Steroid inhibitors of cytoplasmic aldosterone receptor in cortical collecting ducts • reduce K^+ excretion	Excessive K^+ loss when using other diuretics • aldosteronism	Oral	Hyperkalemia • gynecomastia (spironolactone only)
Amiloride	Inhibitor of ENaC epithelial sodium channels in cortical collecting duct, reduces Na^+ reabsorption and K^+ excretion	Excessive K^+ loss when using other diuretics • usually in combination with thiazides	Oral	Hyperkalemia
Triamterene: like amiloride				
Osmotic diuretics				
Mannitol	Osmotically retains water in tubule by reducing reabsorption in proximal tubule, descending limb of Henle's loop, and collecting ducts • in the periphery, mannitol extracts water from cells	Solute overload in rhabdomyolysis, hemolysis • brain edema with coma • acute glaucoma	Intravenous; short duration	Hyponatremia followed by hypernatremia • headache, nausea, vomiting

(Continued)

DRUG SUMMARY TABLE: Diuretic Agents (*Continued*)

Subclass	Mechanism of Action	Clinical Applications	Pharmacokinetics	Toxicities, Interactions
ADH agonists				
Desmopressin, vasopressin	Agonists at V_1 and V_2 ADH receptors, activate insertion of aquaporin water channels in collecting tubule, reduce water excretion • vasoconstriction	Pituitary diabetes insipidus	Subcutaneous, nasal	Hyponatremia • hypertension
ADH antagonists				
Conivaptan	Antagonist at V_{1a}, V_2 receptors	SIADH, hyponatremia	Parenteral	Infusion site reactions
Tolvaptan: like conivaptan, more selective for V_2 receptors *Demeclocycline:* used in SIADH, mechanism unclear				

ADH, antidiuretic hormone; SIADH, syndrome of inappropriate antidiuretic hormone.

PART IV DRUGS WITH IMPORTANT ACTIONS ON SMOOTH MUSCLE

Histamine, Serotonin, & the Ergot Alkaloids

Autacoids are endogenous molecules with powerful pharmacologic effects that do not fall into traditional autonomic groups. **Histamine** and **serotonin** (5-hydroxytryptamine; 5-HT) are the most important amine autacoids. The **ergot alkaloids** are a heterogeneous group of drugs (not autacoids) that interact with serotonin receptors, dopamine receptors, and α receptors. They are included in this chapter because of their effects on serotonin receptors and on smooth muscle. Peptide and eicosanoid autacoids are discussed in Chapters 17 and 18. Nitric oxide is discussed in Chapter 19.

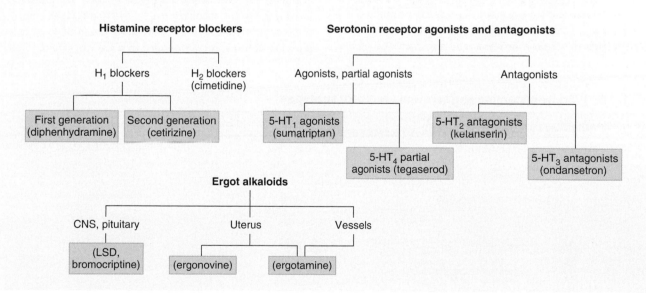

High-Yield Terms to Learn	
Acid-peptic disease	Disease of the upper digestive tract caused by acid and pepsin; includes gastroesophageal reflux, erosions, and ulcers
Autacoids	Endogenous substances with complex physiologic and pathophysiologic functions that have potent nonautonomic pharmacologic effects when administered as drugs; commonly understood to include histamine, serotonin, prostaglandins, and vasoactive peptides
Carcinoid	A neoplasm of the gastrointestinal tract or bronchi that may secrete serotonin and a variety of peptides
Ergotism ("St. Anthony's fire")	Disease caused by excess ingestion of ergot alkaloids; classically an epidemic caused by consumption of grain (eg, in bread) that is contaminated by the ergot fungus
Gastrinoma	A tumor that produces large amounts of gastrin; associated with hypersecretion of gastric acid and pepsin leading to ulceration
IgE-mediated immediate reaction	An allergic response, for example, hay fever, angioedema, caused by interaction of an antigen with IgE antibodies on mast cells; results in the release of histamine and other mediators of allergy
Oxytocic	A drug that causes contraction of the uterus
Zollinger-Ellison syndrome	Syndrome of hypersecretion of gastric acid and pepsin, often caused by gastrinoma; it is associated with severe acid-peptic ulceration and diarrhea

HISTAMINE

Histamine is formed from the amino acid histidine and is stored in high concentrations in vesicles in mast cells, enterochromaffin cells in the gut, some neurons, and a few other cell types. Histamine is metabolized by the enzymes monoamine oxidase and diamine oxidase. Excess production of histamine in the body (eg, in systemic mastocytosis) can be detected by measurement of its major metabolite, imidazole acetic acid, in the urine. Because it is released from mast cells in response to IgE-mediated (immediate) allergic reactions, this autacoid plays a pathophysiologic role in seasonal rhinitis (hay fever), urticaria, and angioneurotic edema.

(The peptide bradykinin also plays an important role in angioneurotic edema, see Chapter 17.) Histamine also plays a physiologic role in the control of acid secretion in the stomach and as a neurotransmitter.

A. Receptors and Effects

Two receptors for histamine, H_1 and H_2, mediate most of the peripheral actions; 2 others (H_3, H_4) have also been identified (Table 16–1). The **triple response**, a classic demonstration of histamine effect, is mediated mainly by H_1 and H_2 receptors. This response involves a small red spot at the center of an intradermal injection of histamine surrounded by a red edematous wheal.

TABLE 16–1 Some histamine and serotonin receptor subtypes.[a]

Receptor Subtype	Distribution	Postreceptor Mechanisms	Prototypic Antagonist
H_1	Smooth muscle	G_q; ↑ IP_3, DAG	Diphenhydramine
H_2	Stomach, heart, mast cells	G_s; ↑ cAMP	Cimetidine
H_3	Nerve endings, CNS	G_i; ↓ cAMP	Clobenpropit[b]
H_4	Leukocytes	G_i; ↓ cAMP	—
5-HT_{1D}	Brain	G_i; ↓ cAMP	—
5-HT_2	Smooth muscle, platelets	G_q; ↑ IP_3, DAG	Ketanserin
5-HT_3	Area postrema (CNS), sensory and enteric nerves	Ligand-gated cation channel	Ondansetron
5-HT_4	Presynaptic nerve terminals in the enteric nervous system	G_s; ↑ cAMP	Tegaserod (partial agonist)

[a]Many other serotonin receptor subtypes are recognized in the CNS. They are discussed in Chapter 21.

[b]Clobenpropit is investigational.

cAMP, cyclic adenosine phosphate; CNS, central nervous system; DAG, diacylglycerol; IP_3, inositol trisphosphate.

1. H$_1$ receptor—This G$_q$-coupled receptor is important in smooth muscle effects, especially those caused by IgE-mediated responses. Inositol trisphosphate (IP$_3$) and diacylglycerol (DAG) are the second messengers. Typical responses include pain and itching in the skin, bronchoconstriction, and vasodilation, the latter caused by release of nitric oxide. Capillary endothelial cells, in addition to releasing nitric oxide (NO) and other vasodilating substances, also contract, opening gaps in the permeability barrier and leading to the formation of local edema. These effects occur in allergic reactions and in mastocytosis.

2. H$_2$ receptor—This G$_s$-coupled receptor mediates gastric acid secretion by parietal cells in the stomach. It also has a cardiac stimulant effect. A third action is to reduce histamine release from mast cells—a negative feedback effect. These actions are mediated by activation of adenylyl cyclase, which increases intracellular cyclic adenosine monophosphate (cAMP).

3. H$_3$ receptor—This G$_i$-coupled receptor appears to be involved mainly in presynaptic modulation of histaminergic neurotransmission in the central nervous system (CNS). Food intake and body weight increase in H$_3$-receptor knockout animals. In the periphery, it appears to be a presynaptic heteroreceptor with modulatory effects on the release of other transmitters (see Chapter 6).

4. H$_4$ receptor—The H$_4$ receptor is located on leukocytes (especially eosinophils) and mast cells and is involved in chemotactic responses by these cells. Like H$_3$, it is G$_i$ coupled.

B. Clinical Use

Histamine has no therapeutic applications, but drugs that block its effects at H$_1$ and at H$_2$ receptors are very important in clinical medicine. No antagonists of H$_3$ or H$_4$ receptors are currently available for clinical use.

HISTAMINE H$_1$ ANTAGONISTS

A. Classification and Prototypes

A wide variety of antihistaminic H$_1$ blockers are available from several different chemical families. Two major subgroups or "generations" have been developed. The older members of the first-generation agents, typified by **diphenhydramine,** are highly sedating agents with significant autonomic receptor-blocking effects. A newer subgroup of first-generation agents is less sedating and has much less autonomic effect. **Chlorpheniramine** and **cyclizine** may be considered prototypes. The second-generation H$_1$ blockers, typified by **cetirizine, fexofenadine,** and **loratadine,** are far less lipid soluble than the first-generation agents and have further reduced sedating and autonomic effects. All H$_1$ blockers are active by the oral route. Several are promoted for topical use in the eye or nose. Most are metabolized extensively in the liver. Half-lives of the older H$_1$ blockers vary from 4 to 12 h. Second-generation agents have half-lives of 12–24 h.

B. Mechanism and Effects

H$_1$ blockers are competitive pharmacologic antagonists at the H$_1$ receptor; these drugs have no effect on histamine release from storage sites. They are more effective if given before histamine release occurs.

Because their structure closely resembles that of muscarinic blockers and α-adrenoceptor blockers, many of the first-generation agents are potent pharmacologic antagonists at these autonomic receptors. A few also block serotonin receptors. As noted, most older first-generation agents are sedating, and some—not all—first-generation agents have anti-motion sickness effects. Many H$_1$ blockers are potent local anesthetics. H$_1$-blocking drugs have negligible effects at H$_2$ receptors.

C. Clinical Use

H$_1$ blockers have major applications in allergies of the immediate type (ie, those caused by antigens acting on IgE antibody-sensitized mast cells). These conditions include hay fever and urticaria.

Diphenhydramine, dimenhydrinate, cyclizine, meclizine, and promethazine are used as anti-motion sickness drugs. Diphenhydramine is also used for management of chemotherapy-induced vomiting.

Adverse effects of the first-generation H$_1$ blockers are sometimes exploited therapeutically (eg, in their use as hypnotics in over-the-counter sleep aids).

D. Toxicity and Interactions

Sedation is common, especially with diphenhydramine and promethazine. It is much less common with second-generation agents, which do not enter the CNS readily. Antimuscarinic effects such as dry mouth and blurred vision occur with some first-generation drugs in some patients. Alpha-adrenoceptor blockade, which is significant with phenothiazine derivatives such as promethazine, may cause orthostatic hypotension.

Interactions occur between older antihistamines and other drugs with sedative effects (eg, benzodiazepines and alcohol). Drugs that inhibit hepatic metabolism may result in dangerously high levels of certain antihistaminic drugs that are taken concurrently. For example, azole antifungal drugs and certain other CYP3A4 inhibitors interfere with the metabolism of astemizole and terfenadine, 2 second-generation agents that have been withdrawn from the US market because high plasma concentrations of either antihistamine can precipitate lethal arrhythmias.

HISTAMINE H$_2$ ANTAGONISTS

A. Classification and Prototypes

Four H$_2$ blockers are available; **cimetidine** is the prototype. **Ranitidine, famotidine,** and **nizatidine** differ only in having fewer adverse effects than cimetidine. These drugs do not resemble H$_1$ blockers structurally. They are orally active, with half-lives of 1–3 h. Because they are all relatively nontoxic, they can be given in large doses, so that the duration of action of a single dose may be 12–24 h. All four agents are available in oral over-the-counter formulations.

B. Mechanism and Effects

H_2 antagonists produce a surmountable pharmacologic blockade of histamine H_2 receptors. They are relatively selective and have no significant blocking actions at H_1 or autonomic receptors. The only therapeutic effect of clinical importance is the reduction of gastric acid secretion, but this is a very useful action. Blockade of cardiovascular and mast cell H_2-receptor-mediated effects can be demonstrated but has no clinical significance.

C. Clinical Use

In acid-peptic disease, especially duodenal ulcer, these drugs reduce nocturnal acid secretion, accelerate healing, and prevent recurrences. Acute ulcer is usually treated with 2 or more doses per day, whereas recurrence of ulcers can often be prevented with a single bedtime dose. H_2 blockers are also effective in accelerating healing and preventing recurrences of gastric peptic ulcers. Intravenous H_2 blockers are useful in preventing gastric erosions and hemorrhage that occur in stressed patients in intensive care units. In Zollinger-Ellison syndrome, which is associated with gastrinoma and characterized by acid hypersecretion, severe recurrent peptic ulceration, gastrointestinal bleeding, and diarrhea, these drugs are helpful, but very large doses are required; proton pump inhibitors are preferred. Similarly, the H_2 blockers have been used in gastroesophageal reflux disease (GERD), but they are not as effective as proton pump inhibitors (see Chapter 60).

SKILL KEEPER: ANTIHISTAMINE ADVERSE EFFECTS (SEE CHAPTERS 8 AND 10)

An elderly dental patient was given promethazine intravenously to reduce anxiety before undergoing an extraction in the dental office. Promethazine is an older first-generation antihistamine. Predict the CNS and autonomic effects of this drug when given intravenously. The Skill Keeper Answer appears at the end of the chapter.

D. Toxicity

Cimetidine is a potent inhibitor of hepatic drug-metabolizing enzymes (see Chapter 4) and may also reduce hepatic blood flow. Cimetidine also has significant antiandrogen effects in patients receiving high doses. Ranitidine has a weaker inhibitory effect on hepatic drug metabolism; neither it nor the other H_2 blockers appear to have any endocrine effects.

SEROTONIN (5-HYDROXYTRYPTAMINE; 5-HT) & RELATED AGONISTS

Serotonin is produced from tryptophan and stored in vesicles in the enterochromaffin cells of the gut and neurons of the CNS and enteric nervous system. After release, it is metabolized by monoamine oxidase. Excess production in the body (eg, in carcinoid syndrome) can be detected by measuring its major metabolite,

5-hydroxyindole acetic acid (5-HIAA), in the urine. Serotonin plays a physiologic role as a neurotransmitter in both the CNS and the enteric nervous system and may have a role as a local hormone that modulates gastrointestinal activity. Serotonin is also stored (but synthesized to only a minimal extent) in platelets. In spite of the very large number of serotonin receptors (14 identified to date), most of the serotonin *agonists* in clinical use act at 5-HT_{1D} receptors. Serotonin antagonists in use or under investigation act at 5-HT_2 and 5-HT_3 receptors (see drug overview figure at the beginning of the chapter).

A. Receptors and Effects

1. 5-HT$_1$ receptors—5-HT_1 receptors are most important in the brain and mediate synaptic inhibition via increased potassium conductance (Table 16–1). Peripheral 5-HT_1 receptors mediate both excitatory and inhibitory effects in various smooth muscle tissues. 5-HT_1 receptors are G_i-protein-coupled.

2. 5-HT$_2$ receptors—5-HT_2 receptors are important in both brain and peripheral tissues. These receptors mediate synaptic excitation in the CNS and smooth muscle contraction (gut, bronchi, uterus, some vessels) or relaxation (other vessels). Several mechanisms are involved, including (in different tissues) increased IP_3, decreased potassium conductance, and decreased cAMP. This receptor probably mediates some of the vasodilation, diarrhea, and bronchoconstriction that occur as symptoms of carcinoid tumor, a neoplasm that releases serotonin and other substances.

3. 5-HT$_3$ receptors—5-HT_3 receptors are found in the CNS, especially in the chemoreceptive area and vomiting center, and in peripheral sensory and enteric nerves. These receptors mediate excitation via a 5-HT-gated cation channel. Antagonists acting at this receptor are extremely useful antiemetic drugs.

4. 5-HT$_4$ receptors—5-HT_4 receptors are found in the gastrointestinal tract and play an important role in intestinal motility.

B. Clinical Uses

Serotonin has no clinical applications, but other more selective agonists are useful.

1. 5-HT$_{1D}$ agonists—**Sumatriptan** is the prototype. **Naratriptan** and other "-triptans" are similar to sumatriptan (see Drug Summary Table). They are the first-line treatment for acute migraine and cluster headache attacks, an observation that strengthens the association of serotonin abnormalities with these headache syndromes. These drugs are active orally; sumatriptan is also available for nasal and parenteral administration. Ergot alkaloids, discussed later, are partial agonists at some 5-HT receptors.

2. 5-HT$_4$ Partial agonist—**Tegaserod** is a newer drug that acts as an agonist in the colon. It was approved and briefly marketed for use in chronic constipation, but because of cardiovascular toxicity, its use is now restricted.

TABLE 16–2 Characteristics of serotonin syndrome and other hyperthermic syndromes.

Syndrome	Precipitating Drugs	Clinical Presentation	Therapy[a]
Serotonin syndrome	SSRIs, second-generation antidepressants, MAOIs, linezolid, tramadol, meperidine, fentanyl, ondansetron, sumatriptan, MDMA, LSD, St. John's wort, ginseng	Hyperthermia, hyperreflexia, tremor, clonus, hypertension, hyperactive bowel sounds, diarrhea, mydriasis, agitation, coma; onset within hours	**Sedation (benzodiazepines), paralysis, intubation and ventilation**[b]**;** consider 5-HT$_2$ block with cyproheptadine or chlorpromazine
Neuroleptic malignant syndrome	D$_2$-blocking antipsychotic drugs	Hyperthermia, acute severe parkinsonism; hypertension, normal or reduced bowel sounds, onset over 1–3 days	**Diphenhydramine (parenteral),** cooling if temperature is very high, sedation with benzodiazepines
Malignant hyperthermia	Volatile anesthetics, succinylcholine	Hyperthermia, muscle rigidity, hypertension, tachycardia; onset within minutes	**Dantrolene,** cooling

[a]Precipitating drugs should be discontinued immediately.

[b]All first-line therapy is in **bold** font.

MAOIs, monoamine oxidase inhibitors; MDMA, methylenedioxy-methamphetamine (ecstasy); SSRIs, selective serotonin reuptake inhibitors.

Modified and reproduced, with permission, from Katzung BG, editor: *Basic & Clinical Pharmacology,* 12th ed. McGraw-Hill, 2012, p. 284.

3. Selective serotonin reuptake inhibitors (SSRI)—A number of important antidepressant drugs act to increase activity at central serotonergic synapses by inhibiting the serotonin reuptake transporter, SERT. These drugs are discussed in Chapter 30. **Dexfenfluramine** (now withdrawn because of cardiotoxicity) was a reuptake inhibitor used exclusively for its appetite-reducing effect. Dexfenfluramine was combined with phentermine, an amphetamine-like anorexiant, in a weight-loss product known as "fen-phen." Because of toxicity, this combination product is also banned.

C. Hyperpyrexic Syndromes

Serotonin and drugs with 5-HT agonist effects are sometimes associated with drug reactions with high fever, skeletal muscle effects, and cardiovascular abnormalities that can be life-threatening. These important syndromes are summarized in Table 16–2.

SEROTONIN ANTAGONISTS

A. Classification and Prototypes

Ketanserin, phenoxybenzamine, and **cyproheptadine** are effective 5-HT$_2$ blockers. **Ondansetron, granisetron, dolasetron,** and **alosetron** are 5-HT$_3$ blockers. The **ergot alkaloids** are partial agonists (and therefore have some antagonist effects) at 5-HT and other receptors (see later discussion).

B. Mechanisms and Effects

Ketanserin and cyproheptadine are competitive pharmacologic 5-HT$_2$ antagonists. Phenoxybenzamine is an irreversible blocker at this receptor.

Ketanserin, cyproheptadine, and phenoxybenzamine are poorly selective agents. In addition to inhibition of serotonin effects, other actions include α-blockade (ketanserin, phenoxybenzamine) or H$_1$-blockade (cyproheptadine).

Ondansetron, granisetron, and dolasetron are selective 5-HT$_3$ receptor blockers and have important antiemetic actions in the area postrema of the medulla and also on peripheral sensory and enteric nerves. Although it acts at the same receptor, alosetron appears to lack these antiemetic effects.

C. Clinical Uses

Ketanserin is used as an antihypertensive drug outside the United States. Ketanserin, cyproheptadine, and phenoxybenzamine may be of value (separately or in combination) in the treatment of carcinoid tumor, a neoplasm that secretes large amounts of serotonin (and peptides) and causes diarrhea, bronchoconstriction, and flushing.

Ondansetron and its congeners are extremely useful in the control of vomiting associated with cancer chemotherapy and postoperative vomiting. Alosetron is used in the treatment of women with irritable bowel syndrome associated with diarrhea.

D. Toxicity

Adverse effects of ketanserin are those of α blockade and H$_1$ blockade. The toxicities of ondansetron, granisetron, and dolasetron include diarrhea and headache. Dolasetron has been associated with QRS and QT$_c$ prolongation in the ECG and should not be used in patients with heart disease. Alosetron causes significant constipation in some patients and has been associated with fatal bowel complications.

ERGOT ALKALOIDS

These complex molecules are produced by a fungus found in wet or spoiled grain. They are responsible for the epidemics of "St. Anthony's fire" (ergotism) described during the Middle Ages and recurring to the present time. There are at least 20 naturally occurring members of the family, but only a few of these and a handful of semisynthetic derivatives are used as therapeutic agents.

TABLE 16–3 **Effects of some ergot alkaloids at several receptors.**

Ergot Alkaloid	Alpha Receptor (α_1)	Dopamine Receptor (D_2)	Serotonin Receptor (5-HT$_2$)	Uterine Smooth Muscle Stimulation
Bromocriptine	–	+++	–	0
Ergonovine	+	+	– (PA)	+++
Ergotamine	– (PA)	0	+ (PA)	+++
Lysergic acid diethylamide (LSD)	+/0	+++	– –/++ in CNS	+

Agonist effects are indicated by +, antagonist by –, no effect by 0. Relative affinity for the receptor is indicated by the number of + or – signs.

PA, partial agonist.

Modified and reproduced, with permission, from Katzung BG, editor: *Basic & Clinical Pharmacology*, 12th ed. McGraw-Hill, 2012, p. 288.

Most ergot alkaloids are partial agonists at α adrenoceptors and 5-HT receptors, and some are potent agonists at dopamine receptors.

A. Classification and Effects

The ergot alkaloids may be divided into 3 major subgroups on the basis of the organ or tissue in which they have their primary effects. The receptor effects of the ergot alkaloids are summarized in Table 16–3 and are most marked in the following tissues:

1. Vessels—Ergot alkaloids can produce marked and prolonged α-receptor-mediated vasoconstriction. **Ergotamine** is the prototype. An overdose can cause ischemia and gangrene of the limbs or bowel. Because they are partial agonists, the drugs may also block the α-agonist effects of sympathomimetics, and ergotamine can cause epinephrine reversal.

2. Uterus—Ergot alkaloids produce powerful contraction in this tissue, especially near term. **Ergonovine** is the prototype. In pregnancy, the uterine contraction is sufficient to cause abortion or miscarriage. Earlier in pregnancy (and in the nonpregnant uterus) much higher doses of ergot alkaloids are needed to cause contraction.

3. Brain—Hallucinations may be prominent with the naturally occurring ergots and with **lysergic acid diethylamide (LSD)**, a semisynthetic prototypical hallucinogenic ergot derivative, but are uncommon with the therapeutic ergot derivatives. Although LSD is a potent 5-HT$_2$ blocker in peripheral tissues, its actions in the CNS are thought to be due to agonist actions at dopamine receptors. In the pituitary, some ergot alkaloids are potent dopamine-like agonists and inhibit prolactin secretion. **Bromocriptine** and **pergolide** are among the most potent semisynthetic ergot derivatives. They act as dopamine D_2 receptors in the pituitary and in the basal ganglia (see Chapter 28).

B. Clinical Uses

1. Migraine—**Ergotamine** has been a mainstay of treatment of acute attacks and is still used in combination with caffeine. Methysergide, dihydroergonovine, and ergonovine have been used for prophylaxis, but methysergide is no longer available in the

United States. The triptan derivatives are now considered preferable to the ergots because of lower toxicity.

2. Obstetric bleeding—**Ergonovine** and ergotamine are effective agents for the reduction of postpartum bleeding. They produce a powerful and long-lasting contraction that reduces bleeding but *must not be given* before delivery of the placenta.

3. Hyperprolactinemia and parkinsonism—**Bromocriptine** and pergolide have been used to reduce prolactin secretion (dopamine is the physiologic prolactin release inhibitor; Chapter 37). Bromocriptine also appears to reduce the size of pituitary tumors of the prolactin-secreting cells. Both drugs have been used in the treatment of Parkinson's disease (see Chapter 28).

C. Toxicity

The toxic effects of ergot alkaloids are quite important, both from a public health standpoint (epidemics of ergotism from spoiled grain) and from the toxicity resulting from overdose or abuse by individuals. Intoxication of grazing animals is sometimes reported by farmers and veterinarians.

1. Vascular effects—Severe prolonged vasoconstriction can result in ischemia and gangrene. The most consistently effective antidote is nitroprusside. When used for long periods, ergot derivatives may produce an unusual hyperplasia of connective tissue. This fibroplasia may be retroperitoneal, retropleural, or subendocardial and can cause hydronephrosis or cardiac valvular and conduction system malfunction. Similar lesions are found in some patients with carcinoid, suggesting that this action is probably mediated by agonist effects at serotonin receptors.

2. Gastrointestinal effects—Ergot alkaloids cause gastrointestinal upset (nausea, vomiting, diarrhea) in many persons.

3. Uterine effects—Marked uterine contractions may be produced. The uterus becomes progressively more sensitive to ergot alkaloids during pregnancy. Although abortion resulting from the use of ergot for migraine is rare, most obstetricians recommend avoidance or very conservative use of these drugs as pregnancy progresses.

4. CNS effects—Hallucinations resembling psychosis are common with LSD but less so with the other ergot alkaloids. Methysergide was occasionally used in the past as an LSD substitute by users of "recreational" drugs.

QUESTIONS

1. Your 37-year-old patient has been diagnosed with a rare metastatic carcinoid tumor. This neoplasm is releasing serotonin, bradykinin, and several unknown peptides. The effects of serotonin in this patient are *most* likely to include which one of the following?
   (A) Constipation
   (B) Episodes of bronchospasm
   (C) Hypersecretion of gastric acid
   (D) Hypotension
   (E) Urinary retention

2. A 23-year-old woman suffers from recurrent episodes of angioneurotic edema with release of histamine and other mediators. Which of the following drugs is the most effective physiologic antagonist of histamine in smooth muscle?
   (A) Cetirizine
   (B) Epinephrine
   (C) Granisetron
   (D) Ranitidine
   (E) Sumatriptan

3. A 20-year-old woman is taking diphenhydramine for severe hay fever. Which of the following adverse effects is she most likely to report?
   (A) Muscarinic increase in bladder tone
   (B) Nausea
   (C) Nervousness, anxiety
   (D) Sedation
   (E) Uterine cramps

4. A laboratory study of new H_2 blockers is planned. Which of the following will result from blockade of H_2 receptors?
   (A) Increased cAMP (cyclic adenosine monophosphate) in cardiac muscle
   (B) Decreased channel opening in enteric nerves
   (C) Decreased cAMP in gastric mucosa
   (D) Increased IP_3 (inositol trisphosphate) in platelets
   (E) Increased IP_3 in smooth muscle

5. You are asked to consult on a series of cases of drug toxicities. Which of the following is a recognized adverse effect of cimetidine?
   (A) Blurred vision
   (B) Diarrhea
   (C) Orthostatic hypotension
   (D) P450 hepatic enzyme inhibition
   (E) Sleepiness

6. A 40-year-old patient is about to undergo cancer chemotherapy with a highly emetogenic (nausea- and vomiting-causing) drug combination. The antiemetic drug most likely to be included in her regimen is
   (A) Bromocriptine
   (B) Cetirizine
   (C) Cimetidine
   (D) Ketanserin
   (E) Ondansetron

7. The hospital Pharmacy Committee is preparing a formulary for staff use. Which of the following is a correct application of the drug mentioned?
   (A) Alosetron: for obstetric bleeding
   (B) Cetirizine: for hay fever
   (C) Ergonovine: for Alzheimer's disease
   (D) Ondansetron: for acute migraine headache
   (E) Ranitidine: for Parkinson's disease

8. A 26-year-old woman presents with amenorrhea and galactorrhea. Her prolactin level is grossly elevated. Which of the following is most useful in the treatment of hyperprolactinemia?
   (A) Bromocriptine
   (B) Cimetidine
   (C) Ergotamine
   (D) Ketanserin
   (E) LSD
   (F) Ondansetron
   (G) Sumatriptan

9. A 28-year-old office worker suffers from intense migraine headaches. Which of the following is a serotonin agonist useful for aborting an acute migraine headache?
   (A) Bromocriptine
   (B) Cimetidine
   (C) Ephedrine
   (D) Ketanserin
   (E) Loratadine
   (F) Ondansetron
   (G) Sumatriptan

10. A 33-year-old woman attempted to induce an abortion using ergotamine. Her legs became cold with absent arterial pulses. Which of the following is the most useful antidote for reversing severe ergot-induced vasospasm?
    (A) Bromocriptine
    (B) Cimetidine
    (C) Ergotamine
    (D) Ketanserin
    (E) LSD
    (F) Nitroprusside
    (G) Sumatriptan
    (H) Ondansetron

ANSWERS

1. Serotonin causes bronchospasm, but the other effects listed are not observed. Carcinoid is associated with diarrhea and hypertension. The answer is **B**.

2. The smooth muscle effects of histamine are mediated mainly by H_1 receptors. Cetirizine is a *pharmacologic* antagonist of histamine. Granisetron is a 5-HT$_3$ antagonist. Sumatriptan is a 5-HT$_{1D}$ agonist. Ranitidine is a histamine antagonist but blocks the H_2 receptor in the stomach and the heart, not H_1 receptors in smooth muscle. Epinephrine has a *physiologic* antagonist action that reverses histamine's effects on smooth muscle. The answer is **B**.

3. H_1 blockers do not activate muscarinic receptors, mediate vasoconstriction, or cause uterine cramping. They do not cause nervousness or anxiety. Diphenhydramine is a potent sedative. The answer is **D**.

4. H_2 receptors are G_s-protein-coupled receptors, like β adrenoceptors. Blockade of this system will cause a decrease in cAMP. The answer is **C.**

5. The older H_1 blockers, not H_2 blockers, cause blurred vision, orthostatic hypotension, and sleepiness. Neither group typically causes diarrhea. Cimetidine (unlike other H_2 blockers) is a potent CYP3A4 inhibitor. The answer is **D.**

6. Ondansetron and other 5-HT_3 antagonists have significant antiemetic effects. Diphenhydramine and prednisone are also used for this purpose. The answer is **E.**

7. Alosetron is indicated in irritable bowel syndrome. Ergonovine is used in uterine bleeding. Ondansetron is useful for chemotherapy-induced emesis. Cetirizine is used in the treatment of hay fever. The answer is **B.**

8. Bromocriptine is an effective dopamine agonist in the CNS with the advantage of oral activity. The drug inhibits prolactin secretion by activating pituitary dopamine receptors. The answer is **A.**

9. Sumatriptan, an agonist at 5-HT_{1D} receptors, is indicated for prevention or treatment of migraine and cluster headaches. Ergotamine (not on the list) is also effective for acute migraine but is produced by the fungus *Claviceps purpurea*. The answer is **G.**

10. A very powerful vasodilator is necessary to reverse ergot-induced vasospasm; nitroprusside is such a drug (see Chapter 11). The answer is **F.**

SKILL KEEPER ANSWER: ANTIHISTAMINE ADVERSE EFFECTS (SEE CHAPTERS 8 AND 10)

Promethazine very effectively alleviated the anxiety of this elderly woman. However, when she attempted to get out of the dental chair after the procedure, she experienced severe orthostatic hypotension and fainted. In the horizontal position on the floor and later on a couch, she rapidly regained consciousness. Supine blood pressure was low normal, and heart rate was elevated. When she sat up, blood pressure dropped and heart rate increased. Promethazine and several other first-generation H_1 antihistamines are effective α (and M_3) blockers (Chapters 8 and 10). After 30 min supine, the patient was able to stand without fainting and experienced only a slight tachycardia. Older antihistaminic agents readily enter the CNS, causing sedation. This patient felt somewhat sleepy for 2 h but had no further signs or symptoms. If she had glaucoma, she might be at risk for an acute angle-closure episode, with markedly increased intraocular pressure as a result of the antimuscarinic action. An elderly man with prostatic hyperplasia might experience urinary retention.

CHECKLIST

When you complete this chapter, you should be able to:

❏ List the major organ system effects of histamine and serotonin.

❏ Describe the pharmacology of the 2 generations and 3 subgroups of H_1 antihistamines; list prototypical agents for each subgroup.

❏ Describe the pharmacology of the H_2 antihistamines; name 2 members of this group.

❏ Describe the action and indication for the use of sumatriptan.

❏ Describe one 5-HT_2 and one 5-HT_3 antagonist and their major applications.

❏ List the major organ system effects of the ergot alkaloids.

❏ Describe the major clinical applications and toxicities of the ergot drugs.

DRUG SUMMARY TABLE: Histamine, Serotonin, & the Ergot Alkaloids

Subclass	Mechanism of Action	Clinical Applications	Pharmacokinetics	Toxicities, Interactions
H₁ blockers, first generation				
Diphenhydramine, dimenhydrinate	Competitive pharmacologic block of peripheral and CNS H₁ receptors plus α- and M-receptor block. Anti-motion sickness effect	Hay fever, angioedema, motion sickness • used orally as OTC sleep aid; used parenterally for dystonias	Oral, parenteral Duration: 6–8 h	Sedation, autonomic block. Rare CNS excitation
Cyclizine: H₁ blocker with more anti-motion sickness action and less sedative and autonomic effect				
Promethazine: H₁ blocker with less anti-motion sickness action and more sedative and autonomic effects				
Chlorpheniramine: H₁ blocker with negligible anti-motion sickness, sedative, and autonomic effects				
H₁ blockers, second generation				
Cetirizine	Competitive pharmacologic block of peripheral H₁ receptors. No autonomic or anti-motion sickness effects	Hay fever, angioedema	Oral Duration: 12 24 h	Minimal toxicities
Fexofenadine, loratadine, desloratadine: very similar to cetirizine				
5-HT₁ agonists				
Sumatriptan	5-HT₁D agonist • causes vasoconstriction • modulates neurotransmitter release	Migraine and cluster headache	Oral, inhaled, parenteral Duration: 2–4 h	Paresthesias, dizziness, chest pain • possible coronary vasospasm
Almotriptan, eletriptan, frovatriptan, naratriptan, rizatriptan, zolmitriptan: very similar to sumatriptan; injectable preparations not available; durations: 2–27 h				
5-HT₂ antagonists				
Ketanserin	Competitive 5-HT₂ and α₁-receptor block	Hypertension, carcinoid tumor (not available in United States)	Oral Duration: 12–24 h	Hypotension
5-HT₃ antagonists				
Ondansetron	Pharmacologic antagonist • blocks chemoreceptor trigger zone and enteric nervous system 5-HT₃ receptors	Chemotherapy and postoperative vomiting	Oral, IV Duration: 3–6 h	QT prolongation, possible arrhythmias
Granisetron, dolasetron, palonosetron: like ondansetron				
Alosetron: approved for treatment of diarrhea-predominant irritable bowel syndrome				
5-HT₄ partial agonist				
Tegaserod	Partial agonist at 5-HT₄ receptors	Constipation-dominant irritable bowel syndrome **(restricted use)**	Oral Duration: 12 h	Diarrhea, ischemic colitis

OTC, over the counter.

Vasoactive Peptides

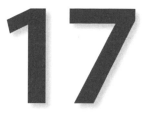

Vasoactive peptides are autacoids with significant actions on vascular smooth muscle as well as other tissues. They include vasoconstrictors, vasodilators, and peptides with mixed effects.

Antagonists of these peptides or the enzymes that produce them have useful clinical properties.

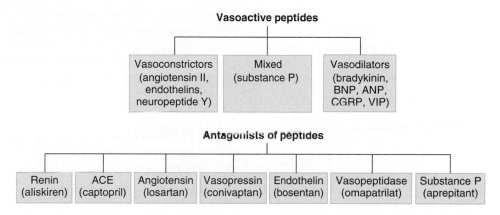

In addition to their actions on smooth muscle, vasoactive peptides function as neurotransmitters and local and systemic hormones. The better-known vasoactive peptides include angiotensin, bradykinin, natriuretic peptides, calcitonin gene-related peptide (CGRP), endothelin, neuropeptide Y (NPY), substance P and vasoactive intestinal peptide (VIP) (discussed in this chapter), and vasopressin (Chapters 15 and 37). Many other endogenous peptides with very important actions (eg, insulin, glucagon, opioid peptides) have less or no direct vascular smooth muscle effects.

Vasoactive peptides probably all act on cell surface receptors. Most act via G-protein-coupled receptors and cause the production of well-known second messengers (Table 17–1); a few may open ion channels.

ANGIOTENSIN & ITS ANTAGONISTS

A. Source and Disposition

Angiotensin I is produced from circulating angiotensinogen by **renin,** an enzyme released from the juxtaglomerular apparatus of the kidney. Angiotensin I is an inactive decapeptide, and is converted into **angiotensin II (ANGII,** also known as **AII),** an active octapeptide, by **angiotensin-converting enzyme (ACE),** also known as peptidyl dipeptidase or kininase II (see Figure 11–3). Angiotensin II, the active form of the peptide, is rapidly degraded by peptidases (angiotensinases).

B. Effects and Clinical Role

ANGII is a potent arteriolar vasoconstrictor and stimulant of aldosterone release. ANGII directly increases peripheral vascular resistance and, through aldosterone, causes renal sodium retention. It also facilitates the release of norepinephrine from adrenergic nerve endings via presynaptic heteroreceptor action (see Chapter 6). All these effects are mediated by the angiotensin AT_1 receptor, a G_q-coupled receptor. The AT_2 receptor appears to mediate vasodilation via nitric oxide and is probably most important during fetal development. ANGII is also mitogenic and plays a role in cardiac remodeling.

ANGII is no longer used for clinical indications. Its major significance is as an endogenous pathophysiologic mediator in

High-Yield Terms to Learn

Kinins	Family of vasoactive peptides associated with tissue injury and inflammation, for example, bradykinin
Natriuretic peptides	Family of peptides synthesized in brain, heart, and other tissues; have vasodilator as well as natriuretic effects
Neuropeptides	Peptides with prominent roles as neurotransmitters or modulators; many also have potent smooth muscle effects
Peptidase	Family of enzymes that activate or inactivate peptides by hydrolysis, for example, angiotensin-converting enzyme (dipeptidyl peptidase), neutral endopeptidase
Tachykinins	Group of 3 potent neuropeptides: substance P, neurokinin A, and neurokinin B

some cases of hypertension (high-renin hypertension) and in heart failure. Regardless of renin levels, ANGII *antagonists* have demonstrated clinical benefits in hypertension and heart failure. Therefore, ANGII antagonists are of considerable clinical importance.

C. Angiotensin Antagonists

As noted in Chapters 11 and 13, 2 types of antagonists are available. **ACE inhibitors** (eg, **captopril, enalapril,** others) are important agents for the treatment of hypertension and heart failure. **ANGII receptor blockers** (eg, **losartan, valsartan,** others) are orally active nonpeptide inhibitors at the ANGII AT$_1$ receptor. Block of angiotensin's effects by either of these drug types is often accompanied by a compensatory increase in renin and angiotensin I. **Aliskiren,** an orally active renin inhibitor, reduces angiotensin I as well as angiotensin II and is approved for use in hypertension.

VASOPEPTIDASE INHIBITORS

The vasopeptidase enzymes include neutral endopeptidase 24.11 and ACE. A class of drugs that block both enzymes is in clinical trials, and these drugs (eg, **omapatrilat**) show considerable efficacy in hypertension and heart failure. They reduce the concentration of ANGII and increase the concentration of natriuretic peptides. Unfortunately, these drugs also cause angioedema in a significant number of patients and have not been approved for clinical use.

BRADYKININ

A. Source and Disposition

Bradykinin is one of several vasodilator **kinins** produced from kininogen by a family of enzymes, the kallikreins. Bradykinin is rapidly degraded by various peptidases, including ACE.

TABLE 17–1 Some vasoactive peptides and their properties.

Peptide	Properties
Angiotensin II (ANGII)	↑ IP$_3$, DAG via AT$_1$ G protein-coupled receptors. Constricts arterioles, increases aldosterone secretion
Bradykinin	↑ IP$_3$, DAG, cAMP, NO. Dilates arterioles, increases capillary permeability, stimulates sensory nerve endings
Natriuretic peptides (ANP, BNP)	↑ cGMP via ANP$_A$ receptors. Dilate vessels, inhibit aldosterone secretion and effects, increase glomerular filtration
Calcitonin gene-related peptide (CGRP)	An extremely potent vasodilator; causes hypotension and reflex tachycardia
Endothelins	↑ IP$_3$, DAG via G protein-coupled ET$_A$ and ET$_B$ receptors. Synthesized in vascular endothelium. Constrict most vessels and contract other smooth muscle
Neuropeptide Y	Causes vasoconstriction and stimulates the heart. Effects mediated in part by IP$_3$
Substance P, neurokinins	Act on neurokinin receptors (NK$_1$, NK$_2$, NK$_3$). Dilate arterioles, contract veins and intestinal and bronchial smooth muscle, cause diuresis; substance P is a transmitter in sensory pain neurons
Vasoactive intestinal peptide (VIP)	↑ cAMP via G protein-coupled receptors VPAC1 and VPAC2. Dilates vessels, relaxes bronchi and intestinal smooth muscle

[a]ANP, atrial natriuretic peptide; BNP, brain natriuretic peptide; cAMP, cyclic adenosine monophosphate; cGMP, cyclic guanosine monophosphate; DAG, diacylglycerol; IP$_3$, inositol trisphosphate.

B. Effects and Clinical Role

Bradykinin acts through at least 2 receptors (B$_1$ and B$_2$) and causes the production of inositol 1,4,5-trisphosphate (IP$_3$), diacylglycerol (DAG), cyclic adenosine monophosphate (cAMP), nitric oxide, and prostaglandins in tissues. Bradykinin is one of the most potent vasodilators known. The peptide is involved in inflammation and causes edema and pain when released or injected into tissue. Bradykinin can be found in saliva and may play a role in stimulating its secretion.

Although it has no therapeutic application, bradykinin may play a role in the antihypertensive action of ACE inhibitors, as previously noted (see Chapter 11; Figure 11–3). Bradykinin also plays a role in hereditary angioedema. **Ecallantide,** a parenteral kallikrein inhibitor, and **icatibant,** an oral bradykinin B$_2$-receptor antagonist, are approved for use in angioedema.

NATRIURETIC PEPTIDES

A. Source and Disposition

Natriuretic peptides (**atrial natriuretic peptide [ANP]** and **brain natriuretic peptide [BNP]**) are synthesized and stored in the cardiac atria of mammals. BNP has also been isolated from brain tissue. They are released from the atria in response to distention of the chambers. A similar peptide, C-type natriuretic peptide, has been isolated from other tissues. BNP appears to be the most important of these peptides.

B. Effects and Clinical Role

Natriuretic peptides activate guanylyl cyclase in many tissues via a membrane-spanning enzyme receptor. They act as vasodilators as well as natriuretic (sodium excretion-enhancing) agents. Their renal action includes increased glomerular filtration, decreased proximal tubular sodium reabsorption, and inhibitory effects on renin secretion. The peptides also inhibit the actions of ANGII and aldosterone. Although they lack positive inotropic action, endogenous natriuretic peptides may play an important compensatory role in congestive heart failure by limiting sodium retention. Blood levels of endogenous BNP have been shown to correlate with the severity of heart failure and can be used as a diagnostic marker.

BNP has shown some benefit in the treatment of acute severe heart failure and is currently available for clinical use as **nesiritide.** This drug is approved for intravenous administration in acute severe heart failure (see Chapter 13) but has very significant toxicity.

ENDOTHELINS

Endothelins are peptide vasoconstrictors formed in and released by endothelial cells in blood vessels. Endothelins appear to function as autocrine and paracrine hormones in the vasculature. Three endothelin peptides (ET-1, ET-2, and ET-3) with minor variations in amino acid sequence have been identified in humans. Two receptors, ET$_A$ and ET$_B$, have been identified, both of which are coupled to their effectors with G proteins. The ET$_A$ receptor appears to be responsible for the vasoconstriction produced by endothelins.

Endothelins are much more potent than norepinephrine as vasoconstrictors and have a relatively long-lasting effect. The peptides also stimulate the heart, increase natriuretic peptide release, and activate smooth muscle proliferation. The peptides may be involved in some forms of hypertension and other cardiovascular disorders. ET$_A$ antagonists available for the treatment of pulmonary hypertension include **bosentan** and **ambrisentan.**

VIP, SUBSTANCE P, CGRP, & NPY

VIP (vasoactive intestinal peptide) is an extremely potent vasodilator but is probably more important as a neurotransmitter. It is found in the central and peripheral nervous systems and in the gastrointestinal tract. No clinical application has been found for this peptide.

The **neurokinins (substance P, neurokinin A,** and **neurokinin B)** act at NK$_1$ and NK$_2$ receptors in the central nervous system (CNS) and the periphery. Substance P has mixed vascular effects. It is a potent arteriolar vasodilator and a potent *stimulant* of veins and intestinal and airway smooth muscle. The peptide may also function as a local hormone in the gastrointestinal tract. Highest concentrations of substance P are found in the parts of the nervous system that contain neurons subserving pain. **Capsaicin,** the "hot" component of chili peppers, releases substance P from its stores in nerve endings and depletes the peptide. Capsaicin has been approved for topical use on arthritic joints and for post-herpetic neuralgia.

Neurokinins appear to be involved in certain CNS conditions, including depression and nausea and vomiting. **Aprepitant** is an oral antagonist at NK$_1$ receptors and is approved for use in chemotherapy-induced nausea and vomiting.

CGRP (calcitonin gene-related peptide) is found (along with calcitonin) in high concentrations in the thyroid but is also present in most smooth muscle tissues. The presence of CGRP in smooth muscle suggests a function as a cotransmitter in autonomic nerve endings. CGRP is the most potent hypotensive agent discovered to date and causes reflex tachycardia. Some evidence suggests that CGRP is involved in migraine headache. Currently, there is no clinical application for this peptide. However, an oral CGRP antagonist, if available, would be of great interest for the treatment of migraine.

NPY (neuropeptide Y) is a potent vasoconstrictor peptide that also stimulates the heart. NPY is found in the CNS and peripheral nerves; it is commonly localized as a cotransmitter in adrenergic nerve endings. In experimental animals, NPY administered in the CNS stimulates feeding and causes hypotension and hypothermia. Peripheral administration causes positive chronotropic and inotropic effects in the heart and hypertension. Several receptor subtypes have been identified, but neither agonists nor antagonists of this peptide have found clinical application.

SKILL KEEPER: ANGIOTENSIN ANTAGONISTS (SEE CHAPTER 11)

Discuss the differences between ACE inhibitors and AT₁-receptor blockers in the context of the peptides described in this chapter. The Skill Keeper Answer appears at the end of the chapter.

QUESTIONS

1. Field workers exposed to a plant toxin develop painful fluid-filled blisters. Analysis of the blister fluid reveals high concentrations of a peptide. Which of the following is a peptide that causes increased capillary permeability and edema?
(A) Angiotensin II
(B) Bradykinin
(C) Captopril
(D) Histamine
(E) Losartan

2. In a laboratory study of several peptides, one is found that decreases peripheral resistance but constricts veins. Which of the following causes arteriolar vasodilation and venoconstriction?
(A) Angiotensin II
(B) Bradykinin
(C) Endothelin-1
(D) Substance P
(E) Vasoactive intestinal peptide

3. Which of the following is elevated in heart failure and is a vasodilator with significant renal toxicity?
(A) Angiotensin I
(B) Angiotensin II
(C) Histamine
(D) Nesiritide
(E) Vasoactive intestinal peptide

4. A 45-year-old painter presents with respiratory symptoms and careful workup reveals idiopathic pulmonary hypertension. Which of the following binds endothelin receptors and is approved for use in pulmonary hypertension?
(A) Aliskiren I
(B) Bosentan
(C) Capsaicin
(D) Losartan
(E) Nesiritide

5. A 60-year-old woman presents with severe pain in a neuronal dermatome region of her chest. This area was previously affected by a herpes zoster rash. Which of the following might be of benefit in controlling this post-herpetic pain?
(A) Aliskiren
(B) Aprepitant
(C) Bosentan
(D) Capsaicin
(E) Captopril
(F) Losartan
(G) Nesiritide

6. In a phase 2 clinical trial in hypertensive patients, an endogenous octapeptide vasoconstrictor was found to increase in the blood of patients treated with large doses of diuretics. Which of the following is the most likely endogenous peptide?
(A) Angiotensin I
(B) Angiotensin II
(C) Atrial natriuretic peptide
(D) Bradykinin
(E) Calcitonin gene-related peptide
(F) Endothelin
(G) Neuropeptide Y
(H) Renin
(I) Substance P
(J) Vasoactive intestinal peptide

7. Which of the following is a vasodilator that increases in the blood or tissues of patients treated with captopril?
(A) Angiotensin II
(B) Bradykinin
(C) Brain natriuretic peptide
(D) Calcitonin gene-related peptide
(E) Endothelin
(F) Neuropeptide Y
(G) Renin

8. Which of the following is an antagonist at NK₁ receptors and is used to prevent or reduce chemotherapy-induced nausea and vomiting?
(A) Angiotensin I
(B) Aprepitant
(C) Bosentan
(D) Bradykinin
(E) Brain natriuretic peptide
(F) Enalapril
(G) Ondansetron

ANSWERS

1. Histamine and bradykinin both cause a marked increase in capillary permeability that is often associated with edema, but histamine is not a peptide. The answer is **B.**

2. Substance P is a potent arterial vasodilator and venoconstrictor. The answer is **D.**

3. BNP is an atrial and brain peptide found in increased amounts in patients with heart failure. The commercial formulation (nesiritide) is approved for use in severe acute heart failure but has significant renal toxicity. The answer is **D.**

4. Aliskiren, captopril, and losartan are used in primary hypertension. Bosentan, an endothelin antagonist, is used in pulmonary hypertension. The answer is **B.**

5. Substance P is an important pain-mediating neurotransmitter peptide and appears to be involved in post-herpetic pain as well as arthritic pain. Capsaicin can be used topically to deplete substance P stores from sensory nerves. The answer is **D.**

6. Angiotensin II, an octapeptide, increases when blood volume decreases (a diuretic effect) because the compensatory response causes an increase in renin secretion. Its precursor, angiotensin I, would also increase, but it is a decapeptide. The answer is **B.**

7. Bradykinin increases because the enzyme inhibited by captopril, converting enzyme, degrades kinins in addition to synthesizing angiotensin II (see Figure 11–3). The answer is **B.**

8. Aprepitant and ondansetron are both used to reduce or prevent chemotherapy-induced nausea and vomiting. Ondansetron is an antagonist at 5-HT$_3$ receptors. The answer is **B.**

SKILL KEEPER ANSWER: ANGIOTENSIN ANTAGONISTS (SEE CHAPTER 11)

Both ACE inhibitors (eg, captopril) and AT$_1$-receptor blockers (eg, losartan) reduce the effects of the renin-angiotensin-aldosterone system and thereby reduce blood pressure. Both result in a compensatory increase in the release of renin and angiotensin I. A major difference between the 2 types of drugs results from the fact that ACE inhibitors increase the circulating levels of bradykinin because bradykinin is normally inactivated by ACE. The increase in bradykinin contributes to the hypotensive action of ACE inhibitors but is probably also responsible for the high incidence of cough associated with ACE inhibitor use. The cough is believed to result from prostaglandins synthesized as a result of the increased bradykinin. AT$_1$-receptor blockers have a lower incidence of cough.

CHECKLIST

When you complete this chapter, you should be able to:

❏ Name an antagonist of angiotensin at its receptor and at least 2 drugs that reduce the formation of angiotensin II.

❏ Outline the major effects of bradykinin and brain natriuretic peptide.

❏ Describe the functions of converting enzyme (peptidyl dipeptidase, kininase II).

❏ List 2 potent vasoconstrictor peptides.

❏ Describe the effects of vasoactive intestinal peptide and substance P.

❏ Describe the clinical applications of bosentan and aprepitant.

DRUG SUMMARY TABLE: Vasoactive Peptides

Subclass	Mechanism of Action	Clinical Applications	Pharmacokinetics	Toxicities, Interactions
Renin-angiotensin antagonists				
Aliskiren	Renin inhibitor • reduces angiotensin I and II and aldosterone secretion	Hypertension	Oral Duration: 12 h	Angioedema, renal impairment
Captopril, enalapril, others	ACE inhibitor • reduces angiotensin II and aldosterone secretion • increases bradykinin	Hypertension, heart failure	Oral Half-life: ~2 h but large doses used for duration of effect ~12 h	Cough, teratogenic, hyperkalemia
Losartan, valsartan, others	AT_1 receptor inhibitor; reduces effects of angiotensin II	Hypertension	Oral Duration: 6–8 h	Teratogenic, hyperkalemia
Natriuretic peptides				
Nesiritide	BNP receptor agonist	Acute heart failure	Parenteral Half-life: 18 min	Renal damage, hypotension
Endothelin antagonists				
Bosentan	ET_A and ET_B receptor antagonist	Pulmonary hypertension	Oral Half-life: 5 h	Hepatic impairment; possible teratogen
Ambrisentan: ET antagonist like bosentan, more selective for ET_A receptor				
Substance P antagonists				
Aprepitant	Tachykinin NK_1 receptor antagonist	Antiemetic for chemotherapy-induced vomiting	Oral Half-life: 9–13 h	Asthenia, hiccups
Capsaicin	Releases substance P from nerve endings	Topical for painful conditions (joints, post-herpetic neuralgia)	Topical Duration: 4–6 h	Burning, stinging, erythema

ACE, angiotensin-converting enzyme; BNP, brain natriuretic peptide.

Prostaglandins & Other Eicosanoids

The eicosanoids are an important group of endogenous fatty acid autacoids that are produced from arachidonic acid, a 20-carbon fatty acid lipid in cell membranes. Major families of eicosanoids include the straight-chain derivatives (leukotrienes) and cyclic derivatives (prostacyclin, prostaglandins, and thromboxane).

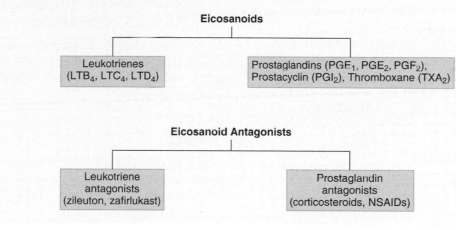

Eicosanoids

Leukotrienes (LTB$_4$, LTC$_4$, LTD$_4$)

Prostaglandins (PGF$_1$, PGE$_2$, PGF$_2$), Prostacyclin (PGI$_2$), Thromboxane (TXA$_2$)

Eicosanoid Antagonists

Leukotriene antagonists (zileuton, zafirlukast)

Prostaglandin antagonists (corticosteroids, NSAIDs)

EICOSANOID AGONISTS

A. Classification

The principal eicosanoid subgroups are the **leukotrienes** and a group of cyclic molecules, including **prostaglandins, prostacyclin**, and **thromboxane**. The leukotrienes retain the straight-chain configuration of arachidonic acid. Prostacyclin, thromboxane, and other members of the prostaglandin group are cyclized derivatives of arachidonic acid. There are several series for most of the principal subgroups, based on different substituents (indicated by letters A, B, etc) and different numbers of double bonds (indicated by a subscript number) in the molecule.

B. Synthesis

Active eicosanoids are synthesized in response to a wide variety of stimuli (eg, physical injury, immune reactions). These stimuli activate phospholipases in the cell membrane or cytoplasm, and arachidonic acid (a tetraenoic [4 double bonds] fatty acid) is released from membrane phospholipids (Figure 18–1). Arachidonic acid is then metabolized by several different enzymes. The 2 most important are **lipoxygenase,** which results in straight-chain leukotrienes, and **cyclooxygenase (COX),** which results in cyclization to prostacyclin, prostaglandins, or thromboxane. COX exists in at least 2 forms. **COX-1** is found in many tissues; the prostaglandins produced by COX-1 appear to be important for a variety of normal physiologic processes (see later discussion). In contrast, **COX-2** is found primarily in inflammatory cells; the products of its actions play a major role in tissue injury (eg, inflammation). In addition to these inflammatory functions, COX-2 is also responsible for synthesis of prostacyclin and of prostaglandins important in renal function. Thromboxane is preferentially synthesized in platelets, whereas prostacyclin is synthesized in the endothelial cells of vessels. Naturally occurring eicosanoids have very short half-lives (seconds to minutes) and are inactive when given orally.

High-Yield Terms to Learn

Abortifacient	A drug used to cause an abortion. Example: prostaglandin $F_{2\alpha}$
Cyclooxygenase	Enzyme that converts arachidonic acid to PGG and PGH, the precursors of the prostaglandins, including PGE, PGF, prostacyclin, and thromboxane
Dysmenorrhea	Painful uterine cramping caused by prostaglandins released during menstruation
Great vessel transposition	Congenital anomaly in which the pulmonary artery exits from the left ventricle and the aorta from the right ventricle. Incompatible with life after birth unless a large patent ductus or ventricular septal defect is present
Lipoxygenase	Enzyme that converts arachidonic acid to leukotriene precursors
NSAID	Nonsteroidal anti-inflammatory drug, for example, aspirin, ibuprofen, celecoxib. NSAIDs are cyclooxygenase inhibitors
Oxytocic	A substance that causes uterine contraction
Patent ductus arteriosus	Abnormal persistence after birth of the shunt between the pulmonary artery and the aorta; normal in the fetus
Phospholipase A_2	Enzyme in the cell membrane that generates arachidonic acid from membrane lipid constituents
Slow-reacting substance of anaphylaxis (SRS-A)	Material originally identified by bioassay from tissues of animals in anaphylactic shock; now recognized as a mixture of leukotrienes, especially LTC_4 and LTD_4

Replacement of tetraenoic fatty acids in the diet with trienoic (3 double bonds) or pentaenoic (5 double bonds) precursors results in the synthesis of much less active prostaglandin and leukotriene products. Thus, dietary therapy with fatty oils from plant or cold-water fish sources can be useful in conditions involving eicosanoids.

C. Mechanism of Action

Most eicosanoid effects are brought about by activation of cell surface receptors (Table 18–1) that are coupled by the G_s protein to adenylyl cyclase (producing cyclic adenosine monophosphate [cAMP]) or by the G_q protein to the phosphatidylinositol cascade (producing inositol 1,4,5-trisphosphate [IP_3] and diacylglycerol [DAG] second messengers).

D. Effects

A vast array of effects are produced in smooth muscle, platelets, the central nervous system, and other tissues. Some of the most important effects are summarized in Table 18–1. Eicosanoids

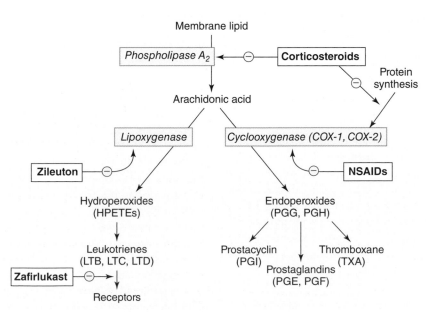

FIGURE 18–1 Synthesis of eicosanoid autacoids. Arachidonic acid is released from membrane lipids by phospholipase A_2 and then converted into straight-chain derivatives by lipoxygenase or into cyclized derivatives by cyclooxygenase. Because many of the effects of these products are pathogenic, drugs that inhibit synthesis or prevent the actions of the products are clinically useful.

TABLE 18–1 Effects of some important eicosanoids.

Effect	PGE_2	$PGF_{2\alpha}$	PGI_2	TXA_2	LTB_4	LTC_4	LTD_4
Major receptors	EP_{1-4}	$FP_{A,B}$	IP	$TP_{\alpha,\beta}$	$BLT_{1,2}$	$CysLT_2$	$CysLT_1$
Coupling protein	G_s, G_q	G_q	G_s	G_q	G_q	G_q	G_q, G_i
Vascular tone	↓	↑ or ↓	↓↓	↑↑↑	?	↑ or ↓	↑ or ↓
Bronchial tone	↓↓	↑↑	↓	↑↑↑	?	↑↑↑↑	↑↑↑↑
Uterine tone	↑, ↓[a]	↑↑↑	↓	↑↑	?	?	?
Platelet aggregation	↑ or ↓		↓↓↓	↑↑↑	?	?	?
Leukocyte chemotaxis	?	?	?	?	↑↑↑↑	↑↑	↑↑

[a]Low concentrations cause contraction; higher concentrations cause relaxation.

?, unknown effect.

most directly involved in pathologic processes include prostaglandin (PG) $F_{2\alpha}$, thromboxane A_2 (TXA_2), and the leukotrienes LTC_4 and LTD_4. LTC_4 and LTD_4 are components of the important mediator of bronchoconstriction, **slow-reacting substance of anaphylaxis (SRS-A).** Leukotriene LTB_4 is a chemotactic factor important in inflammation. PGE_2 and prostacyclin may act as endogenous vasodilators. PGE_1 and its derivatives have significant protective effects on the gastric mucosa. The mechanism may involve increased secretion of bicarbonate and mucus, decreased acid secretion, or both. PGE_1 and PGE_2 relax vascular and other smooth muscle. PGE_2 appears to be the natural vasodilator that maintains patency of the ductus arteriosus during fetal development. Prostaglandins are important modulators of glomerular filtration and act on the afferent and efferent arterioles and mesangial cells. Suppression of prostaglandin production with nonsteroidal anti-inflammatory drugs (NSAIDs, see following text) can markedly reduce the efficacy of diuretic agents (see Chapter 15). PGE_2 and $PGF_{2\alpha}$ are released in large amounts from the endometrium during menstruation and can cause dysmenorrhea. PGE_2 appears to be involved in the physiologic softening of the cervix at term; PGE_2 and $PGF_{2\alpha}$ may play a physiologic role in labor. Platelet aggregation is strongly activated by thromboxane. $PGF_{2\alpha}$ reduces intraocular pressure (see later discussion), but it is not known whether this is a physiologic effect of endogenous $PGF_{2\alpha}$.

E. Clinical Uses

1. Obstetrics—PGE_2 and $PGF_{2\alpha}$ cause contraction of the uterus. PGE_2 (as **dinoprostone**) is approved for use to soften the cervix at term before induction of labor with oxytocin. Both PGE_2 and $PGF_{2\alpha}$ have been used as abortifacients in the second trimester of pregnancy. Although effective in inducing labor at term, they produce more adverse effects (nausea, vomiting, diarrhea) than do other oxytocics (eg, oxytocin) used for this application. The PGE_1 analog **misoprostol** has been used with the progesterone antagonist mifepristone (RU 486) as an extremely effective

and safe abortifacient combination. Misoprostol has been used for this purpose in combination with either methotrexate or mifepristone in the United States. Misoprostol may cause diarrhea.

2. Pediatrics—PGE_1 is given as an infusion to maintain patency of the ductus arteriosus in infants with transposition of the great vessels until surgical correction can be undertaken.

3. Pulmonary hypertension and dialysis—Prostacyclin (PGI_2) is approved for use (as **epoprostenol**) in severe pulmonary hypertension and to prevent platelet aggregation in dialysis machines.

4. Peptic ulcer associated with NSAID use—Misoprostol is approved in the United States for the prevention of peptic ulcers in patients who must take high doses of NSAIDs for arthritis and who have a history of ulcer associated with this use.

5. Urology—PGE_1 (as **alprostadil**) is used in the treatment of impotence by injection into the cavernosa.

6. Ophthalmology—**Latanoprost,** a $PGF_{2\alpha}$ derivative, is used extensively for the topical treatment of glaucoma. **Bimatoprost, travoprost,** and **unoprostone** are newer, related drugs. These agents apparently increase the outflow of aqueous humor, thus reducing intraocular pressure.

EICOSANOID ANTAGONISTS

Phospholipase A_2 and cyclooxygenase can be inhibited by drugs and some of these inhibitors are mainstays in the treatment of inflammation (Figure 18–1 and Chapter 36). **Zileuton** is a selective inhibitor of lipoxygenase and some cyclooxygenase inhibitors exert a mild inhibitory effect on leukotriene synthesis. Inhibitors of the receptors for the prostaglandins and the leukotrienes are being actively sought. **Zafirlukast** and **montelukast,** inhibitors at the LTD_4 receptor, are currently available for the treatment of asthma (Chapter 20).

A. Corticosteroids

As indicated in Figure 18–1, corticosteroids inhibit the production of arachidonic acid by phospholipases in the membrane. This effect is mediated by intracellular steroid receptors that, when activated by an appropriate steroid, increase expression of specific proteins capable of inhibiting phospholipase. Steroids also inhibit the synthesis of COX-2. These effects are thought to be the major mechanisms of the important anti-inflammatory action of corticosteroids (see Chapter 39).

B. NSAIDs

Aspirin and other nonsteroidal anti-inflammatory drugs inhibit cyclooxygenase and the production of the thromboxane, prostaglandin, and prostacyclin (see Fig. 18–1). Most of the currently available NSAIDs nonselectively inhibit both COX-1 and COX-2. In fact, many inhibit COX-1 somewhat more effectively than COX-2, the isoform thought to be responsible for synthesis of inflammatory eicosanoids. **Celecoxib** is the most selective COX-2 inhibitor available in the United States; meloxicam is also slightly COX-2-selective. The highly COX-2-selective **rofecoxib** and **valdecoxib** were withdrawn from the US market because of reports of cardiovascular toxicity (see Chapter 36).

Inhibition of cyclooxygenase by aspirin, unlike that by other NSAIDs, is irreversible. Aspirin allergy may result from diversion of arachidonic acid to the leukotriene pathway when the cyclooxygenase-catalyzed prostaglandin pathway is blocked. The resulting increase in leukotriene synthesis causes the bronchoconstriction that is typical of aspirin allergy. For unknown reasons, this form of aspirin allergy is more common in persons with nasal polyps.

The antiplatelet action of aspirin results from the fact that the drug's inhibition of thromboxane synthesis is essentially permanent in platelets; they lack the machinery for new protein synthesis. In contrast, inhibition of prostacyclin synthesis in the vascular endothelium is temporary because these cells can synthesize new enzyme. Inhibition of prostaglandin synthesis also results in important anti-inflammatory effects. Inhibition of synthesis of fever-inducing prostaglandins in the brain produces the antipyretic action of NSAIDs. Closure of a patent ductus arteriosus in an otherwise normal infant can be accelerated with an NSAID such as indomethacin or ibuprofen.

C. Leukotriene Antagonists

As noted, an inhibitor of lipoxygenase (**zileuton**) and LTD_4 and LTE_4 receptor antagonists (**zafirlukast, montelukast**) are available for clinical use. Currently, these agents are approved only for use in asthma (see Chapter 20).

QUESTIONS

1. You have been treating a 50-year-old woman with moderately severe arthritis with nonsteroidal anti-inflammatory drugs for 6 months. She now complains of heartburn and indigestion. You give her a prescription for a drug to be taken along with the anti-inflammatory agent, but 2 days later she calls the office complaining that your last prescription has caused severe diarrhea. Which of the following is most likely to be associated with increased gastrointestinal motility and diarrhea?
   (A) Aspirin
   (B) Corticosteroids
   (C) Leukotriene LTB_4
   (D) Misoprostol
   (E) Zileuton

2. Which of the following drugs inhibits thromboxane synthesis much more effectively than prostacyclin synthesis?
   (A) Aspirin
   (B) Hydrocortisone
   (C) Ibuprofen
   (D) Indomethacin
   (E) Zileuton

3. A 57-year-old man has severe pulmonary hypertension and right ventricular hypertrophy. Which of the following agents causes vasodilation and may be useful in pulmonary hypertension?
   (A) Angiotensin II
   (B) Ergotamine
   (C) Prostaglandin $PGF_{2\alpha}$
   (D) Prostacyclin
   (E) Thromboxane

4. A 19-year-old woman complains of severe dysmenorrhea. A uterine stimulant derived from membrane lipid in the endometrium is
   (A) Angiotensin II
   (B) Oxytocin
   (C) Prostacyclin (PGI_2)
   (D) Prostaglandin PGE_2
   (E) Serotonin

5. Inflammation is a complex tissue reaction that includes the release of cytokines, leukotrienes, prostaglandins, and peptides. Prostaglandins involved in inflammatory processes are typically produced from arachidonic acid by which of the following enzymes?
   (A) Cyclooxygenase-1
   (B) Cyclooxygenase-2
   (C) Glutathione-S-transferase
   (D) Lipoxygenase
   (E) Phospholipase A_2

6. A newborn infant is diagnosed with transposition of the great vessels, wherein the aorta exits from the right ventricle and the pulmonary artery from the left ventricle. Which of the following drugs is likely to be used in preparation for surgical correction of this anomaly?
   (A) Aspirin
   (B) Leukotriene LTC_4
   (C) Prednisone
   (D) Prostaglandin PGE_2
   (E) Prostaglandin $PGF_{2\alpha}$

7. A patient with a bleeding tendency presents in the hematology clinic. He is apparently taking large amounts of an unidentified drug that inhibits platelet activity. Which of the following *directly* and *reversibly* inhibits platelet cyclooxygenase?
   (A) Alprostadil
   (B) Aspirin
   (C) Ibuprofen
   (D) Leukotriene LTC$_4$
   (E) Misoprostol
   (F) Prednisone
   (G) Prostacyclin
   (H) Zafirlukast
   (I) Zileuton

8. Which of the following is a component of slow-reacting substance of anaphylaxis (SRS-A)?
   (A) Alprostadil
   (B) Aspirin
   (C) Leukotriene LTB$_4$
   (D) Leukotriene LTC$_4$
   (E) Misoprostol
   (F) Prednisone
   (G) Prostacyclin
   (H) Zafirlukast
   (I) Zileuton

9. A 17-year-old patient complains that he develops wheezing and severe shortness of breath whenever he takes aspirin for headache. Increased levels of which of the following may be responsible, in part, for some cases of aspirin hypersensitivity?
   (A) Alprostadil
   (B) Hydrocortisone
   (C) Ibuprofen
   (D) Leukotriene LTC$_4$
   (E) Misoprostol
   (F) PGE$_2$
   (G) Prostacyclin
   (H) Thromboxane
   (I) Zileuton

10. Which of the following is a leukotriene receptor blocker?
   (A) Alprostadil
   (B) Aspirin
   (C) Ibuprofen
   (D) Leukotriene LTC$_4$
   (E) Misoprostol
   (F) Prednisone
   (G) Prostacyclin
   (H) Zafirlukast
   (I) Zileuton

ANSWERS

1. Aspirin, corticosteroids, and zileuton do not cause diarrhea. LTB$_4$ is a chemotactic factor. The answer is **D**.

2. Hydrocortisone and other corticosteroids inhibit phospholipase. Ibuprofen and indomethacin inhibit cyclooxygenase reversibly, whereas zileuton inhibits lipoxygenase. Because aspirin inhibits cyclooxygenase irreversibly, its action is more effective in platelets, which lack the ability to synthesize new enzyme, than in the endothelium. The answer is **A**.

3. Prostacyclin (PGI$_2$) is a very potent vasodilator. All the other choices in the list are vasoconstrictors. The answer is **D**.

4. Although serotonin and, in some species, histamine may cause uterine stimulation, these substances are not derived from membrane lipid. Similarly, oxytocin causes uterine contraction, but it is a peptide hormone secreted by the posterior pituitary. Prostacyclin relaxes the uterus (Table 18–1). The answer is **D**.

5. See Figure 18–1. Phospholipase A$_2$ converts membrane phospholipid to arachidonic acid. Cyclooxygenases convert arachidonic acid to prostaglandins. COX-2 is the enzyme believed to be responsible for this reaction in inflammatory cells. The answer is **B**.

6. Infants with great vessel transposition pump venous blood to the aorta and oxygenated blood back to the lungs. Therefore, they require surgical correction as soon as they are strong enough to withstand the procedure. In the meantime, they are dependent on a patent ductus arteriosus to allow some oxygenated blood to flow from the left ventricle via the pulmonary artery to the aorta. The ductus can be prevented from closing by infusing the vasodilator PGE$_2$. The answer is **D**.

7. Aspirin is a direct but *irreversible* inhibitor of cyclooxygenase. NSAIDs other than aspirin (such as ibuprofen) are reversible inhibitors of COX. Corticosteroids reduce the synthesis of cyclooxygenase. The answer is **C**.

8. The leukotriene C and D series are major components of SRS-A. Leukotriene LTB$_4$ is a chemotactic eicosanoid. The answer is **D**.

9. When cyclooxygenase is blocked, leukotrienes may be produced in increased amounts by diversion of prostaglandin precursors into the lipoxygenase pathway (Figure 18–1). In patients with aspirin hypersensitivity, this might precipitate the bronchoconstriction often observed in this condition. The answer is **D**.

10. Zileuton blocks the synthesis of leukotrienes. Zafirlukast and montelukast block LTD$_4$ receptors. The answer is **H**.

CHECKLIST

When you complete this chapter, you should be able to:

❏ List the major effects of PGE_2, $PGF_{2\alpha}$, PGI_2, LTB_4, LTC_4, and LTD_4.

❏ List the cellular sites of synthesis and the effects of thromboxane and prostacyclin in the vascular system.

❏ List the currently available antagonists of leukotrienes and prostaglandins and their targets (receptors or enzymes).

❏ Explain the different effects of aspirin on prostaglandin, thromboxane, and leukotriene synthesis.

DRUG SUMMARY TABLE: Prostaglandins & Other Eicosanoids

Subclass	Mechanism of Action	Clinical Applications	Pharmacokinetics	Toxicities, Interactions
Leukotrienes				
LTB_4	Chemotactic factor in inflammation	None	Local release Duration: seconds	Inflammatory mediator
LTC_4, LTD_4	Bronchoconstrictors important in anaphylaxis • cause edema	None	Local release Duration: seconds	Inflammatory mediators
Leukotriene antagonists				
Lipoxygenase inhibitor: zileuton	Blocks synthesis of leukotrienes	Asthma prophylaxis	Oral Duration: ~3 h	Liver enzyme elevation
Leukotriene receptor inhibitors: montelukast, zafirlukast	Block $CysLT_1$ receptor • reduce bronchoconstriction in asthma	Asthma prophylaxis	Oral Duration: 3–10 h	Liver enzyme elevation
Thromboxane				
TXA_2	Activates $TP_{\alpha,\beta}$ receptors, causes platelet aggregation, vasoconstriction	None	Local release Duration: seconds	See Mechanism of Action
Prostacyclin				
PGI_2: epoprostenol	Activates IP receptors, causes vasodilation, reduces platelet aggregation	Vasodilator in pulmonary hypertension, antiplatelet agent in extracorporeal dialysis	Infusion Duration: minutes	Hypotension, flushing, headache
PGI_2 analog, treprostinil: parenteral for pulmonary hypertension				
Prostaglandins				
PGE_1 derivative: misoprostol	Activates EP receptors, causes increased HCO_3^- and mucus secretion in stomach • uterine contraction	Protective agent in peptic ulcer disease • abortifacient	Oral Duration: minutes	Diarrhea, uterine cramping
PGE_1 analog, alprostadil: injectable form for erectile dysfunction				
PGE_1	Relaxes smooth muscle in ductus arteriosus	Transposition of great vessels, to maintain patent ductus until surgery	Infusion Duration: minutes	Hypotension
PGE_2: dinoprostone	Low concentrations contract, higher concentrations relax uterine and cervical smooth muscle	Abortifacient, cervical ripening	Vaginal Duration: 3–5 h	Cramping, fetal trauma
PGF_2 derivative: latanoprost	Increases outflow of aqueous humor, reduces intraocular pressure	Glaucoma	Topical Duration: 4–8 h	Color change in iris

(Continued)

DRUG SUMMARY TABLE: Prostaglandins & Other Eicosanoids (*Continued*)

Subclass	Mechanism of Action	Clinical Applications	Pharmacokinetics	Toxicities, Interactions
Cyclooxygenase inhibitors (NSAIDs)				
Nonselective COX-1, COX-2 inhibitors: ibuprofen, indomethacin, naproxen, others	Reversibly inhibit COX-1 and COX-2 • reduce synthesis of prostaglandins	See Chapter 36		
Aspirin	Irreversibly inhibits COX-1 and COX-2 • reduces synthesis of prostaglandins	See Chapter 36		
Selective COX-2 inhibitor: celecoxib	Selectively reversibly inhibits COX-2	See Chapter 36		
Phospholipase A$_2$ inhibitors				
Corticosteroids	Reversibly inhibit phospholipase A$_2$ and reduce synthesis of COX enzymes	See Chapter 39		

Nitric Oxide, Donors, & Inhibitors

Nitric oxide is an autacoid produced from arginine in the body, and the active metabolite of drugs that release it (NO donors); it is available as a drug in itself (NO gas). It interacts with iron in hemoglobin and can be inhibited by hemoglobin.

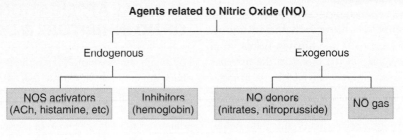

Agents related to Nitric Oxide (NO)

Endogenous

Exogenous

NOS activators
(ACh, histamine, etc)

Inhibitors
(hemoglobin)

NO donors
(nitrates, nitroprusside)

NO gas

Nitric oxide (NO) is a product of the metabolism of arginine in many tissues. It is thought to be an important paracrine vasodilator, and it may also play a role in cell death and in neurotransmission; it therefore qualifies as an autacoid. NO is also released from several important vasodilator drug molecules.

ENDOGENOUS NO

Endogenous NO is synthesized by a family of enzymes collectively called **nitric oxide synthase (NOS)**, Figure 19–1. These intracellular enzymes are activated by calcium influx or by cytokines. Arginine, the primary substrate, is converted by NOS to citrulline and NO. Three forms of NO synthase are known: isoform 1 (bNOS, cNOS, or nNOS, a constitutive form found in epithelial and neuronal cells); isoform 2 (iNOS or mNOS, an inducible form found in macrophages and smooth muscle cells); and isoform 3 (eNOS, a constitutive form found in endothelial cells). NOS can be inhibited by arginine analogs such as N^G-monomethyl-L-arginine (L-NMMA). Under some circumstances (eg, ischemia), NO may be formed from endogenous nitrate ion. NO is not stored in cells. Because it is a gas at body temperature, NO very rapidly diffuses from its site of synthesis to surrounding tissues. Drugs that cause endogenous NO release do so by stimulating its synthesis by NOS. Such drugs include muscarinic agonists, histamine, and certain other vasodilators (bradykinin, hydralazine).

High-Yield Terms to Learn	
Endothelium-derived relaxing factor, EDRF	A mixture of nitric oxide and other vasodilator substances synthesized in vascular endothelium
Nitric oxide donor	A molecule from which nitric oxide can be released (eg, arginine, nitroprusside, nitroglycerin)
cNOS, iNOS, eNOS	Naturally occurring isoforms of nitric oxide synthase: respectively, constitutive (NOS-1), inducible (NOS-2), and endothelial (NOS-3) isoforms

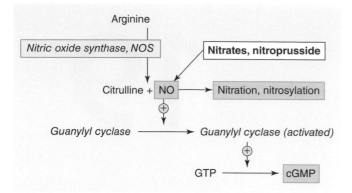

FIGURE 19–1 The pathway for nitric oxide (NO) synthesis and release from NO-containing drugs and the mechanism of stimulation of cGMP (cyclic guanosine monophosphate) synthesis. The action of cGMP on smooth muscle relaxation is shown in Figure 12–3.

EXOGENOUS NO DONORS

NO is released from several important drugs, including **nitroprusside** (Chapter 11), **nitrates** (Chapter 12), and **nitrites.** Release from nitroprusside occurs spontaneously in the blood in the presence of oxygen, whereas release from nitrates and nitrites is intracellular and requires the presence of the mitochondrial enzyme ALD2 and thiol compounds such as cysteine (see Chapter 12). Tolerance may develop to nitrates and nitrites if endogenous thiol compounds are depleted.

EFFECTS OF NO

A. Smooth Muscle

NO is a powerful vasodilator in all vascular beds and a potent relaxant in most other smooth muscle tissues. The mechanism of this effect involves activation of guanylyl cyclase (Figure 19–1) and the synthesis of cyclic guanosine monophosphate (cGMP). This cGMP, in turn, facilitates the dephosphorylation and inactivation of myosin light chains, which results in relaxation of smooth muscle (see Figure 12–3). NO plays a physiologic role in erectile tissue function, in which smooth muscle relaxation is required to bring about the influx of blood that causes erection. NO appears to be a pathophysiologic contributor to hypotension in septic shock.

B. Cell Adhesion

NO has effects on cell adhesion that result in reduced platelet aggregation and reduced neutrophil adhesion to vascular endothelium. The latter effect is probably due to reduced expression of adhesion molecules, for example, integrins, by endothelial cells.

C. Inflammation

Tissue injury causes NO synthesis, and NO appears to facilitate inflammation both directly and through the stimulation of prostaglandin synthesis by cyclooxygenase 2.

D. Other Effects

Some evidence suggests that NO may act as a neurotransmitter. NO also may be involved in some types of apoptosis and cell death and in host reactions to parasites.

CLINICAL APPLICATIONS OF NO INHIBITORS & DONORS

Although *inhibitors* of NO synthesis are of great research interest, none are currently in clinical use. NO can be *inactivated* by heme and hemoglobin, but application of this approach is investigational.

In contrast, drugs that activate endogenous NO synthesis and donors of the molecule were in use long before NO was discovered and continue to be very important in clinical medicine. The cardiovascular applications of nitroprusside (Chapter 11) and the nitrates and nitrites (Chapter 12) have been discussed. The treatment of preeclampsia, pulmonary hypertension, and acute respiratory distress syndrome are currently under clinical investigation. Early results from pulmonary disease studies appear promising, and one preparation of NO gas (INOmax) has been approved for use in neonates with hypoxic respiratory failure and adults with pulmonary hypertension.

Preclinical studies suggest that chronic use of NO donor drugs or dietary supplementation with arginine may assist in slowing atherosclerosis, especially in grafted organs. In contrast, *acute rejection* of grafts may involve upregulation of NOS enzymes, and inhibition of these enzymes may prolong graft survival.

QUESTIONS

1. Which one of the following is not a nitric oxide donor but causes it to be released from endogenous precursors, resulting in vasodilation?
    (A) Acetylcholine
    (B) Arginine
    (C) Isosorbide mononitrate
    (D) Nitroglycerin
    (E) Nitroprusside

2. A molecule that releases nitric oxide in the blood is
 (A) Citrulline
 (B) Histamine
 (C) Isoproterenol
 (D) Nitroglycerin
 (E) Nitroprusside

3. The inducible isoform of nitric oxide synthase (iNOS, isoform 2) is found primarily in which of the following?
 (A) Cartilage
 (B) Eosinophils
 (C) Macrophages
 (D) Platelets
 (E) Vascular endothelial cells

4. The primary endogenous substrate for the enzyme nitric oxide synthase (NOS) is
 (A) Acetylcholine
 (B) Angiotensinogen
 (C) Arginine
 (D) Citrulline
 (E) Heme

5. Which of the following is a recognized effect of nitric oxide (NO)?
 (A) Arrhythmia
 (B) Bronchoconstriction
 (C) Constipation
 (D) Inhibition of acute graft rejection
 (E) Pulmonary vasodilation

6. Which of the following is an approved application for nitric oxide administered as a gas?
 (A) Asthma
 (B) Dysmenorrhea
 (C) Patent ductus arteriosus
 (D) Pulmonary hypertension
 (E) Transposition of the great vessels in newborns

ANSWERS

1. Nitroprusside and organic nitrites (eg, amyl nitrite) and nitrates (eg, nitroglycerin, isosorbide dinitrate, and isosorbide mononitrate) contain NO groups that can be released as NO. Arginine is the normal source of endogenous NO. Acetylcholine stimulates the production of NO from arginine. The answer is **A.**

2. Nitroprusside is the only molecule in this list that releases NO in the bloodstream. The answer is **E.**

3. The inducible form of NOS is associated with inflammation, and the enzyme is found in highest concentration in macrophages, cells that are particularly involved in inflammation. The answer is **C.**

4. Arginine is the substrate and citrulline and NO are the products of NOS. The answer is **C.**

5. NO does not cause arrhythmias or constipation. It causes bronchodilation and may hasten graft rejection. NO does cause pulmonary vasodilation. The answer is **E.**

6. Thus far, NO gas has been approved for use by inhalation in neonatal hypoxic respiratory failure and adult pulmonary hypertension. The answer is **D.**

SKILL KEEPER ANSWER: NONINNERVATED RECEPTORS (SEE CHAPTER 6)

Endothelial cells lining blood vessels have noninnervated muscarinic receptors. These M_3 receptors use the G_q-coupling protein to activate phospholipase C, which releases inositol 1,4,5-trisphosphate and diacylglycerol from membrane lipids. eNOS is activated and NO is released, causing vasodilation. Histamine H_1 receptors are also found in the vascular endothelium and similarly cause vasodilation through the synthesis and release of NO. Other noninnervated (or poorly innervated) receptors found in blood vessels include α_2 and β_2 receptors. The α_2 receptors use G_i to inhibit adenylyl cyclase, reducing cyclic adenosine monophosphate (cAMP) and causing contraction in the vessel. (Recall that the blood pressure-lowering action of α_2 agonists is mediated by actions in the CNS, not in the vessels.) Conversely, β_2 receptors activate adenylyl cyclase via G_s and increase cAMP, resulting in relaxation.

CHECKLIST

When you complete this chapter, you should be able to:

❑ Name the enzyme responsible for the synthesis of NO in tissues.

❑ List the major beneficial and toxic effects of endogenous NO.

❑ List 2 drugs that cause release of endogenous NO.

❑ List 2 drugs that spontaneously or enzymatically break down in the body to release NO.

DRUG SUMMARY TABLE: Nitric Oxide, Donors, & Inhibitors

Subclass	Mechanism of Action	Clinical Applications	Pharmacokinetics	Toxicities, Interactions
Nitric oxide (NO)				
Nitric oxide gas	Activates guanylyl cyclase, increases cGMP synthesis, causes smooth muscle relaxation	Pulmonary hypertension	Inhaled gas administered continuously	Methemoglobinemia, conversion to nitrogen dioxide (a pulmonary irritant)
Nitric oxide synthase (NOS) activators				
Acetylcholine, histamine, others	Increased $IP_3 \rightarrow \uparrow$ intracellular $Ca^{2+} \rightarrow$ activates NOS, resulting in conversion of arginine to citrulline plus NO	See Chapters 7 and 16		
Nitric oxide donors				
Nitroglycerin, other nitrates, nitroprusside	Release NO in smooth muscle (nitrates) or in blood (nitroprusside) • increase cGMP synthesis and cause relaxation in smooth muscle	See Chapters 11 and 12		

cGMP, cyclic guanosine monophosphate.

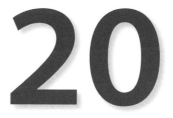

Drugs Used in Asthma & Chronic Obstructive Pulmonary Disease

Asthma is a disease characterized by airway inflammation and episodic, reversible bronchospasm. Drugs useful in asthma include bronchodilators (smooth muscle relaxants) and anti-inflammatory drugs. Bronchodilators include sympathomimetics, especially β_2-selective agonists, muscarinic antagonists, methylxanthines, and leukotriene receptor blockers. Anti-inflammatory drugs used

in asthma include corticosteroids, mast cell stabilizers, and an anti-IgE antibody. Leukotriene antagonists play a dual role. Chronic obstructive pulmonary disease (COPD) is characterized by airflow limitation that is less reversible than in asthma and by a progressive course. However, many of the same drugs are used.

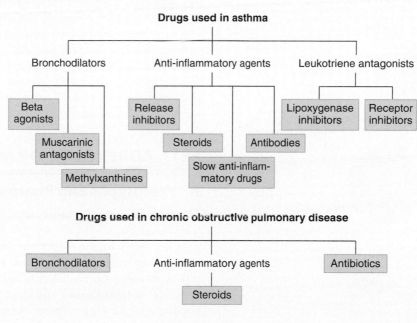

PATHOPHYSIOLOGY OF ASTHMA

The immediate cause of asthmatic bronchoconstriction is the release of several mediators from IgE-sensitized mast cells and other cells involved in immunologic responses (Figure 20–1). These mediators include the leukotrienes LTC_4 and LTD_4. In addition, chemotactic

mediators such as LTB_4 attract inflammatory cells to the airways. Finally, several cytokines and some enzymes are released, leading to chronic inflammation. Chronic inflammation leads to marked bronchial hyperreactivity to various inhaled substances, including antigens, histamine, muscarinic agonists, and irritants such as sulfur dioxide (SO_2) and cold air. This reactivity is partially mediated by

High-Yield Terms to Learn

Bronchial hyperreactivity	Pathologic increase in the bronchoconstrictor response to antigens and irritants; caused by bronchial inflammation
IgE-mediated disease	Disease caused by excessive or misdirected immune response mediated by IgE antibodies. Example: asthma
Mast cell degranulation	Exocytosis of granules from mast cells with release of mediators of inflammation and bronchoconstriction
Phosphodiesterase (PDE)	Family of enzymes that degrade cyclic nucleotides to nucleotides, for example, cAMP (active) to AMP (inactive); various isoforms, some degrade cGMP to GMP
Tachyphylaxis	Rapid loss of responsiveness to a stimulus (eg, a drug)

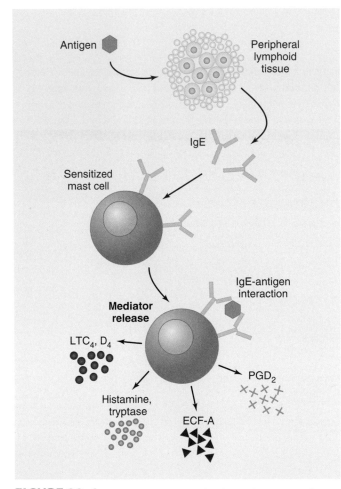

FIGURE 20–1 Immunologic model for the pathogenesis of asthma. Exposure to antigen causes synthesis of IgE, which binds to and sensitizes mast cells and other inflammatory cells. When such sensitized cells are challenged with antigen, a variety of mediators are released that can account for most of the signs of the early bronchoconstrictor response in asthma. LTC_4, D_4, leukotrienes C_4 and D_4; ECF-A, eosinophil chemotactic factor-A; PGD_2, prostaglandin D_2. (Modified and reproduced, with permission, from Gold WW: Cholinergic pharmacology in asthma. In: *Asthma Physiology, Immunopharmacology, and Treatment.* Austen KF, Lichtenstein LM, editors. Academic Press, 1974.)

vagal reflexes. COPD is often triggered by upper respiratory infection (like asthma) but occurs in older patients (usually long-term smokers) and is poorly reversible with bronchodilators.

STRATEGIES OF ASTHMA THERAPY

Acute bronchospasm must be treated promptly and effectively with bronchodilators ("reliever" drugs). **Beta₂ agonists, muscarinic antagonists,** and **theophylline** and its derivatives are available for this indication. Long-term preventive treatment requires control of the inflammatory process in the airways ("controller" drugs). The most important anti-inflammatory drugs in the treatment of chronic asthma are the **corticosteroids.** Long-acting β_2 agonists can improve the response to corticosteroids. Anti-IgE antibodies also appear promising for chronic therapy. The **leukotriene antagonists** have effects on both bronchoconstriction and inflammation but are used only for prophylaxis.

BETA-ADRENOCEPTOR AGONISTS

A. Prototypes and Pharmacokinetics

The most important sympathomimetics used to reverse asthmatic bronchoconstriction are the direct-acting **β₂-selective agonists** (see Chapter 9). Of the indirect-acting sympathomimetics, ephedrine was once used, but it is now obsolete for this application. Of the selective agents, **albuterol, terbutaline,** and **metaproterenol**[*] are short-acting and are the most important in the United States. **Salmeterol, formoterol,** and **indacaterol** are long-acting β₂-selective agonists, but indacaterol is currently approved only for COPD. Beta agonists are given almost exclusively by inhalation, usually from pressurized aerosol canisters but occasionally by nebulizer. The inhalational route decreases the systemic dose (and adverse effects) while delivering an effective dose locally to the airway smooth muscle. The older drugs have durations of action of 6 h or less; salmeterol, formoterol, and indacaterol act for 12–24 h.

---

[*]Do not confuse metaproterenol, a β_2 agonist, with metoprolol, a β-blocker.

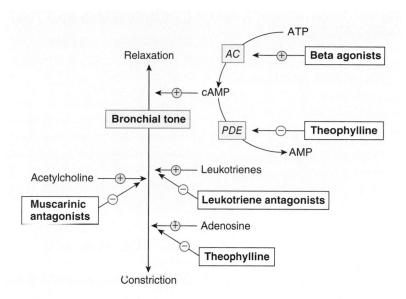

FIGURE 20–2 Possible mechanisms of β agonists, muscarinic antagonists, theophylline, and leukotriene antagonists in altering bronchial tone in asthma. AC, adenylyl cyclase; PDE, phosphodiesterase.

B. Mechanism and Effects

Beta-adrenoceptor agonists stimulate adenylyl cyclase (via the β_2-adrenoceptor–G_s-coupling protein-adenylyl cyclase pathway) and increase cyclic adenosine monophosphate (cAMP) in smooth muscle cells (Figure 20–2). The increase in cAMP results in a powerful bronchodilator response.

C. Clinical Use and Toxicity

Sympathomimetics are first-line therapy in acute asthma. Shorter acting sympathomimetics (albuterol, metaproterenol, terbutaline) are the drugs of choice for acute episodes of bronchospasm. Their effects last for 4 h or less, and they are not effective for prophylaxis. The long-acting agents (salmeterol, formoterol) should be used for prophylaxis, in which their 12-h duration of action is useful. They should not be used for acute episodes because their onset of action is too slow. Furthermore, used alone, they increase asthma mortality, whereas in combination with corticosteroids, they improve control. In almost all patients, the shorter-acting β agonists are the most effective bronchodilators available and are life-saving for acute asthma. Many patients with chronic obstructive pulmonary disease (COPD) also benefit, although the risk of toxicity is increased in this condition.

Skeletal muscle tremor is a common adverse β_2 effect. Beta$_2$ selectivity is relative. At high clinical dosage, these agents have significant β_1 effects. Even when they are given by inhalation, some cardiac effect (tachycardia) is common. Other adverse effects are rare. When the agents are used excessively, arrhythmias may occur. Loss of responsiveness (tolerance, tachyphylaxis) is an unwanted effect of excessive use of the short-acting sympathomimetics. Patients with COPD often have concurrent cardiac disease and may have arrhythmias even at normal dosage.

METHYLXANTHINES

A. Prototypes and Pharmacokinetics

The methylxanthines are purine derivatives. Three major methylxanthines are found in plants and provide the stimulant effects of 3 common beverages: **caffeine** (in coffee), **theophylline** (tea), and **theobromine** (cocoa). Theophylline is the only member of this group that is important in the treatment of asthma. This drug and several analogs are orally active and available as various salts and as the base. Theophylline is available in both prompt-release and slow-release forms. Theophylline is eliminated by P450 drug-metabolizing enzymes in the liver. Clearance varies with age (highest in young adolescents), smoking status (higher in smokers), and concurrent use of other drugs that inhibit or induce hepatic enzymes.

B. Mechanism of Action and Effects

The methylxanthines inhibit phosphodiesterase (PDE), the enzyme that degrades cAMP to AMP (Figure 20–2), and thus increase cAMP. This anti-PDE effect, however, requires high concentrations of the drug. Methylxanthines also block adenosine receptors in the central nervous system (CNS) and elsewhere, but a relation between this action and the bronchodilating effect has not been clearly established. It is possible that bronchodilation is caused by a third as yet unrecognized action.

In asthma, bronchodilation is the most important therapeutic action of theophylline. Increased strength of contraction of the diaphragm has been demonstrated in some patients, an effect particularly useful in COPD. Other effects of therapeutic doses include CNS stimulation, cardiac stimulation, vasodilation, a slight increase in blood pressure (probably caused by the release of norepinephrine from adrenergic nerves), diuresis, and increased gastrointestinal motility.

C. Clinical Use and Toxicity

The major clinical use of methylxanthines is asthma and COPD. Slow-release theophylline (for control of nocturnal asthma) is the most commonly used methylxanthine. **Aminophylline** is a salt of theophylline that is sometimes prescribed. Another methylxanthine derivative, **pentoxifylline,** is promoted as a remedy for intermittent claudication; this effect is said to result from decreased viscosity of the blood. Of course, the nonmedical use of the methylxanthines in coffee, tea, and cocoa is far greater, in total quantities consumed, than the medical uses of the drugs.

The common adverse effects of methylxanthines include gastrointestinal distress, tremor, and insomnia. Severe nausea and vomiting, hypotension, cardiac arrhythmias, and seizures may result from overdosage. Very large overdoses (eg, in suicide attempts) are potentially lethal because of arrhythmias and seizures. Beta blockers are useful in reversing severe cardiovascular toxicity from theophylline.

MUSCARINIC ANTAGONISTS

A. Prototypes and Pharmacokinetics

Atropine and other naturally occurring belladonna alkaloids were used for many years in the treatment of asthma but have been replaced by **ipratropium,** a quaternary antimuscarinic agent designed for aerosol use. This drug is delivered to the airways by pressurized aerosol and has little systemic action. **Tiotropium** is a longer-acting analog.

B. Mechanism of Action and Effects

When given by aerosol, ipratropium and tiotropium competitively block muscarinic receptors in the airways and effectively prevent bronchoconstriction mediated by vagal discharge. If given systemically (not an approved use), these drugs are indistinguishable from other short-acting muscarinic blockers.

Muscarinic antagonists reverse bronchoconstriction in some asthma patients (especially children) and in many patients with COPD. They have no effect on the chronic inflammatory aspects of asthma.

C. Clinical Use and Toxicity

Ipratropium and tiotropium are useful in one third to two thirds of asthmatic patients; β_2 agonists are effective in almost all. For acute bronchospasm, therefore, the β agonists are usually preferred. However, in COPD, which is often associated with acute episodes of bronchospasm, the antimuscarinic agents may be more effective and less toxic than β agonists.

Because these agents are delivered directly to the airway and are minimally absorbed, systemic effects are small. When given in excessive dosage, minor atropine-like toxic effects may occur (see Chapter 8). In contrast to the β_2 agonists, muscarinic antagonists do not cause tremor or arrhythmias.

CROMOLYN & NEDOCROMIL

A. Prototypes and Pharmacokinetics

Cromolyn (disodium cromoglycate) and nedocromil are unusually insoluble chemicals, so that even massive doses given orally or by aerosol result in minimal systemic blood levels. They are given by aerosol for asthma but are now rarely used in the United States. **Cromolyn** is the prototype of this group.

B. Mechanism of Action and Effects

The mechanism of action of these drugs is poorly understood but may involve a decrease in the release of mediators (such as leukotrienes and histamine). The drugs have no bronchodilator action but can prevent bronchoconstriction caused by a challenge with antigen to which the patient is allergic. Cromolyn and nedocromil are capable of preventing both early and late responses to challenge (Figure 20–3).

Because they are not absorbed from the site of administration, cromolyn and nedocromil have only local effects. When administered orally, cromolyn has some efficacy in preventing food allergy. Similar actions have been demonstrated after local application in the conjunctiva and the nasopharynx for allergic IgE-mediated reactions in these tissues.

C. Clinical Uses and Toxicity

Asthma (especially in children) was the most important use for cromolyn and nedocromil. Nasal and eyedrop formulations of cromolyn are available for hay fever, and an oral formulation is used for food allergy.

Cromolyn and nedocromil may cause cough and irritation of the airway when given by aerosol. Rare instances of drug allergy have been reported.

CORTICOSTEROIDS

A. Prototypes and Pharmacokinetics

All the corticosteroids are potentially beneficial in severe asthma (see Chapter 39). However, because of their toxicity,

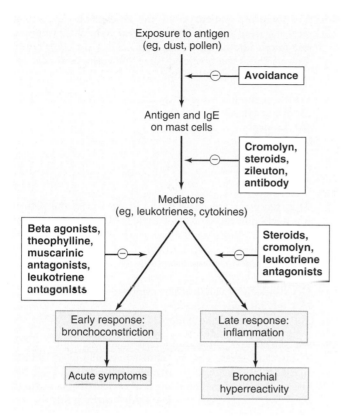

Exposure to antigen
(eg, dust, pollen)

⊖ Avoidance

Antigen and IgE
on mast cells

⊖ Cromolyn,
steroids,
zileuton,
antibody

Mediators
(eg, leukotrienes, cytokines)

Beta agonists,
theophylline,
muscarinic
antagonists,
leukotriene
antagonists ⊖

⊖ Steroids,
cromolyn,
leukotriene
antagonists

Early response:
bronchoconstriction

Late response:
inflammation

Acute symptoms

Bronchial
hyperreactivity

FIGURE 20–3 Summary of treatment strategies in asthma. (This article was published in *Allergy Asthma Immunol*, Vol 55, Cockcroft DW, The bronchial late response in the pathogenesis of asthma and its modulation by therapy, Page 857, Copyright Elsevier, 1985.)

systemic (oral) corticosteroids (usually **prednisone**) are used chronically only when other therapies are unsuccessful. In contrast, local aerosol administration of surface-active corticosteroids (eg, **beclomethasone, budesonide, dexamethasone, flunisolide, fluticasone, mometasone**) is relatively safe, and inhaled corticosteroids have become common first-line therapy for individuals with moderate to severe asthma. Important intravenous corticosteroids for status asthmaticus include **prednisolone** (the active metabolite of prednisone) and **hydrocortisone**.

B. Mechanism of Action and Effects

Corticosteroids reduce the synthesis of arachidonic acid by phospholipase A_2 and inhibit the expression of COX-2, the inducible form of cyclooxygenase (see Chapter 18). It has also been suggested that corticosteroids increase the responsiveness of β adrenoceptors in the airway and they probably act by other mechanisms as well.

Glucocorticoids bind to intracellular receptors and activate glucocorticoid response elements (GREs) in the nucleus, resulting in synthesis of substances that prevent the full expression of inflammation and allergy. See Chapter 39 for

details. Reduced activity of phospholipase A_2 is thought to be particularly important in asthma because the leukotrienes that result from eicosanoid synthesis are extremely potent bronchoconstrictors and may also participate in the late inflammatory response (Figure 20–3).

C. Clinical Use and Toxicity

Inhaled glucocorticoids are now considered appropriate (even for children) in most cases of moderate asthma that are not fully responsive to aerosol β agonists. It is believed that such early use may prevent the severe, progressive inflammatory changes characteristic of long-standing asthma. This is a shift from earlier beliefs that steroids should be used only in severe refractory asthma. In such cases of severe asthma, patients are usually hospitalized and stabilized on daily systemic prednisone and then switched to inhaled or alternate-day oral therapy before discharge. In status asthmaticus, parenteral steroids are lifesaving and apparently act more promptly than in ordinary asthma. Patients with COPD tend to be more resistant to the beneficial effects of steroids. Their mechanism of action in these conditions is not fully understood. (See Chapter 39 for other uses.)

Frequent aerosol administration of glucocorticoids can occasionally result in a very small degree of adrenal suppression, but this is rarely significant. More commonly, changes in oropharyngeal flora result in candidiasis. If oral therapy is required, adrenal suppression can be reduced by using alternate-day therapy (ie, giving the drug in slightly higher dosage every other day rather than smaller doses every day). The major systemic toxicities of the glucocorticoids described in Chapter 39 are much more likely to occur when systemic treatment is required for more than 2 weeks, as in severe refractory asthma. Regular use of inhaled steroids *does* cause mild growth retardation in children, but these children eventually reach full predicted adult stature.

LEUKOTRIENE ANTAGONISTS

These drugs interfere with the synthesis or the action of the leukotrienes (see also Chapter 18). Although their value has been established, they are not as effective as corticosteroids in severe asthma.

A. Leukotriene Receptor Blockers

Zafirlukast and **montelukast** are antagonists at the LTD_4 leukotriene receptor (see Table 18–1). The LTE_4 receptor is also blocked. These drugs are orally active and have been shown to be effective in preventing exercise-, antigen-, and aspirin-induced bronchospasm. They are not recommended for acute episodes of asthma. Toxicity is generally low. Rare reports of Churg-Strauss syndrome, allergic granulomatous angiitis, have appeared, but an association with these drugs has not been established.

B. Lipoxygenase Inhibitor

Zileuton is an orally active drug that selectively inhibits 5-lipoxygenase, a key enzyme in the conversion of arachidonic acid to leukotrienes. The drug is effective in preventing both exercise- and antigen-induced bronchospasm. It is also effective against "aspirin allergy," the bronchospasm that results from ingestion of aspirin by individuals who apparently divert all eicosanoid production to leukotrienes when the cyclooxygenase pathway is blocked (Chapter 18). The toxicity of zileuton includes occasional elevation of liver enzymes, and this drug is therefore less popular than the receptor blockers.

ANTI-IgE ANTIBODY

Omalizumab is a humanized murine monoclonal antibody to human IgE. It binds to the IgE on sensitized mast cells and prevents activation by asthma triggers and subsequent release of inflammatory mediators. Although approved in 2003 for the prophylactic management of asthma, experience with this drug is limited because it is very expensive and must be administered parenterally.

QUESTIONS

1. One effect that theophylline, nitroglycerin, isoproterenol, and histamine have in common is
   (A) Direct stimulation of cardiac contractile force
   (B) Tachycardia
   (C) Bronchodilation
   (D) Postural hypotension
   (E) Throbbing headache

2. A 23-year-old woman is using an albuterol inhaler for frequent acute episodes of asthma and complains of symptoms that she ascribes to the albuterol. Which of the following is *not* a recognized action of albuterol?
   (A) Diuretic effect
   (B) Positive inotropic effect
   (C) Skeletal muscle tremor
   (D) Smooth muscle relaxation
   (E) Tachycardia

3. A 10-year-old child has severe asthma and was hospitalized 5 times between the ages of 7 and 9. He is now receiving outpatient medications that have greatly reduced the frequency of severe attacks. Which of the following is most likely to have adverse effects when used daily over long periods for severe asthma?
   (A) Albuterol by aerosol
   (B) Beclomethasone by aerosol
   (C) Cromolyn by inhaler
   (D) Prednisone by mouth
   (E) Theophylline in long-acting oral form

4-5. A 16-year-old patient is in the emergency department receiving nasal oxygen. She has a heart rate of 125 bpm, a respiratory rate of 40 breaths/min, and a peak expiratory flow <50% of the predicted value. Wheezing and rales are audible without a stethoscope.

4. Which of the following drugs does *not* have a direct bronchodilator effect?
   (A) Epinephrine
   (B) Terbutaline
   (C) Prednisone
   (D) Theophylline
   (E) Ipratropium

5. After successful treatment of the acute attack, the patient was referred to the outpatient clinic for follow-up treatment for asthma. Which of the following is *not* an established prophylactic strategy for asthma?
   (A) Avoidance of antigen exposure
   (B) Blockade of histamine receptors
   (C) Blockade of leukotriene receptors
   (D) IgE antibody blockade
   (E) Inhibition of phospholipase A_2

6. Mr Green is a 60-year-old former smoker with cardiac disease and severe chronic obstructive pulmonary disease (COPD) associated with frequent episodes of bronchospasm. Which of the following is a bronchodilator useful in COPD and least likely to cause cardiac arrhythmia?
   (A) Aminophylline
   (B) Cromolyn
   (C) Epinephrine
   (D) Ipratropium
   (E) Metaproterenol
   (F) Metoprolol
   (G) Prednisone
   (H) Salmeterol
   (I) Zafirlukast
   (J) Zileuton

7. A 22-year-old man is brought to the emergency department after suffering seizures resulting from an overdose of a drug he has been taking. His friends state that he took the drug orally and sometimes had insomnia after taking it. Which of the following is a direct bronchodilator that is most often used in asthma by the oral route and is capable of causing insomnia and seizures?
   (A) Cromolyn
   (B) Epinephrine
   (C) Ipratropium
   (D) Metaproterenol
   (E) Metoprolol
   (F) Prednisone
   (G) Salmeterol
   (H) Theophylline
   (I) Zileuton

8. Which of the following in its parenteral form is life-saving in severe status asthmaticus and acts, at least in part, by inhibiting phospholipase A$_2$?
   (A) Aminophylline
   (B) Cromolyn
   (C) Epinephrine
   (D) Ipratropium
   (E) Metaproterenol
   (F) Metoprolol
   (G) Prednisone
   (H) Salmeterol
   (I) Zafirlukast
   (J) Zileuton

9. Which of the following has a slow onset but long duration of action and is always used in combination with a corticosteroid by inhalation?
   (A) Aminophylline
   (B) Cromolyn
   (C) Epinephrine
   (D) Ipratropium
   (E) Metaproterenol
   (F) Metoprolol
   (G) Prednisone/prednisolone
   (H) Salmeterol
   (I) Zafirlukast
   (J) Zileuton

10. Oral medications are popular for the treatment of asthma in children because young children may have difficulty with the proper use of aerosol inhalers. Which of the following is an orally active inhibitor of leukotriene receptors?
    (A) Albuterol
    (B) Aminophylline
    (C) Ipratropium
    (D) Montelukast
    (E) Zileuton

ANSWERS

1. Theophylline does not ordinarily cause headache or postural hypotension. Nitroglycerin does not cause direct cardiac stimulation but does evoke a compensatory sympathetic reflex. Histamine does not cause bronchodilation. The answer is **B.**

2. Albuterol is a β$_2$-selective receptor agonist, but in moderate to high doses it induces β$_1$ cardiac effects as well as β$_2$-mediated smooth and skeletal muscle effects. It does not cause diuresis. The answer is **A.**

3. If oral corticosteroids must be used, alternate-day therapy is preferred because it interferes less with normal growth in children. The answer is **D.**

4. Although extremely important in severe chronic asthma and status asthmaticus, corticosteroids do not have a demonstrable direct bronchodilator action. The answer is **C.**

5. Histamine does not appear to play a significant role in asthma, and antihistaminic drugs, even in high doses, are of little or no value. Antigen avoidance is well established. Blockade of leukotriene receptors with montelukast; inhibition of phospholipase with corticosteroids; and inhibition of mediator release with the IgE antibody are also useful. The answer is **B.**

6. Ipratropium is the bronchodilator that is most likely to be useful in COPD without causing arrhythmias. Tiotropium is similar. The answer is **D.**

7. Theophylline is a bronchodilator that is active by the oral route. It causes insomnia in therapeutic doses and seizures in overdosage. The answer is **H.**

8. Parenteral corticosteroids such as prednisolone (the active metabolite of prednisone) are lifesaving in status asthmaticus. They probably act by reducing production of leukotrienes (see Chapter 18). The answer is **G.**

9. Salmeterol is a β$_2$-selective agonist that has a slow onset and long duration of action. Used alone, it increases asthma mortality, but in combination with inhaled corticosteroids it improves asthma control. The answer is **H.**

10. Zileuton is an inhibitor of the lipoxygenase enzyme involved in the synthesis of leukotrienes. Montelukast and zafirlukast are leukotriene antagonists at the leukotriene receptor. The answer is **D.**

SKILL KEEPER ANSWER: SYMPATHOMIMETICS IN ASTHMA (SEE CHAPTER 9)

Direct-acting sympathomimetics are usually rapid in onset and short acting (eg, epinephrine, albuterol; exceptions: salmeterol, formoterol, indacaterol). Most direct-acting sympathomimetics have poor oral bioavailability.

Indirect-acting sympathomimetics (eg, ephedrine) are usually longer acting and have good bioavailability. An important disadvantage of the indirect-acting group is their CNS activity: Most enter the CNS and produce undesirable stimulation. Even more important in asthma is the lack of receptor selectivity of the indirect-acting group. Because they release norepinephrine and epinephrine from stores, they produce all the α- and β$_1$-adrenoceptor-mediated effects of these catecholamines, most of which are undesirable in asthma. In contrast, the direct-acting agents can be tailored for selective β$_2$ activity. Furthermore, local application by aerosol administration is convenient and greatly reduces the systemic toxicity associated with oral or other systemic routes.

CHECKLIST

When you complete this chapter, you should be able to:

- ❑ Describe the strategies of drug treatment of asthma and COPD.
- ❑ List the major classes of drugs used in asthma and COPD.
- ❑ Describe the mechanisms of action of these drug groups.
- ❑ List the major adverse effects of the prototype drugs used in airways disease.

DRUG SUMMARY TABLE: Bronchodilators & Other Drugs Used in Asthma & COPD

Subclass	Mechanism of Action	Clinical Applications	Pharmacokinetics	Toxicities, Interactions
Short-acting β agonists				
Albuterol	Beta$_2$-selective agonist • bronchodilation	Asthma acute attack relief **drug of choice** (not for prophylaxis)	Inhalation (aerosol) Duration: 2–4 h	Tremor, tachycardia
Metaproterenol, terbutaline: similar to albuterol; terbutaline also available as oral and parenteral formulations				
Long-acting β agonists				
Salmeterol, formoterol, indacaterol	Beta$_2$-selective agonists; bronchodilation; potentiation of corticosteroid action	Asthma prophylaxis (not for acute relief) • indacaterol for COPD	Inhalation (aerosol) Duration: 12–24 h	Tremor, tachycardia, cardiovascular events
Nonselective sympathomimetics				
Epinephrine, isoproterenol	Nonselective β activation • epinephrine also an α agonist	Asthma (obsolete)	Inhalation (aerosol, nebulizer) Duration: 1–2 h	Excess sympathomimetic effect (Chapter 9)
Indirect-acting sympathomimetic				
Ephedrine	Releases stored catecholamines • causes nonselective sympathetic effects	Asthma (obsolete)	Oral Duration: 6–8 h	Insomnia, tremor, anorexia, arrhythmias
Methylxanthines				
Theophylline	Phosphodiesterase inhibition, adenosine receptor antagonist • other effects poorly understood	Asthma, especially prophylactic against nocturnal attacks	Oral slow-release Duration: 12 h	Insomnia, tremor, anorexia, seizures, arrhythmias
Caffeine: similar to theophylline with increased CNS effect *Theobromine:* similar to theophylline with increased cardiac effect				
Antimuscarinic agents				
Ipratropium, tiotropium	Competitive pharmacologic muscarinic antagonists	Asthma and chronic obstructive pulmonary disease	Inhalation (aerosol) Duration: several hours	Dry mouth, cough

(Continued)

DRUG SUMMARY TABLE: Bronchodilators & Other Drugs Used in Asthma & COPD (*Continued*)

Subclass	Mechanism of Action	Clinical Applications	Pharmacokinetics	Toxicities, Interactions
Unknown mechanism, possibly mast cell stabilizers				
Cromolyn, nedocromil	Reduce release of inflammatory and bronchoconstrictor mediators from sensitized mast cells	Rarely used prophylaxis of asthma; cromolyn also used for ophthalmic, nasopharyngeal, and gastrointestinal allergy	Inhaled aerosol for asthma • cromolyn local application for other applications Duration: 3–6 h	Cough
Leukotriene antagonists				
Montelukast, zafirlukast	Pharmacologic antagonists at LTD_4 receptors	Prophylaxis of asthma	Oral Duration: 12–24 h	Minimal
Zileuton	Inhibitor of lipoxygenase • reduces synthesis of leukotrienes	Prophylaxis of asthma	Oral Duration: 12 h	Elevation of liver enzymes
Corticosteroids				
Inhaled Beclomethasone, others	Inhibition of phospholipase A_2 • reduces expression of cyclooxygenase	Prophylaxis of asthma: **drugs of choice**	Inhalation Duration: 10–12 h	Pharyngeal candidiasis • minimal systemic steroid toxicity (eg, adrenal suppression)
Systemic Prednisone	Like inhaled corticosteroids	Treatment of severe refractory chronic asthma	Oral Duration: 12–24 h	See Chapter 39
Prednisolone: parenteral for status asthmaticus; similar to prednisone				
Antibodies				
Omalizumab	Binds IgE antibodies on mast cells; reduces reaction to inhaled antigen	Prophylaxis of severe, refractory asthma not responsive to all other drugs	Parenteral • administered as several courses of injections	Extremely expensive • long-term toxicity not yet well documented

C H A P T E R

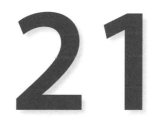

Introduction to CNS Pharmacology

TARGETS OF CNS DRUG ACTION

Most drugs that act on the central nervous system (CNS) appear to do so by changing ion flow through transmembrane channels of nerve cells.

A. Types of Ion Channels

Ion channels of neuronal membranes are of 2 major types: voltage gated and ligand gated (Figure 21–1). Voltage-gated ion channels respond to changes in membrane potential. They are concentrated on the axons of nerve cells and include the sodium channels responsible for action potential propagation. Cell bodies and dendrites also have voltage-sensitive ion channels for potassium and calcium. Ligand-gated ion channels, also called ionotropic receptors, respond to chemical neurotransmitters that bind to receptor subunits present in their macromolecular structure. Neurotransmitters also bind to G protein-coupled receptors (metabotropic receptors) that can modulate voltage-gated ion channels. Neurotransmitter-coupled ion channels are found on cell bodies and on both the presynaptic and postsynaptic sides of synapses.

B. Types of Receptor-Channel Coupling

In the case of ligand-gated ion channels, activation (or inactivation) is initiated by the interaction between chemical neurotransmitters and their receptors (Figure 21–1). Coupling may be (1) through a receptor that acts directly on the channel protein (B),

(2) through a receptor that is coupled to the ion channel through a G protein (C), or (3) through a receptor coupled to a G protein that modulates the formation of diffusible second messengers, including cyclic adenosine monophosphate (cAMP), inositol trisphosphate (IP_3), and diacylglycerol (DAG), which secondarily modulate ion channels (D).

C. Role of the Ion Current Carried by the Channel

Excitatory postsynaptic potentials (EPSPs) are usually generated by the opening of sodium or calcium channels. In some synapses, similar depolarizing potentials result from the *closing* of potassium channels. Inhibitory postsynaptic potentials (IPSPs) are usually generated by the opening of potassium or chloride channels. For example, activation of postsynaptic metabotropic receptors increases the efflux of potassium. Presynaptic inhibition can occur via a decrease in calcium influx elicited by activation of metabotropic receptors.

SITES & MECHANISMS OF DRUG ACTION

A small number of neuropharmacologic agents exert their effects through direct interactions with molecular components of ion channels on axons. Examples include certain anticonvulsants (eg, carbamazepine, phenytoin), local anesthetics, and some drugs used in general anesthesia. However, the effects of most therapeutically important CNS drugs are exerted mainly at synapses.

High-Yield Terms to Learn

Voltage-gated ion channels	Transmembrane ion channels regulated by changes in membrane potential
Ligand-gated ion channels	Transmembrane ion channels that are regulated by interactions between neurotransmitters and their receptors (also called ionotropic receptors)
Metabotropic receptors	G protein-coupled receptors that respond to neurotransmitters either by a direct action of G proteins on ion channels or by G protein-enzyme activation that leads to formation of diffusible second messengers
EPSP	Excitatory postsynaptic potential; a depolarizing potential change
IPSP	Inhibitory postsynaptic potential; a hyperpolarizing potential change
Synaptic mimicry	Ability of an administered chemical to mimic the actions of the natural neurotransmitter: a criterion for identification of a putative neurotransmitter

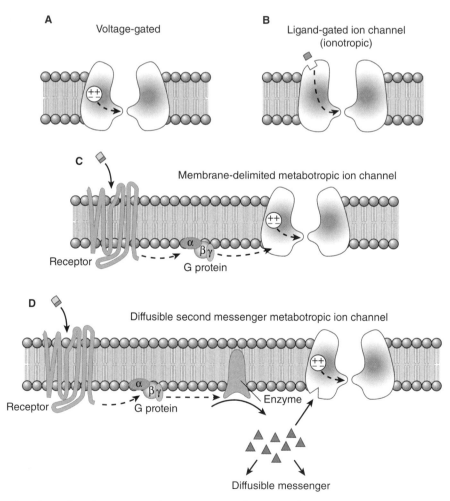

FIGURE 21−1 Types of ion channels and neurotransmitter receptors in the CNS: **A** shows a voltage-gated ion channel in which the voltage sensor controls the gating (*broken arrow*). **B** shows a ligand-gated ion channel in which binding of the neurotransmitter to the ionotropic channel receptor controls the gating. **C** shows a metabotropic receptor coupled to a G protein that can interact directly with an ion channel. **D** shows a receptor coupled to a G protein that activates an enzyme; the activated enzyme generates a diffusible second messenger, for example, cAMP, which interacts to modulatean ion channel. (Reproduced, with permission, from Katzung BG, editor: *Basic & Clinical Pharmacology*, 12th ed. McGraw-Hill, 2012: Fig. 21–2.)

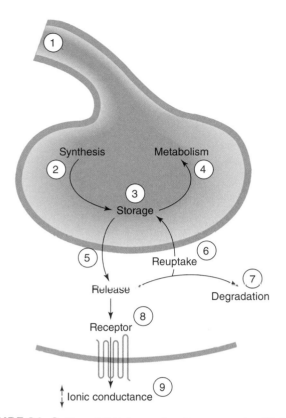

FIGURE 21–2 Sites of CNS drug action. Drugs may alter (1) the action potential in the presynaptic fiber; (2) synthesis of transmitter; (3) storage; (4) metabolism; (5) release; (6) reuptake; (7) degradation; (8) receptor for the transmitter; or (9) receptor-induced decrease or increase in ionic conduction. (Reproduced, with permission, from Katzung BG, editor: *Basic & Clinical Pharmacology,* 10th ed. McGraw-Hill, 2007: Fig. 21–2.)

Possible mechanisms are indicated in Figure 21–2. Thus, drugs may act presynaptically to alter the synthesis, storage, release, reuptake, or metabolism of transmitter chemicals. Other drugs can activate or block both pre- and postsynaptic receptors for specific transmitters or can interfere with the actions of second messengers. The selectivity of CNS drug action is largely based on the fact that different groups of neurons use different neurotransmitters and that they are segregated into networks that subserve different CNS functions.

A few neurotoxic substances damage or kill nerve cells. For example, 1-methyl-4-phenyl-1,2,3,6-tetrahydropyridine (MPTP) is cytotoxic to neurons of the nigrostriatal dopaminergic pathway.

ROLE OF CNS ORGANIZATION

The CNS contains 2 types of neuronal systems: hierarchical and diffuse.

A. Hierarchical Systems

These systems are delimited in their anatomic distribution and generally contain large myelinated, rapidly conducting fibers. Hierarchical systems control major sensory and motor functions.

The major excitatory transmitters in these systems are aspartate and glutamate. These systems also include numerous small inhibitory interneurons, which use γ-aminobutyric acid (GABA) or glycine as transmitters. Drugs that affect hierarchical systems often have profound effects on the overall excitability of the CNS.

B. Diffuse Systems

Diffuse or nonspecific systems are broadly distributed, with single cells frequently sending processes to many different areas. The axons are fine and branch repeatedly to form synapses with many cells. Axons commonly have periodic enlargements (varicosities) that contain transmitter vesicles. The transmitters in diffuse systems are often amines (norepinephrine, dopamine, serotonin) or peptides that commonly exert actions on metabotropic receptors. Drugs that affect these systems often have marked effects on such CNS functions as attention, appetite, and emotional states.

TRANSMITTERS AT CENTRAL SYNAPSES

A. Criteria for Transmitter Status

To be accepted as a neurotransmitter, a candidate chemical must (1) be present in higher concentration in the synaptic area than in other areas (ie, must be localized in appropriate areas), (2) be released by electrical or chemical stimulation via a calcium-dependent mechanism, and (3) produce the same sort of postsynaptic response that is seen with physiologic activation of the synapse (ie, must exhibit synaptic mimicry). Table 21–1 lists the most important chemicals currently accepted as neurotransmitters in the CNS.

B. Acetylcholine

Approximately 5% of brain neurons have receptors for acetylcholine (ACh). Most CNS responses to ACh are mediated by a large family of G protein-coupled muscarinic M_1 receptors that lead to slow excitation when activated. The ionic mechanism of slow excitation involves a *decrease* in membrane permeability to potassium. Of the nicotinic receptors present in the CNS (they are less common than muscarinic receptors), those on the Renshaw cells activated by motor axon collaterals in the spinal cord are the best characterized. Drugs affecting the activity of cholinergic systems in the brain include the acetylcholinesterase inhibitors used in Alzheimer's disease (eg, tacrine) and the muscarinic blocking agents used in parkinsonism (eg, benztropine).

C. Dopamine

Dopamine exerts slow inhibitory actions at synapses in specific neuronal systems commonly via G protein-coupled activation of potassium channels (postsynaptic) or inactivation of calcium channels (presynaptic). The D_2 receptor is the main dopamine subtype in basal ganglia neurons, and it is widely distributed at the supraspinal level. Dopaminergic pathways include the nigrostriatal, mesolimbic, and tuberoinfundibular tracts. In addition to the 2 receptors listed in Table 21–1, 3 other dopamine receptor subtypes have been identified (D_3, D_4, and D_5). Drugs that block

TABLE 21–1 Neurotransmitter pharmacology in the CNS.

Transmitter	Anatomical Distribution	Receptor Subtypes	Receptor Mechanisms
Acetylcholine	Cell bodies at all levels, short and long axons	Muscarinic, M_1; blocked by pirenzepine and atropine	Excitatory; $\downarrow K^+$ conductance; $\uparrow IP_3$ and DAG
		Muscarinic, M_2; blocked by atropine	Inhibitory; $\uparrow K^+$ conductance; $\downarrow$ cAMP
	Motoneuron-Renshaw cell synapse	Nicotinic, N	Excitatory; $\uparrow$ cation conductance
Dopamine	Cell bodies at all levels, short, medium, and long axons	D_1; blocked by phenothiazines	Inhibitory; $\uparrow$cAMP
		D_2; blocked by phenothiazines and haloperidol	Inhibitory (presynaptic); $\downarrow Ca^{2+}$ conductance;
			Inhibitory (postsynaptic); $\uparrow K^+$ conductance; cAMP
Norepinephrine	Cell bodies in pons and brain stem project to all levels	Alpha$_1$; blocked by prazosin	Excitatory; $\downarrow K^+$ conductance; $\uparrow IP_3$ and DAG
		Alpha$_2$; activated by clonidine	Inhibitory (presynaptic); $\downarrow Ca^{2+}$ conductance
			Inhibitory (postsynaptic); $\uparrow K^+$ conductance; cAMP
		Beta$_1$; blocked by propranolol	Excitatory; $\downarrow K^+$ conductance; $\uparrow$ cAMP
		Beta$_2$; blocked by propranolol	Inhibitory; $\uparrow$ electrogenic sodium pump
Serotonin (5-hydroxy-tryptamine)	Cell bodies in midbrain and pons project to all levels	5-HT$_{1A}$; buspirone is a partial agonist	Inhibitory; $\uparrow K^+$ conductance
		5-HT$_{2A}$; blocked by clozapine, risperidone, and olanzapine	Excitatory; $\downarrow K^+$ conductance; $\uparrow IP_3$ and DAG
		5-HT$_3$; blocked by ondansetron	Excitatory; $\uparrow$ cation conductance
		5-HT$_4$	Excitatory; $\downarrow K^+$ conductance; $\uparrow$ cAMP
GABA	Supraspinal interneurons; spinal interneurons involved in presynaptic inhibition	GABA$_A$; facilitated by benzodiazepines and zolpidem	Inhibitory; $\uparrow Cl^-$ conductance
		GABA$_B$; activated by baclofen	Inhibitory (presynaptic); $\downarrow Ca^{2+}$ conductance
			Inhibitory (postsynaptic); $\uparrow K^+$ conductance
Glutamate, aspartate	Relay neurons at all levels	Four subtypes; NMDA subtype blocked by phencyclidine, ketamine, and memantine	Excitatory; $\uparrow Ca^{2+}$ or cation conductance
		Metabotropic subtypes	Inhibitory (presynaptic); $\downarrow Ca^{2+}$ conductance $\downarrow$ cAMP
			Excitatory (postsynaptic); $\downarrow K^+$ conductance, $\uparrow IP^3$ and DAG
Glycine	Interneurons in spinal cord and brain stem	Single subtype; blocked by strychnine	Inhibitory; $\uparrow Cl^-$ conductance
Opioid peptides	Cell bodies at all levels	Three major subtypes: μ, δ, κ	Inhibitory (presynaptic); $\downarrow Ca^{2+}$ conductance; $\downarrow$cAMP
			Inhibitory (postsynaptic); $\uparrow K^+$ conductance; $\downarrow$cAMP

Adapted, with permission, from Katzung BG, editor: *Basic & Clinical Pharmacology*, 12th ed. McGraw-Hill, 2012.

the activity of dopaminergic pathways include older antipsychotics (eg, chlorpromazine, haloperidol), which may cause parkinsonian symptoms. Drugs that increase brain dopaminergic activity include CNS stimulants (eg, amphetamine), and commonly used antiparkinsonism drugs (eg, levodopa).

D. Norepinephrine

Noradrenergic neuron cell bodies are mainly located in the brain stem and the lateral tegmental area of the pons. These neurons fan out broadly to provide most regions of the CNS with diffuse noradrenergic input. Excitatory effects are produced by activation of α_1 and β_1 receptors. Inhibitory effects are caused by activation of α_2 and β_2 receptors. CNS stimulants (eg, amphetamines, cocaine), monoamine oxidase inhibitors (eg, phenelzine), and tricyclic antidepressants (eg, amitriptyline) are examples of drugs that enhance the activity of noradrenergic pathways.

E. Serotonin

Most serotonin (5-hydroxytryptamine; 5-HT) pathways originate from cell bodies in the raphe or midline regions of the pons and upper brain stem; these pathways innervate most regions of the CNS. Multiple 5-HT receptor subtypes have been identified and, with the exception of the $5-HT_3$ subtype, all are metabotropic. $5-HT_{1A}$ receptors and $GABA_B$ receptors share the same potassium channel. Serotonin can cause excitation or inhibition of CNS neurons depending on the receptor subtype activated. Both excitatory and inhibitory actions can occur on the same neuron if appropriate receptors are present. Most of the agents used in the treatment of major depressive disorders affect serotonergic pathways (eg, tricyclic antidepressants, selective serotonin reuptake inhibitors). The actions of some CNS stimulants and newer antipsychotic drugs (eg, olanzapine) also appear to be mediated via effects on serotonergic transmission. Reserpine, which may cause severe depression of mood, depletes vesicular stores of both serotonin and norepinephrine in CNS neurons.

F. Glutamic Acid

Most neurons in the brain are excited by glutamic acid. High concentrations of glutamic acid in synaptic vesicles is achieved by the vesicular glutamate transporter (VGLUT). Both ionotropic and metabotropic receptors have been characterized. Subtypes of glutamate receptors include the N-methyl-D-aspartate (NMDA) receptor, which is blocked by phencyclidine (PCP) and ketamine. NMDA receptors appear to play a role in synaptic plasticity related to learning and memory. Memantine is an NMDA antagonist introduced for treatment of Alzheimer's dementia. Excessive activation of NMDA receptors after neuronal injury may be responsible for cell death. Glutamate metabotropic receptor activation can result in G protein-coupled activation of phospholipase C or inhibition of adenylyl cyclase.

G. GABA and Glycine

GABA is the primary neurotransmitter mediating IPSPs in neurons in the brain; it is also important in the spinal cord. $GABA_A$ receptor activation opens chloride ion channels. $GABA_B$ receptors (activated by baclofen, a centrally acting muscle relaxant) are coupled to G proteins that either open potassium channels or close calcium channels. Fast IPSPs are blocked by $GABA_A$ receptor antagonists, and slow IPSPs are blocked by $GABA_B$ receptor antagonists. Drugs that influence $GABA_A$ receptor systems include sedative-hypnotics (eg, barbiturates, benzodiazepines, zolpidem) and some anticonvulsants (eg, gabapentin, tiagabine, vigabatrin). Glycine receptors, which are more numerous in the cord than in the brain, are blocked by strychnine, a spinal convulsant.

H. Peptide Transmitters

Many peptides have been identified in the CNS, and some meet most or all of the criteria for acceptance as neurotransmitters. The best-defined peptides are the opioid peptides (beta-endorphin, met- and leu-enkephalin, and dynorphin), which are distributed at all levels of the neuraxis. Some of the important therapeutic actions of opioid analgesics (eg, morphine) are mediated via activation of receptors for these endogenous peptides. Another peptide substance P is a mediator of slow EPSPs in neurons involved in nociceptive sensory pathways in the spinal cord and brain stem. Peptide transmitters differ from nonpeptide transmitters in that (1) the peptides are synthesized in the cell body and transported to the nerve ending via axonal transport, and (2) no reuptake or specific enzyme mechanisms have been identified for terminating their actions.

I. Endocannabinoids

These are widely distributed brain lipid derivatives (eg, 2-arachidonyl-glycerol) that bind to receptors for cannabinoids found in marijuana. They are synthesized and released postsynaptically after membrane depolarization but travel backward acting presynaptically (retrograde) to decrease transmitter release, via their interaction with a specific cannabinoid receptor CB1.

SKILL KEEPER: BIODISPOSITION OF CNS DRUGS (SEE CHAPTER 1)

1. *What characteristics of drug molecules afford access to the CNS?*

2. *What concerns do you have regarding CNS drug use in the pregnant patient?*

3. *How are most CNS drugs usually eliminated from the body?*

The Skill Keeper Answers appear at the end of the chapter.

QUESTIONS

1. Which of the following chemicals does *not* satisfy the criteria for a neurotransmitter role in the CNS?
   (A) Acetylcholine
   (B) Cyclic AMP
   (C) Dopamine
   (D) Glutamic acid
   (E) Serotonin

2. Neurotransmitters may
   (A) Increase chloride conductance to cause inhibition
   (B) Increase potassium conductance to cause inhibition
   (C) Increase sodium conductance to cause excitation
   (D) Increase calcium conductance to cause excitation
   (E) Exert all of the above actions

3. All of the listed neurotransmitters change membrane excitability by decreasing K^+ conductance EXCEPT
   (A) Acetylcholine
   (B) Dopamine
   (C) Glutamic acid
   (D) Norepinephrine
   (E) Serotonin

4. Which of the following receptors shares the same potassium channel as the $5\text{-}HT_{1A}$ receptor?
   (A) Dopamine D_2 receptor
   (B) $GABA_B$ receptor
   (C) Mu opioid receptor
   (D) Muscarinic M_1 receptor
   (E) Substance P receptor

5. Which of the following chemicals is most likely to function as a neurotransmitter in hierarchical systems?
   (A) Dopamine
   (B) Glutamate
   (C) Met-enkephalin
   (D) Nitric oxide
   (E) Norepinephrine

6. Activation of metabotropic receptors located presynaptically causes inhibition by decreasing the inward flux of
   (A) Calcium
   (B) Chloride
   (C) Potassium
   (D) Sodium
   (E) All of the above

7. This transmitter is mostly located in diffuse neuronal systems in the CNS, with cell bodies particularly in the raphe nuclei. It appears to play a major role in the expression of mood states, and many antidepressant drugs are thought to increase its functional activity.
   (A) Acetylcholine
   (B) Dopamine
   (C) Glutamate
   (D) Serotonin
   (E) Substance P

8. Cyclic adenosine monophosphate (cAMP) functions as a diffusible second messenger after activation of
   (A) Acetylcholine M_1 receptors
   (B) $Beta_1$ adrenoceptors
   (C) $5\text{-}HT_3$ receptors
   (D) $GABA_A$ receptors
   (E) Glutamate NMDA receptors

9. One of the first neurotransmitter receptors to be identified in the CNS is located on the Renshaw cell in the spinal cord. Activation of this receptor results in excitation via an increase in cation conductance independently of G protein-coupled mechanisms. Which of the following compounds is most likely to activate this receptor?
   (A) Aspartate
   (B) Dopamine
   (C) GABA
   (D) Nicotine
   (E) Serotonin

10. This neurotransmitter, found in high concentrations in cell bodies in the pons and brain stem, can exert both excitatory and inhibitory actions. Multiple receptor subtypes have been identified, some of which are targets for drugs that can exert both CNS and peripheral actions.
    (A) Acetylcholine
    (B) Beta-endorphin
    (C) Glycine
    (D) Glutamate
    (E) Norepinephrine

ANSWERS

1. Cyclic AMP (cAMP) is a mediator in many receptor mechanisms in the CNS, including those for acetylcholine (M_2), and norepinephrine (β_1). However, the characteristics of cAMP do not satisfy the criteria for a neurotransmitter role (see A. Criteria for Transmitter Status). The answer is **B.**

2. Activation of chloride or potassium ion channels commonly generates inhibitory postsynaptic potentials (IPSPs). Activation of sodium and calcium channels (and *inhibition* of potassium ion channels) generate excitatory postsynaptic potentials (EPSPs). The answer is **E.**

3. A decrease in K^+ conductance is associated with neuronal excitation. With the exception of dopamine, all of the neurotransmitters listed are able to cause excitation by this mechanism via their activation of specific receptors: acetylcholine (M_1), glutamate (metabotropic), norepinephrine (α_1 and β_1), and serotonin ($5\text{-}HT_{2A}$). The answer is **B.**

4. $GABA_B$ receptors and $5\text{-}HT_{1A}$ receptors share the same potassium ion channel, with a G protein involved in the coupling mechanism. The spasmolytic drug baclofen is an activator of $GABA_B$ receptors in the spinal cord. The anxiolytic drug buspirone may act as a partial agonist at brain $5\text{-}HT_{1A}$ receptors. The answer is **B.**

5. Catecholamines (dopamine, norepinephrine), opioid peptides, and serotonin act as neurotransmitters in nonspecific or diffuse neuronal systems. Glutamate is the primary excitatory transmitter in hierarchical neuronal systems. These systems also contain numerous inhibitory neurons, which use GABA and glycine. Nitric oxide, though present in many brain regions, does not meet the critera for a CNS neurotransmitter. The answer is **B.**

6. Activation of metabotropic receptors located presynaptically results in the inhibition of calcium influx with a resultant decrease in the release of neurotransmitter from nerve endings. This type of presynaptic inhibition occurs after activation of dopamine D_2, norepinephrine α_2, glutamate, and mu opioid peptide receptors. The answer is **A.**

7. Amine transmitters thought to be involved in the control of mood states include norepinephrine and serotonin. Cell bodies of serotonergic neurons are found in the raphe nuclei. Many of the drugs used for the treatment of major depressive disorders act to increase serotonergic activity in the CNS. The answer is **D**.

8. Metabotropic receptors modulate voltage-gated ion channels directly (membrane-delimited action) and also by the formation of diffusible second messengers through G-protein-mediated effects on enzymes involved in their synthesis. An example of the latter type of action is provided by the β_1 adrenoceptor, which generates cAMP via the activation of adenylyl cyclase. The answer is **B**.

9. Nicotinic receptors on the Renshaw cell are activated by the release of ACh from motor neuron collaterals. This results in the release of glycine, which, via interaction with its receptors on the motor neuron, causes membrane hyperpolarization, an example of feedback inhibition. The receptors were so named because of their activation by nicotine. The answer is **D**.

10. The brief description might apply to several CNS neurotransmitters, including serotonin and possibly dopamine (neither of which is listed). Cell bodies of noradrenergic neurons located in the pons and brain stem project to all levels of the CNS. Most of the subclasses of adrenergic receptors that occur in peripheral tissues are present in the CNS. Agents that activate presynaptic α_2 receptors on such neurons (eg, clonidine, methyldopa) decrease central noradrenergic activity, an action thought to result in decreased vasomotor outflow. The answer is **E**.

SKILL KEEPER ANSWERS: BIODISPOSITION OF CNS DRUGS (SEE CHAPTER 1)

1. *Lipid solubility is an important characteristic of most CNS drugs in terms of their ability to cross the blood-brain barrier. Access to the CNS of water-soluble (polar) molecules is limited to those of low molecular weight such as lithium ion and ethanol.*

2. *CNS drugs readily cross the placental barrier and enter the fetal circulation. Concerns during pregnancy include possible effects on fetal development and the potential for drug effects on the neonate if CNS drugs are used near the time of delivery.*

3. *With the notable exception of lithium, almost all CNS drugs require metabolism to more water-soluble (polar) metabolites for their elimination. Thus, drugs that modify the activities of drug-metabolizing enzymes may have an impact on the clearance of CNS drugs, possibly affecting the intensity or duration of their effects.*

CHECKLIST

When you complete this chapter, you should be able to:

❑ Explain the difference between voltage-gated and ligand-gated ion channels.

❑ List the criteria for accepting a chemical as a neurotransmitter.

❑ Identify the major excitatory and inhibitory CNS neurotransmitters in the CNS.

❑ Identify the sites of drug action at synapses and the mechanisms by which drugs modulate synaptic transmission.

❑ Give an example of a CNS drug that influences neurotransmitter functions at the level of (a) synthesis, (b) metabolism, (c) release, (d) reuptake, and (e) receptor.

Sedative-Hypnotic Drugs

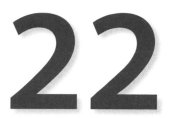

The sedative-hypnotics belong to a chemically heterogeneous class of drugs, almost all of which produce dose-dependent CNS depressant effects. A major subgroup is the benzodiazepines, but representatives of other subgroups, including barbiturates, and miscellaneous agents (carbamates, alcohols, and cyclic ethers) are still in use. Newer drugs with distinctive characteristics include the anxiolytic buspirone, several widely used hypnotics (zolpidem, zaleplon, eszopiclone), and ramelteon, a novel drug used in sleep disorders.

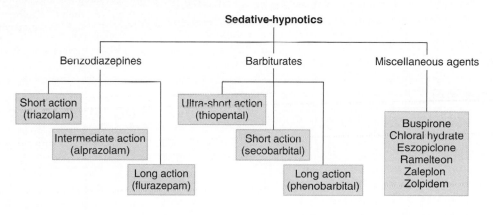

PHARMACOKINETICS

A. Absorption and Distribution

Most sedative-hypnotic drugs are lipid-soluble and are absorbed well from the gastrointestinal tract, with good distribution to the brain. Drugs with the highest lipid solubility (eg, **thiopental**) enter the CNS rapidly and can be used as induction agents in anesthesia. The CNS effects of thiopental are terminated by rapid **redistribution** of the drug from brain to other highly perfused tissues, including skeletal muscle. Other drugs with a rapid onset of CNS action include eszopiclone, zaleplon, and zolpidem.

B. Metabolism and Excretion

Sedative-hypnotics are metabolized before elimination from the body, mainly by hepatic enzymes. Metabolic rates and pathways vary among different drugs. Many benzodiazepines are converted initially to **active metabolites** with long half-lives. After several days of therapy with some drugs (eg, diazepam, flurazepam), accumulation of active metabolites can lead to excessive sedation. Lorazepam and oxazepam undergo extrahepatic conjugation and do not form active metabolites. With the exception of phenobarbital, which is excreted partly unchanged in the urine, the barbiturates are extensively metabolized. Chloral hydrate is oxidized to trichloroethanol, an active metabolite. Rapid metabolism by liver enzymes is responsible for the short duration of action of zolpidem. A biphasic release form of zolpidem extends its plasma half-life. Zaleplon undergoes even more rapid hepatic metabolism by aldehyde oxidase and cytochrome P450. Eszopiclone is also metabolized by cytochrome P450 with a half-life of 6 h. The duration of CNS actions of sedative-hypnotic drugs ranges from just a few hours (eg, zaleplon < zolpidem = triazolam = eszopiclone < chloral hydrate) to more than 30 h (eg, chlordiazepoxide, clorazepate, diazepam, phenobarbital).

High-Yield Terms to Learn

Sedation	Reduction of anxiety
Addiction	The state of response to a drug whereby the drug taker feels compelled to use the drug and suffers anxiety when separated from it
Anesthesia	Loss of consciousness associated with absence of response to pain
Anxiolytic	A drug that reduces anxiety, a sedative
Dependence	The state of response to a drug whereby removal of the drug evokes unpleasant, possibly life-threatening symptoms, often the opposite of the drug's effects
Hypnosis	Induction of sleep
REM sleep	Phase of sleep associated with rapid eye movements; most dreaming takes place during REM sleep
Sedation	Reduction of anxiety
Tolerance	Reduction in drug effect requiring an increase in dosage to maintain the same response

MECHANISMS OF ACTION

No single mechanism of action for sedative-hypnotics has been identified, and the different chemical subgroups may have different actions. Certain drugs (eg, benzodiazepines) facilitate neuronal membrane inhibition by actions at specific receptors.

A. Benzodiazepines

Receptors for benzodiazepines (BZ receptors) are present in many brain regions, including the thalamus, limbic structures, and the cerebral cortex. The BZ receptors form part of a $GABA_A$ receptor-chloride ion channel macromolecular complex, a pentameric structure assembled from 5 subunits each with 4 transmembrane domains. A major isoform of the $GABA_A$ receptor consists of 2 α_1, 2 β_2, and 1 γ_2 subunits. In this isoform, the binding site for benzodiazepines is between an α_1 and the γ_2 subunit. However, benzodiazepines also bind to other $GABA_A$ receptor isoforms that contain α_2, α_3, and α_5 subunits. Binding of benzodiazepines facilitates the inhibitory actions of GABA, which are exerted through increased chloride ion conductance (Figure 22–1).

Benzodiazepines increase the *frequency* of GABA-mediated chloride ion channel opening. **Flumazenil** reverses the CNS effects of benzodiazepines and is classified as an **antagonist** at BZ receptors. Certain β-carbolines have a high affinity for BZ receptors and can elicit anxiogenic and convulsant effects. These drugs are classified as **inverse agonists.**

B. Barbiturates

Barbiturates depress neuronal activity in the midbrain reticular formation, facilitating and prolonging the inhibitory effects of GABA and glycine. Barbiturates also bind to multiple isoforms of the $GABA_A$ receptor but at different sites from those with which benzodiazepines interact. Their actions are not antagonized by flumazenil. Barbiturates increase the *duration* of GABA-mediated chloride ion channel opening. They may also block the excitatory transmitter glutamic acid, and, at high concentration, sodium channels.

C. Other Drugs

The hypnotics **zolpidem**, **zaleplon**, and **eszopiclone** are not benzodiazepines but appear to exert their CNS effects via interaction with certain benzodiazepine receptors, classified as BZ_1 or ω_1 subtypes.

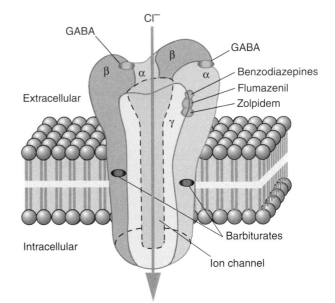

FIGURE 22–1 A model of the $GABA_A$ receptor-chloride ion channel macromolecular complex. A hetero-oligomeric glycoprotein, the complex consists of 5 or more membrane-spanning subunits. Multiple forms of α, β, and γ subunits are arranged in various pentameric combinations so that $GABA_A$ receptors exhibit molecular heterogeneity. GABA appears to interact at two sites between α and β subunits, triggering chloride channel opening with resulting membrane hyperpolarization. Binding of benzodiazepines and the newer hypnotic drugs such as zolpidem occurs at a single site between α and γ subunits, facilitating the process of chloride ion channel opening. The benzodiazepine antagonist flumazenil also binds at this site and can reverse the hypnotic effects of zolpidem. Note that these binding sites are distinct from those of the barbiturates. (Reproduced, with permission, from Katzung BG, editor: *Basic & Clinical Pharmacology*, 12th ed. McGraw-Hill, 2012: Fig. 22–6.)

In contrast to benzodiazepines, these drugs bind more selectively, interacting only with GABA$_A$ receptor isoforms that contain α_1 subunits. Their CNS depressant effects can be antagonized by flumazenil.

PHARMACODYNAMICS

The CNS effects of most sedative-hypnotics depend on dose, as shown in Figure 22–2. These effects range from sedation and relief of anxiety (anxiolysis), through hypnosis (facilitation of sleep), to anesthesia and coma. Depressant effects are additive when 2 or more drugs are given together. The steepness of the dose-response curve varies among drug groups; those with flatter curves, such as benzodiazepines and the newer hypnotics (eg, zolpidem), are safer for clinical use.

A. Sedation

Sedative actions, with relief of anxiety, occur with all drugs in this class. Anxiolysis is usually accompanied by some impairment of psychomotor functions, and behavioral disinhibition may also occur. In animals, most conventional sedative-hypnotics release punishment-suppressed behavior.

B. Hypnosis

Sedative-hypnotics can promote sleep onset and increase the duration of the sleep state. Rapid eye movement (REM) sleep duration is usually decreased at high doses; a rebound increase in REM sleep may occur on withdrawal from chronic drug use. Effects on sleep patterns occur infrequently with newer hypnotics such as zaleplon and zolpidem.

C. Anesthesia

At high doses of most older sedative-hypnotics, loss of consciousness may occur, with amnesia and suppression of reflexes. Anterograde amnesia is more likely with benzodiazepines than with other sedative-hypnotics. Anesthesia can be produced by most barbiturates (eg, thiopental) and certain benzodiazepines (eg, midazolam).

D. Anticonvulsant Actions

Suppression of seizure activity occurs with high doses of most of the barbiturates and some of the benzodiazepines, but this is usually at the cost of marked sedation. Selective anticonvulsant action (ie, suppression of convulsions at doses that do not cause severe sedation) occurs with only a few of these drugs (eg, phenobarbital, clonazepam). High doses of intravenous diazepam, lorazepam, or phenobarbital are used in status epilepticus. In this condition, heavy sedation is desirable.

E. Muscle Relaxation

Relaxation of skeletal muscle occurs only with high doses of most sedative-hypnotics. However, diazepam is effective at sedative dose levels for specific spasticity states, including cerebral palsy. Meprobamate also has some selectivity as a muscle relaxant.

F. Medullary Depression

High doses of conventional sedative-hypnotics, especially alcohols and barbiturates, can cause depression of medullary neurons, leading to respiratory arrest, hypotension, and cardiovascular collapse. These effects are the cause of death in suicidal overdose.

G. Tolerance and Dependence

Tolerance—a decrease in responsiveness—occurs when sedative-hypnotics are used chronically or in high dosage. Cross-tolerance may occur among different chemical subgroups. Psychological dependence occurs frequently with most sedative-hypnotics and is manifested by the compulsive use of these drugs to reduce anxiety. Physiologic dependence constitutes an altered state that leads to an abstinence syndrome (withdrawal state) when the drug is discontinued. Withdrawal signs, which may include anxiety, tremors, hyperreflexia, and seizures, occur more commonly

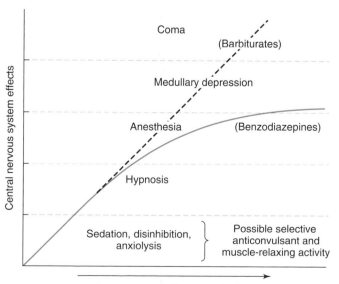

FIGURE 22–2 Relationships between dose of benzodiazepines and barbiturates and their CNS effects.

with shorter-acting drugs. The dependence liability of zolpidem, zaleplon, and eszopiclone may be less than that of the benzodiazepines since withdrawal symptoms are minimal after their abrupt discontinuance.

CLINICAL USES

Most of these uses can be predicted from the pharmacodynamic effects outlined previously.

A. Anxiety States

Benzodiazepines are favored in the drug treatment of acute anxiety states and for rapid control of panic attacks. Although it is difficult to demonstrate the superiority of one drug over another, alprazolam and clonazepam have greater efficacy than other benzodiazepines in the longer term treatment of panic and phobic disorders. *Note the increasing use of newer antidepressants in the treatment of chronic anxiety states (see Chapter 30).*

B. Sleep Disorders

Benzodiazepines, including estazolam, flurazepam, and triazolam, have been widely used in primary insomnia and for the management of certain other sleep disorders. Lower doses should be used in elderly patients who are more sensitive to their CNS depressant effects. More recently there has been increasing use of zolpidem, zaleplon, and eszopiclone in insomnia, since they have rapid onset with minimal effects on sleep patterns and cause less daytime cognitive impairment than benzodiazepines. Note that sedative-hypnotic drugs are not recommended for breathing-related sleep disorders.

C. Other Uses

Thiopental is commonly used for the induction of anesthesia, and certain benzodiazepines (eg, diazepam, midazolam) are used as components of anesthesia protocols including those used in day surgery. Special uses include the management of seizure disorders (eg, clonazepam, phenobarbital) and bipolar disorder (eg, clonazepam) and treatment of muscle spasticity (eg, diazepam). Longer acting benzodiazepines (eg, chlordiazepoxide, diazepam) are used in the management of withdrawal states in persons physiologically dependent on ethanol and other sedative-hypnotics.

TOXICITY

A. Psychomotor Dysfunction

This includes cognitive impairment, decreased psychomotor skills, and unwanted daytime sedation. These adverse effects are more common with benzodiazepines that have active metabolites with long half-lives (eg, diazepam, flurazepam), but can also occur after a single dose of a short-acting benzodiazepine such as triazolam. The dosage of a sedative-hypnotic should be reduced in elderly patients, who are more susceptible to drugs that cause

psychomotor dysfunction. In such patients excessive daytime sedation has been shown to increase the risk of falls and fractures. Anterograde amnesia may also occur with benzodiazepines, especially when used at high dosage, an action that forms the basis for their criminal use in cases of "date rape." Zolpidem and the newer hypnotics cause modest day-after psychomotor depression with few amnestic effects. However, all prescription drugs used as sleep aids may cause functional impairment, including "sleep driving," defined as "driving while not fully awake after ingestion of a sedative-hypnotic product, with no memory of the event."

B. Additive CNS Depression

This occurs when sedative-hypnotics are used with other drugs in the class as well as with alcoholic beverages, antihistamines, antipsychotic drugs, opioid analgesics, and tricyclic antidepressants. This is the most common type of drug interaction involving sedative-hypnotics.

C. Overdosage

Overdosage of sedative-hypnotic drugs causes severe respiratory and cardiovascular depression; these potentially lethal effects are more likely to occur with alcohols, barbiturates, and carbamates than with benzodiazepines or the newer hypnotics such as zolpidem. Management of intoxication requires maintenance of a patent airway and ventilatory support. Flumazenil may reverse CNS depressant effects of benzodiazepines, eszopiclone, zolpidem, and zaleplon but has no beneficial actions in overdosage with other sedative-hypnotics.

D. Other Adverse Effects

Barbiturates and carbamates (but not benzodiazepines, eszopiclone, zolpidem, or zaleplon) induce the formation of the liver microsomal enzymes that metabolize drugs. This enzyme induction may lead to multiple drug interactions. Barbiturates may also precipitate acute intermittent porphyria in susceptible patients. Chloral hydrate may displace coumarins from plasma protein binding sites and increase anticoagulant effects.

ATYPICAL SEDATIVE-HYPNOTICS

A. Buspirone

Buspirone is a selective anxiolytic, with minimal CNS depressant effects (it does not affect driving skills) and has no anticonvulsant or muscle relaxant properties. The drug interacts with the 5-HT$_{1A}$ subclass of brain serotonin receptors as a partial agonist, but the precise mechanism of its anxiolytic effect is unknown. Buspirone has a slow onset of action (>1 week) and is used in generalized anxiety disorder(s), but is less effective in panic disorders. Tolerance development is minimal with chronic use, and there is little rebound anxiety or withdrawal symptoms on discontinuance. Buspirone is metabolized by CYP3A4, and its plasma levels are markedly increased by drugs such as erythromycin and ketoconazole. Side effects of buspirone include tachycardia, paresthesias, pupillary constriction, and gastrointestinal distress. Buspirone has minimal abuse liability and is not a schedule-controlled drug. The drug appears to be safe in pregnancy.

B. Ramelteon

This novel hypnotic drug that activates melatonin receptors in the suprachiasmatic nuclei of the CNS decreases the latency of sleep onset with minimal rebound insomnia or withdrawal symptoms. Ramelteon has no direct effects on GABA-ergic neurotransmission in the CNS. Unlike conventional hypnotics, ramelteon appears to have minimal abuse liability, and it is not a controlled substance. The drug is metabolized by hepatic cytochrome P450 forming an active metabolite. The CYP inducer rifampin markedly reduces plasma levels of ramelteon and its metabolite. Conversely, inhibitors of CYP1A2 (eg, fluvoxamine) or CYP2C9 (eg, fluconazole) increase plasma levels of ramelteon. The adverse effects of the drug include dizziness, fatigue, and endocrine changes including decreased testosterone and increased prolactin.

QUESTIONS

1. A 43-year-old very overweight man complains of not sleeping well and feeling tired during the day. He tells his physician that his wife is the cause of the problem because she wakes him up several times during the night because of his loud snores. This appears to be a breathing-related sleep disorder, so you should probably write a prescription for
   (A) Buspirone
   (B) Eszopiclone
   (C) Flurazepam
   (D) Secobarbital
   (E) None of the above

2. Which statement concerning the barbiturates is accurate?
   (A) Abstinence syndromes are more severe during withdrawal from phenobarbital than from secobarbital
   (B) Alkalinization of the urine accelerates the elimination of phenobarbital
   (C) Barbiturates may increase the half-lives of drugs metabolized by the liver
   (D) Compared with barbiturates, the benzodiazepines exhibit a steeper dose-response relationship
   (E) Respiratory depression caused by barbiturate overdosage can be reversed by flumazenil

3. A 24-year-old stockbroker has developed a "nervous disposition." He is easily startled, worries about inconsequential matters, and sometimes complains of stomach cramps. At night he grinds his teeth in his sleep. There is no history of drug abuse. Diagnosed as suffering from generalized anxiety disorder, he is prescribed buspirone. His physician should inform the patient to anticipate
   (A) A need to continually increase drug dosage because of tolerance
   (B) A significant effect of the drug on memory
   (C) Additive CNS depression with alcoholic beverages
   (D) That the drug is likely to take a week or more to begin working
   (E) That if he stops taking the drug abruptly, he will experience withdrawal signs

4. Which of the following best describes the mechanism of action of benzodiazepines?
   (A) Activate GABA$_B$ receptors in the spinal cord
   (B) Block glutamate receptors in hierarchical neuronal pathways in the brain
   (C) Increase frequency of opening of chloride ion channels coupled to GABA$_A$ receptors
   (D) Inhibit GABA transaminase to increase brain levels of GABA
   (E) Stimulate release of GABA from nerve endings in the brain

5. An 82-year-old woman, otherwise healthy for her age, has difficulty sleeping. Triazolam is prescribed for her at one half of the conventional adult dose. Which statement about the use of triazolam in this elderly patient is accurate?
   (A) Ambulatory dysfunction does not occur in elderly patients taking one half of the conventional adult dose
   (B) Hypertension is a common adverse effect of benzodiazepines in elderly patients
   (C) Over-the-counter cold medications may antagonize the hypnotic effects of the drug
   (D) The patient may experience amnesia, especially if she also consumes alcoholic beverages
   (E) Triazolam is distinctive in that it does not cause rebound insomnia on abrupt discontinuance

6. The most likely explanation for the increased sensitivity of elderly patients after administration of a single dose of a benzodiazepine is
   (A) Changes in brain function accompanying aging
   (B) Changes in plasma protein binding
   (C) Decreased hepatic metabolism of lipid-soluble drugs
   (D) Decreases in renal function
   (E) Increased cerebral blood flow

7. A 28-year-old woman has sporadic attacks of intense anxiety with marked physical symptoms, including hyperventilation, tachycardia, and sweating. If she is diagnosed as suffering from a panic disorder, the most appropriate drug to use is
   (A) Clonazepam
   (B) Eszopiclone
   (C) Flurazepam
   (D) Propranolol
   (E) Ramelteon

8. Which drug used in the maintenance treatment of patients with tonic-clonic or partial seizure states increases the hepatic metabolism of many drugs including both warfarin and phenytoin?
   (A) Buspirone
   (B) Chlordiazepoxide
   (C) Eszopiclone
   (D) Phenobarbital
   (E) Triazolam

9. A patient with liver dysfunction is scheduled for a surgical procedure. Lorazepam or oxazepam can be used for preanesthetic sedation in this patient without special concern regarding excessive CNS depression because these drugs are
   (A) Actively secreted in the renal proximal tubule
   (B) Eliminated via the lungs
   (C) Metabolized via conjugation extrahepatically
   (D) Reversible by administration of naloxone
   (E) Selective anxiolytics like buspirone

10. This drug used in the management of insomnia facilitates the inhibitory actions of GABA, but it lacks anticonvulsant or muscle-relaxing properties and has minimal effect on sleep architecture. Its actions are antagonized by flumazenil.

(A) Buspirone
(B) Chlordiazepoxide
(C) Eszopiclone
(D) Ramelteon
(E) Phenobarbital

ANSWERS

1. Benzodiazepines and barbiturates are contraindicated in breathing-related sleep disorders because they further compromise ventilation. In obstructive sleep apnea (pickwickian syndrome), obesity is a major risk factor. Buspirone is a selective anxiolytic not a hypnotic. The best prescription you can give this patient is to lose weight. The answer is **E.**

2. Withdrawal symptoms from use of the shorter-acting barbiturate secobarbital are more severe than with phenobarbital. The dose-response curve for benzodiazepines is flatter than that for barbiturates. Induction of liver drug-metabolizing enzymes occurs with barbiturates and may lead to *decreases* in half-life of other drugs. Flumazenil is an antagonist at BZ receptors and is used to reverse CNS depressant effects of benzodiazepines. As a weak acid (pK_a, 7), phenobarbital will be more ionized (nonprotonated) in the urine at alkaline pH and less reabsorbed in the renal tubule. The answer is **B.**

3. Buspirone is a selective anxiolytic with pharmacologic characteristics different from those of sedative-hypnotics. Buspirone has minimal effects on cognition or memory; it is not an additive with ethanol in terms of CNS depression; tolerance is minimal; and it has no dependence liability. Buspirone is not effective in *acute* anxiety because it has a slow onset of action. The answer is **D.**

4. Benzodiazepines exert most of their CNS effects by increasing the inhibitory effects of GABA, interacting with components of the $GABA_A$ receptor-chloride ion channel macromolecular complex to increase the frequency of chloride ion channel opening. Benzodiazepines do not affect GABA metabolism or release, and they are not GABA receptor agonists because they do not interact directly with the binding site for GABA. The answer is **C.**

5. In elderly patients taking benzodiazepines, hypotension is far more likely than an increase in blood pressure. Elderly patients are more prone to the CNS depressant effects of hypnotics; a dose reduction of 50% may still cause excessive sedation with possible ambulatory impairment. Additive CNS depression occurs commonly with drugs used in over-the-counter cold medications, and rebound insomnia can occur with abrupt discontinuance of benzodiazepines used as sleeping pills. Alcohol enhances psychomotor depression and the amnestic effects of the benzodiazepines. The answer is **D.**

6. Decreased blood flow to vital organs, including the liver and kidney, occurs during the aging process. These changes may contribute to cumulative effects of sedative-hypnotic drugs. However, this does not explain the enhanced sensitivity of the elderly patient to a **single** dose of a central depressant, which appears to be due to changes in brain function that accompany aging. The answer is **A.**

7. Alprazolam (not listed) and clonazepam are the most effective of the benzodiazepines for the treatment of panic disorders. Eszopiclone and flumazenil are hypnotics. Propranolol is commonly used to attenuate excessive sympathomimetic activity in persons who suffer from performance anxiety ("stage fright"). The answer is **A.**

8. Chronic administration of phenobarbital increases the activity of hepatic drug-metabolizing enzymes, including several cytochrome P450 isozymes. This can increase the rate of metabolism of drugs administered concomitantly, resulting in decreases in the intensity and duration of their effects. The answer is **D.**

9. The elimination of most benzodiazepines involves their metabolism by liver enzymes, including cytochrome P450 isozymes. In a patient with liver dysfunction, lorazepam and oxazepam, which are metabolized extrahepatically, are less likely to cause excessive CNS depression. Benzodiazepines are not eliminated via the kidneys or lungs. Flumazenil is used to reverse excessive CNS depression caused by benzodiazepines. The answer is **C.**

10. Only two of the drugs listed are used for insomnia, eszopiclone and ramelteon. Eszopiclone, zaleplon, and zolpidem are related hypnotics that, though structurally different from benzodiazepines, appear to have a similar mechanism of action. However, these drugs are not effective in seizures or in muscle spasticity states. Compared with benzodiazepines, the newer hypnotics are less likely to alter sleep patterns. Ramelteon activates melatonin receptors in the suprachiasmatic nuclei. Buspirone is not a hypnotic! The answer is **C.**

SKILL KEEPER ANSWER: LOADING DOSE (SEE CHAPTER 3)

Because the half-life of diazepam is 2 days, one may assume that the plasma concentration 3 h after drug ingestion is of an order of magnitude similar to that of the peak plasma level. If so, and assuming 100% bioavailability, then

Dose ingested = Plasma concentration $\times V_d$

$\qquad\qquad$ = 2 mg/L $\times$ 80 L

$\qquad\qquad$ = 160 mg

CHECKLIST

When you complete this chapter, you should be able to:

❏ Identify major drugs in each sedative-hypnotic subgroup.

❏ Recall the significant pharmacokinetic features of the sedative-hypnotic drugs commonly used for treatment of anxiety and sleep disorders.

❏ Describe the proposed mechanisms of action of benzodiazepines, barbiturates, and zolpidem.

❏ List the pharmacodynamic actions of major sedative-hypnotics in terms of their clinical uses and their adverse effects.

❏ Identify the distinctive properties of buspirone, eszopiclone, ramelteon, zaleplon, and zolpidem.

❏ Describe the symptoms and management of overdose of sedative-hypnotics and withdrawal from physiologic dependence.

DRUG SUMMARY TABLE: Sedative-Hypnotics

Subclass	Mechanism of Action	Clinical Applications	Pharmacokinetics and Drug Interactions	Toxicities
Benzodiazepines				
Alprazolam Chlordiazepoxide Clorazepate Clonazepam Diazepam Flurazepam Lorazepam Midazolam, etc	Bind GABA$_A$ receptor subunits to facilitate chloride channel opening • membrane hyperpolarization	Acute anxiety states, panic attacks, generalized anxiety disorder, insomnia; skeletal muscle relaxation • seizure disorders	Hepatic metabolism • active metabolites. Additive CNS depression with many drugs Half-lives: 2–4 h	Extension of CNS depressant actions • tolerance • dependence liability
Benzodiazepine antagonist				
Flumazenil	Antagonist at benzodiazepine sites on GABA$_A$ receptor	Management of benzodiazepine overdose	IV form Short half-life	Agitation, confusion • possible withdrawal syndrome
Barbiturates				
Amobarbital Butabarbital Pentobarbital Phenobarbital Secobarbital Thiopental	Bind to GABA$_A$ receptor sites (distinct from benzodiazepines) • facilitate chloride channel opening	Anesthesia (thiopental) • insomnia and sedation (secobarbital) • seizure disorders (phenobarbital)	Oral activity • hepatic metabolism; induction of metabolism of many drugs Half-lives: 4–60 h	Extension of CNS depressant actions • tolerance • dependence liability > benzodiazepines
Newer hypnotics				
Eszopiclone Zaleplon Zolpidem	Bind to GABA$_A$ receptor sites (close to benzodiazepine site) • facilitate chloride channel opening	Sleep disorders, esp when sleep onset is delayed	Oral activity, CYP substrates Additive CNS depression with ethanol and other depressants Short half-lives	Extension of CNS depressant effects • dependence liability

(Continued)

DRUG SUMMARY TABLE: Sedative-Hypnotics (*Continued*)

Subclass	Mechanism of Action	Clinical Applications	Pharmacokinetics and Drug Interactions	Toxicities
Melatonin receptor agonist				
Ramelteon	Activates MT1 and MT2 receptors in suprachiasmatic nucleus	Sleep disorders, esp when sleep onset is delayed Not a controlled substance	Oral activity; forms active metabolite via CYP1A2 • fluvoxamine inhibits metabolism	Dizziness, fatigue, endocrine changes
5-HT agonist				
Buspirone	Partial agonist at 5-HT receptors and possibly D2 receptors	Generalized anxiety states	Oral activity • forms active metabolite • interactions with CYP3A4 inducers and inhibitors; short half-life	GI distress, tachycardia • paresthesias

Alcohols

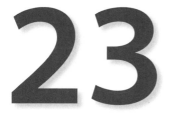

Ethanol, a sedative-hypnotic drug, is the most important alcohol of pharmacologic interest. Its abuse causes major medical and socioeconomic problems. Other alcohols of toxicologic importance are methanol and ethylene glycol. Several drugs discussed in this chapter are used to prevent the potentially life-threatening ethanol withdrawal syndrome, to treat chronic alcohol use disorders, or to treat acute methanol and ethylene glycol poisoning.

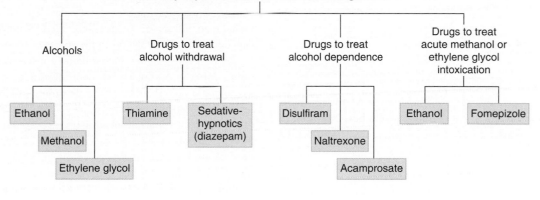

Clinically important alcohols and their antagonists

Alcohols: Ethanol, Methanol, Ethylene glycol

Drugs to treat alcohol withdrawal: Thiamine, Sedative-hypnotics (diazepam)

Drugs to treat alcohol dependence: Disulfiram, Naltrexone, Acamprosate

Drugs to treat acute methanol or ethylene glycol intoxication: Ethanol, Fomepizole

ETHANOL

A. Pharmacokinetics

After ingestion, ethanol is rapidly and completely absorbed; the drug is then distributed to most body tissues. Two enzyme systems metabolize ethanol to acetaldehyde (Figure 23–1).

1. Alcohol dehydrogenase (ADH)—This family of cytosolic, NAD⁺-dependent enzymes, found mainly in the liver and gut, accounts for the metabolism of low to moderate doses of ethanol. Because of the limited supply of the coenzyme NAD⁺, the reaction has *zero-order kinetics,* resulting in a fixed capacity for ethanol metabolism of 7–10 g/h. Gastrointestinal metabolism of ethanol is lower in women than in men. Genetic variation in ADH affects the rate of ethanol metabolism and vulnerability to alcohol-use disorders.

2. Microsomal ethanol-oxidizing system (MEOS)—At blood ethanol levels higher than 100 mg/dL, the liver microsomal mixed function oxidase system that catalyzes most phase I drug-metabolizing reactions (see Chapter 2) contributes significantly to ethanol metabolism (Figure 23–1). Chronic ethanol consumption induces cytochrome P450 enzyme synthesis and MEOS activity; this is partially responsible for the development of tolerance to ethanol. The primary isoform of cytochrome P450 induced by ethanol—2E1 (see Table 4–3)—converts acetaminophen to a hepatotoxic metabolite.

Acetaldehyde formed from the oxidation of ethanol by either ADH or MEOS is rapidly metabolized to acetate by aldehyde dehydrogenase, a mitochondrial enzyme found in the liver and many other tissues. Aldehyde dehydrogenase is inhibited by **disulfiram** and other drugs, including **metronidazole, oral hypoglycemics,** and some **cephalosporins.** Some individuals, primarily of Asian descent, have genetic deficiency of aldehyde dehydrogenase.

High-Yield Terms to Learn

Alcohol abuse	An alcohol-use disorder characterized by compulsive use of ethanol in dangerous situations (eg, driving, combined with other CNS depressants) or despite adverse consequences directly related to the drinking
Alcohol dependence	An alcohol-use disorder characterized by alcohol abuse plus physical dependence on ethanol
Alcohol withdrawal syndrome	The characteristic syndrome of insomnia, tremor, agitation, seizures, and autonomic instability engendered by deprivation in an individual who is physically dependent on ethanol
Delirium tremens (DTs)	Severe form of alcohol withdrawal whose main symptoms are sweating, tremor, confusion, and hallucinations
Fetal alcohol syndrome	A syndrome of craniofacial dysmorphia, heart defects, and mental retardation caused by the teratogenic effects of ethanol consumption during pregnancy
Wernicke-Korsakoff syndrome	A syndrome of ataxia, confusion, and paralysis of the extraocular muscles that is associated with chronic alcoholism and thiamine deficiency

After consumption of even small quantities of ethanol, these individuals experience nausea and a flushing reaction from accumulation of acetaldehyde.

B. Acute Effects

1. CNS—The major acute effects of ethanol on the CNS are sedation, loss of inhibition, impaired judgment, slurred speech, and ataxia. In nontolerant persons, impairment of driving ability is thought to occur at ethanol blood levels between 60 and 80 mg/dL. Blood levels of 120 to 160 mg/dL are usually associated with gross drunkenness. Levels greater than 300 mg/dL may lead to loss of consciousness, anesthesia, and coma sometimes with fatal respiratory and cardiovascular depression. Blood levels higher than 500 mg/dL are usually lethal. Individuals with alcohol dependence who are tolerant to the effects of ethanol can function almost normally at much higher blood concentrations than occasional drinkers. Additive CNS depression occurs with concomitant ingestion of ethanol and a wide variety of CNS depressants, including sedative-hypnotics, opioid agonists, and many drugs that block muscarinic and H_1 histamine receptors. The molecular mechanisms underlying the complex CNS effects of ethanol are not fully understood. Specific receptors for ethanol have not been identified. Rather, ethanol appears to modulate the function of a number of signaling proteins. It facilitates the action of GABA at $GABA_A$ receptors, inhibits the ability of glutamate to activate NMDA (*N*-methyl-D-aspartate) receptors, and modifies the activities of adenylyl cyclase, phospholipase C, and ion channels.

2. Other organ systems—Ethanol, even at relatively low blood concentrations, significantly depresses the heart. Vascular smooth muscle is relaxed, which leads to vasodilation, sometimes with marked hypothermia.

C. Chronic Effects

1. Tolerance and dependence—Tolerance occurs mainly as a result of CNS adaptation and to a lesser extent by an increased rate of ethanol metabolism. There is cross-tolerance to sedative-hypnotic drugs that facilitate GABA activity (eg, benzodiazepines and barbiturates). Both psychological and physical dependence are marked.

2. Liver—Liver disease is the most common medical complication of chronic alcohol abuse. Progressive loss of liver function occurs with reversible fatty liver progressing to irreversible hepatitis, cirrhosis, and liver failure. Hepatic dysfunction is often more severe in women than in men and in both men and women infected with hepatitis B or C virus.

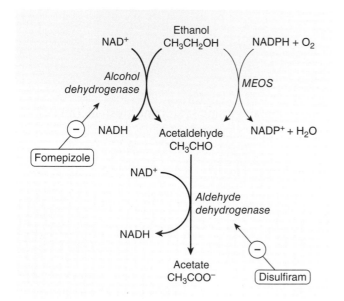

FIGURE 23–1 Metabolism of ethanol by alcohol dehydrogenase (ADH) and the microsomal ethanol-oxidizing system (MEOS). Alcohol dehydrogenase and aldehyde dehydrogenase are inhibited by fomepizole and disulfiram, respectively. (Reproduced, with permission, from Katzung BG, Masters SB, Trevor AT, editors: *Basic & Clinical Pharmacology*, 12th ed. McGraw-Hill, 2012: Fig. 23–1.)

3. Gastrointestinal system—Irritation, inflammation, bleeding, and scarring of the gut wall occur after chronic heavy use of ethanol and may cause absorption defects and exacerbate nutritional deficiencies. Chronic alcohol abuse greatly increases the risk of pancreatitis.

4. CNS—Peripheral neuropathy is the most common neurologic abnormality in chronic alcohol abuse. More rarely, thiamine deficiency, along with alcohol abuse, leads to **Wernicke-Korsakoff** syndrome, which is characterized by ataxia, confusion, and paralysis of the extraocular muscles. Prompt treatment with parenteral thiamine is essential to prevent a permanent memory disorder known as Korsakoff's psychosis.

5. Endocrine system—Gynecomastia, testicular atrophy, and salt retention can occur, partly because of altered steroid metabolism in the cirrhotic liver.

6. Cardiovascular system—Excessive chronic ethanol use is associated with an increased incidence of hypertension, anemia, and dilated cardiomyopathy. Acute drinking for several days ("binge" drinking) can cause arrhythmias. However, the ingestion of modest quantities of ethanol (10–15 g/day) raises serum levels of high-density lipoprotein (HDL) cholesterol and may *protect* against coronary heart disease.

7. Fetal alcohol syndrome—Ethanol use in pregnancy is associated with teratogenic effects that include mental retardation (most common), growth deficiencies, microcephaly, and a characteristic underdevelopment of the midface region.

8. Neoplasia—Ethanol is not a primary carcinogen, but its chronic use is associated with an increased incidence of neoplastic diseases in the gastrointestinal tract and a small increase in the risk of breast cancer.

9. Immune system—Chronic alcohol abuse has complex effects on immune functions because it enhances inflammation in the liver and pancreas and inhibits immune function in other tissues. Heavy use predisposes to infectious pneumonia.

SKILL KEEPER: ELIMINATION HALF-LIFE (SEE CHAPTER 1)

Search "high and low" through drug information resources and you will not find data on the elimination half-life of ethanol! Can you explain why this is the case? The Skill Keeper Answer appears at the end of the chapter.

D. Treatment of Acute and Chronic Alcoholism

1. Excessive CNS depression—Acute ethanol intoxication is managed by maintenance of vital signs and prevention of aspiration after vomiting. Intravenous dextrose is standard. Thiamine administration is used to protect against Wernicke-Korsakoff syndrome, and correction of electrolyte imbalance may be required.

2. Alcohol withdrawal syndrome—In individuals physically dependent on ethanol, discontinuance can lead to a withdrawal syndrome characterized by insomnia, tremor, anxiety, and, in severe cases, life-threatening seizures and delirium tremens (DTs). Peripheral effects include nausea, vomiting, diarrhea, and arrhythmias. The withdrawal syndrome is managed by correction of electrolyte imbalance, and administration of thiamine and a sedative-hypnotic. A long-acting benzodiazepine (eg, diazepam, chlordiazepoxide) is preferred unless the patient has compromised liver function, in which case a short-acting benzodiazepine with less complex metabolism (eg, lorazepam) is preferred.

3. Treatment of alcoholism—Alcoholism is a complex sociomedical problem, characterized by a high relapse rate. Several CNS neurotransmitter systems appear to be targets for drugs that reduce the craving for alcohol. The opioid receptor antagonist **naltrexone** has proved to be useful in some patients, presumably through its ability to decrease the effects of endogenous opioid peptides in the brain (see Chapters 31 and 32). **Acamprosate,** an NMDA glutamate receptor antagonist, is also FDA approved for treatment of alcoholism. The aldehyde dehydrogenase inhibitor disulfiram is used adjunctively in some treatment programs. If ethanol is consumed by a patient who has taken **disulfiram,** acetaldehyde accumulation leads to nausea, headache, flushing, and hypotension (Figure 23–1).

OTHER ALCOHOLS

A. Methanol

Methanol (wood alcohol), a constituent of windshield cleaners and "canned heat," is sometimes ingested intentionally. Intoxication causes visual dysfunction, gastrointestinal distress, shortness of breath, loss of consciousness, and coma. Methanol is metabolized to formaldehyde and formic acid, which causes severe acidosis, retinal damage, and blindness. The formation of formaldehyde is reduced by prompt intravenous administration of **fomepizole,** an inhibitor of alcohol dehydrogenase, or ethanol, which competitively inhibits alcohol dehydrogenase oxidation of methanol (Figure 23–2).

B. Ethylene Glycol

Industrial exposure to ethylene glycol (by inhalation or skin absorption) or self-administration (eg, by drinking antifreeze products) leads to severe acidosis and renal damage from the metabolism of ethylene glycol to oxalic acid. Prompt treatment with intravenous fomepizole or ethanol may slow or prevent formation of this toxic metabolite (Figure 23–2).

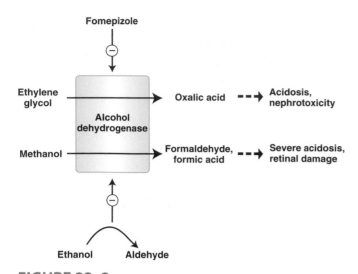

FIGURE 23–2 The oxidation of ethylene glycol and methanol by alcohol dehydrogenase (ADH) creates metabolites that cause serious toxicity. Fomepizole, an inhibitor of alcohol dehydrogenase, is used in methanol or ethylene glycol poisoning to slow the rate of formation of toxic metabolites. Ethanol, a substrate with higher affinity for ADH than ethylene glycol or methanol, also slows the formation of toxic metabolites and is an alternative to fomepizole.

QUESTIONS

1. A 45-year-old moderately obese man has been drinking heavily for 72 h. This level of drinking is much higher than his regular habit of drinking 1 alcoholic drink per day. His only significant medical problem is mild hypertension, which is adequately controlled by metoprolol. With this history, this man is at significant risk for
   (A) Arrhythmia
   (B) Bacterial pneumonia
   (C) Hyperthermia
   (D) Tonic-clonic seizures
   (E) Wernicke-Korsakoff syndrome

2. A 42-year-old man with a history of alcoholism is brought to the emergency department in a confused and delirious state. He has truncal ataxia and ophthalmoplegia. The most appropriate immediate course of action is to administer diazepam plus
   (A) Chlordiazepoxide
   (B) Disulfiram
   (C) Folic acid
   (D) Fomepizole
   (E) Thiamine

3. The cytochrome P450-dependent microsomal ethanol oxidizing system (MEOS) pathway of ethanol metabolism is *most* likely to be maximally activated under the condition of low concentrations of
   (A) Acetaldehyde
   (B) Ethanol
   (C) NAD$^+$
   (D) NADPH
   (E) Oxygen

4. A freshman student (weight 70 kg) attends a college party where he rapidly consumes a quantity of an alcoholic beverage that results in a blood level of 500 mg/dL. Assuming that this young man has not had an opportunity to develop tolerance to ethanol, his present condition is *best* characterized as
   (A) Able to walk, but not in a straight line
   (B) Alert and competent to drive a car
   (C) Comatose and near death
   (D) Sedated with increased reaction times
   (E) Slightly inebriated

Questions 5 and 6. A homeless middle-aged male patient presents in the emergency department in a state of intoxication. You note that he is behaviorally disinhibited and rowdy. He tells you that he has recently consumed about a pint of a red-colored liquid that his friends were using to "get high." He complains that his vision is blurred and that it is "like being in a snowstorm." His breath smells a bit like formaldehyde. He is acidotic.

5. Which of the following is the most likely cause of this patient's intoxicated state?
   (A) Ethanol
   (B) Ethylene glycol
   (C) Isopropanol
   (D) Hexane
   (E) Methanol

6. After assessing and stabilizing the patient's airway, respiration, and circulatory status, fomepizole was administered intravenously. Which of the following most accurately describes the therapeutic purpose of the fomepizole administration?
   (A) Accelerate the rate of elimination of the toxic liquid that he consumed
   (B) Combat his acidosis
   (C) Inhibit the metabolic production of a toxic metabolite of the poison
   (D) Prevent alcohol withdrawal seizures
   (E) Sedate the patient

7. The regular ingestion of moderate or heavy amounts of alcohol predisposes to hepatic damage after overdose of acetaminophen because of chronic ethanol ingestion
   (A) Blocks acetaminophen metabolism
   (B) Causes thiamine deficiency
   (C) Displaces acetaminophen from plasma proteins
   (D) Induces liver drug-metabolizing enzymes
   (E) Inhibits renal clearance of acetaminophen

8. A 23-year-old pregnant woman with alcoholism presented to the emergency department in the early stages of labor. She had consumed large amounts of alcohol throughout her pregnancy. This patient's infant is at high risk of a syndrome that includes
   (A) Ambiguous genitalia in a male fetus and normal genitalia in a female fetus
   (B) Failure of closure of the atrial septum or ventricular septum
   (C) Limb or digit malformation
   (D) Mental retardation and craniofacial abnormalities
   (E) Underdevelopment of the lungs

9. The combination of ethanol and disulfiram results in nausea and hypotension as a result of the accumulation of which of the following?
   (A) Acetaldehyde
   (B) Acetate
   (C) Methanol
   (D) NADH
   (E) Pyruvate

10. The intense craving experienced by those who are trying to recover from chronic alcohol abuse can be ameliorated by a drug that is an
   (A) Agonist of α_1 adrenoceptors
   (B) Agonist of serotonin receptors
   (C) Antagonist of β_2 adrenoceptors
   (D) Antagonist of opioid receptors
   (E) Inhibitor of cyclooxygenase

ANSWERS

1. This man's regular rate of alcohol consumption is not high enough to put him at risk of long-term consequences such as Wernicke-Korsakoff syndrome, increased susceptibility to bacterial pneumonia, or alcohol withdrawal seizures. This pattern of "binge drinking" does put him at increased risk of cardiac arrhythmia. The answer is **A.**

2. This patient has symptoms of Wernicke's encephalopathy, including delirium, gait disturbances, and paralysis of the external eye muscles. The condition results from thiamine deficiency but is rarely seen in the absence of alcoholism. The diazepam is administered to prevent the alcohol withdrawal syndrome. The answer is **E.**

3. The microsomal ethanol-oxidizing system (MEOS) contributes most to ethanol metabolism at relatively high blood alcohol concentrations (>100 mg/dL), when the alcohol dehydrogenase pathway is saturated due to depletion of NAD^+. So, the MEOS system contributes most when the NAD^+ concentration is low. NADPH and oxygen are cofactors for MEOS reactions. The concentration of acetaldehyde does not appear to affect the rate of either the ADH or the MEOS reactions. The answer is **C.**

4. The blood level of ethanol achieved in this individual is extremely high and likely to result in coma and possibly death due to respiratory arrest in a person who lacks tolerance to ethanol. The answer is **C.**

5. Behavioral disinhibition is a feature of early intoxication from ethanol and most other alcohols but not the solvent, hexane. Ocular dysfunction, including horizontal nystagmus and diplopia, is also a common finding in poisoning with alcohols, but the complaint of "flickering white spots before the eyes" or "being in a snowstorm" is highly suggestive of methanol intoxication. In some cases, the odor of formaldehyde may be present on the breath. In this patient, blood methanol levels should be determined as soon as possible. The answer is **E.**

6. In patients with suspected methanol intoxication, fomepizole is given intravenously to inhibit the ADH-catalyzed formation of toxic metabolites. The answer is **C.**

7. Chronic use of ethanol induces a cytochrome P450 2E1 isozyme that converts acetaminophen to a cytotoxic metabolite. This appears to be the explanation for the increased susceptibility to acetaminophen-induced hepatotoxicity found in individuals who regularly ingest alcohol. The answer is **D.**

8. This woman's infant is at risk for fetal alcohol syndrome, a syndrome associated with mental retardation, abnormalities of the head and face, and growth deficiency. This syndrome is a leading cause of mental retardation. The answer is **D.**

9. Nausea, hypotension, and ill feeling that result from drinking ethanol while also taking disulfiram stems from acetaldehyde accumulation. Disulfiram inhibits acetaldehyde dehydrogenase, the enzyme that converts acetaldehyde to acetate. The answer is **A.**

10. Naltrexone, a competitive inhibitor of opioid receptors, decreases the craving for alcohol in patients who are recovering from alcoholism. The answer is **D.**

SKILL KEEPER ANSWER: ELIMINATION HALF-LIFE (SEE CHAPTER 1)

*Drug information resources do not provide data on the elimination half-life of ethanol because, in the case of this drug, it is not constant. Ethanol elimination follows **zero-order kinetics** because the drug is metabolized at a constant rate irrespective of its concentration in the blood (see Chapter 3). The pharmacokinetic relationship between elimination half-life, volume of distribution, and clearance, given by*

$$t_{1/2} = \frac{0.693 \times V_d}{CL}$$

is not applicable to ethanol. Its rate of metabolism is constant, but its clearance decreases with an increase in blood level. The arithmetic plot of ethanol blood level versus time follows a straight line (not exponential decay).

CHECKLIST

When you complete this chapter, you should be able to:

❑ Sketch the biochemical pathways for ethanol metabolism and indicate where fomepizole and disulfiram act.

❑ Summarize characteristic pharmacodynamic and pharmacokinetic properties of ethanol.

❑ Relate blood alcohol levels in a nontolerant person to CNS depressant effects of acute alcohol ingestion.

❑ Identify the toxic effects of chronic ethanol ingestion.

❑ Describe the fetal alcohol syndrome.

❑ Describe the treatment of ethanol overdosage.

❑ Outline the pharmacotherapy of (1) the alcohol withdrawal syndrome and (2) alcohol-use disorders.

❑ Describe the toxicity and treatment of acute poisoning with (1) methanol and (2) ethylene glycol.

DRUG SUMMARY TABLE: Alcohols

Subclass	Mechanism of Action	Clinical Applications	Pharmacokinetics	Toxicities, Interactions
Alcohols				
Ethanol	Multiple effects on neurotransmitter receptors, ion channels, and signaling pathways	Antidote in methanol and ethylene glycol poisoning	Zero-order metabolism, duration depends on dose	Toxicity: Acute, CNS depression and respiratory failure. Chronic, damage to many systems, including liver, pancreas, gastrointestinal tract, and central and peripheral nervous systems. Interactions: Induction of CYP2E1 • increased conversion of acetaminophen to toxic metabolite

Methanol: poisoning result in toxic levels of formate, which causes characteristic visual disturbance plus coma, seizures, acidosis, and death due to respiratory failure
Ethylene glycol: poisoning creates toxic aldehydes and oxalate, which causes kidney damage and severe acidosis

Drugs used in acute ethanol withdrawal				
Benzodiazepines Diazepam	BDZ receptor agonist that facilitates GABA-mediated activation of GABA$_A$ receptors	Prevention and treatment of acute ethanol withdrawal syndrome • see Chapter 22	See Chapter 22	See Chapter 22

Other long-acting benzodiazepines and barbiturates are also effective (see Chapter 22)

Thiamine (vitamin B$_1$)	Essential vitamin required for synthesis of the coenzyme thiamine pyrophosphate	Administered to patients suspected of alcohol dependence to prevent the Wernicke-Korsakoff syndrome	Parenteral administration	None

(Continued)

DRUG SUMMARY TABLE: Alcohols (*Continued*)

Subclass	Mechanism of Action	Clinical Applications	Pharmacokinetics	Toxicities, Interactions
Drugs used in chronic alcoholism				
Opioid receptor antagonist Naltrexone	Nonselective competitive antagonist of opioid receptors	Reduced risk of relapse in individuals with alcohol-use disorders	Available as an oral or long-acting parenteral formulation (see Chapters 31 and 32)	Gastrointestinal effects and liver toxicity • rapid antagonism of all opioid actions
Other				
Acamprosate	Poorly understood NMDA receptor antagonist and GABA$_A$ agonist effects	Reduced risk of relapse in individuals with alcohol-use disorders	Oral administration	Gastrointestinal effects and rash
Enzyme inhibitor				
Disulfiram	Inhibits aldehyde dehydrogenase • causes aldehyde accumulation during ethanol ingestion	Deterrent to relapse in individuals with alcohol-use disorders	Oral administration	Little effect on its own but severe flushing, headache, nausea, vomiting, and hypotension when combined with ethanol
Drugs used in acute methanol or ethylene glycol toxicity				
Fomepizole	Inhibits alcohol dehydrogenase • prevents conversion of methanol and ethylene glycol to toxic metabolites	Methanol and ethylene glycol poisoning	Parenteral administration	Headache, nausea, dizziness, rare allergic reactions
Ethanol: higher affinity for alcohol dehydrogenase; used to reduce metabolism to toxic products				

Antiseizure Drugs

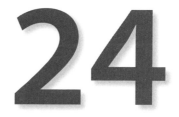

Epilepsy comprises a group of chronic syndromes that involve the recurrence of seizures (ie, limited periods of abnormal discharge of cerebral neurons). Effective antiseizure drugs have, to varying degrees, selective depressant actions on such abnormal neuronal activity. However, they vary in terms of their mechanisms of action and in their effectiveness in specific seizure disorders.

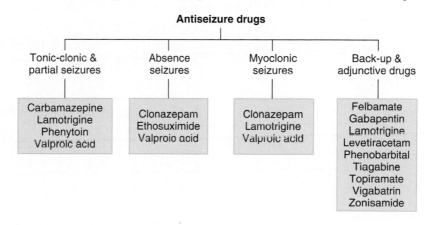

PHARMACOKINETICS

Antiseizure drugs are commonly used for long periods of time, and consideration of their pharmacokinetic properties is important for avoiding toxicity and drug interactions. For some of these drugs (eg, phenytoin), determination of plasma levels and clearance in individual patients may be necessary for optimum therapy. In general, antiseizure drugs are well absorbed orally and have good bioavailability. Most antiseizure drugs are metabolized by hepatic enzymes (exceptions include gabapentin and vigabatrin), and in some cases active metabolites are formed. Resistance to antiseizure drugs may involve increased expression of drug transporters at the level of the blood-brain barrier.

Pharmacokinetic drug interactions are common in this drug group. In the presence of drugs that inhibit antiseizure drug metabolism or that displace anticonvulsants from plasma protein binding sites, plasma concentrations of the antiseizure agents may reach toxic levels. On the other hand, drugs that induce hepatic drug-metabolizing enzymes (eg, rifampin) may result in

plasma levels of the antiseizure agents that are inadequate for seizure control. Several antiseizure drugs are themselves capable of inducing hepatic drug metabolism, especially carbamazepine and phenytoin.

A. Phenytoin

The oral bioavailability of phenytoin is variable because of individual differences in first-pass metabolism. Rapid-onset and extended-release forms are available. Phenytoin metabolism is nonlinear; elimination kinetics shift from first-order to zero-order at moderate to high dose levels. The drug binds extensively to plasma proteins (97–98%), and free (unbound) phenytoin levels in plasma are increased transiently by drugs that compete for binding (eg, carbamazepine, sulfonamides, valproic acid). The metabolism of phenytoin is enhanced in the presence of inducers of liver metabolism (eg, phenobarbital, rifampin) and inhibited by other drugs (eg, cimetidine, isoniazid). Phenytoin itself induces hepatic drug metabolism, decreasing the effects of

Seizures	Finite episodes of brain dysfunction resulting from abnormal discharge of cerebral neurons
Partial seizures, simple	Consciousness preserved; manifested variously as convulsive jerking, paresthesias, psychic symptoms (altered sensory perception, illusions, hallucinations, affect changes), and autonomic dysfunction
Partial seizures, complex	Impaired consciousness that is preceded, accompanied, or followed by psychological symptoms
Tonic-clonic seizures, generalized	Tonic phase (less than 1 min) involves abrupt loss of consciousness, muscle rigidity, and respiration arrest; clonic phase (2–3 min) involves jerking of body muscles, with lip or tongue biting, and fecal and urinary incontinence; formerly called grand mal
Absence seizures, generalized	Impaired consciousness (often abrupt onset and brief), sometimes with automatisms, loss of postural tone, or enuresis; begin in childhood (formerly, petit mal) and usually cease by age 20 yrs
Myoclonic seizures	Single or multiple myoclonic muscle jerks
Status epilepticus	A series of seizures (usually tonic-clonic) without recovery of consciousness between attacks; it is a life-threatening emergency

other antiepileptic drugs including carbamazepine, clonazepam, and lamotrigine. **Fosphenytoin** is a water-soluble prodrug form of phenytoin that is used parenterally.

B. Carbamazepine

Carbamazepine induces formation of liver drug-metabolizing enzymes that increase metabolism of the drug itself and may increase the clearance of many other anticonvulsant drugs including clonazepam, lamotrigine, and valproic acid. Carbamazepine metabolism can be inhibited by other drugs (eg, propoxyphene, valproic acid). A related drug, oxcarbazepine, is less likely to be involved in drug interactions.

C. Valproic Acid

In addition to competing for phenytoin plasma protein binding sites, valproic acid inhibits the metabolism of carbamazepine, ethosuximide, phenytoin, phenobarbital, and lamotrigine. Hepatic biotransformation of valproic acid leads to formation of a toxic metabolite that has been implicated in the hepatotoxicity of the drug.

D. Other Drugs

Gabapentin, pregabalin, levetiracetam, and vigabatrin are unusual in that they are eliminated by the kidney, largely in unchanged form. These agents have virtually no drug-drug interactions. Tiagabine, topiramate, and zonisamide undergo both hepatic metabolism and renal elimination of intact drug. Lamotrigine is eliminated via hepatic glucuronidation.

MECHANISMS OF ACTION

The general effect of antiseizure drugs is to suppress repetitive action potentials in epileptic foci in the brain. Many different mechanisms are involved in achieving this effect. In some cases, several mechanisms may contribute to the antiseizure activity of an individual drug. Some of the recognized mechanisms are described next.

A. Sodium Channel Blockade

At therapeutic concentrations, **phenytoin**, **carbamazepine**, **lamotrigine**, and **zonisamide** block voltage-gated sodium channels in neuronal membranes. This action is rate-dependent (ie, dependent on the frequency of neuronal discharge) and results in prolongation of the inactivated state of the Na^+ channel and the refractory period of the neuron. **Phenobarbital** and **valproic acid** may exert similar effects at high doses.

B. GABA-Related Targets

As described in Chapter 22, **benzodiazepine**s interact with specific receptors on the $GABA_A$ receptor–chloride ion channel macromolecular complex. In the presence of benzodiazepines, the *frequency* of chloride ion channel opening is increased; these drugs facilitate the inhibitory effects of GABA. **Phenobarbital** and other barbiturates also enhance the inhibitory actions of GABA but interact with a different receptor site on chloride ion channels that results in an increased *duration* of chloride ion channel opening.

GABA aminotransaminase (GABA-T) is an important enzyme in the termination of action of GABA. The enzyme is irreversibly inactivated by **vigabatrin** at therapeutic plasma levels and can also be inhibited by valproic acid at very high concentrations. **Tiagabine** inhibits a GABA transporter (GAT-1) in neurons and glia prolonging the action of the neurotransmitter. **Gabapentin** is a structural analog of GABA, but it does not activate GABA receptors directly. Other drugs that may facilitate the inhibitory actions of GABA include **felbamate, topiramate,** and **valproic acid.**

C. Calcium Channel Blockade

Ethosuximide inhibits low-threshold (T type) Ca^{2+} currents, especially in thalamic neurons that act as pacemakers to generate rhythmic cortical discharge. A similar action is reported for **valproic acid**, as well as for both **gabapentin** and **pregabalin**, and it may be the primary action of the latter drugs.

D. Other Mechanisms

In addition to its action on calcium channels, **valproic acid** causes neuronal membrane hyperpolarization, possibly by enhancing K^+ channel permeability. Although **phenobarbital** acts on both sodium channels and GABA-chloride channels, it also acts as an antagonist at some glutamate receptors. **Felbamate** blocks glutamate NMDA receptors. **Topiramate** blocks sodium channels and potentiates the actions of GABA and may also block glutamate receptors.

SKILL KEEPER: ANTIARRHYTHMIC DRUG ACTIONS (SEE CHAPTER 14)

1. *Which of the mechanisms of action of antiseizure drugs have theoretical implications regarding their activity in cardiac arrhythmias?*
2. *Can you recall any clinical uses of antiseizure drugs in the management of cardiac arrhythmias?*

The Skill Keeper Answers appear at the end of the chapter.

CLINICAL USES

Diagnosis of a specific seizure type is important for prescribing the most appropriate antiseizure drug (or combination of drugs). Drug choice is usually made on the basis of established efficacy in the specific seizure state that has been diagnosed, the prior responsiveness of the patient, and the anticipated toxicity of the drug. Treatment may involve combinations of drugs, following the principle of adding known effective agents if the preceding drugs are not sufficient.

A. Generalized Tonic-Clonic Seizures

Valproic acid, carbamazepine, and phenytoin are the drugs of choice for generalized tonic-clonic (grand mal) seizures. Phenobarbital (or primidone) is now considered to be an alternative agent in adults but continues to be a primary drug in infants. Lamotrigine and topiramate are also approved drugs for this indication, and several others may be used adjunctively in refractory cases.

B. Partial Seizures

The drugs of first choice are carbamazepine (or oxcarbazepine) or lamotrigine or phenytoin. Alternatives include felbamate, phenobarbital, topiramate, and valproic acid. Many of the newer anticonvulsants can be used adjunctively including gabapentin and pregabalin, a structural congener.

C. Absence Seizures

Ethosuximide or valproic acid are the preferred drugs because they cause minimal sedation. Ethosuximide is often used in uncomplicated absence seizures if patients can tolerate its gastrointestinal side effects. Valproic acid is particularly useful in patients who have concomitant generalized tonic-clonic or myoclonic seizures. Clonazepam is effective as an alternative drug but has the disadvantages of causing sedation and tolerance. Lamotrigine, levetiracetam, and zonisamide are also effective in absence seizures.

D. Myoclonic and Atypical Absence Syndromes

Myoclonic seizure syndromes are usually treated with valproic acid; lamotrigine is approved for adjunctive use, but is commonly used as monotherapy. Clonazepam can be effective, but the high doses required cause drowsiness. Levetiracetam, topiramate, and zonisamide are also used as backup drugs in myoclonic syndromes. Felbamate has been used adjunctively with the primary drugs but has both hematotoxic and hepatotoxic potential.

E. Status Epilepticus

Intravenous diazepam or lorazepam is usually effective in terminating attacks and providing short-term control. For prolonged therapy, intravenous phenytoin has often been used because it is highly effective and less sedating than benzodiazepines or barbiturates. However, phenytoin may cause cardiotoxicity (perhaps because of its solvent propylene glycol), and fosphenytoin (water-soluble) is a safer parenteral agent. Phenobarbital has also been used in status epilepticus, especially in children. In very severe status epilepticus that does not respond to these measures, general anesthesia may be used.

F. Other Clinical Uses

Several antiseizure drugs are effective in the management of bipolar affective disorders, especially valproic acid, which is now often used as a first-line drug in the treatment of mania. Carbamazepine and lamotrigine have also been used successfully in bipolar disorder. Carbamazepine is the drug of choice for trigeminal neuralgia, and its congener oxcarbazepine may provide similar analgesia with fewer adverse effects. Gabapentin has efficacy in pain of neuropathic origin, including postherpetic neuralgia, and, like phenytoin, may have some value in migraine. Topiramate is also used in the treatment of migraine. Pregabalin is also approved for neuropathic pain.

TOXICITY

Chronic therapy with antiseizure drugs is associated with specific toxic effects, the most important of which are listed in Table 24–1.

A. Teratogenicity

Children born of mothers taking anticonvulsant drugs have an increased risk of congenital malformations. Neural tube defects (eg, spina bifida) are associated with the use of valproic acid;

TABLE 24–1 Adverse effects and complications of antiepileptic drugs.

Antiepileptic Drug	Adverse Effects
Benzodiazepines	Sedation, tolerance, dependence
Carbamazepine	Diplopia, cognitive dysfunction, drowsiness, ataxia; rare occurrence of severe blood dyscrasias and Stevens-Johnson syndrome; teratogenic potential
Ethosuximide	Gastrointestinal distress, lethargy, headache, behavioral changes
Felbamate	Aplastic anemia, hepatic failure
Gabapentin	Dizziness, sedation, ataxia, nystagmus; does not affect drug metabolism (pregabalin is similar)
Lamotrigine	Dizziness, ataxia, nausea, rash, rare Stevens-Johnson syndrome
Levetiracetam	Dizziness, sedation, weakness, irritability, hallucinations, and psychosis have occurred
Oxcarbazepine	Similar to carbamazepine, but hyponatremia is more common; unlike carbamazepine, does not induce drug metabolism
Phenobarbital	Sedation, cognitive dysfunction, tolerance, dependence, induction of hepatic drug metabolism; primidone is similar
Phenytoin	Nystagmus, diplopia, sedation, gingival hyperplasia, hirsutism, anemias, peripheral neuropathy, osteoporosis, induction of hepatic drug metabolism
Tiagabine	Abdominal pain, nausea, dizziness, tremor, asthenia; drug metabolism is not induced
Topiramate	Drowsiness, dizziness, ataxia, psychomotor slowing and memory impairment; paresthesias, weight loss, acute myopia
Valproic acid	Drowsiness, nausea, tremor, hair loss, weight gain, hepatotoxicity (infants), inhibition of hepatic drug metabolism
Vigabatrin	Sedation, dizziness, weight gain; visual field defects with long-term use, which may not be reversible
Zonisamide	Dizziness, confusion, agitation, diarrhea, weight loss, rash, Stevens-Johnson syndrome

carbamazepine has been implicated as a cause of craniofacial anomalies and spina bifida; and a fetal hydantoin syndrome has been described after phenytoin use by pregnant women.

B. Overdosage Toxicity

Most of the commonly used anticonvulsants are CNS depressants, and respiratory depression may occur with overdosage. Management is primarily supportive (airway management, mechanical ventilation), and flumazenil may be used in benzodiazepine overdose.

C. Life-Threatening Toxicity

Fatal hepatotoxicity has occurred with valproic acid, with greatest risk to children younger than 2 years and patients taking multiple anticonvulsant drugs. Lamotrigine has caused skin rashes and life-threatening Stevens-Johnson syndrome or toxic epidermal necrolysis. Children are at higher risk (1–2% incidence), especially if they are also taking valproic acid. Zonisamide may also cause severe skin reactions. Reports of aplastic anemia and acute hepatic failure have limited the use of felbamate to severe, refractory seizure states.

D. Withdrawal

Withdrawal from antiseizure drugs should be accomplished gradually to avoid increased seizure frequency and severity. In general,

withdrawal from anti-absence drugs is more easily accomplished than withdrawal from drugs used in partial or generalized tonic-clonic seizure states.

QUESTIONS

1. A 9-year-old child is having learning difficulties at school. He has brief lapses of awareness with eyelid fluttering that occur every 5–10 min. Electroencephalogram (EEG) studies reveal brief 3-Hz spike and wave discharges appearing synchronously in all leads. Which drug would be effective in this child without the disadvantages of excessive sedation or tolerance development?
   (A) Clonazepam
   (B) Ethosuximide
   (C) Gabapentin
   (D) Felbamate
   (E) Phenobarbital

2. Which statement concerning the proposed mechanisms of action of anticonvulsant drugs is inaccurate?
   (A) Diazepam facilitates GABA-mediated inhibitory actions
   (B) Ethosuximide selectively blocks potassium ion (K^+) channels in thalamic neurons
   (C) Phenobarbital has multiple actions, including enhancement of the effects of GABA, antagonism of glutamate receptors, and blockade of sodium ion (Na^+) channels
   (D) Phenytoin prolongs the inactivated state of the Na^+ channel
   (E) Zonisamide blocks voltage-gated Na^+ channels

3. Which drug used in management of seizure disorders is most likely to elevate the plasma concentration of other drugs administered concomitantly?
(A) Carbamazepine
(B) Clonazepam
(C) Gabapentin
(D) Valproic acid
(E) Vigabatrin

4. A young female patient suffers from absence seizures. Which of the following statements about her proposed drug management is NOT accurate?
(A) Ethosuximide and valproic acid are preferred drugs
(B) Gastrointestinal side effects are common with ethosuximide
(C) She should be examined every 2 or 3 mo for deep tendon reflex activity
(D) The use of valproic acid in pregnancy may cause congenital malformations
(E) Weight gain is common in patients on valproic acid

5. Which statement concerning the pharmacokinetics of antiseizure drugs is accurate?
(A) Administration of phenytoin to patients in methadone maintenance programs has led to symptoms of opioid overdose, including respiratory depression
(B) Although ethosuximide has a half-life of approximately 40 h, the drug is usually taken twice a day
(C) At high doses, phenytoin elimination follows first-order kinetics
(D) Valproic acid may increase the synthesis of porphyrins
(E) Treatment with vigabatrin reduces the effectiveness of oral contraceptives

6. With chronic use in seizure states, the adverse effects of this drug include coarsening of facial features, hirsutism, and gingival hyperplasia.
(A) Carbamazepine
(B) Felbamate
(C) Phenytoin
(D) Phenobarbital
(E) Valproic acid

7. Abrupt withdrawal of antiseizure drugs can result in increases in seizure frequency and severity. Withdrawal is most easily accomplished if the patient is being treated with
(A) Carbamazepine
(B) Diazepam
(C) Ethosuximide
(D) Phenobarbital
(E) Phenytoin

8. The mechanism of antiseizure activity of carbamazepine is
(A) Block of sodium ion channels
(B) Block of calcium ion channels
(C) Facilitation of GABA actions on chloride ion channels
(D) Glutamate receptor antagonism
(E) Inhibition of GABA transaminase

9. Which statement about phenytoin is accurate?
(A) Displaces sulfonamides from plasma proteins
(B) Drug of choice in myoclonic seizures
(C) Half-life is increased if used with phenobarbital
(D) Isoniazid (INH) decreases steady-state blood levels of phenytoin
(E) Toxic effects may occur with only small increments in dose

10. A young male patient suffers from a seizure disorder characterized by tonic rigidity of the extremities followed in 15–30 s of tremor progressing to massive jerking of the body. This clonic phase lasts for 1 or 2 min, leaving the patient in a stuporous state. Of the following drugs, which is most suitable for long-term management of this patient?
(A) Carbamazepine
(B) Clonazepam
(C) Ethosuximide
(D) Felbamate
(E) Tiagabine

ANSWERS

1. This child suffers from absence seizures, and 2 of the drugs listed are effective in this seizure disorder. Clonazepam is effective but exerts troublesome CNS-depressant effects, and tolerance develops with chronic use. Ethosuximide is not excessively sedating, and tolerance does not develop to its antiseizure activity. Valproic acid (not listed) is also used in absence seizures. The answer is **B.**

2. The mechanism of action of phenylsuccinimides such as ethosuximide involves blockade of T-type Ca^{2+} channels in thalamic neurons. Ethosuximide does not block K^+ channels, which in any case would be likely to result in an increase (rather than a decrease) in neuronal excitability. The answer is **B.**

3. With chronic use, carbamazepine induces the formation of hepatic drug-metabolizing enzymes (as do phenobarbital and phenytoin). This action may lead to a *decrease* in the plasma concentration of other drugs used concomitantly. Valproic acid, an inhibitor of drug metabolism, can increase the plasma levels of many drugs, including carbamazepine, lamotrigine, phenobarbital, and phenytoin. Benzodiazepines (including clonazepam and diazepam), as well as gabapentin and vigabatrin, have no major effects on the metabolism of other drugs. The answer is **D.**

4. Ethosuximide and valproic acid are preferred drugs in absence seizures because they cause minimal sedation. However, valproic acid causes gastrointestinal distress and weight gain and is potentially hepatotoxic. In addition, its use in pregnancy has been associated with teratogenicity (neural tube defects). Peripheral neuropathy, including diminished deep tendon reflexes in the lower extremities, occurs with the chronic use of phenytoin, not valproic acid. The answer is **C.**

5. The enzyme-inducing activity of phenytoin has led to symptoms of opioid *withdrawal*, presumably because of an increase in the rate of metabolism of methadone. Monitoring of plasma concentration of phenytoin may be critical in establishing an effective dosage because of nonlinear elimination kinetics at high doses. Valproic acid has no effect on porphyrin synthesis. Vigabatrin does not affect the metabolism

of oral contraceptives. Twice-daily dosage of ethosuximide reduces the severity of adverse gastrointestinal effects. The answer is **B**.

6. Common adverse effects of phenytoin include nystagmus, diplopia, and ataxia. With chronic use, abnormalities of vitamin D metabolism, coarsening of facial features, gingival overgrowth, and hirsutism may also occur. The answer is **C**.

7. Dose tapering is an important principle in antiseizure drug withdrawal. As a rule, withdrawal from drugs used for absence seizures is easier than withdrawal from drugs used for partial and tonic-clonic seizures. Withdrawal is most difficult in patients who have been treated with barbiturates and benzodiazepines. The answer is **C**.

8. The mechanism of action of carbamazepine is similar to that of phenytoin, blocking sodium ion channels. Ethosuximide blocks calcium channels; benzodiazepines and barbiturates facilitate the inhibitory actions of GABA; topiramate may block glutamate receptors; and vigabatrin inhibits GABA metabolism. The answer is **A**.

9. Sulfonamides can displace phenytoin from its binding sites, increasing the plasma-free fraction of the drug. Induction of liver drug-metabolizing enzymes by phenobarbital results in a *decreased* half-life of phenytoin, and isoniazid *increases* plasma levels of phenytoin by inhibiting its metabolism. Because of the dose-dependent elimination kinetics of phenytoin, some toxicity may occur with only small increments in dose. The answer is **E**.

10. This patient is suffering from generalized tonic-clonic seizures. For many years, the drugs of choice in this seizure disorder have been carbamazepine or phenytoin or valproic acid. However, many newer drugs are also effective, including gabapentin, lamotrigine, levetiracetem, topiramate, and zonisamide. Clonazepam and ethosuximide are not effective in this type of seizure disorder. Fosphenytoin is available for parenteral use in the management of status epilepticus. Tiagabine is approved for adjunctive use only in partial seizures. The answer is **A**.

SKILL KEEPER ANSWERS: ANTIARRHYTHMIC DRUG ACTIONS (SEE CHAPTER 14)

1. *Close similarities of structure and function exist between voltage-gated sodium channels in neurons and in cardiac cells. Drugs that exert antiseizure actions via their blockade of sodium channels in the CNS have the potential for a similar action in the heart. Delayed recovery of sodium channels from their inactivated state subsequently slows the rising phase of the action potential in Na^+-dependent fibers and is characteristic of group I antiarrhythmic drugs. In theory, antiseizure drugs that block calcium ion channels might also have properties akin to those of group IV antiarrhythmic drugs.*

2. *In practice, the only antiseizure drug that has been used in cardiac arrhythmias is phenytoin, which has characteristics similar to those of group IB antiarrhythmic drugs. Phenytoin has been used for arrhythmias resulting from cardiac glycoside overdose and for ventricular arrhythmias unresponsive to lidocaine.*

CHECKLIST

When you complete this chapter, you should be able to:

❑ List the drugs of choice for partial seizures, generalized tonic-clonic seizures, absence and myoclonic seizures, and status epilepticus.

❑ Identify the mechanisms of antiseizure drug action at the levels of specific ion channels and/or neurotransmitter systems.

❑ Describe the main pharmacokinetic features, and list the adverse effects of carbamazepine, phenytoin, and valproic acid.

❑ Identify the distinctive toxicities of new antiseizure drugs.

❑ Describe the important pharmacokinetic and pharmacodynamic considerations relevant to the long-term use of antiseizure drugs.

DRUG SUMMARY TABLE: Antiseizure Drugs

Subclass	Mechanism of Action	Clinical Applications	Pharmacokinetics and Interactions	Toxicities
Cyclic ureides				
Phenytoin	Blocks voltage-gated Na^+ channels	Generalized tonic-clonic and partial seizures	Variable absorption, dose-dependent elimination; protein binding; many drug interactions	Ataxia, diplopia, gingival hyperplasia, hirsutism, neuropathy
Phenobarbital	Enhances $GABA_A$ receptor responses	Same as above	Long half-life, inducer of P450 • many interactions	Sedation, ataxia
Ethosuximide	Decreases Ca^{2+} currents (T-type)	Absence seizures	Long half-life	GI distress, dizziness, headache
Tricyclics				
Carbamazepine	Blocks voltage-gated Na^+ channels and decreases glutamate release	Generalized tonic-clonic and partial seizures	Well absorbed, active metabolite • many drug interactions	Ataxia, diplopia, headache, nausea
Benzodiazepines				
Diazepam	Enhance $GABA_A$ receptor responses	Status epilepticus	See Chapter 22	Sedation
Clonazepam		Absence and myoclonic seizures, infantile spasms	Similar to above	Similar to above
GABA derivatives				
Gabapentin	Blocks Ca^{2+} channels	Generalized tonic-clonic and partial seizures	Variable bioavailability • renal elimination	Ataxia, dizziness, somnolence
Pregabalin	Same as above	Partial seizures	Renal elimination	Same as above
Vigabatrin	Inhibits GABA transaminase	Same as above	Renal elimination	Drowsiness, dizziness, psychosis, ocular effects
Miscellaneous				
Valproate	β Blocks high-frequency firing	Generalized tonic-clonic, partial, and myoclonic seizures	Extensive protein binding and metabolism; many drug interactions	Nausea, alopecia, weight gain, teratogenic
Lamotrigine	Blocks Na^+ and Ca^{2+} channels, decreases glutamate	Generalized tonic-clonic, partial, myoclonic, and absence seizures	Not protein-bound, extensive metabolism • many drug interactions	Dizzines, diplopia, headache, rash
Leveliracetam	Binds synaptic protein	Generalized tonic-clonic and partial seizures	Well absorbed, extensive metabolism • some drug interactions	Dizziness, nervousness, depression, seizures
Tiagabine	Blocks GABA reuptake	Partial seizures	Extensive protein binding and metabolism • some drug interactions	Dizziness, nervousness, depression, seizures
Topiramate	Unknown	Generalized tonic-clonic, absence, and partial seizures, migraine	Both hepatic and renal clearance	Sleepiness, cognitive slowing, confusion, paresthesias
Zonisamide	Blocks Na^+ channels	Generalized tonic-clonic, partial, and myoclonic seizures	Both hepatic and renal clearance	Sleepiness, cognitive slowing, poor concentration, paresthesias

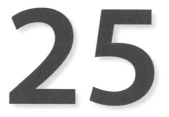

General Anesthetics

General anesthesia is a state characterized by unconsciousness, analgesia, amnesia, skeletal muscle relaxation, and loss of reflexes. Drugs used as general anesthetics are CNS depressants with actions that can be induced and terminated more rapidly than those of conventional sedative-hypnotics.

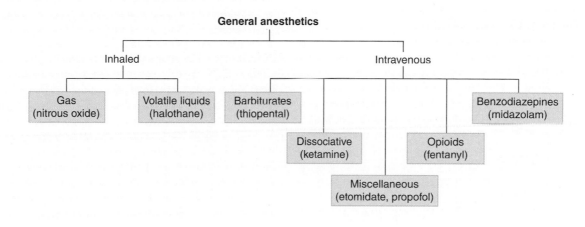

General anesthetics
- Inhaled
  - Gas (nitrous oxide)
  - Volatile liquids (halothane)
- Intravenous
  - Barbiturates (thiopental)
  - Dissociative (ketamine)
  - Miscellaneous (etomidate, propofol)
  - Opioids (fentanyl)
  - Benzodiazepines (midazolam)

STAGES OF ANESTHESIA

Modern anesthetics act very rapidly and achieve deep anesthesia quickly. With older and more slowly acting anesthetics, the progressively greater depth of central depression associated with increasing dose or time of exposure is traditionally described as **stages of anesthesia.**

A. Stage 1: Analgesia

In stage 1, the patient has decreased awareness of pain, sometimes with amnesia. Consciousness may be impaired but is not lost.

B. Stage 2: Disinhibition

In stage 2, the patient appears to be delirious and excited. Amnesia occurs, reflexes are enhanced, and respiration is typically irregular; retching and incontinence may occur.

C. Stage 3: Surgical Anesthesia

In stage 3, the patient is unconscious and has no pain reflexes; respiration is very regular, and blood pressure is maintained.

D. Stage 4: Medullary Depression

In stage 4, the patient develops severe respiratory and cardiovascular depression that requires mechanical and pharmacologic support.

ANESTHESIA PROTOCOLS

Anesthesia protocols vary according to the proposed type of diagnostic, therapeutic, or surgical intervention. For minor procedures, **conscious sedation** techniques that combine intravenous agents with local anesthetics (see Chapter 26) are often used. These can provide profound analgesia, with retention of the patient's ability to maintain a patent airway and respond to verbal commands. For more extensive surgical procedures, anesthesia protocols commonly include intravenous drugs to induce the anesthetic state, inhaled anesthetics (with or without intravenous agents) to maintain an anesthetic state, and neuromuscular blocking agents to effect muscle relaxation (see Chapter 27). Vital sign monitoring remains the standard method of assessing "depth of anesthesia" during surgery. Cerebral monitoring, automated techniques based on quantification of anesthetic effects on the electroencephalograph (EEG), is also useful.

MECHANISMS OF ACTION

The mechanisms of action of general anesthetics are varied. As CNS depressants, these drugs usually increase the threshold for firing of CNS neurons. The potency of inhaled anesthetics is roughly proportional to their lipid solubility. Mechanisms of action include effects on ion channels by interactions of anesthetic drugs with membrane lipids or proteins with subsequent effects on central neurotransmitter mechanisms. Inhaled anesthetics, barbiturates, benzodiazepines, etomidate, and propofol facilitate γ-aminobutyric acid (GABA)-mediated inhibition at $GABA_A$ receptors. These receptors are sensitive to clinically relevant concentrations of the anesthetic agents and exhibit the appropriate stereospecific effects in the case of enantiomeric drugs. Ketamine does not produce its effects via facilitation of $GABA_A$ receptor functions, but possibly via its antagonism of the action of the excitatory neurotransmitter glutamic acid on the *N*-methyl-D-aspartate (NMDA) receptor. Most inhaled anesthetics also inhibit nicotinic acetylcholine (ACh) receptor isoforms at moderate to high concentrations. The strychnine-sensitive glycine receptor is another ligand-gated ion channel that may function as a "target" for certain inhaled anesthetics. CNS neurons in different regions of the brain have different sensitivities to general anesthetics; inhibition of neurons involved in pain pathways occurs before inhibition of neurons in the midbrain reticular formation.

INHALED ANESTHETICS

A. Classification and Pharmacokinetics

The agents currently used in inhalation anesthesia are nitrous oxide (a gas) and several easily vaporized liquid halogenated hydrocarbons, including halothane, desflurane, enflurane, isoflurane, sevoflurane, and methoxyflurane. They are administered as gases; their partial pressure, or "tension," in the inhaled air or in blood or other tissue is a measure of their concentration. Because the standard pressure of the total inhaled mixture is atmospheric

pressure (760 mm Hg at sea level), the partial pressure may also be expressed as a percentage. Thus, 50% nitrous oxide in the inhaled air would have a partial pressure of 380 mm Hg. The speed of induction of anesthetic effects depends on several factors, discussed next.

1. Solubility—The more rapidly a drug equilibrates with the blood, the more quickly the drug passes into the brain to produce anesthetic effects. Drugs with a low blood:gas partition coefficient (eg, nitrous oxide) equilibrate more rapidly than those with a higher blood solubility (eg, halothane), as illustrated in Figure 25–1. Partition coefficients for inhalation anesthetics are shown in Table 25–1.

2. Inspired gas partial pressure—A high partial pressure of the gas in the lungs results in more rapid achievement of anesthetic levels in the blood. This effect can be taken advantage of by the initial administration of gas concentrations higher than those required for maintenance of anesthesia.

3. Ventilation rate—The greater the ventilation, the more rapid is the rise in alveolar and blood partial pressure of the agent and the onset of anesthesia (Figure 25–2). This effect is taken advantage of in the induction of the anesthetic state.

4. Pulmonary blood flow—At high pulmonary blood flows, the gas partial pressure rises at a slower rate; thus, the speed of onset of anesthesia is reduced. At low flow rates, onset is faster. In circulatory shock, this effect may accelerate the rate of onset of anesthesia with agents of high blood solubility.

5. Arteriovenous concentration gradient—Uptake of soluble anesthetics into highly perfused tissues may decrease gas tension in mixed venous blood. This can influence the rate of onset of anesthesia because achievement of equilibrium is dependent on the difference in anesthetic tension between arterial and venous blood.

B. Elimination

Anesthesia is terminated by redistribution of the drug from the brain to the blood and elimination of the drug through the lungs. The rate of recovery from anesthesia using agents with low blood:gas partition coefficients is faster than that of anesthetics

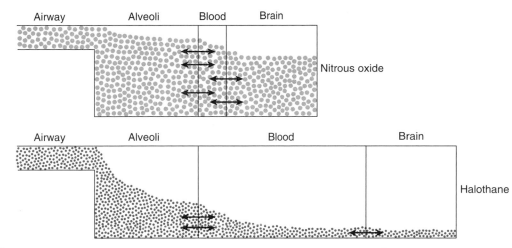

FIGURE 25–1 Why induction of anesthesia is slower with more soluble anesthetic gases and faster with less soluble ones. In this schematic diagram, solubility is represented by the size of the blood compartment (the more soluble the gas, the larger is the compartment). For a given concentration or partial pressure of the 2 anesthetic gases in the inspired air, it will take much longer with halothane than with nitrous oxide for the blood partial pressure to rise to the same partial pressure as in the alveoli. Because the concentration in the brain can rise no faster than the concentration in the blood, the onset of anesthesia will be much slower with halothane than with nitrous oxide. (Reproduced, with permission, from Katzung BG, editor: *Basic & Clinical Pharmacology,* 12th ed. McGraw-Hill, 2012: Fig. 25–3.)

with high blood solubility. This important property has led to the introduction of several newer inhaled anesthetics (eg, desflurane, sevoflurane), which, because of their low blood solubility, are characterized by recovery times that are considerably shorter than is the case with older agents. Halothane and methoxyflurane are metabolized by liver enzymes to a significant extent (Table 25–1). Metabolism of halothane and methoxyflurane has only a minor influence on the speed of recovery from their anesthetic effect but does play a role in potential toxicity of these anesthetics.

C. Minimum Alveolar Anesthetic Concentration

The potency of inhaled anesthetics is best measured by the minimum alveolar anesthetic concentration (MAC), defined as

the alveolar concentration required to eliminate the response to a standardized painful stimulus in 50% of patients. Each anesthetic has a defined MAC (Table 25–1), but this value may vary among patients depending on age, cardiovascular status, and use of adjuvant drugs. Estimations of MAC value suggest a relatively "steep" dose-response relationship for inhaled anesthetics. MACs for infants and elderly patients are lower than those for adolescents and young adults. When several anesthetic agents are used simultaneously, their MAC values are additive.

D. Effects of Inhaled Anesthetics

1. CNS effects—Inhaled anesthetics decrease brain metabolic rate. They reduce vascular resistance and thus increase cerebral blood flow. This may lead to an increase in intracranial pressure.

TABLE 25–1 Properties of inhalation anesthetics.

Anesthetic	Blood:Gas Partition Coefficient	Minimum Alveolar Concentration (%)[a]	Metabolism
Nitrous oxide	0.47	>100	None
Desflurane	0.42	6.5	<0.1%
Sevoflurane	0.69	2.0	2–5% (fluoride)
Isoflurane	1.40	1.4	<2%
Enflurane	1.80	1.7	8%
Halothane	2.30	0.75	>40%
Methoxyflurane	12	0.16	>70% (fluoride)

[a]Minimum alveolar concentration (MAC) is the anesthetic concentration that eliminates the response in 50% of patients exposed to a standardized painful stimulus. In this table, MAC is expressed as a percentage of the inspired gas mixture.

Modified and reproduced, with permission, from Katzung BG, editor: *Basic & Clinical Pharmacology,* 10th ed. McGraw-Hill, 2007.

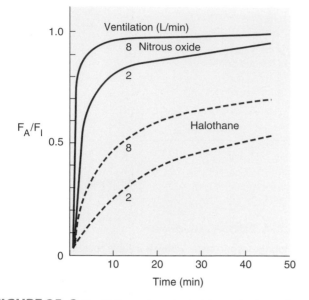

FIGURE 25–2 Ventilation rate and arterial anesthetic tensions. Increased ventilation (8 versus 2 L/min) has a much greater effect on equilibration of halothane than nitrous oxide. (Reproduced, with permission, from Katzung BG, editor: *Basic & Clinical Pharmacology*, 12th ed. McGraw-Hill, 2012: Fig. 25–5.)

High concentrations of enflurane may cause spike-and-wave activity and muscle twitching, but this effect is unique to this drug. Although nitrous oxide has low anesthetic potency (ie, a high MAC), it exerts marked analgesic and amnestic actions.

2. Cardiovascular effects—Most inhaled anesthetics decrease arterial blood pressure moderately. Enflurane and halothane are myocardial depressants that decrease cardiac output, whereas isoflurane, desflurane, and sevoflurane cause peripheral vasodilation. Nitrous oxide is less likely to lower blood pressure than are other inhaled anesthetics. Blood flow to the liver and kidney is decreased by most inhaled agents. Inhaled anesthetics depress myocardial function—nitrous oxide least. Halothane, and to a lesser degree isoflurane, may sensitize the myocardium to the arrhythmogenic effects of catecholamines.

3. Respiratory effects—Although the rate of respiration may be increased, all inhaled anesthetics cause a dose-dependent decrease in tidal volume and minute ventilation, leading to an increase in arterial CO_2 tension. Inhaled anesthetics decrease ventilatory response to hypoxia even at subanesthetic concentrations (eg, during recovery). Nitrous oxide has the smallest effect on respiration. Most inhaled anesthetics are bronchodilators, but desflurane is a pulmonary irritant and may cause bronchospasm. The pungency of enflurane causing breath-holding limits its use in anesthesia induction.

4. Toxicity—Postoperative hepatitis has occurred (rarely) after halothane anesthesia in patients experiencing hypovolemic shock or other severe stress. The mechanism of hepatotoxicity is unclear but may involve formation of reactive metabolites that cause

direct toxicity or initiate immune-mediated responses. Fluoride released by metabolism of methoxyflurane (and possibly both enflurane and sevoflurane) may cause renal insufficiency after prolonged anesthesia. Prolonged exposure to nitrous oxide decreases methionine synthase activity and may lead to megaloblastic anemia. Susceptible patients may develop **malignant hyperthermia** when anesthetics are used together with neuromuscular blockers (especially succinylcholine). This rare condition is thought in some cases to be due to mutations in the gene loci corresponding to the ryanodine receptor (RyR1). Other chromosomal loci for malignant hyperthermia include mutant alleles of the gene-encoding skeletal muscle L-type calcium channels. The uncontrolled release of calcium by the sarcoplasmic reticulum of skeletal muscle leads to muscle spasm, hyperthermia, and autonomic lability. Dantrolene is indicated for the treatment of this life-threatening condition, with supportive management.

SKILL KEEPER: SIGNALING MECHANISMS (SEE CHAPTER 2)

*Like most drugs, general anesthetics appear to act via interactions with specific receptor molecules involved in cell signaling. For review purposes, try to recall the major types of **signaling mechanisms** relevant to the actions of drugs that act via receptors. The Skill Keeper Answers appear at the end of the chapter.*

INTRAVENOUS ANESTHETICS

A. Barbiturates

Thiopental and **methohexital** have high lipid solubility, which promotes rapid entry into the brain and results in surgical anesthesia in one circulation time (<1 min). These drugs are used for induction of anesthesia and for short surgical procedures. The anesthetic effects of thiopental are terminated by redistribution from the brain to other highly perfused tissues (Figure 25–3), but hepatic metabolism is required for elimination from the body. Barbiturates are respiratory and circulatory depressants; because they depress cerebral blood flow, they can also decrease intracranial pressure.

B. Benzodiazepines

Midazolam is widely used adjunctively with inhaled anesthetics and intravenous opioids. The onset of its CNS effects is slower than that of thiopental, and it has a longer duration of action. Cases of severe postoperative respiratory depression have occurred. The benzodiazepine receptor antagonist, flumazenil, accelerates recovery from midazolam and other benzodiazepines.

C. Ketamine

This drug produces a state of "dissociative anesthesia" in which the patient remains conscious but has marked catatonia, analgesia,

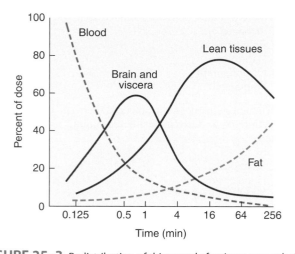

FIGURE 25-3 Redistribution of thiopental after intravenous bolus administration. Note that the time axis is not linear. (Reproduced, with permission, from Katzung BG, editor: *Basic & Clinical Pharmacology*, 12th ed. McGraw-Hill, 2012: Fig. 25–7.)

and amnesia. Ketamine is a chemical congener of the psychotomimetic agent, phencyclidine (PCP). The drug is a cardiovascular stimulant, and this action may lead to an increase in intracranial pressure. Emergence reactions, including disorientation, excitation, and hallucinations, which occur during recovery from ketamine anesthesia, can be reduced by the preoperative use of benzodiazepines.

D. Opioids

Morphine and **fentanyl** are used with other CNS depressants (nitrous oxide, benzodiazepines) in anesthesia regimens and are especially valuable in high-risk patients who might not survive a full general anesthetic. Intravenous opioids may cause chest wall rigidity, which can impair ventilation. Respiratory depression with these drugs may be reversed postoperatively with naloxone. **Neuroleptanesthesia** is a state of analgesia and amnesia is produced when fentanyl is used with droperidol and nitrous oxide. Newer opioids related to fentanyl have been introduced for intravenous anesthesia. Alfentanil and remifentanil have been used for induction of anesthesia. Recovery from the actions of remifentanil is faster than recovery from other opioids used in anesthesia because of its rapid metabolism by blood and tissue esterases.

E. Propofol

Propofol produces anesthesia as rapidly as the intravenous barbiturates, and recovery is more rapid. Propofol has antiemetic actions, and recovery is not delayed after prolonged infusion. The drug is commonly used as a component of balanced anesthesia and as an anesthetic in outpatient surgery. Propofol is also effective in producing prolonged sedation in patients in critical care settings. Propofol may cause marked hypotension during induction of anesthesia, primarily through decreased peripheral resistance. Total body clearance of propofol is greater than hepatic

blood flow, suggesting that its elimination includes other mechanisms in addition to metabolism by liver enzymes. Fospropofol, a water-soluble prodrug form, is broken down in the body by alkaline phosphatase to form propofol. However, onset and recovery are both slower than with propofol. While fospropofol appears to cause less pain at injection sites than the standard form of the drug, many patients experience paresthesias.

F. Etomidate

This imidazole derivative affords rapid induction with minimal change in cardiac function or respiratory rate and has a short duration of action. The drug is not analgesic, and its primary advantage is in anesthesia for patients with limited cardiac or respiratory reserve. Etomidate may cause pain and myoclonus on injection and nausea postoperatively. Prolonged administration may cause adrenal suppression.

G. Dexmedetomidine

This centrally acting α_2-adrenergic agonist has analgesic and hypnotic actions when used intravenously. Its characteristics include rapid clearance resulting in a short elimination half-life. Dexmedetomidine is used mainly for short-term sedation in an ICU setting. When used in general anesthesia, the drug decreases dose requirements for both inhaled and intravenous anesthetics

QUESTIONS

1. A new halogenated gas anesthetic has a blood:gas partition coefficient of 0.5 and a MAC value of 1%. Which prediction about this agent is most accurate? (Refer to Table 25–1 for comparison of agents.)
   (A) Equilibrium between arterial and venous gas tension will be achieved very slowly
   (B) It will be metabolized by the liver to release fluoride ions
   (C) It will be more soluble in the blood than isoflurane
   (D) Speed of onset will be similar to that of nitrous oxide
   (E) The new agent will be more potent than halothane

2. Which statement concerning the effects of anesthetic agents is false?
   (A) Bronchiolar smooth muscle occurs during halothane anesthesia
   (B) Chest muscle rigidity often follows the administration of fentanyl
   (C) Mild, generalized muscle twitching occurs at high doses of enflurane
   (D) Severe hepatitis has been reported after the use of desflurane
   (E) The use of midazolam with inhalation anesthetics may prolong the postanesthesia recovery period

3. A 23-year-old man has a pheochromocytoma, blood pressure of 190/120 mm Hg, and hematocrit of 50%. Pulmonary function and renal function are normal. His catecholamines are elevated, and he has a well-defined abdominal tumor on MRI. He has been scheduled for surgery. Which one of the following agents should be avoided in the anesthesia protocol?
(A) Desflurane
(B) Fentanyl
(C) Isoflurane
(D) Midazolam
(E) Sevoflurane

4. Which statement concerning nitrous oxide is accurate?
(A) A useful component of anesthesia protocols because it lacks cardiovascular depression
(B) Anemia is a common adverse effect in patients exposed to nitrous oxide for periods longer than 2 h
(C) It is the most potent of the inhaled anesthetics
(D) There is a direct association between the use of nitrous oxide and malignant hyperthermia
(E) Up to 50% of nitrous oxide is eliminated via hepatic metabolism

5. Which statement concerning anesthetic MAC (minimum anesthetic concentration) value is accurate?
(A) Anesthetics with low MAC value have low potency
(B) MAC values increase in elderly patients
(C) MAC values give information about the slope of the dose-response curve
(D) Methoxyflurane has an extremely low MAC value
(E) Simultaneous use of opioid analgesics increases the MAC for inhaled anesthetics

6. Total intravenous anesthesia with fentanyl has been selected for a frail elderly woman about to undergo cardiac surgery. Which statement about this anesthesia protocol is accurate?
(A) Intravenous fentanyl will provide useful cardiostimulatory effects
(B) Marked relaxation of skeletal muscles is anticipated
(C) Opioids such as fentanyl control the hypertensive response to surgical stimulation
(D) Patient awareness may occur during surgery, with recall after recovery
(E) The patient is likely to experience pain during surgery

Questions 7 and 8. A 20-year-old male patient scheduled for hernia surgery was anesthetized with halothane and nitrous oxide; tubocurarine was provided for skeletal muscle relaxation. The patient rapidly developed tachycardia and became hypertensive. Generalized skeletal muscle rigidity was accompanied by marked hyperthermia. Laboratory values revealed hyperkalemia and acidosis.

7. This unusual complication of anesthesia is most likely caused by
(A) Acetylcholine release from somatic nerve endings at skeletal muscle
(B) Activation of brain dopamine receptors by halothane
(C) Block of autonomic ganglia by tubocurarine
(D) Pheochromocytoma
(E) Release of calcium from the sarcoplasmic reticulum

8. The patient should be treated immediately with
(A) Atropine
(B) Baclofen
(C) Dantrolene
(D) Edrophonium
(E) Flumazenil

9. If ketamine is used as the sole anesthetic in the attempted reduction of a dislocated shoulder joint, its actions will include
(A) Analgesia
(B) Bradycardia
(C) Hypotension
(D) Muscle rigidity
(E) Respiratory depression

10. For which of these drugs is the following true? Postoperative vomiting is uncommon with this intravenous agent, and patients are often able to ambulate sooner than those who receive other anesthetics.
(A) Enflurane
(B) Etomidate
(C) Propofol
(D) Remifentanil
(E) Thiopental

ANSWERS

1. The partition coefficient of an inhaled anesthetic is a determinant of its kinetic characteristics. Agents with low blood:gas solubility have a fast onset of action and a short duration of recovery. The new agent described here resembles nitrous oxide but is more potent, as indicated by its low MAC value. Not all halogenated anesthetics undergo significant hepatic metabolism or release fluoride ions. The answer is **D**.

2. Hepatitis after general anesthesia has been linked to use of *halothane* although the incidence is very low (1 in 20,00–35,000). Hepatotoxicity has not been reported after administration of desflurane, or other inhaled anesthetics. The answer is **D**.

3. Isoflurane sensitizes the myocardium to catecholamines, as does halothane (not listed). Arrhythmias may occur in patients with cardiac disease who have high circulating levels of epinephrine and norepinephrine (eg, patients with pheochromocytoma). Newer inhaled anesthetics are considerably less arrhythmogenic. The answer is **C**.

4. Anemia has *not* been reported in patients exposed to nitrous oxide anesthesia for periods as long as 6 h. Nitrous oxide is the least potent of the inhaled anesthetics, and the compound has not been implicated in malignant hyperthermia. More than 98% of the gas is eliminated via exhalation. The answer is **A**.

5. MAC value is inversely related to potency; a *low* MAC means *high* potency. MAC gives no information about the slope of the dose-response curve. Use of opioid analgesics or other CNS depressants with inhaled anesthetics lowers the MAC value. As with most CNS depressants, the elderly patient is more sensitive, so MAC values are lower. Methoxyflurane has the lowest MAC value of the inhaled anesthetics. The answer is **D**.

6. Intravenous opioids (eg, fentanyl) are widely used in anesthesia for cardiac surgery because they provide full analgesia and cause less cardiac depression than inhalation of anesthetic agents. They are not cardiac stimulants, and fentanyl is more likely to cause skeletal muscle rigidity than relaxation. Disadvantages of this technique are patient recall (which can be decreased by concomitant use of a benzodiazepine) and the occurrence of hypertensive responses to surgical stimulation. The addition of vasodilators (eg, nitroprusside) or a β blocker (eg, esmolol) may be needed to prevent intraoperative hypertension. The answer is **D**.

7. Malignant hyperthermia is a rare but life-threatening reaction that may occur during general anesthesia with halogenated anesthetics and skeletal muscle relaxants, particularly succinylcholine and tubocurarine. Release of calcium from skeletal muscle leads to muscle spasms, hyperthermia, and autonomic instability. Predisposing genetic factors include clinical myopathy associated with mutations in the gene loci for the skeletal muscle ryanodine receptor or L-type calcium receptors. The answer is **E**.

8. The drug of choice in malignant hyperthermia is dantrolene, which prevents release of calcium from the sarcoplasmic reticulum of skeletal muscle cells. Appropriate measures must be taken to lower body temperature, control hypertension, and restore acid-base and electrolyte balance. The answer is **C**.

9. Ketamine is a cardiovascular stimulant, increasing heart rate and blood pressure. This results in part from central sympathetic stimulation and from inhibition of norepinephrine reuptake at sympathetic nerve endings. Analgesia and amnesia occur, with preservation of muscle tone and minimal depression of respiration. The answer is **A**.

10. Propofol is used extensively in anesthesia protocols, including those for day surgery. The favorable properties of the drug include an antiemetic effect and recovery more rapid than that after use of other intravenous drugs. Propofol does not cause cumulative effects, possibly because of its short half-life (2–8 min) in the body. The drug is also used for prolonged sedation in critical care settings. The answer is **C**.

SKILL KEEPER ANSWER: SIGNALING MECHANISMS (SEE CHAPTER 2)

1. Receptors that modify gene transcription: adrenal and gonadal steroids
2. Receptors on membrane-spanning enzymes: insulin
3. Receptors activating Janus kinases that modulate STAT molecules: cytokines
4. Receptors directly coupled to ion channels: nicotinic (ACh), GABA, glycine
5. Receptors coupled to enzymes via G proteins: many endogenous compounds (eg, ACh, NE, serotonin) and drugs
6. Receptors that are enzymes or transporters: acetylcholinesterase, angiotensin-converting enzyme, carbonic anhydrase, H^+/K^+ antiporter, and so on

CHECKLIST

When you complete this chapter, you should be able to:

❑ Name the inhalation anesthetic agents and identify their pharmacodynamic and pharmacokinetic properties.

❑ Describe what is meant by the terms (1) blood:gas partition coefficient and (2) minimum alveolar anesthetic concentration.

❑ Identify proposed molecular targets for the actions of anesthetic drugs.

❑ Describe how the blood:gas partition coefficient of an inhalation anesthetic influences its speed of onset of anesthesia and its recovery time.

❑ Identify the commonly used intravenous anesthetics and point out their main pharmacokinetic and pharmacodynamic characteristics.

DRUG SUMMARY TABLE: General Anesthetics

Subclass	Possible Mechanism	Pharmacologic Effects	Pharmacokinetics	Toxicities and Interactions
Inhaled anesthetics				
Desflurane Enflurane Halothane Isoflurane Sevoflurane Nitrous oxide	Facilitate GABA-mediated inhibition • block brain NMDA and ACh-N receptors	Increase cerebral blood flow • enflurane and halothane decrease cardiac output. Others cause vasodilation • all decrease respiratory functions—lung irritation (desflurane)	Rate of onset and recovery vary by blood:gas partition coefficient • recovery mainly due to redistribution from brain to other tissues	Toxicity: extensions of effects on brain, heart/ vasculature, lungs Drug interactions: additive CNS depression with many agents, especially opioids and sedative-hypnotics
Intravenous anesthetics				
Barbiturates				
Thiopental, Thioamylal, Methohexital	Barbiturates, benzodiazepines, etomidate, and propofol facilitate GABA-mediated inhibition at GABA$_A$ receptors	Barbiturates: circulatory and respiratory depression • decrease intracranial pressure	Barbiturates: high lipid solubility—fast onset and short action due to redistribution	Barbiturates: extensions of CNS depressant actions • additive CNS depression with many drugs
Benzodiazepines				
Midazolam		Benzodiazepines: less depressant than barbiturates	Slower onset, but longer duration than barbiturates	Postoperative respiratory depression reversed by flumazenil
Dissociative				
Ketamine	Blocks excitation by glutamate at NMDA receptors	Analgesia, amnesia and catatonia but "consciousness" retained • cardiovascular (CV) stimulation!	Moderate duration of action—hepatic metabolism	Increased intracranial pressure • emergence reactions
Imidazole				
Etomidate		Minimal effects on CV and respiratory functions	Short duration due to redistribution	No analgesia, pain on injection (may need opioid), myoclonus, nausea, and vomiting
Opioids				
Fentanyl Alfentanil Remifentanil Morphine	Interact with μ, κ, and δ receptors for endogenous opioid peptides	Marked analgesia, respiratory depression (see Chapter 31)	Alfentanil and remifentanil fast onset (induction)	Respiratory depression—reversed by naloxone
Phenols				
Propofol, Fospropofol		Propofol: vasodilation and hypotension • negative inotropy. Fospropofol water-soluble	Propofol: fast onset and fast recovery due to inactivation	Propofol: hypotension (during induction), cardiovascular depression

ACh, acetylcholine; NMDA, N-methyl-D-aspartate.

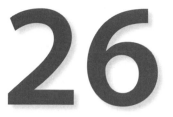

Local Anesthetics

Local anesthesia is the condition that results when sensory transmission from a local area of the body to the CNS is blocked. The local anesthetics constitute a group of chemically similar agents (esters and amides) that block the sodium channels of excitable membranes.

Because these drugs can be administered by injection in the target area, or by topical application in some cases, the anesthetic effect can be restricted to a localized area (eg, the cornea or an arm). When given intravenously, local anesthetics have effects on other tissues.

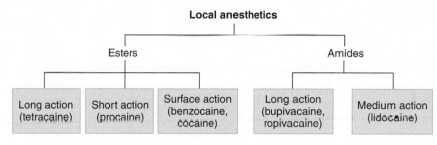

CHEMISTRY

Most local anesthetic drugs are esters or amides of simple benzene derivatives. Subgroups within the local anesthetics are based on this chemical characteristic and on duration of action. The commonly used local anesthetics are weak bases with at least 1 ionizable amine function that can become charged through the gain of a proton (H^+). As discussed in Chapter 1, the degree of ionization is a function of the pK_a of the drug and the pH of the medium. Because the pH of tissue may differ from the physiologic 7.4 (eg, it may be as low as 6.4 in infected tissue), the degree of ionization of the drug will vary. Because the pK_a of most local anesthetics is between 8.0 and 9.0 (benzocaine is an exception), variations in pH associated with infection can have significant effects on the proportion of ionized to nonionized drug. The question of the active form of the drug (ionized versus nonionized) is discussed later.

PHARMACOKINETICS

Many shorter-acting local anesthetics are readily absorbed into the blood from the injection site after administration. The duration of local action is therefore limited unless blood flow to the area is reduced. This can be accomplished by administration of a vasoconstrictor (usually an α-agonist sympathomimetic) with the local anesthetic agent. Cocaine is an important exception because it has intrinsic sympathomimetic action due to its inhibition of norepinephrine reuptake into nerve terminals. The longer-acting agents (eg, bupivicaine, ropivicaine, tetracain) are also less dependent on the coadministration of vasoconstrictors. Surface activity (ability to reach superficial nerves when applied to the surface of mucous membranes) is a property of certain local anesthetics, especially cocaine and benzocaine (both only available as topical forms), lidocaine, and tetracaine.

Metabolism of ester local anesthetics is carried out by plasma cholinesterases (pseudocholinesterases) and is very rapid for procaine (half-life, 1–2 min), slower for cocaine, and very slow for tetracaine. The amides are metabolized in the liver, in part by cytochrome P450 isozymes. The half-lives of lidocaine and prilocaine are approximately 1.5 h. Bupivacaine and ropivacaine are the longest-acting amide local anesthetics with half-lives of 3.5 and 4.2 h, respectively. Liver dysfunction may increase the elimination half-life of amide local anesthetics (and increase the risk of toxicity).

Acidification of the urine promotes ionization of local anesthetics; the charged forms of such drugs are more rapidly excreted than nonionized forms.

MECHANISM OF ACTION

Local anesthetics block voltage-dependent sodium channels and reduce the influx of sodium ions, thereby preventing depolarization

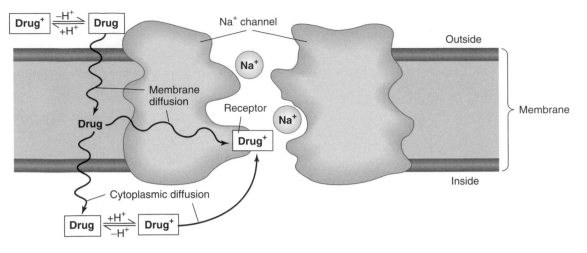

FIGURE 26–1 Schematic diagram of the sodium channel in an excitable membrane (eg, an axon) and the pathways by which a local anesthetic molecule (*Drug*) may reach its receptor. Sodium ions are not able to pass through the channel when the drug is bound to the receptor. The local anesthetic diffuses within the membrane in its uncharged form. In the aqueous extracellular and intracellular spaces, the charged form (*Drug*$^+$) is also present.

of the membrane and blocking conduction of the action potential. Local anesthetics gain access to their receptors from the cytoplasm or the membrane (Figure 26–1). Because the drug molecule must cross the lipid membrane to reach the cytoplasm, the more lipid-soluble (nonionized, uncharged) form reaches effective intracellular concentrations more rapidly than does the ionized form. On the other hand, once inside the axon, the ionized (charged) form of the drug is the more effective blocking entity. Thus, both the nonionized and the ionized forms of the drug play important roles—the first in reaching the receptor site and the second in causing the effect. The affinity of the receptor site within the sodium channel for the local anesthetic is a function of the state of the channel, whether it is resting, open, or inactivated, and therefore follows the same rules of use dependence and voltage

dependence that were described for the sodium channel-blocking antiarrhythmic drugs (see Chapter 14). In particular, if other factors are equal, rapidly firing fibers are usually blocked before slowly firing fibers. High concentrations of extracellular K$^+$ may enhance local anesthetic activity, whereas elevated extracellular Ca^{2+} may antagonize it.

PHARMACOLOGIC EFFECTS

A. Nerves

Differential sensitivity of various types of nerve fibers to local anesthetics depends on fiber diameter, myelination, physiologic firing rate, and anatomic location (Table 26–1). In general, smaller

TABLE 26–1 Susceptibility to block of types of nerve fibers.

Fiber Type	Function	Diameter (µm)	Myelination	Conduction Velocity (m/s)	Sensitivity to Block
Type A					
Alpha	Proprioception, motor	12–20	Heavy	70–120	+
Beta	Touch, pressure	5–12	Heavy	30–70	++
Gamma	Muscle spindles	3–6	Heavy	15–30	++
Delta	Pain, temperature	2–5	Heavy	12–30	+++
Type B	Preganglionic, autonomic	<3	Light	3–15	++++
Type C					
Dorsal root	Pain	0.4–1.2	None	0.5–2.3	++++
Sympathetic	Postganglionic	0.3–1.3	None	0.7–2.3	++++

Reproduced, with permission, from Katzung BG, editor: *Basic & Clinical Pharmacology*, 12th ed. McGraw-Hill, 2012.

fibers are blocked more easily than larger fibers, and myelinated fibers are blocked more easily than unmyelinated fibers. Activated pain fibers fire rapidly; thus, pain sensation appears to be selectively blocked by local anesthetics. Fibers located in the periphery of a thick nerve bundle are blocked sooner than those in the core because they are exposed earlier to higher concentrations of the anesthetic.

B. Other Tissues

The effects of these drugs on the heart are discussed in Chapter 14 (see group I antiarrhythmic agents). Most local anesthetics also have weak blocking effects on skeletal muscle neuromuscular transmission, but these actions have no clinical application. The mood elevation induced by cocaine reflects actions on dopamine or other amine-mediated synaptic transmission in the CNS rather than a local anesthetic action on membranes.

CLINICAL USE

The local anesthetics are commonly used for minor surgical procedures often in combination with vasoconstrictors such as epinephrine. Onset of action may be accelerated by the addition of sodium bicarbonate, which enhances intracellular access of these weakly basic compounds. Articaine has the fastest onset of action. Local anesthetics are also used in spinal anesthesia and to produce autonomic blockade in ischemic conditions. Slow epidural infusion at low concentrations has been used successfully for postoperative analgesia (in the same way as epidural opioid infusion; Chapter 31). Repeated epidural injection in anesthetic doses may lead to tachyphylaxis, however. Intravenous local anesthetics may be used for reducing pain in the perioperative period. Oral and parenteral forms of local anesthetics are sometimes used adjunctively in neuropathic pain states.

TOXICITY

A. CNS Effects

The important toxic effects of most local anesthetics are in the CNS. All local anesthetics are capable of producing a spectrum of central effects, including light-headedness or sedation, restlessness, nystagmus, and tonic-clonic convulsions. Severe convulsions may be followed by coma with respiratory and cardiovascular depression.

B. Cardiovascular Effects

With the exception of cocaine, all local anesthetics are vasodilators. Patients with preexisting cardiovascular disease may develop heart block and other disturbances of cardiac electrical function at high plasma levels of local anesthetics. Bupivacaine, a racemic mixture of two isomers may produce severe cardiovascular toxicity, including arrhythmias and hypotension. The (S)isomer, levobupivicaine, is less cardiotoxic. Cardiotoxicity has also been reported for ropivicaine when used for peripheral nerve block. The ability of cocaine to block norepinephrine reuptake at

sympathetic neuroeffector junctions and the drug's vasoconstricting actions contribute to cardiovascular toxicity. When cocaine is used as a drug of abuse, its cardiovascular toxicity includes severe hypertension with cerebral hemorrhage, cardiac arrhythmias, and myocardial infarction.

C. Other Toxic Effects

Prilocaine is metabolized to products that include *o*-toluidine, an agent capable of converting hemoglobin to methemoglobin. Though tolerated in healthy persons, even moderate methemoglobinemia can cause decompensation in patients with cardiac or pulmonary disease. The ester-type local anesthetics are metabolized to products that can cause antibody formation in some patients. Allergic responses to local anesthetics are rare and can usually be prevented by using an agent from the amide subclass. In high concentrations, local anesthetics may cause a local neurotoxic action that includes histologic damage and permanent impairment of function.

> **SKILL KEEPER: CARDIAC TOXICITY OF LOCAL ANESTHETICS (SEE CHAPTER 14)**
>
> *Explain how hyperkalemia facilitates the cardiac toxicity of local anesthetics.* The Skill Keeper Answer appears at the end of the chapter.

D. Treatment of Toxicity

Severe toxicity is treated symptomatically; there are no antidotes. Convulsions are usually managed with intravenous diazepam or a short-acting barbiturate such as thiopental. Hyperventilation with oxygen is helpful. Occasionally, a neuromuscular blocking drug may be used to control violent convulsive activity. The cardiovascular toxicity of bupivacaine overdose is difficult to treat and has caused fatalities in healthy young adults.

QUESTIONS

1. Characteristic properties of local anesthetics include all of the following EXCEPT
   (A) An increase in membrane refractory period
   (B) Blockade of voltage-dependent sodium channels
   (C) Effects on vascular tone
   (D) Preferential binding to resting channels
   (E) Slowing of axonal impulse conduction

2. The pK_a of bupivicaine is 8.3. In infected tissue, which can be acidic, for example, at pH 6.3, the percentage of the drug in the nonionized form will be
   (A) 1%
   (B) 10%
   (C) 50%
   (D) 90%
   (E) 99%

3. Which statement about the speed of onset of nerve blockade with local anesthetics is correct?
(A) Faster in hypocalcemia
(B) Faster in myelinated fibers
(C) Faster in tissues that are infected
(D) Slower in hyperkalemia
(E) Slower in the periphery of a nerve bundle than in the center of a bundle

4. The most important effect of inadvertent intravenous administration of a large dose of an amide local anesthetic is
(A) Bronchoconstriction
(B) Hepatic damage
(C) Renal failure
(D) Seizures
(E) Tachycardia

5. All of the following factors influence the action of local anesthetics EXCEPT
(A) Acetylcholinesterase activity in the region of the injection site
(B) Blood flow through the tissue in which the injection is made
(C) Dose of local anesthetic injected
(D) The use of vasoconstrictors
(E) Tissue pH

6. You have a vial containing 5 mL of a 1% solution of lidocaine. How much lidocaine is present in 1 mL?
(A) 2 mg
(B) 5 mg
(C) 10 mg
(D) 20 mg
(E) 50 mg

7. Which statement about the toxicity of local anesthetics is correct?
(A) Cyanosis may occur after injection of large doses of lidocaine, especially in patients with pulmonary disease
(B) In overdosage, hyperventilation (with oxygen) is helpful to correct acidosis and lower extracellular potassium
(C) Intravenous injection of local anesthetics may stimulate ectopic cardiac pacemaker activity
(D) Most local anesthetics cause vasoconstriction
(E) Serious cardiovascular reactions are more likely to occur with tetracaine than with bupivacaine

8. A vasoconstrictor added to a solution of lidocaine for a peripheral nerve block will
(A) Decrease the risk of a seizure
(B) Increase the duration of anesthetic action of the local anesthetic
(C) Both A and B
(D) Neither A nor B

9. A child requires multiple minor surgical procedures in the nasopharynx. Which drug has high surface local anesthetic activity and intrinsic vasoconstrictor actions that reduce bleeding in mucous membranes?
(A) Bupivacaine
(B) Cocaine
(C) Lidocaine
(D) Procaine
(E) Tetracaine

10. Prilocaine is relatively contraindicated in patients with cardiovascular of pulmonary disease because the drug
(A) Acts as an agonist at β adrenoceptors in the heart and the lung
(B) Causes decompensation through formation of methemoglobin
(C) Inhibits cyclooxygenase in cardiac and pulmonary cells
(D) Is a potent bronchoconstrictor
(E) None of the above

ANSWERS

1. Local anesthetics bind preferentially to sodium channels in the open and inactivated states. Recovery from drug-induced block is 10–1000 times slower than recovery of channels from normal inactivation. Resting channels have a lower affinity for local anesthetics. The answer is **D.**

2. Because the drug is a weak base, it is more ionized (protonated) at pH values lower than its pK_a. Because the pH given is 2 log units lower (more acid) than the pK_a, the ratio of ionized to nonionized drug will be approximately 99:1. The answer is **A.** (Recall from Chapter 1 that at a pH equal to pK_a, the ratio is 1:1; at 1 log unit difference, the ratio is approximately 90:10; at 2 log units difference, 99:1; and so on).

3. Myelinated nerve fibers are blocked by local anesthetics more readily than unmyelinated ones. See the Skill Keeper Answer for an explanation of the effects of hypocalcemia and hyperkalemia on nerve blockade by local anesthetics. The answer is **B.**

4. Of the effects listed, the most important in local anesthetic overdose (of both amide and ester types) concern the CNS. Such effects can include sedation or restlessness, nystagmus, coma, respiratory depression, and seizures. Intravenous diazepam is commonly used for seizures caused by local anesthetics. The answer is **D.**

5. Local anesthetics are poor substrates for acetylcholinesterase, and the activity of this enzyme does not play a part in terminating the actions of local anesthetics. Ester-type local anesthetics are hydrolyzed by plasma (and tissue) pseudo-cholinesterases. Persons with genetically based defects in pseudocholinesterase activity are unusually sensitive to procaine and other esters. The answer is **A.**

6. The fact that you have 5 mL of the solution of lidocaine is irrelevant. A 1% solution of any drug contains 1 g per 100 mL. The amount of lidocaine in 1 mL of a 1% solution is thus 0.01 g, or 10 mg. The answer is **C.**

7. Acidosis resulting from tissue hypoxia favors local anesthetic toxicity because these drugs bind more avidly (or dissociate more slowly) from the sodium channel binding site when they are in the charged state. (Note that *onset* of therapeutic effect may be slower because charged local anesthetics penetrate the membrane less rapidly; see text.) Hyperkalemia depolarizes the membrane, which also favors local anesthetic binding. Oxygenation reduces both acidosis and hyperkalemia. The answer is **B.**

8. Epinephrine increases the duration of a nerve block when it is administered with short- and medium-duration local anesthetics. As a result of the vasoconstriction that prolongs the duration of this block, less local anesthetic is required, so the risk of toxicity (eg, a seizure) is reduced. The answer is **C**.

9. Cocaine is the only local anesthetic with intrinsic vasoconstrictor activity owing to its action to block the reuptake of norepinephrine released from sympathetic nerve endings (Chapter 9). Cocaine also has significant surface local anesthetic activity and is favored for head, neck, and pharyngeal surgery. The answer is **B**.

10. Large doses of prilocaine may cause accumulation of *o*-toluidine, a metabolite that converts hemoglobin to methemoglobin. Patients may become cyanotic with blood "chocolate colored." High blood levels of methemoglobin have resulted in decompensation in patients who have cardiac or pulmonary diseases. The answer is **B**.

SKILL KEEPER: CARDIAC TOXICITY OF LOCAL ANESTHETICS (SEE CHAPTER 14)

Sodium channel blockers (eg, local anesthetics) bind more readily to open (activated) or inactivated sodium channels. Hyperkalemia depolarizes the resting membrane potential, so more sodium channels are in the inactivated state. Conversely, hypercalcemia tends to hyperpolarize the resting potential and reduces the block of sodium channels.

CHECKLIST

When you complete this chapter, you should be able to:

❑ Describe the mechanism of action of local anesthetics.

❑ Know what is meant by the terms "use-dependent blockade" and "state-dependent blockade."

❑ Explain the relationship among tissue pH, drug pK_a, and the rate of onset of local anesthetic action.

❑ List 4 factors that determine the susceptibility of nerve fibers to local anesthetic blockade.

❑ Describe the major toxic effects of the local anesthetics.

DRUG SUMMARY TABLE: Drugs Used for Local Anesthesia

Subclass	Mechanism of Action	Pharmacokinetics	Clinical Applications	Toxicities
Amides				
Articaine Bupivacaine Levobupivacaine Lidocaine[a] Mepivacaine Prilocaine Ropivacaine	Blockade of Na^+ channels slows, then prevents axon potential propagation	Hepatic metabolism via CYP450 in part Half-lives: lidocaine, prilocaine < 2 h, others 3–4 h	Analgesia via topical use, or injection (perineural, epidural, subarachnoid) • rarely IV	CNS: excitation, seizures CV: vasodilation, hypotension, arrhythmias (bupivacaine)
Esters				
Benzocaine[a] Cocaine[a] Procaine Tetracaine[a]	As above, plus cocaine has intrinsic sympathomimetic actions	Rapid metabolism via plasma esterases • short half-lives	Analgesia, topical only for cocaine and benzocaine	As above re CNS actions • cocaine vasoconstricts When abused has caused hypertension and cardiac arrhythmias

[a]*Topical fomulations available.*

Skeletal Muscle Relaxants

The drugs in this chapter are divided into 2 dissimilar groups. The neuromuscular blocking drugs, which act at the skeletal myoneural junction, are used to produce muscle paralysis to facilitate surgery or assisted ventilation. The spasmolytic drugs, most of which act in the CNS, are used to reduce abnormally elevated tone caused by neurologic or muscle end plate disease.

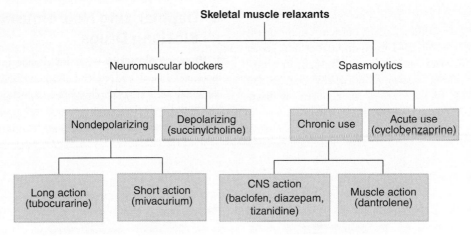

NEUROMUSCULAR BLOCKING DRUGS

A. Classification and Prototypes

Skeletal muscle contraction is evoked by a nicotinic cholinergic transmission process. Blockade of transmission at the end plate (the postsynaptic structure bearing the nicotinic receptors) is clinically useful in producing muscle relaxation, a requirement for surgical relaxation, tracheal intubation and control of ventilation. The neuromuscular blockers are quaternary amines structurally related to acetylcholine (ACh). Most are antagonists (nondepolarizing type), and the prototype is **tubocurarine.** One neuromuscular blocker used clinically, **succinylcholine,** is an agonist at the nicotinic end plate receptor (depolarizing type).

B. Nondepolarizing Neuromuscular Blocking Drugs

1. Pharmacokinetics—All agents are given parenterally. They are highly polar drugs and do not cross the blood-brain barrier. Drugs that are metabolized (eg, mivacurium, by plasma cholinesterase) or eliminated in the bile (eg, vecuronium) have shorter durations of action (10–20 min) than those eliminated by the kidney (eg, metocurine, pancuronium, pipecuronium, and tubocurarine), which usually have durations of action of less than 35 min. In addition to hepatic metabolism, atracurium clearance involves rapid spontaneous breakdown (Hofmann elimination) to form laudanosine and other products. At high blood levels, laudanosine may cause seizures. Cisatracurium, a stereoisomer of atracurium, is also inactivated spontaneously but forms less laudanosine and currently is one of the most commonly used muscle relaxants in clinical practice.

2. Mechanism of action—Nondepolarizing drugs prevent the action of ACh at the skeletal muscle end plate (Figure 27–1). They act as surmountable blockers. (That is, the blockade can be overcome by increasing the amount of agonist [ACh] in the synaptic cleft.) They behave as though they compete with ACh at the receptor, and their effect is reversed by cholinesterase inhibitors. Some drugs in this group may also act directly to plug the ion

High-Yield Terms to Learn

Depolarizing blockade	Neuromuscular paralysis that results from persistent depolarization of the end plate (eg, by succinylcholine)
Desensitization	A phase of blockade by a depolarizing blocker during which the end plate repolarizes but is less than normally responsive to agonists (acetylcholine or succinylcholine)
Malignant hyperthermia	Hyperthermia that results from massive release of calcium from the sarcoplasmic reticulum, leading to uncontrolled contraction and stimulation of metabolism in skeletal muscle
Nondepolarizing blockade	Neuromuscular paralysis that results from pharmacologic antagonism at the acetylcholine receptor of the end plate (eg, by tubocurarine)
Spasmolytic	A drug that reduces abnormally elevated muscle tone (spasm) without paralysis (eg, baclofen, dantrolene)
Stabilizing blockade	Synonym for nonpolarizing blockade

channel operated by the ACh receptor. Post-tetanic potentiation is preserved in the presence of these agents, but tension during the tetanus fades rapidly. See Table 27–1 for additional details. Larger muscles (eg, abdominal, diaphragm) are more resistant to neuromuscular blockade, but they recover more rapidly than smaller muscles (eg, facial, hand). Of the available nondepolarizing drugs, rocuronium (60–120 s) has the most rapid onset time.

C. Depolarizing Neuromuscular Blocking Drugs

1. Pharmacokinetics—Succinylcholine is composed of 2 ACh molecules linked end to end. Succinylcholine is metabolized by cholinesterase (butyrylcholinesterase or pseudocholinesterase) in the liver and plasma. It has a duration of action of only a few minutes if given as a single dose. Blockade may be prolonged in patients with

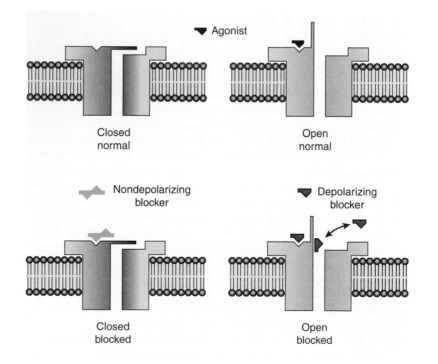

FIGURE 27–1 Drug interactions with the acetylcholine (ACh) receptor on the skeletal muscle end plate. **Top:** ACh, the normal agonist, opens the sodium channel. **Bottom left:** Nondepolarizing blockers bind to the receptor to prevent opening of the channel. **Bottom right:** Succinylcholine causes initial depolarization (fasciculation) and then persistent depolarization of the channel, which leads to muscle relaxation. (Reproduced, with permission, from Katzung BG, editor: *Basic & Clinical Pharmacology*, 12th ed. McGraw-Hill, 2012: Fig. 27–6.)

TABLE 27–1 Comparison of a typical nondepolarizing neuromuscular blocker (tubocurarine) and a depolarizing blocker (succinylcholine).

Process	Tubocurarine	Succinylcholine Phase I	Phase II
Administration of tubocurarine	Additive	Antagonistic	Augmented[a]
Administration of succinylcholine	Antagonistic	Additive	Augmented[a]
Effect of neostigmine	Antagonistic	Augmented[a]	Antagonistic
Initial excitatory effect on skeletal muscle	None	Fasciculations	None
Response to tetanic stimulus	Unsustained ("fade")	Sustained[b]	Unsustained
Post-tetanic facilitation	Yes	No	Yes

[a]It is not known whether this interaction is additive or synergistic (superadditive).

[b]The amplitude is decreased, but the response is sustained.

Adapted, with permission, from Katzung BG, editor: *Basic & Clinical Pharmacology*, 12th ed. McGraw-Hill, 2012.

genetic variants of plasma cholinesterase that metabolize succinylcholine very slowly. Such variant cholinesterases are resistant to the inhibitory action of dibucaine. Succinylcholine is not rapidly hydrolyzed by acetylcholinesterase.

2. Mechanism of action—Succinylcholine acts like a nicotinic agonist and depolarizes the neuromuscular end plate (Figure 27–1).

The initial depolarization is often accompanied by twitching and fasciculations (prevented by pretreatment with small doses of a nondepolarizing blocker). Because tension cannot be maintained in skeletal muscle without periodic repolarization and depolarization of the end plate, continuous depolarization results in muscle relaxation and paralysis. Succinylcholine may also plug the end plate channels.

When given by continuous infusion, the effect of succinylcholine changes from continuous depolarization (phase I) to gradual repolarization with resistance to depolarization (phase II) (ie, a curare-like block; see Table 27–1).

D. Reversal of Blockade

The action of nondepolarizing blockers is readily reversed by increasing the concentration of normal transmitter at the receptors. This is best accomplished by administration of cholinesterase inhibitors such as neostigmine or pyridostigmine. In contrast, the paralysis produced by the depolarizing blocker succinylcholine is *increased* by cholinesterase inhibitors during phase I. During phase II, the block produced by succinylcholine is usually reversible by cholinesterase inhibitors.

E. Toxicity

1. Respiratory paralysis—The action of full doses of neuromuscular blockers leads directly to respiratory paralysis. If mechanical ventilation is not provided, the patient will asphyxiate.

2. Autonomic effects and histamine release—Autonomic ganglia are stimulated by succinylcholine and weakly blocked by tubocurarine. Succinylcholine activates cardiac muscarinic receptors, whereas pancuronium is a moderate blocking agent and causes tachycardia. Tubocurarine and mivacurium are the most likely of these agents to cause histamine release, but it may also occur to a slight extent with atracurium and succinylcholine. Vecuronium and several newer nondepolarizing drugs (cisatracurium, doxacurium, pipecuronium, rocuronium) have no significant effects on autonomic functions or histamine release. A summary of the autonomic effects of neuromuscular drugs is shown in Table 27–2.

3. Specific effects of succinylcholine—Muscle pain is a common postoperative complaint, and muscle damage may occur. Succinylcholine may cause hyperkalemia, especially in patients with burn or spinal cord injury, peripheral nerve dysfunction, or muscular dystrophy. Increases in intragastric pressure caused by fasciculations may promote regurgitation with possible aspiration of gastric contents.

4. Drug interactions—Inhaled anesthetics, especially isoflurane, strongly potentiate and prolong neuromuscular blockade. A rare interaction of succinylcholine (and possibly tubocurarine) with inhaled anesthetics can result in malignant hyperthermia. A very early sign of this potentially life-threatening condition is contraction of the jaw muscles (trismus). Aminoglycoside antibiotics and antiarrhythmic drugs may potentiate and prolong the relaxant action of neuromuscular blockers to a lesser degree.

5. Effects of aging and diseases—Older patients (>75 years) and those with myasthenia gravis are more sensitive to the actions of the nondepolarizing blockers, and doses should be reduced in these patients. Conversely, patients with severe burns or who suffer from upper motor neuron disease are less responsive to these agents, probably as a result of proliferation of extrajunctional nicotinic receptors.

TABLE 27–2 Autonomic effects of neuromuscular drugs.

Drug	Effect on Autonomic Ganglia	Effect on Cardiac Muscarinic Receptors	Ability to Release Histamine
Nondepolarizing			
Atracurium	None	None	Slight
Cisatracurium	None	None	None
Mivacurium	None	None	Moderate
Pancuronium	None	Moderate block	None
Tubocurarine	Weak block	None	Moderate
Vecuronium	None	None	None
Depolarizing			
Succinylcholine	Stimulation	Stimulation	Slight

Modified and reproduced with permission from Katzung BG, editor: *Basic & Clinical Pharmacology*, 12th ed. McGraw-Hill, 2012.

SPASMOLYTIC DRUGS

Certain chronic diseases of the CNS (eg, cerebral palsy, multiple sclerosis, stroke) are associated with abnormally high reflex activity in the neuronal pathways that control skeletal muscle; the result is painful spasm. Bladder control and anal sphincter control are also affected in most cases and may require autonomic drugs for management. In other circumstances, acute injury or inflammation of muscle leads to spasm and pain. Such temporary spasm can sometimes be reduced with appropriate drug therapy.

The goal of spasmolytic therapy in both chronic and acute conditions is reduction of excessive skeletal muscle tone without reduction of strength. Reduced spasm results in reduction of pain and improved mobility.

A. Drugs for Chronic Spasm

1. Classification—The spasmolytic drugs do not resemble ACh in structure or effect. They act in the CNS and in one case in the skeletal muscle cell rather than at the neuromuscular end plate. The spasmolytic drugs used in treatment of the chronic conditions mentioned previously include **diazepam,** a benzodiazepine (see Chapter 22); **baclofen,** a γ-aminobutyric acid (GABA) agonist; **tizanidine,** a congener of clonidine; and **dantrolene,** an agent that acts on the sarcoplasmic reticulum of skeletal muscle. These agents are usually administered by the oral route. Refractory cases may respond to chronic intrathecal administration of baclofen. **Botulinum toxin** injected into selected muscles can reduce pain caused by severe spasm (see Chapter 6) and also has application for ophthalmic purposes and in more generalized spastic disorders (eg, cerebral palsy). **Gabapentin** and **pregabalin,** antiseizure drugs, have been shown to be effective spasmolytics in patients with multiple sclerosis.

2. Mechanisms of action—The spasmolytic drugs act by several mechanisms. Three of the drugs (baclofen, diazepam, and tizanidine) act in the spinal cord (Figure 27–2).

Baclofen acts as a GABA$_B$ agonist at both presynaptic and postsynaptic receptors, causing membrane hyperpolarization. Presynaptically, baclofen, by reducing calcium influx, decreases the release of the excitatory transmitter glutamic acid; at postsynaptic receptors, baclofen facilitates the inhibitory action of GABA. Diazepam facilitates GABA-mediated inhibition via its interaction with GABA$_A$ receptors (see Chapter 22). Tizanidine, an imidazoline related to clonidine with significant α$_2$ agonist activity, reinforces presynaptic inhibition in the spinal cord. All 3 drugs reduce the tonic output of the primary spinal motoneurons.

Dantrolene acts in the skeletal muscle cell to reduce the release of activator calcium from the sarcoplasmic reticulum via interaction with the ryanodine receptor (RyR1) channel. Cardiac muscle and smooth muscle are minimally depressed. Dantrolene is also effective in the treatment of **malignant hyperthermia,** a disorder characterized by massive calcium release from the sarcoplasmic reticulum of skeletal muscle. Though rare, malignant hyperthermia can be triggered by general anesthesia protocols that include succinylcholine or tubocurarine (see Chapter 25). In this emergency condition, dantrolene is given intravenously to block calcium release.

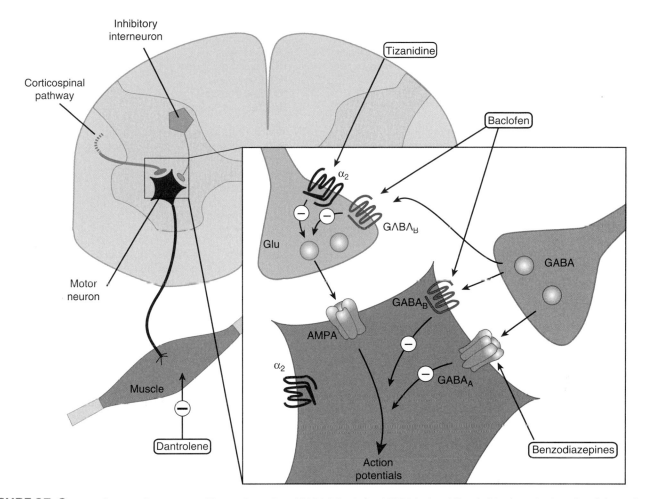

FIGURE 27–2 Sites of spasmolytic action of benzodiazepines (GABA_A), baclofen (GABA_B), tizanidine (α_2) in the spinal cord and dantrolene (skeletal muscle). AMPA, amino-hydroxyl-methyl-isosoxazole-proprionic acid, a ligand for a glutamate receptor subtype; Glu, glutamatergic neuron. (Reproduced, with permission, from Katzung BG, editor: *Basic & Clinical Pharmacology*, 12th ed. McGraw-Hill, 2012: Fig. 27–11.)

3. Toxicity—The sedation produced by diazepam is significant but milder than that produced by other sedative-hypnotic drugs at doses that induce equivalent muscle relaxation. Baclofen causes somewhat less sedation than diazepam, and tolerance occurs with chronic use—withdrawal should be accomplished slowly. Tizanidine may cause asthenia, drowsiness, dry mouth, and hypotension. Dantrolene causes significant muscle weakness but less sedation than either diazepam or baclofen.

B. Drugs for Acute Muscle Spasm

Many drugs (eg, cyclobenzaprine, metaxalone, methocarbamol, orphenadrine) are promoted for the treatment of acute spasm resulting from muscle injury. Most of these drugs are sedatives or act in the brain stem. **Cyclobenzaprine,** a typical member of this group, is believed to act in the brain stem, possibly by interfering with polysynaptic reflexes that maintain skeletal muscle tone. The drug is active by the oral route and has marked sedative and antimuscarinic actions. Cyclobenzaprine may cause confusion and visual hallucinations in some patients. None of these drugs used for acute spasm is effective in muscle spasm resulting from cerebral palsy or spinal cord injury.

Patients with renal failure often have decreased levels of plasma cholinesterase, thus prolonging the duration of action of mivacurium or succinylcholine.

QUESTIONS

1. Characteristics of phase I depolarizing neuromuscular blockade due to succinylcholine include
   (A) Easy reversibility with nicotinic receptor antagonists
   (B) Marked muscarinic blockade
   (C) Muscle fasciculations only in the later stages of block
   (D) Reversibility by acetylcholinesterase (AChE) inhibitors
   (E) Sustained tension during a period of tetanic stimulation

Questions 2 and 3. A patient underwent a surgical procedure of 2 h. Anesthesia was provided by isoflurane, supplemented by intravenous midazolam and a nondepolarizing muscle relaxant. At the end of the procedure, a low dose of glycopyrrolate was administered followed by pyridostigmine.

2. The main reason for administering the muscarinic receptor antagonist was to
   (A) Enhance the action of pyridostigmine
   (B) Prevent spasm of gastrointestinal smooth muscle
   (C) Prevent activation of cardiac muscarinic receptors
   (D) Provide postoperative analgesia
   (E) Reverse the effects of the muscle relaxant

3. A muscarinic receptor antagonist would probably not be needed for reversal of the skeletal muscle relaxant actions of a nondepolarizing drug if the agent used was
   (A) Cisatracurium
   (B) Mivacurium
   (C) Pancuronium
   (D) Tubocurarine
   (E) Vecuronium

4. Which of the following drugs is the most effective in the emergency management of malignant hyperthermia?
   (A) Baclofen
   (B) Dantrolene
   (C) Gabapentin
   (D) Secobarbital
   (E) Vecuronium

5. The clinical use of succinylcholine, especially in patients with diabetes, is associated with
   (A) Antagonism by pyridostigmine during the early phase of blockade
   (B) Aspiration of gastric contents
   (C) Decreased intragastric pressure
   (D) Histamine release in a genetically determined population
   (E) Metabolism at the neuromuscular junction by acetylcholinesterase

6. Which drug is most often associated with hypotension caused by histamine release?
   (A) Baclofen
   (B) Pancuronium
   (C) Tizanidine
   (D) Tubocurarine
   (E) Vecuronium

7. Regarding the spasmolytic drugs, which of the following statements is *not* accurate?
   (A) Baclofen acts on GABA receptors in the spinal cord to increase chloride ion conductance
   (B) Cyclobenzaprine decreases both oropharyngeal secretions and gut motility
   (C) Dantrolene has no significant effect on the release of calcium from cardiac muscle
   (D) Diazepam causes sedation at doses commonly used to reduce muscle spasms
   (E) Intrathecal use of baclofen is effective in some refractory cases of muscle spasticity

8. Which drug is most likely to cause hyperkalemia leading to cardiac arrest in patients with extensive burns?
   (A) Baclofen
   (B) Cyclobenzaprine
   (C) Dantrolene
   (D) Rocuronium
   (E) Succinylcholine

9. Which drug has spasmolytic activity and could also be used in the management of seizures caused by overdose of a local anesthetic?
   (A) Baclofen
   (B) Cyclobenzaprine
   (C) Diazepam
   (D) Gabapentin
   (E) Tizanidine

10. Myalgias are a common postoperative complaint of patients who receive large doses of succinylcholine, possibly the result of muscle fasciculations caused by depolarization. Which drug administered in the operating room can be used to prevent postoperative pain caused by succinylcholine?
    (A) Baclofen
    (B) Cisatracurium
    (C) Dantrolene
    (D) Lidocaine
    (E) Morphine

ANSWERS

1. Phase I depolarizing blockade caused by succinylcholine is not associated with antagonism at muscarinic receptors, nor is it reversible with cholinesterase inhibitors. Muscle fasciculations occur at the start of the action of succinylcholine. The answer is **E.**

2. Acetylcholinesterase inhibitors used for reversing the effects of nondepolarizing muscle relaxants cause increases in ACh at all sites where it acts as a neurotransmitter. To offset the resulting side effects, including bradycardia, a muscarinic blocking agent is used concomitantly. Although atropine is effective, glycopyrrolate is usually preferred because it lacks CNS effects. The answer is **C.**

3. One of the distinctive characteristics of pancuronium is that it can block muscarinic receptors, especially those in the heart. It has sometimes caused tachycardia and hypertension and may cause dysrhythmias in predisposed individuals. The answer is **C.**

4. Prompt treatment is essential in malignant hyperthermia to control body temperature, correct acidosis, and prevent calcium release. Dantrolene interacts with the RyR1 channel to block the release of activator calcium from the sarcoplasmic reticulum, which prevents the tension-generating interaction of actin with myosin. The answer is **B.**

5. Fasciculations associated with succinylcholine may **increase** intragastric pressure with possible complications of regurgitation and aspiration of gastric contents. The complication is more likely in patients with delayed gastric emptying such as those with esophageal dysfunction or diabetes. Histamine release resulting from succinylcholine is not genetically determined. The answer is **B.**

6. Hypotension may occur with tubocurarine and with the spasmolytic drug tizanidine. In the case of tubocurarine, the decrease in blood pressure may be due partly to histamine release and to ganglionic blockade. Tizanidine causes hypotension via α_2-adrenoceptor activation like its congener clonidine. The answer is **D.**

7. Baclofen activates $GABA_B$ receptors in the spinal cord. However, these receptors are coupled to K^+ channels (see Chapter 21). $GABA_A$ receptors in the CNS modulate chloride ion channels, an action facilitated by diazepam and other benzodiazepines. The answer is **A.**

8. Skeletal muscle depolarization by succinylcholine releases potassium from the cells, and the ensuing hyperkalemia can be life-threatening in terms of cardiac arrest. Patients most susceptible include those with extensive burns, spinal cord injuries, neurologic dysfunction, or intra-abdominal infection. The answer is **E.**

9. Diazepam is both an effective antiseizure drug and a spasmolytic. The spasmolytic action of diazepam is thought to be exerted partly in the spinal cord because it reduces spasm of skeletal muscle in patients with cord transection. Cyclobenzaprine is used for acute local spasm and has no antiseizure activity. The answer is **C.**

10. The depolarizing action of succinylcholine at the skeletal muscle end plate can be antagonized by small doses of depolarizing blockers. To prevent skeletal muscle fasciculations and the resulting postoperative pain caused by succinylcholine, a small nonparalyzing dose of a nondepolarizing drug is often given immediately before succinylcholine. The answer is **B.**

SKILL KEEPER ANSWER: AUTONOMIC CONTROL OF HEART RATE (SEE CHAPTER 6)

Reflex changes in heart rate involve ganglionic transmission. Activation of α_1 receptors on blood vessels by phenylephrine elicits a reflex bradycardia because mean blood pressure is increased. One of the characteristic effects of tubocurarine is its block of autonomic ganglia; this action can interfere with reflex changes in heart rate. Tubocurarine would not prevent bradycardia resulting from neostigmine (an inhibitor of acetylcholinesterase) because this occurs via stimulation by ACh of cardiac muscarinic receptors.

CHECKLIST

When you complete this chapter, you should be able to:

❑ Describe the transmission process at the skeletal neuromuscular end plate and the points at which drugs can modify this process.

❑ Identify the major nondepolarizing neuromuscular blockers and 1 depolarizing neuromuscular blocker; compare their pharmacokinetics.

❑ Describe the differences between depolarizing and nondepolarizing blockers from the standpoint of tetanic and post-tetanic twitch strength.

❑ Describe the method of reversal of nondepolarizing blockade.

❑ List drugs for treatment of skeletal muscle spasticity and identify their sites of action and their adverse effects.

DRUG SUMMARY TABLE: Skeletal Muscle Relaxants

Subclass	Mechanism of Action	Receptor Interactions	Pharmacokinetics	Adverse Effects
Depolarizing				
Succinylcholine	Agonist at ACh-N receptors causing initial twitch then persistent depolarization	Stimulates ANS ganglia and M receptors	Parenteral: short action, inactivated by plasma esterases	Muscle pain, hyperkalemia, increased intragastric and intraocular pressure
Nondepolarizing				
d-Tubocurarine Atracurium Cistracurium Mivacurium Rocuronium Vecuronium	Competitive antagonists at skeletal muscle ACh-N receptors	ANS ganglion block (tubocurarine) Cardiac M block (pancuronium)	Parenteral use, variable disposition Spontaneous inactivation (atracurium, cisatracurium) Plasma ChE (mivacurium) Hepatic metabolism (rocuronium, vecuronium) Renal elimination (doxacurium, pancuronium, tubocurarine)	Histamine release (mivacurium, tubocurarine) Laudanosine formation (atracurium) Muscle relaxation is potentiated by inhaled anesthetics, aminoglycosides and possibly quinidine
Centrally acting				
Baclofen	Facilitates spinal inhibition of motor neurons	GABA$_B$ receptor activation: pre- and postsynaptic	Oral and intrathecal for severe spasticity	Sedation, muscle weakness
Cyclobenzaprine (many others; see text)	Inhibition of spinal stretch reflex	Mechanism unknown	Oral for acute muscle spasm due to injury or inflammation	M block, sedation, confusion, and ocular effects
Diazepam	Facilitates GABA-ergic transmission in CNS	GABA$_A$ receptor activation—postsynaptic	Oral and parenteral for acute and chronic spasms	Sedation, additive with other CNS depressants • abuse potential
Tizanidine	Pre- and postsynaptic inhibition	α_2 Agonist in spinal cord	Oral for acute and chronic spasms	Muscle weakness, sedation, hypotension
Direct-acting				
Dantrolene	Weakens muscle contraction by reducing myosin-actin interaction	Blocks RyR1 Ca^{2+} channels in skeletal muscle	Oral for acute and chronic spasms • IV for malignant hyperthermia	Muscle weakness

ACh, acetylcholine; ANS, autonomic nervous system; ChE, cholinesterase.

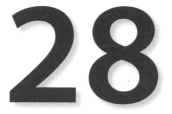
Drugs Used in Parkinsonism & Other Movement Disorders

Movement disorders constitute a number of heterogeneous neurologic conditions with very different therapies. They include parkinsonism, Huntington's disease, Wilson's disease, and Gilles de la Tourette's syndrome. Movement disorders, including athetosis, chorea, dyskinesia, dystonia, tics, and tremor, can be caused by a variety of general medical conditions, neurologic dysfunction, and drugs.

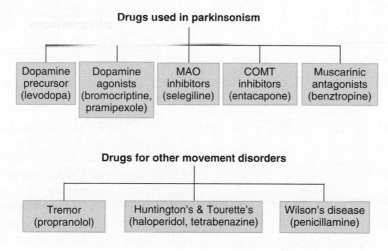

Drugs used in parkinsonism

| Dopamine precursor (levodopa) | Dopamine agonists (bromocriptine, pramipexole) | MAO inhibitors (selegiline) | COMT inhibitors (entacapone) | Muscarinic antagonists (benztropine) |

Drugs for other movement disorders

| Tremor (propranolol) | Huntington's & Tourette's (haloperidol, tetrabenazine) | Wilson's disease (penicillamine) |

PARKINSONISM

A. Pathophysiology

Parkinsonism (paralysis agitans) is a common movement disorder that involves dysfunction in the basal ganglia and associated brain structures. Signs include rigidity of skeletal muscles, akinesia (or bradykinesia), flat facies, and tremor at rest (mnemonic **RAFT**).

1. Naturally occurring parkinsonism—The naturally occurring disease is of uncertain origin and occurs with increasing frequency during aging from the fifth or sixth decade of life onward. Pathologic characteristics include a decrease in the levels of striatal dopamine and the degeneration of dopaminergic neurons in the nigrostriatal tract that normally *inhibit* the activity of striatal GABAergic neurons (Figure 28–1). Most of the postsynaptic dopamine receptors on GABAergic neurons are of the D_2 subclass (negatively coupled to adenylyl cyclase). The reduction of normal dopaminergic neurotransmission leads to excessive *excitatory* actions of cholinergic neurons on striatal GABAergic neurons; thus, dopamine and acetylcholine activities are out of balance in parkinsonism (Figure 28–1).

2. Drug-induced parkinsonism—Many drugs can cause parkinsonian symptoms; these effects are usually reversible. The most important drugs are the butyrophenone and phenothiazine

High-Yield Terms to Learn

Athetosis	Involuntary slow writhing movements, especially severe in the hands; "mobile spasm"
Chorea	Irregular, unpredictable, involuntary muscle jerks that impair voluntary activity
Dystonia	Prolonged muscle contractions with twisting and repetitive movements or abnormal posture; may occur in the form of rhythmic jerks
Huntingdon's disease	An inherited adult-onset neurologic disease characterized by dementia and bizarre involuntary movements
Parkinsonism	A progressive neurologic disease characterized by shuffling gait, stooped posture, resting tremor, speech impediments, movement difficulties, and an eventual slowing of mental processes and dementia
Tics	Sudden coordinated abnormal movements, usually repetitive, especially about the face and head
Tourette's syndrome	A neurologic disease of unknown cause that presents with multiple tics associated with snorting, sniffing, and involuntary vocalizations (often obscene)
Wilson's disease	An inherited (autosomal recessive) disorder of copper accumulation in liver, brain, kidneys, and eyes; symptoms include jaundice, vomiting, tremors, muscle weakness, stiff movements, liver failure, and dementia

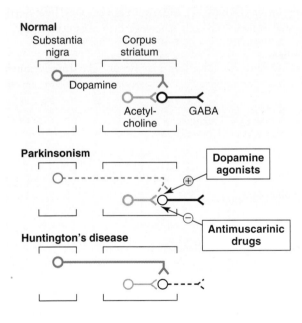

FIGURE 28–1 Schematic representation of the sequence of neurons involved in parkinsonism and Huntington's chorea. **Top:** Neurons in the normal brain. **Middle:** Neurons in parkinsonism. The dopaminergic neuron is lost. **Bottom:** Neurons in Huntington's disease. The GABAergic neuron is lost. (Reproduced, with permission, from Katzung BG, editor: *Basic & Clinical Pharmacology*, 9th ed. McGraw-Hill, 2004: Fig. 28–1).

antipsychotic drugs, which block brain dopamine receptors. At high doses, **reserpine** causes similar symptoms, presumably by depleting brain dopamine. **MPTP** (1-methyl-4-phenyl-1,2,3,6-tetrahydropyridine), a by-product of the attempted synthesis of an illicit meperidine analog, causes irreversible parkinsonism through destruction of dopaminergic neurons in the nigrostriatal tract. Treatment with type B monoamine oxidase inhibitors (MAOIs) protects against MPTP neurotoxicity in animals.

DRUG THERAPY OF PARKINSONISM

Strategies of drug treatment of parkinsonism involve increasing dopamine activity in the brain, decreasing muscarinic cholinergic activity in the brain, or both.

Although several dopamine receptor subtypes are present in the substantia nigra, the benefits of most antiparkinson drugs appear to depend on activation of the D_2 receptor subtype.

A. Levodopa

1. Mechanisms—Because dopamine has low bioavailability and does not readily cross the blood-brain barrier, its precursor, L-dopa (levodopa), is used. This amino acid enters the brain via an L-amino acid transporter (LAT) and is converted to dopamine by the enzyme aromatic L-amino acid decarboxylase (dopa decarboxylase), which is present in many body tissues, including the brain. Levodopa is usually given with **carbidopa,** a drug that does not cross the blood-brain barrier but inhibits dopa decarboxylase in peripheral tissues (Figure 28–2). With this combination, the plasma half-life is prolonged, lower doses of levodopa are effective, and there are fewer peripheral side effects.

2. Pharmacologic effects—Levodopa ameliorates the signs of parkinsonism, particularly bradykinesia; moreover, the mortality rate is decreased. However, the drug does not cure parkinsonism, and responsiveness fluctuates and gradually decreases with time, which may reflect progression of the disease. Clinical response fluctuations may, in some cases, be related to the timing of levodopa dosing. In other cases, unrelated to dosing, off-periods of akinesia may alternate over a few hours with on-periods of improved mobility but often with dyskinesias (on-off phenomena). In some case, off-periods may respond to apomorphine. Although drug holidays sometimes reduce toxic effects, they rarely affect response fluctuations. However, catechol-O-methyltransferase (COMT) inhibitors used adjunctively may improve fluctuations in levodopa responses in some patients (see below).

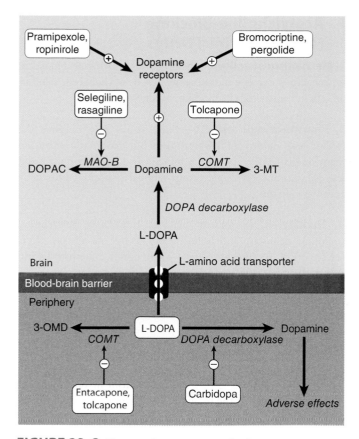

FIGURE 28–2 Pharmacologic strategies for dopaminergic therapy of Parkinson's disease. The actions of the drugs are described in the text. MAO, monoamine oxidase; COMT, catechol-*O*-methyltransferase; DOPAC, dihydroxyphenylacetic acid; L-DOPA, levodopa; 3-OMD, 3-*O*-methyldopa. (Reproduced, with permission, from Katzung BG, editor: *Basic & Clinical Pharmacology*, 12th ed. McGraw-Hill, 2012: Fig. 28–5.)

3. Toxicity—Most adverse effects are dose dependent. Gastrointestinal effects include anorexia, nausea, and emesis and can be reduced by taking the drug in divided doses. Tolerance to the emetic action of levodopa usually occurs after several months.

Postural hypotension is common, especially in the early stage of treatment. Other cardiac effects include tachycardia, asystole, and cardiac arrhythmias (rare).

Dyskinesias occur in up to 80% of patients, with choreoathetosis of the face and distal extremities occurring most often. Some patients may exhibit chorea, ballismus, myoclonus, tics, and tremor.

Behavioral effects may include anxiety, agitation, confusion, delusions, hallucinations, and depression. Levodopa is contraindicated in patients with a history of psychosis.

B. Dopamine Agonists

1. Bromocriptine—An ergot alkaloid bromocriptine acts as a partial agonist at dopamine D$_2$ receptors in the brain. The drug increases the functional activity of dopamine neurotransmitter

pathways, including those involved in extrapyramidal functions (Figure 28–2).

Bromocriptine has been used as an individual drug, in combinations with levodopa (and with anticholinergic drugs), and in patients who are refractory to or cannot tolerate levodopa. Common adverse effects include anorexia, nausea and vomiting, dyskinesias, and postural hypotension. Behavioral effects, which occur more commonly with bromocriptine than with newer dopamine agonists, include confusion, hallucinations, and delusions. Ergot-related effects include erythromelalgia and pulmonary infiltrates. Use of bromocriptine in patients with Parkinson's disease has declined with the introduction of non-ergot dopamine receptor agonists.

2. Pramipexole—This non-ergot has high affinity for the dopamine D$_3$ receptor. It is effective as monotherapy in mild parkinsonism and can be used together with levodopa in more advanced disease. Pramipexole is administered orally 3 times daily and is excreted largely unchanged in the urine. The dose of pramipexole may need to be reduced in renal dysfunction. Adverse effects include anorexia, nausea and vomiting, postural hypotension, and dyskinesias. Mental disturbances (confusion, delusions, hallucinations, impulsivity) are more common with pramipexole than with levodopa. In rare cases, an uncontrollable tendency to fall asleep may occur. The drug is contraindicated in patients with active peptic ulcer disease, psychotic illness, or recent myocardial infarction. Pramipexole may be neuroprotective because it is reported to act as a scavenger for hydrogen peroxide.

3. Ropinirole—Another non-ergot, this drug has high affinity for the dopamine D$_2$ receptor. It is effective as monotherapy and can be used with levodopa to smooth out response fluctuations. The standard form is given 3 times daily, but a prolonged release form can be taken once daily. Ropinirole is metabolized by hepatic CYP1A2, and other drugs metabolized by this isoform (eg, caffeine, warfarin) may reduce its clearance. Adverse effects and contraindications are similar to those of pramipexole.

4. Apomorphine—A potent dopamine receptor agonist, apomorphine injected subcutaneously may provide rapid (within 10 min) but temporary relief (1–2 h) of "off-periods" of akinesia in patients on optimized dopaminergic therapy. Because of severe nausea, pretreatment for 3 days with antiemetics (eg, trimethobenzamide) is necessary. Other side effects of apomorphine include dyskinesias, hypotension, drowsiness, and sweating.

C. Monoamine Oxidase Inhibitors

1. Mechanism—Selegiline and rasagiline are selective inhibitors of monoamine oxidase type B, the form of the enzyme that metabolizes dopamine (Figure 28–2). Hepatic metabolism of selegiline results in the formation of desmethylselegiline (possibly neuroprotective) and amphetamine.

2. Clinical use—Selegiline has minimal efficacy in parkinsonism if given alone but can be used adjunctively with levodopa. Rasagiline is more potent and has been used as monotherapy in early symptomatic parkinsonism as well as in combinations with levodopa.

3. Toxicity and drug interactions—Adverse effects and interactions of monoamine oxidase inhibitors include insomnia, mood changes, dyskinesias, gastrointestinal distress, and hypotension. Combinations of these drugs with meperidine have resulted in agitation, delirium, and mortality. Selegiline has been implicated in the serotonin syndrome when used with serotonin selective reuptake inhibitors (SSRIs).

D. Catechol-*O*-methyltransferase (COMT) Inhibitors

1. Mechanism of action—Entacapone and tolcapone are inhibitors of COMT, the enzyme in both the CNS and peripheral tissues (Figure 28–2) that converts levodopa to 3-*O*-methyldopa (3-OMD). Increased plasma levels of 3-OMD are associated with poor response to levodopa partly because the compound competes with levodopa for active transport into the CNS. Entacapone acts only in the periphery.

2. Clinical uses—The drugs are used individually as adjuncts to levodopa-carbidopa, decreasing fluctuations, improving response, and prolonging "on-time." Tolcapone is taken 3 times daily, entacapone 5 times daily. A formulation combining levodopa, carbidopa, and entacapone is available, simplifying the drug regimen.

3. Toxicity—Adverse effects related partly to increased levels of levodopa include dyskinesias, gastrointestinal distress, and postural hypotension. Levodopa dose reductions may be needed for the first few days of COMT inhibitor use. Other side effects include sleep disturbances and orange discoloration of the urine. Tolcapone increases liver enzymes and has caused acute hepatic failure, necessitating routine monitoring of liver function tests and signed patient consent for use in the United States.

E. Amantadine

1. Mechanism of action—Amantadine enhances dopaminergic neurotransmission by unknown mechanisms that may involve increasing synthesis or release of dopamine or inhibition of dopamine reuptake. The drug also has muscarinic blocking actions.

2. Pharmacologic effects—Amantadine may improve bradykinesia, rigidity, and tremor but is usually effective for only a few weeks. Amantadine also has antiviral effects.

3. Toxicity—**Behavioral effects** include restlessness, agitation, insomnia, confusion, hallucinations, and acute toxic psychosis. **Dermatologic reactions** include livedo reticularis. **Miscellaneous effects** may include gastrointestinal disturbances, urinary retention, and postural hypotension. Amantadine also causes peripheral edema, which responds to diuretics.

F. Acetylcholine-Blocking (Antimuscarinic) Drugs

1. Mechanism of action—The drugs (eg, benztropine, biperiden, orphenadrine) decrease the excitatory actions of cholinergic neurons on cells in the striatum by blocking muscarinic receptors.

2. Pharmacologic effects—These drugs may improve the tremor and rigidity of parkinsonism but have little effect on bradykinesia. They are used adjunctively in parkinsonism and also alleviate the reversible extrapyramidal symptoms caused by antipsychotic drugs.

3. Toxicity—CNS toxicity includes drowsiness, inattention, confusion, delusions, and hallucinations. Peripheral adverse effects are typical of atropine-like drugs. These agents exacerbate tardive dyskinesias that result from prolonged use of antipsychotic drugs.

> ### SKILL KEEPER: AUTONOMIC DRUG SIDE EFFECTS (SEE CHAPTERS 8 AND 9)
>
> *Based on your understanding of the receptors affected by drugs used in Parkinson's disease, what types of autonomic side effects can you anticipate? The Skill Keeper Answers appear at the end of the chapter.*

DRUG THERAPY OF OTHER MOVEMENT DISORDERS

A. Tremor

Physiologic and essential tremor are clinically similar conditions characterized by postural tremor. The conditions may be accentuated by anxiety, fatigue, and certain drugs, including bronchodilators, tricyclic antidepressants, and lithium. They may be alleviated by β-blocking drugs including **propranolol.** Beta blockers should be used with caution in patients with congestive heart failure, asthma, diabetes, or hypoglycemia. **Metoprolol,** a β_1-selective antagonist, is also effective, and its use is preferred in patients with concomitant pulmonary disease. Antiepileptic drugs including gabapentin, primidone, and topiramate, as well as intramuscular injection of botulinum toxin, have also been used to treat essential tremor.

B. Huntington's Disease and Tourette's Syndrome

Huntington's disease, an inherited disorder, results from a brain neurotransmitter imbalance such that GABA functions are diminished and dopaminergic functions are enhanced (Figure 28–1). There may also be a cholinergic deficit because choline acetyltransferase is decreased in the basal ganglia of patients with this disease. However, pharmacologic attempts to enhance brain

GABA and acetylcholine activities have not been successful in patients with this disease. Drug therapy usually involves the use of amine-depleting drugs (eg, **reserpine, tetrabenazine**), the latter having less troublesome adverse effects. Dopamine receptor antagonists (eg, **haloperidol, perphenazine**) are also sometimes effective, and recent reports suggest that olanzapine is also useful.

Tourette's syndrome is a disorder of unknown cause that frequently responds to haloperidol and other dopamine D_2 receptor blockers, including pimozide. Though less effective overall, carbamazepine, clonazepam, and clonidine have also been used.

C. Drug-Induced Dyskinesias

Parkinsonism symptoms caused by antipsychotic agents (see Chapter 29) are usually reversible by lowering drug dosage, changing the therapy to a drug that is less toxic to extrapyramidal function, or treating with a muscarinic blocker. In acute dystonias, parenteral administration of benztropine or diphenhydramine is helpful. Levodopa and bromocriptine are not useful because dopamine receptors are blocked by the antipsychotic drugs. **Tardive dyskinesias** that develop from therapy with older antipsychotic drugs are possibly a form of denervation supersensitivity. They are not readily reversed; no specific drug therapy is available.

D. Wilson's Disease

This recessively inherited disorder of copper metabolism results in deposition of copper salts in the liver and other tissues. Hepatic and neurologic damage may be severe or fatal. Treatment involves use of the chelating agent **penicillamine** (dimethylcysteine), which removes excess copper. Toxic effects of penicillamine include gastrointestinal distress, myasthenia, optic neuropathy, and blood dyscrasias.

E. Restless Legs Syndrome

This syndrome, of unknown cause, is characterized by an unpleasant creeping discomfort in the limbs that occurs particularly when the patient is at rest. The disorder is more common in pregnant women and in uremic and diabetic patients. Dopaminergic therapy is the preferred treatment, and both **pramipexole** and **ropinirole** are approved for this condition. Opioid analgesics, benzodiazepines, and certain anticonvulsants (eg, gabapentin) are also used.

QUESTIONS

Questions 1 and 2. Bradykinesia has made drug treatment necessary in a 60-year-old male patient with Parkinson's disease, and therapy is to be initiated with levodopa.

1. Regarding the anticipated actions of levodopa, the patient would *not* be informed that
   (A) A netlike reddish to blue discoloration of the skin is a possible side effect
   (B) Dizziness may occur upon standing up
   (C) He should take the drug in divided doses to avoid nausea
   (D) The drug will probably improve his symptoms for a period of time but not indefinitely
   (E) Uncontrollable muscle jerks may occur

2. The prescribing physician will (or should) know that levodopa
   (A) Causes less severe behavioral side effects if given together with a drug that inhibits hepatic dopa decarboxylase
   (B) Fluctuates in its effectiveness with increasing frequency as treatment continues
   (C) Prevents extrapyramidal adverse effects of antipsychotic drugs
   (D) Protects against cancer in patients with melanoma
   (E) Has toxic effects, which include pulmonary infiltrates

3. Which statement about ropinirole is accurate?
   (A) Effectiveness of the drug in Parkinson's disease requires its metabolic conversion to an active metabolite
   (B) It should not be administered to patients taking antimuscarinic drugs
   (C) Ropinirole causes less mental disturbances than levodopa
   (D) Ropinirole specifically activates the dopamine D_3 receptor subtype
   (E) Warfarin may enhance the actions of ropinirole

4. A patient with parkinsonism is being treated with levodopa. He suffers from irregular, involuntary muscle jerks that affect the proximal muscles of the limbs. Which of the following statements about these symptoms is accurate?
   (A) Coadministration of muscarinic blockers prevents the occurrence of dyskinesias during treatment with levodopa
   (B) Dyskinesias are less likely to occur if levodopa is administered with carbidopa
   (C) Other drugs that activate dopamine receptors can exacerbate dyskinesias in a patient taking levodopa
   (D) The symptoms are likely to be alleviated by continued treatment with levodopa
   (E) The symptoms are usually reduced if the dose of levodopa is increased

5. A 51-year-old patient with parkinsonism is being maintained on levodopa-carbidopa with adjunctive use of low doses of entacapone, but continues to have off-periods of akinesia. The most appropriate drug to "rescue" the patient but that will only provide temporary relief is
   (A) Apomorphine
   (B) Benztropine
   (C) Carbidopa
   (D) Ropinirole
   (E) Selegiline

6. Concerning the drugs used in parkinsonism, which statement is accurate?
   (A) Dopamine receptor agonists should never be used in Parkinson's disease before a trial of levodopa
   (B) Levodopa causes mydriasis and may precipitate an acute attack of glaucoma
   (C) Selegiline is a selective inhibitor of COMT
   (D) The primary benefit of antimuscarinic drugs in parkinsonism is their ability to relieve bradykinesia
   (E) Therapeutic effects of amantadine continue for several years

7. A previously healthy 40-year-old woman begins to suffer from slowed mentation, lack of coordination, and brief writhing movements of her hands that are not rhythmic. In addition, she has delusions of being persecuted. The woman has no history of psychiatric or neurologic disorders. Although further diagnostic assessment should be made, it is very likely that the most appropriate drug for treatment will be
(A) Amantadine
(B) Bromocriptine
(C) Diazepam
(D) Levodopa
(E) Tetrabenazine

8. With respect to ropinirole, which of the following is accurate?
(A) Activates brain dopamine D_3 receptors
(B) Effective as monotherapy in mild parkinsonism
(C) May cause postural hypotension
(D) Not an ergot derivative
(E) All of the above

9. Entacapone may be of value in patients being treated with levodopa-carbidopa because it
(A) Activates COMT
(B) Decreases the formation of 3-O-methyldopa
(C) Inhibits monoamine oxidase type B
(D) Inhibits neuronal reuptake of dopamine
(E) Releases dopamine from nerve endings

10. Which of the following drugs is most suitable for management of tremor in a patient who has pulmonary disease?
(A) Diazepam
(B) Levodopa
(C) Metoprolol
(D) Propranolol
(E) Terbutaline

ANSWERS

1. In prescribing levodopa, the patient should be informed about adverse effects, including gastrointestinal distress, postural hypotension, and dyskinesias. It is reasonable to advise the patient that therapeutic benefits cannot be expected to continue indefinitely. Livedo reticularis (a netlike rash) is an adverse effect of treatment with amantadine. The answer is **A.**

2. Levodopa causes less peripheral toxicity but more CNS or behavioral side effects when its conversion to dopamine is inhibited outside the CNS. The drug is not effective in antagonizing the akinesia, rigidity, and tremor caused by treatment with antipsychotic agents. Levodopa is a precursor of melanin and may *activate* malignant melanoma. Use of levodopa is not associated with pulmonary dysfunction. The answer is **B.**

3. Ropinirole is a dopamine D_2 receptor activator and does not require bioactivation. Confusion, delusions, and hallucinations occur more frequently with dopamine receptor activators than with levodopa. The use of dopaminergic agents in combination with antimuscarinic drugs is common in the treatment of parkinsonism. Ropinirole is metabolized by hepatic CYP1A2, and its plasma levels may be increased by other substrates of this enzyme including caffeine and warfarin. The answer is **E.**

4. The form and severity of dyskinesias resulting from levodopa may vary widely in individual patients. Dyskinesias occur in up to 80% of patients receiving levodopa for long periods. With continued treatment, dyskinesias may develop at a dose of levodopa that was previously well tolerated. Muscarinic receptor blockers do not prevent their occurrence. They occur more commonly in patients treated with levodopa in combination with carbidopa or with other dopamine receptor agonists. The answer is **C.**

5. Apomorphine, via subcutaneous injection, is used for temporary relief of off-periods of akinesia ("rescue") in parkinsonian patients on dopaminergic drug therapy. Pretreatment with the antiemetic trimethobenzamide for 3 days is essential to prevent severe nausea. The answer is **A.**

6. The non-ergot dopamine agonists (pramipexole, ropinirole) are commonly used prior to levodopa in mild parkinsonism. The mydriatic action of levodopa may increase intraocular pressure; the drug should be used cautiously in patients with open-angle glaucoma and is contraindicated in those with angle-closure glaucoma. Antimuscarinic drugs may improve the tremor and rigidity of parkinsonism but have little effect on bradykinesia. Selegiline is a selective inhibitor of MAO type B. The answer is **B.**

7. Although further diagnosis is desirable, choreoathetosis with decreased mental abilities and psychosis (paranoia) suggests that this patient has the symptoms of Huntington's disease. Drugs that are partly ameliorative include agents that deplete dopamine (eg, tetrabenazine) or that block dopaminergic receptors (eg, haloperidol). The answer is **E.**

8. Ropinirole is a non-ergot agonist at dopamine receptors and has greater selectivity for D_2 receptors in the striatum. Ropinirole (or the D_3 receptor antagonist pramipexole) is often chosen for monotherapy of mild parkinsonism, and these drugs sometimes have value in patients who have become refractory to levodopa. Adverse effects of these drugs include dyskinesias, postural hypotension, and somnolence. The answer is **E.**

9. Entacapone is an inhibitor of COMT used adjunctively in patients treated with levodopa-carbidopa. The drug decreases the formation of 3-O-methyldopa (3-OMD) from levodopa. This can improve patient response by increasing levodopa levels and by decreasing competition between 3-OMD and levodopa for active transport into the brain by L-amino acid carrier mechanism. The answer is **B.**

10. Increased activation of β adrenoceptors has been implicated in essential tremor, and management commonly involves administration of propranolol. However, the more selective β_1 blocker metoprolol is equally effective and is more suitable in a patient with pulmonary disease. The answer is **C.**

SKILL KEEPER ANSWERS: AUTONOMIC DRUG SIDE EFFECTS (SEE CHAPTERS 8 AND 9)

Pharmacologic strategy in Parkinson's disease involves attempts to enhance dopamine functions or antagonize acetylcholine at muscarinic receptors. Thus, peripheral adverse effects must be anticipated.

1. *Adverse effects referable to activation of peripheral dopamine (or adrenoceptors in the case of levodopa) include postural hypotension, tachycardia (possible arrhythmias), mydriasis, and emetic responses.*

2. *Adverse effects referable to antagonism of peripheral muscarinic receptors include dry mouth, mydriasis, urinary retention, and cardiac arrhythmias.*

CHECKLIST

When you complete this chapter, you should be able to:

❑ Describe the neurochemical imbalance underlying the symptoms of Parkinson's disease.

❑ Identify the mechanisms by which levodopa, dopamine receptor agonists, selegiline, and muscarinic blocking drugs alleviate parkinsonism.

❑ Describe the therapeutic and toxic effects of the major antiparkinsonism agents.

❑ Identify the compounds that inhibit dopa decarboxylase and COMT and describe their use in parkinsonism.

❑ Identify the chemical agents and drugs that cause parkinsonism symptoms.

❑ Identify the most important drugs used in the management of tremor, Huntington's disease, drug-induced dyskinesias, restless legs syndrome, and Wilson's disease.

DRUG SUMMARY TABLE: Drugs Used for Movement Disorders

Subclass	Mechanism of Action	Clinical Applications	Pharmacokinetics	Toxicities
Levodopa (+/– carbidopa)	Precursor of dopamine Carbidopa inhibits peripheral metabolism via dopa decarboxylase	Primary drug used in Parkinson's disease	Oral, COMT and MAO type B inhibitors diminish doses and prolong actions Duration of effects: 6–8 h	GI upsets, dyskinesias, behavioral effects • on-off phenomena
Dopamine agonists				
Pramipexole Ropinirole Apomorphine Bromocriptine (rarely used)	D_2 agonists (apomorphine bromocriptine, and ropinirole) • D_3 agonist (pramipexole)	Pramipexole and ropinirole used as sole agents in early Parkinson's disease and adjunct to L-dopa • apomorphine "rescue" therapy	Oral • pramipexole: short half-life (tid dosing), renal elimination Ropinirole, CYP1A2 metabolism • drug interactions possible	Anorexia, nausea, constipation postural hypotension, dyskinesias, mental disturbances
MAO inhibitors				
Rasagiline Selegiline	Inhibit MAO type B	Rasagiline for early PD Both drugs adjunctive with L-dopa	Oral • half-lives permit bid dosing	Serotonin syndrome with meperidine and possibly SSRIs and TCAs

(Continued)

DRUG SUMMARY TABLE: Drugs Used for Movement Disorders (*Continued*)

Subclass	Mechanism of Action	Clinical Applications	Pharmacokinetics	Toxicities
COMT inhibitors				
Entacapone Tolcapone	Block L-dopa metabolism in periphery (both) and CNS (tolcapone)	Prolong L-dopa actions Oral		Relates to increased levels of L-dopa
Antimuscarinic agents				
Benztropine, and others	Block M receptors	Improve tremor and rigidity *not* bradykinesia	Oral: once daily	Typical atropine-like side effects
Drugs for Huntington's disease				
Tetrabenazine, reserpine Haloperidol	Tetrabenazine and reserpine: deplete amines Haloperidol: D_2 antagonist	Reduce symptom (eg, chorea) severity	Oral (see Chapter 11) Oral (see Chapter 29)	Tetrabenazine: depression, hypotension, sedation Haloperidol: extrapyramidal dysfunction
Drugs for Tourette's syndrome				
Haloperidol Clonidine	Haloperidol: D_2 receptor blocker Clonidine: α_2 blocker	Reduce vocal and motor tic frequency and severity	Oral Oral	Haloperidol: extrapyramidal dysfunction

COMT, catechol-O-methyltransferase; MAO, monoamine oxidase; SSRIs, selective serotonin reuptake inhibitors; TCAs, tricyclic antidepressants.

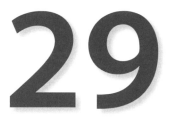

Antipsychotic Agents & Lithium

The antipsychotic drugs (neuroleptics) are used in schizophrenia and are also effective in the treatment of other psychoses and agitated states. Older drugs have high affinity for dopamine D_2 receptors, whereas newer antipsychotic drugs have greater affinity for serotonin $5\text{-}HT_2$ receptors. Although schizophrenia is not cured by drug therapy, the symptoms, including thought disorder, emotional withdrawal, and hallucinations or delusions, may be ameliorated by antipsychotic drugs. Unfortunately, protracted therapy (years) is often needed and can result in severe toxicity in some patients. In bipolar affective disorder, although lithium has been the mainstay of treatment for many years, the use of newer antipsychotic agents and of several antiseizure drugs is increasing.

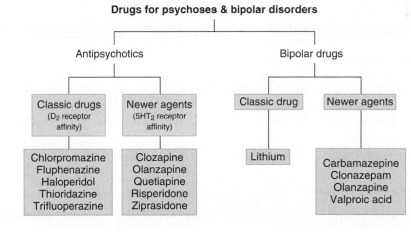

ANTIPSYCHOTIC DRUGS

A. Classification

The major chemical subgroups of older antipsychotic drugs are the **phenothiazines** (eg, chlorpromazine, thioridazine, fluphenazine), the **thioxanthenes** (eg, thiothixene), and the **butyrophenones** (eg, haloperidol).

Newer "second generation" drugs of varied **heterocyclic** structure are also effective in schizophrenia, including clozapine, loxapine, olanzapine, risperidone, quetiapine, ziprasidone, and aripiprazole. In some cases, these atypical antipsychotic drugs may be somewhat more effective and less toxic than the older drugs. However, they are much more costly than standard older drugs, most of which are prescribed generically.

B. Pharmacokinetics

The antipsychotic drugs are well absorbed when given orally, and because they are lipid soluble, they readily enter the central nervous system (CNS) and most other body tissues. Many are bound extensively to plasma proteins. These drugs require metabolism by liver enzymes before elimination and have long plasma half-lives that permit once-daily dosing. In some cases, other drugs that inhibit cytochrome P450 enzymes can prolong the half-lives of antipsychotic agents. Parenteral forms of many agents (eg, fluphenazine, haloperidol) are available for both rapid initiation of therapy and depot treatment.

C. Mechanism of Action

1. The dopamine hypothesis—The dopamine hypothesis of schizophrenia proposes that the disorder is caused by a relative

255

excess of functional activity of the neurotransmitter dopamine in specific neuronal tracts in the brain. This hypothesis is based on several observations. First, many antipsychotic drugs block brain dopamine receptors (especially D_2 receptors). Second, dopamine agonist drugs (eg, amphetamine, levodopa) exacerbate schizophrenia. Third, an increased density of dopamine receptors has been detected in certain brain regions of untreated schizophrenics. The dopamine hypothesis of schizophrenia is not fully satisfactory because antipsychotic drugs are only partly effective in most patients and because many effective drugs have a much higher affinity for other receptors, including serotonin receptors, than for D_2 receptors.

2. Dopamine receptors—Five different dopamine receptors (D_1–D_5) have been characterized. Each is G protein-coupled and contains 7 transmembrane domains. The D_2 receptor, found in the caudate putamen, nucleus accumbens, cerebral cortex, and hypothalamus, is negatively coupled to adenylyl cyclase. The therapeutic efficacy of the older antipsychotic drugs correlates with their relative affinity for the D_2 receptor. Unfortunately, there is also a correlation between blockade of D_2 receptors and extrapyramidal dysfunction.

3. Other receptors—Most of the newer atypical antipsychotic agents have higher affinities for other receptors than for the D_2 receptor. For example, α adrenoceptor-blocking action correlates well with antipsychotic effect for many of the drugs (Table 29–1). Clozapine, a drug with significant D_4 and 5-HT$_2$ receptor-blocking actions, has virtually no affinity for D_2 receptors. Most of the newer atypical drugs (eg, olanzapine, quetiapine, and risperidone) also have high affinity for 5-HT$_{2A}$ receptors, although they may also interact with D_2 and other receptors. Ziprasidone is an antagonist at the D_2, 5-HT$_{2A}$, and 5-HT$_{1D}$ receptors and an agonist at the 5-HT$_{1A}$ receptor.

The newer antipsychotic agent aripiprazole is a partial agonist at D_2 and 5-HT$_{1A}$ receptors but is a strong antagonist at 5-HT$_{2A}$ receptors. The receptor-binding characteristics of the newer antipsychotic drugs have led to a serotonin hypothesis as an alternative to the dopamine hypothesis of the nature of schizophrenia. Most of the atypical drugs cause less extrapyramidal dysfunction than standard drugs. With the exception of haloperidol, all antipsychotic drugs block H_1 receptors to some degree.

D. Effects

Dopamine receptor blockade is the major effect that correlates with therapeutic benefit for older antipsychotic drugs. Dopaminergic tracts in the brain include the mesocortical-mesolimbic pathways (regulating mentation and mood), nigrostriatal tract (extrapyramidal function), tuberoinfundibular pathways (control of prolactin release), and chemoreceptor trigger zone (emesis). Mesocortical-mesolimbic dopamine receptor blockade presumably underlies antipsychotic effects, and a similar action on the chemoreceptor trigger zone leads to the useful antiemetic properties of some antipsychotic drugs. Adverse effects resulting from receptor blockade in the other dopaminergic tracts, a major problem with older antipsychotic drugs, include extrapyramidal dysfunction and hyperprolactinemia (see later discussion). Note that almost all antipsychotic agents block both α_1 and histamine H_1 receptors to some extent. The relative receptor-blocking actions of various antipsychotic drugs are shown in Table 29–1.

E. Clinical Use

1. Treatment of schizophrenia—Antipsychotic drugs reduce some of the positive symptoms of schizophrenia, including hyperactivity, bizarre ideation, hallucinations, and delusions. Consequently,

TABLE 29–1 Relative receptor-blocking actions of neuroleptic drugs.

Drug	D_2 Block	D_4 Block	Alpha$_1$ Block	5-HT$_2$ Block	M Block	H_1 Block
Most phenothiazines and thioxanthines	++	–	++	+	+	+
Thioridazine	++	–	++	+	+++	+
Haloperidol	+++	–	+	–	–	–
Clozapine	–	++	++	++	++	+
Molindone	++	–	+	–	+	+
Olanzapine	+	–	+	++	+	+
Quetiapine	+	–	+	++	+	+
Risperidone	++	–	+	++	+	+
Ziprasidone	++	–	++	++	–	+
Aripiprazole[a]	+	+	+	++	–	+

[a]Partial agonist at D_2 and 5-HT$_{1A}$ receptors and antagonist activity at 5-HT$_{2A}$ receptors.

+, blockade; –, no effect. The number of plus signs indicates the intensity of receptor blockade.

they can facilitate functioning in both inpatient and outpatient environments. Beneficial effects may take several weeks to develop. Overall efficacy of the antipsychotic drugs is, for the most part, equivalent in terms of the management of the floridly psychotic forms of the illness, although individual patients may respond best to a specific drug. However, clozapine is effective in some schizophrenic patients resistant to treatment with other antipsychotic drugs. Older drugs are still commonly used partly because of their low cost compared with newer agents. However, none of the traditional drugs has much effect on negative symptoms of schizophrenia. Newer atypical drugs are reported to improve some of the negative symptoms of schizophrenia, including emotional blunting, social withdrawal, and lack of motivation.

2. Other psychiatric and neurologic indications—The newer antipsychotic drugs are often used with lithium in the initial treatment of mania. Several second-generation drugs are approved for treatment of acute mania; two of these (aripiprazole and olanzapine) are approved for maintenance treatment of bipolar disorder. The antipsychotic drugs are also used in the management of psychotic symptoms of schizoaffective disorders, in Gilles de la Tourette syndrome, and for management of toxic psychoses caused by overdosage of certain CNS stimulants. Molindone is used mainly in Tourette's syndrome; it is rarely used in schizophrenia. The newer atypical antipsychotics have also been used to allay psychotic symptoms in patients with Alzheimer's disease and in parkinsonism.

3. Nonpsychiatric indications—With the exception of thioridazine, most phenothiazines have antiemetic actions; prochlorperazine is promoted solely for this indication. H_1-receptor blockade, most often present in short side-chain phenothiazines, provides the basis for their use as antipruritics and sedatives and contributes to their antiemetic effects.

F. Toxicity

1. Reversible neurologic effects—Dose-dependent extrapyramidal effects include a Parkinson-like syndrome with bradykinesia, rigidity, and tremor. This toxicity may be reversed by a decrease in dose and may be antagonized by concomitant use of muscarinic blocking agents. Extrapyramidal toxicity occurs most frequently with haloperidol and the more potent piperazine side-chain phenothiazines (eg, fluphenazine, trifluoperazine). Parkinsonism occurs infrequently with clozapine and is much less common with the newer drugs. Other reversible neurologic dysfunctions that occur more frequently with older agents include akathisia and dystonias; these usually respond to treatment with diphenhydramine or muscarinic blocking agents.

2. Tardive dyskinesias—This important toxicity includes choreoathetoid movements of the muscles of the lips and buccal cavity and may be irreversible. Tardive dyskinesias tend to develop after several years of antipsychotic drug therapy but have appeared as early as 6 mo. Antimuscarinic drugs that usually ameliorate other extrapyramidal effects generally *increase* the severity of tardive dyskinesia symptoms. There is no effective drug treatment for tardive dyskinesia. Switching to clozapine does not exacerbate the condition. Tardive dyskinesia may be attenuated *temporarily* by increasing neuroleptic dosage; this suggests that tardive dyskinesia may be caused by dopamine receptor sensitization.

3. Autonomic effects—Autonomic effects result from blockade of peripheral muscarinic receptors and α adrenoceptors and are more difficult to manage in elderly patients. Tolerance to some of the autonomic effects occurs with continued therapy. Of the older antipsychotic agents, thioridazine has the strongest autonomic effects and haloperidol the weakest. Clozapine and most of the atypical drugs have intermediate autonomic effects.

Regarding muscarinic receptor blockade, atropine-like effects (dry mouth, constipation, urinary retention, and visual problems) are often pronounced with the use of thioridazine and phenothiazines with aliphatic side chains (eg, chlorpromazine). These effects also occur with clozapine and most of the atypical drugs but not with ziprasidone or aripiprazole. CNS effects from block of M receptors may include a toxic confusional state similar to that produced by atropine and the tricyclic antidepressants.

Regarding α-receptor blockade, postural hypotension caused by α blockade is a common manifestation of many of the older drugs, especially phenothiazines. In the elderly, measures must be taken to avoid falls resulting from postural fainting. The atypical drugs, especially clozapine and ziprasidone, also block α receptors and can cause orthostatic hypotension. Failure to ejaculate is common in men treated with the phenothiazines.

4. Endocrine and metabolic effects—Endocrine and metabolic effects include hyperprolactinemia, gynecomastia, the amenorrhea-galactorrhea syndrome, and infertility. Most of these side effects are predictable manifestations of dopamine D_2 receptor blockade in the pituitary; dopamine is the normal inhibitory regulator of prolactin secretion. Elevated prolactin is prominent with risperidone. Significant weight gain and hyperglycemia due to a diabetogenic action occur with several of the atypical agents, especially clozapine and olanzapine. These effects may be especially problematic in pregnancy. Aripiprazole and ziprasidone have little or no tendency to cause hyperglycemia, hyperprolactinemia, or weight gain.

5. Neuroleptic malignant syndrome—Patients who are particularly sensitive to the extrapyramidal effects of antipsychotic drugs may develop a malignant hyperthermic syndrome. The symptoms include muscle rigidity, impairment of sweating, hyperpyrexia, and autonomic instability, which may be life threatening. Drug treatment involves the prompt use of dantrolene, diazepam, and dopamine agonists.

6. Sedation—This is more marked with phenothiazines (especially chlorpromazine) than with other antipsychotics; this

TABLE 29–2 Adverse pharmacologic effects antipsychotic drugs.

Type	Manifestations	Mechanism
Autonomic nervous system	Loss of accommodation, dry mouth, difficulty urinating, constipation Orthostatic hypotension, impotence, failure to ejaculate	Muscarinic cholinoceptor blockade α-Adrenoceptor blockade
Central nervous system	Parkinson's syndrome, akathisia, dystonias Tardive dyskinesia Toxic-confusional state	Dopamine-receptor blockade Supersensitivity of dopamine receptors Muscarinic blockade
Endocrine system	Amenorrhea-galactorrhea, infertility, impotence	Dopamine-receptor blockade resulting in hyperprolactinemia
Other	Weight gain	Possibly combined H_1 and 5-HT_2 blockade

Reproduced, with permission, from Katzung BG, editor: *Basic & Clinical Pharmacology*, 12th ed. McGraw-Hill, 2012.

effect is usually perceived as unpleasant by nonpsychotic persons. Fluphenazine and haloperidol are the least sedating of the older drugs; aripiprazole appears to be the least sedating of the newer agents.

7. Miscellaneous toxicities—Visual impairment caused by retinal deposits has occurred with **thioridazine**; at high doses, this drug may also cause severe conduction defects in the heart resulting in fatal ventricular arrhythmias. Most of the atypicals, especially **quetiapine** and **ziprasidone,** prolong the QT interval of the electrocardiogram (ECG); the underlying myocardial effect could lead to cardiac arrhythmias (eg, torsades) in some patients. **Clozapine** causes a small but important (1–2%) incidence of agranulocytosis and at high doses has caused seizures.

8. Overdosage toxicity—Poisoning with antipsychotics other than thioridazine is not usually fatal, although the FDA has warned of an increased risk of death in elderly patients with dementia. Hypotension often responds to fluid replacement. Most neuroleptics lower the convulsive threshold and may cause seizures, which are usually managed with diazepam or phenytoin. Thioridazine (and possibly ziprasidone) overdose, because of cardiotoxicity, is more difficult to treat.

Table 29–2 is a summary of the adverse pharmacologic effects of the antipsychotic drugs.

LITHIUM & OTHER DRUGS USED IN BIPOLAR (MANIC-DEPRESSIVE) DISORDER

Lithium is effective in treatment of the manic phase of bipolar disorder and continues to be used for acute-phase illness and for prevention of recurrent manic and depressive episodes.

A. Pharmacokinetics

Lithium is absorbed rapidly and completely from the gut. The drug is distributed throughout the body water and cleared by the kidneys at a rate one-fifth that of creatinine. The half-life of lithium is about 20 h. Plasma levels should be monitored, especially during the first weeks of therapy, to establish an effective and safe dosage regimen. For acute symptoms, the target therapeutic plasma concentration is 0.8–1.2 mEq/L and for maintenance 0.4–0.7 mEq/L. Plasma levels of the drug may be altered by changes in body water. Dehydration, or treatment with thiazides, nonsteroidal anti-inflammatory drugs (NSAIDs), angiotensin-converting enzyme inhibitors (ACEIs), and loop diuretics, may result in an increase of lithium in the blood to toxic levels. Caffeine and theophylline increase the renal clearance of lithium.

B. Mechanism of Action

The mechanism of action of lithium is not well defined. The drug inhibits several enzymes involved in the recycling of neuronal membrane phosphoinositides. This action may result in depletion of the second messenger source, phosphatidylinositol bisphosphate (PIP_2), which, in turn, would decrease generation of inositol trisphosphate (IP_3) and diacylglycerol (DAG). These second messengers are important in amine neurotransmission, including that mediated by central adrenoceptors and muscarinic receptors (Figure 29–1).

C. Clinical Use

Lithium carbonate continues to be used for the treatment of bipolar disorder (manic-depressive disease) although other drugs including valproic acid and carbamazepine are equally effective (see text that follows). Maintenance therapy with lithium decreases manic behavior and reduces both the frequency and the magnitude of mood swings. Antipsychotic agents and/or benzodiazepines are commonly required at the initiation of treatment because both lithium and valproic acid have a slow onset of action. Olanzapine and quetiapine are both approved as monotherapy for acute mania.

Although lithium has protective effects against suicide and self-harm, antidepressant drugs are often used concurrently during maintenance. Note that monotherapy with antidepressants can precipitate mania in bipolar patients.

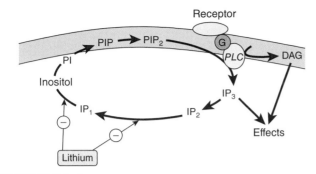

FIGURE 29–1 Postulated effect of lithium on the inositol trisphosphate (IP₃) and diacylglycerol (DAG) second messenger system. The schematic diagram shows the synaptic membrane of a neuron in the brain. PLC, phospholipase C; G, coupling protein; PI, PIP, PIP₂, IP₂, IP₁, intermediates in the production of IP₃. By interfering with this cycle, lithium may cause a use-dependent reduction of synaptic transmission (Reproduced, with permission, from Katzung BG, editor: *Basic & Clinical Pharmacology*, 12th ed. McGraw-Hill, 2012: Fig. 29–4.)

D. Toxicity

Adverse neurologic effects of lithium include tremor, sedation, ataxia, and aphasia. Thyroid enlargement may occur, but hypothyroidism is rare. Reversible nephrogenic diabetes insipidus occurs commonly at therapeutic drug levels. Edema is a common adverse effect of lithium therapy; acneiform skin eruptions occur; and leukocytosis is always present. The issue of dysmorphogenesis is not settled. The use of lithium during pregnancy is thought to increase the incidence of congenital cardiac anomalies (Ebstein's anomaly). Recent analyses suggest that the teratogenic risk is low, but in pregnancy it appears to contribute to low Apgar scores in the neonate. Consequently, lithium should be withheld 24–48 h before delivery, and its use is contraindicated in nursing mothers.

E. Other Drugs Used in Bipolar Disorder

The manic phase in bipolar disorder can be treated with antipsychotic drugs, and both olanzapine and quetiapine are approved as monotherapy for this indication. Several antiseizure drugs are used in bipolar disorder. Valproic acid has antimanic effects equivalent to those of lithium and is now widely used in the Unites States for this indication, often as a first choice in acute illness. Valproic acid may be effective in patients who fail to respond to lithium, and in some instances it has been used in combination with lithium. The antiseizure drugs carbamazepine and lamotrigine are also used both in acute mania and for prophylaxis in the depressive phase. For more information on antiseizure drugs, see Chapter 24.

QUESTIONS

1. Concerning hypotheses for the pathophysiologic basis of schizophrenia, which statement is accurate?
   (A) All clinically effective antipsychotic drugs have high affinity for dopamine D₂ receptors
   (B) Dopamine receptor-blocking drugs are used to alleviate psychotic symptoms in parkinsonism
   (C) Drug-induced psychosis can occur without activation of brain dopamine receptors
   (D) Serotonin receptors are present at lower than normal levels in the brains of untreated schizophrenics
   (E) The clinical potency of clozapine correlates well with its dopamine receptor-blocking activity

2. Trifluoperazine was prescribed for a young male patient diagnosed as suffering from schizophrenia. He complains about the side effects of his medication. Which of the following is *not* likely to be on his list?
   (A) Constipation
   (B) Disinterest in sexual activity
   (C) Dizziness if he stands up too quickly
   (D) Excessive salivation
   (E) Small print in the newspaper is hard to see

3. Which statement concerning the adverse effects of antipsychotic drugs is accurate?
   (A) Acute dystonic reactions occur very infrequently with olanzapine
   (B) Akathisias due to antipsychotic drugs are managed by increasing the drug dose
   (C) Blurring of vision and urinary retention are common adverse effects of haloperidol
   (D) Retinal pigmentation is a dose-dependent toxic effect of clozapine
   (E) The late-occurring choreoathetoid movements caused by conventional antipsychotic drugs are alleviated by atropine

4. Haloperidol is *not* an appropriate drug for management of
   (A) Acute mania
   (B) The amenorrhea-galactorrhea syndrome
   (C) Phencyclidine intoxication
   (D) Schizoaffective disorders
   (E) Tourette's syndrome

5. Which statement concerning the use of lithium in the treatment of bipolar affective disorder is accurate?
   (A) Excessive intake of sodium chloride enhances the toxicity of lithium
   (B) Lithium alleviates the manic phase of bipolar disorder within 12 h
   (C) Lithium dosage may need to be decreased in patients taking thiazides
   (D) Since lithium does not cross the placental barrier, it is quite safe in pregnancy
   (E) The elimination rate of lithium is equivalent to that of creatinine

6. A 30-year-old male patient is on drug therapy for a psychiatric problem. He complains that he feels "flat" and that he gets confused at times. He has been gaining weight and has lost his sex drive. As he moves his hands, you notice a slight tremor. He tells you that since he has been on medication he is always thirsty and frequently has to urinate. The drug he is most likely to be taking is
(A) Carbamazepine
(B) Clozapine
(C) Fluphenazine
(D) Lithium
(E) Valproic acid

7. A young male patient recently diagnosed as schizophrenic develops severe muscle cramps with torticollis a short time after drug therapy is initiated with haloperidol. The best course of action would be to
(A) Add risperidone to the drug regimen
(B) Discontinue haloperidol and observe the patient
(C) Give oral diphenhydramine
(D) Inject benztropine
(E) Switch the patient to fluphenazine

8. Which of the following drugs is established to be both effective and safe to use in a pregnant patient suffering from bipolar disorder?
(A) Carbamazepine
(B) Chlorpromazine
(C) Lithium
(D) Quetiapine
(E) Valproic acid

9. In comparing the characteristics of thioridazine with other older antipsychotic drugs, which of the following statements is accurate?
(A) Most likely to cause extrapyramidal dysfunction
(B) Least likely to cause urinary retention
(C) Most likely to be safe in patients with history of cardiac arrhythmias
(D) Most likely to cause ocular dysfunction
(E) The safest antipsychotic drug in overdose

10. Which of the following drugs has a high affinity for 5-HT$_2$ receptors in the brain, does not cause extrapyramidal dysfunction or hematotoxicity, and is reported to increase the risk of significant QT prolongation?
(A) Clozapine
(B) Haloperidol
(C) Molindone
(D) Olanzapine
(E) Ziprasidone

ANSWERS

1. Although most older antipsychotic drugs block D$_2$ receptors, this action is not a requirement for antipsychotic action. Aripiprazole, clozapine, and most newer second-generation drugs have a very low affinity for such receptors, but a high affinity for serotonin 5-HT$_2$ receptors. There are no reports of changed levels of serotonin in the brains of schizophrenics. The CNS effects of phencyclidine (PCP) closely parallel an acute schizophrenic episode, but PCP has no actions on brain dopamine receptors. Dopamine receptor blockers *cause* extrapyramidal dysfunction. The answer is **C.**

2. Phenothiazines such as trifluoperazine cause sedation and are antagonists at muscarinic and α adrenoceptors. Postural hypotension, blurring of vision, and dry mouth are common autonomic adverse effects, as is constipation Effects on the male libido may result from increased prolactin or from increased peripheral conversion of androgens to estrogens. The answer is **D.**

3. Olanzapine has minimal dopamine receptor-blocking action and is unlikely to cause acute dystonias. Muscarinic blockers such as atropine exacerbate tardive dyskinesias. Akathisias (uncontrollable restlessness) resulting from antipsychotic drugs may be relieved by a *reduction* in dosage. Retinal pigmentation may occur with thioridazine, not clozapine. The answer is **A.**

4. In addition to its use in schizophrenia and acute mania, haloperidol has been used in the management of intoxication due to phencyclidine (PCP) and in Tourette's syndrome. Hyperprolactinemia and the amenorrhea-galactorrhea syndrome may occur as *adverse* effects during treatment with antipsychotic drugs, especially those like haloperidol that strongly antagonize dopamine receptors in the tuberoinfundibular tract. The answer is **B.**

5. Clinical effects of lithium are slow in onset and may not be apparent before 1 or 2 weeks of daily treatment. High urinary levels of sodium inhibit renal tubular reabsorption of lithium, thus *decreasing* its plasma levels. Lithium clearance is decreased by distal tubule diuretics (eg, thiazides) because natriuresis stimulates a reflex increase in the proximal tubule reabsorption of both lithium and sodium. Any drug that can cross the blood-brain barrier can cross the placental barrier! Teratogenic risk is low, but use of lithium during pregnancy may contribute to low Apgar score in the neonate. The answer is **C**.

6. Confusion, mood changes, decreased sexual interest, and weight gain are symptoms that may be unrelated to drug administration. On the other hand, psychiatric drugs are often responsible for such symptoms. Tremor and symptoms of nephrogenic diabetes insipidus are characteristic adverse effects of lithium that may occur at blood levels within the therapeutic range. The answer is **D**.

7. Acute dystonic reactions are usually very painful and should be treated immediately with parenteral administration of a drug that blocks muscarinic receptors such as benztropine. Adding risperidone is not protective, and fluphenazine is as likely as haloperidol to cause acute dystonia. Oral administration of diphenhydramine is a possibility, but the patient may find it difficult to swallow and it would take a longer time to act. The answer is **D**.

8. Carbamazepine and valproic acid are effective in bipolar disorder but are contraindicated in the pregnant patient because of possible effects on fetal development. Although the potential for dysmorphogenesis due to lithium is probably low, the most conservative approach would be to treat the patient with quetiapine or olanzapine. Chlorpromazine has no proven efficacy in bipolar disorder. The answer is **D**.

9. Atropine-like side effects are more prominent with thioridazine than with other phenothiazines, but the drug is less likely to cause extrapyramidal dysfunction. The drug has quinidine-like actions on the heart and, in overdose, may cause arrhythmias and cardiac conduction block with fatality. At high doses, thioridazine causes retinal deposits, which in advanced cases resemble retinitis pigmentosa. The patient may complain of browning of vision. The answer is **D**.

10. Many of the newer antipsychotic drugs have a greater affinity for 5-HT$_2$ receptors than dopamine receptors. However, because clozapine is hematotoxic, the choice comes down to olanzapine and ziprasidone, both of which block 5-HT receptors. Of the currently available atypical antipsychotic drugs, ziprasidone carries the greatest risk of QT prolongation. The answer is **E**.

SKILL KEEPER ANSWERS: RECEPTOR MECHANISMS (SEE CHAPTERS 2, 6, AND 21)

1. D_2: G_i linked ↓ cAMP
2. M_3: G_q linked ↑ IP$_3$ and DAG
3. Alpha$_1$: G_q linked ↑ IP$_3$ and DAG
4. 5-HT$_{2A}$: G_q linked ↑ IP$_3$ and DAG

CHECKLIST

When you complete this chapter, you should be able to:

❑ Describe the "dopamine hypothesis" of schizophrenia.

❑ Identify 4 receptors blocked by antipsychotic drugs.

❑ Describe the relationship of receptor-blocking actions to the pharmacodynamics of both the older and the newer (atypical) antipsychotics.

❑ Identify the established toxicities of each of the following drugs: chlorpromazine, clozapine, haloperidol, thioridazine, ziprasidone.

❑ Describe tardive dyskinesia and the neuroleptic malignant syndrome.

❑ Identify the distinctive pharmacokinetic features of lithium, and list its adverse effects and toxicities.

❑ List the "alternative" drugs used in bipolar disorder.

DRUG SUMMARY TABLE: Antipsychotics and Lithium

Subclass	Mechanism of Action	Effects	Clinical Applications	Pharmacokinetics and Interactions	Toxicities
Phenothiazines					
Chlorpromazine Fluphenazine Thioridazine **Thioxanthene** Thiothixene	Block of D_2 receptors >> $5\text{-}HT_2$ receptors	Block α, M, and H_1 receptors • sedation, decreased seizure threshold	Schizophrenia • bipolar disorder (manic phase), antiemesis, preop sedation	Oral and parenteral forms, hepatic metabolism, long half-life	Extensions of α- and M receptor-blocking actions • extrapyramidal dysfunction, tardive dyskinesias, hyperprolactinemia
Butyrophenone					
Haloperidol	Block of D_2 receptors >> $5\text{-}HT_2$ receptors	Some α block • less M block and sedation than phenothiazines	Schizophrenia; bipolar disorder (manic phase), Huntington's chorea, Tourette's syndrome	Oral and parenteral forms • hepatic metabolism	Extrapyramidal dysfunction (major)
Atypicals					
Aripiprazole Clozapine Olanzapine Quetiapine Risperidone Ziprasidone	Block of $5\text{-}HT_2$ receptors >> D_2 receptors	Some α block (clozapine, risperidone, ziprasidone) and M block (clozapine, olanzapine), variable H_1 block	Schizophrenia (positive and negative symptoms) • bipolar disorder (olanzapine, risperidone), major depression (aripiprazole), agitation in Alzheimer's and Parkinson's	Oral and parenteral forms • hepatic metabolism	Agranulocytosis (clozapine) • diabetes and weight gain (clozapine, olanzapine), hyperprolactinemia (risperidone) • QT prolongation (ziprasidone)
Lithium					
	Uncertain, suppresses IP_3 and DAG signaling	No specific actions on ANS receptors or specific CNS receptors • no sedation	Bipolar affective disorder • prevents mood swings (prophylaxis)	Renal elimination, half-life 20 h • narrow therapeutic window— monitor blood levels • clearance decreased by thiazides and NSAIDs	Tremor, edema, hypothyroidism, renal dysfunction • pregnancy category D
Newer drugs for bipolar affective disorder					
Carbamazepine Lamotrigine Valproic acid	Unclear re: bipolar disorder • see Chapter 24 for antiepileptic drug mechanism	Ataxia and diplopia (carbamazepine) • nausea, dizziness, and headache (lamotrigine) • gastrointestinal distress, weight gain, alopecia (valproic acid)	Valproic acid competes with lithium as first choice in bipolar disorder, acute phase • others also used in acute phase and for prophylaxis in depressive phase	Carbamazepine forms active metabolite (phase I); lamotrigine and valproic acid form conjugates (phase II)	Hematotoxicity and induction of drug metabolism (carbamazepine) • rash (lamotrigine) • hepatic dysfunction, weight gain, and inhibition of drug metabolism (valproic acid)

ANS, autonomic nervous system; DAG, diacylglycerol; $5\text{-}HT_2$, serotonin type 2; IP_3, inositol triphosphate; NSAIDs, nonsteroidal anti-inflammatory drugs.

Antidepressants

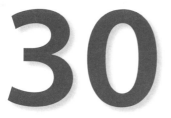

Major depressive disorder, or endogenous depression, is a depression of mood without any obvious medical or situational causes, manifested by an inability to cope with ordinary events or experience pleasure. The drugs used in major depressive disorder are of varied chemical structures; many have effects that enhance the CNS actions of norepinephrine, serotonin, or both.

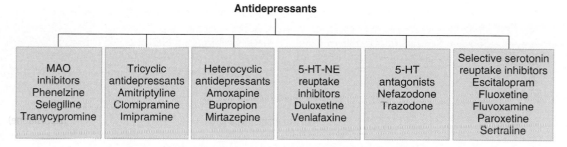

THE AMINE HYPOTHESIS OF MOOD

The **amine hypothesis of mood** postulates that brain amines, particularly norepinephrine (NE) and serotonin (5-HT), are neurotransmitters in pathways that function in the expression of mood. According to the hypothesis, a functional decrease in the activity of such amines is thought to result in depression; a functional increase of activity results in mood elevation. The amine hypothesis is largely based on studies showing that many drugs capable of alleviating symptoms of major depressive disorders enhance the actions of the central nervous system (CNS) neurotransmitters 5-HT and NE. Difficulties with this hypothesis include the facts that (1) postmortem studies do not reveal any decreases in the brain levels of NE or 5-HT in patients suffering from depression; (2) although antidepressant drugs may cause changes in brain amine activity within hours, weeks may be required for them to achieve clinical effects; (3) most antidepressants ultimately cause a *down*regulation of amine receptors; and (4) at least 1 effective antidepressant, bupropion, has minimal effects on brain NE or 5-HT.

DRUG CLASSIFICATION & PHARMACOKINETICS

A. Tricyclic Antidepressants

Tricyclic antidepressants (TCAs; eg, **imipramine, amitriptyline**) are structurally related to the phenothiazine antipsychotics and share certain of their pharmacologic effects. The TCAs are well absorbed orally but may undergo first-pass metabolism. They have high volumes of distribution and are not readily dialyzable. Extensive hepatic metabolism is required before their elimination; plasma half-lives of 8–36 h usually permit once-daily dosing. Both amitriptyline and imipramine form active metabolites, nortriptyline and desipramine, respectively.

B. Selective Serotonin Reuptake Inhibitors

Fluoxetine is the prototype of a group of drugs that are selective serotonin reuptake inhibitors (SSRIs). All of them require hepatic metabolism and have half-lives of 18–24 h. However, fluoxetine forms an active metabolite with a half-life of several days (the basis for a once-weekly formulation). Other members of this

Amine hypothesis of mood	The hypothesis that major depressive disorders result from a functional deficiency of norepinephrine or serotonin at synapses in the CNS
MAO inhibitors (MAOIs)	Drugs inhibiting monoamine oxidases that metabolize norepinephrine and serotonin MAO type A) and dopamine (MAO type B)
Tricyclic antidepressants (TCAs)	Structurally related drugs that block reuptake transporters of both norepinephrine (NE) and serotonin (5-HT)
Selective serotonin reuptake inhibitors (SSRIs)	Drugs that selectively inhibit serotonin (5-HT) transporters with only modest effects on other neurotransmitters
Serotonin-norepinephrine reuptake inhibitors (SNRIs)	Heterocyclic drugs that block NE and 5-HT transporters, but lack the alpha blocking, anticholinergic and antihistaminic actions of TCAs
5-HT$_2$ receptor antagonists	Structurally related drugs that block this subgroup of serotonin receptors with only minor effects on amine transporters
Heterocyclics	Term used for antidepressants of varying chemical structures, the characteristics of which do not strictly conform to any of the above designations

group (eg, **citalopram, escitalopram, fluvoxamine, paroxetine,** and **sertraline**) do not form long-acting metabolites.

C. Heterocyclics

These drugs have varied structures and include drugs that are serotonin-norepinephrine reuptake inhibitors (SNRIs, **duloxetine, venlafaxine**), 5-HT$_2$ receptor antagonists (**nefazodone, trazodone**) and miscellaneous other heterocyclic agents including **amoxapine, bupropion, maprotiline,** and **mirtazapine.** The pharmacokinetics of most of these agents are similar to those of the TCAs. Nefazodone and trazodone are exceptions; their half-lives are short and usually require administration 2 or 3 times daily.

D. Monoamine Oxidase Inhibitors

Monoamine oxidase inhibitors (MAOIs; eg, **phenelzine, tranylcypromine**) are structurally related to amphetamines and are orally active. The older, standard drugs inhibit both MAO-A (monoamine oxidase type A), which metabolizes NE, 5-HT, and tyramine, and MAO-B (monoamine oxidase type A), which metabolizes dopamine. Tranylcypromine is the fastest in onset of effect but has a shorter duration of action (about 1 week) than other MAOIs (2–3 weeks). In spite of these prolonged actions, the MAOIs are given daily. They are inhibitors of hepatic drug-metabolizing enzymes and cause drug interactions. Selegiline, a selective inhibitor of MAO type B, was recently approved for treatment of depression.

MECHANISMS OF ANTIDEPRESSANT ACTION

Potential sites of action of antidepressants at CNS synapses are shown in Figure 30–1. By means of several mechanisms, most antidepressants cause potentiation of the neurotransmitter actions of NE, 5-HT, or both. However, nefazodone and trazodone are weak inhibitors of NE and 5-HT transporters, and their main action appears to be antagonism of the 5-HT$_{2A}$ receptor. Long-term use of tricyclics and MAOIs, but not SSRIs, leads to *down-regulation* of β receptors.

A. TCAs

The acute effect of tricyclic drugs is to inhibit the reuptake mechanisms (transporters) responsible for the termination of the synaptic actions of both NE and 5-HT in the brain. This presumably results in potentiation of their neurotransmitter actions at postsynaptic receptors.

B. SSRIs

The acute effect of SSRIs is a highly selective action on the serotonin transporter (SERT). SSRIs allosterically inhibit the transporter, binding at a site other than that of serotonin. They have minimal inhibitory effects on the NE transporter, or blocking actions on adrenergic and cholinergic receptors.

C. SNRIs

SNRIs bind to transporters for both serotonin and NE, presumably enhancing the actions of both neurotransmitters. Venlafaxine has less affinity for the NE transporter than desvenlafaxine or duloxetine. The SNRIs differ from the TCAs in lacking significant blocking effects on peripheral receptors including histamine H$_1$, muscarinic, or α-adrenergic receptors.

D. Serotonin 5-HT$_2$ Receptor Antagonists

The major antidepressant actions of nefazodone and trazodone appear to result from block of the 5-HT$_{2A}$ receptor, a G protein-coupled receptor located in several CNS regions including the neocortex. Antagonism of this receptor is equated with both the antianxiety and antidepressant actions of these drugs.

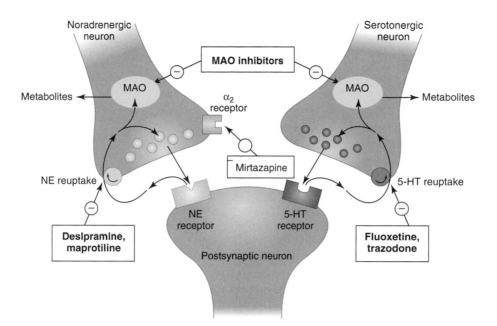

FIGURE 30–1 Possible sites of action of antidepressant drugs. Inhibition of neuronal uptake of norepinephrine (NE) and serotonin (5-HT) increases the synaptic activities of these neurotransmitters. Inhibition of monoamine oxidase increases the presynaptic stores of both NE and 5-HT, which leads to increased neurotransmitter effects. Blockade of the presynaptic α$_2$ autoreceptor prevents feedback inhibition of the release of NE. **Note:** *These are acute actions of antidepressants.*

E. Other Heterocyclic Antidepressants

Mirtazapine has a unique action to increase amine release from nerve endings by antagonism of presynaptic α$_2$ adrenoceptors involved in feedback inhibition. The drug is also an antagonist at serotonin 5-HT$_2$ receptors. The mechanism of antidepressant action of bupropion is unknown—the drug has no effect on either 5-HT or NE receptors or on amine transporters.

F. MAOIs

The MAOIs increase brain amine levels by interfering with their metabolism in the nerve endings, resulting in an increase in the vesicular stores of NE and 5-HT. When neuronal activity discharges the vesicles, increased amounts of the amines are released, presumably enhancing the actions of these neurotransmitters.

PHARMACOLOGIC EFFECTS

A. Amine Uptake Blockade

The drugs that block NE transporters in the CNS (eg, tricyclics, maprotiline, venlafaxine) also inhibit the reuptake of NE at nerve endings in the autonomic nervous system. Likewise, MAOIs increase NE in sympathetic nerve terminals. In both cases, this can lead to peripheral autonomic sympathomimetic effects. However, long-term use of MAOIs can decrease blood pressure.

B. Sedation

Sedation is a common CNS effect of tricyclic drugs and some heterocyclic agents, especially mirtazapine and the 5-HT$_2$ receptor

antagonists nefazodone and trazodone (Table 30–1), the latter commonly prescribed for this purpose and as a sleeping aid. MAOIs, SSRIs, and bupropion are more likely to cause CNS-stimulating effects.

C. Muscarinic Receptor Blockade

Antagonism of muscarinic receptors occurs with all tricyclics and is particularly marked with amitriptyline and doxepin (Table 30–1). Atropine-like adverse effects may also occur with nefazodone, amoxapine, and maprotiline. Atropine-like effects are minimal with the other heterocyclics, the SSRIs, and bupropion.

D. Cardiovascular Effects

Cardiovascular effects occur most commonly with tricyclics and include hypotension from α-adrenoceptor blockade and depression of cardiac conduction. The latter effect may lead to arrhythmias. There have been reports of cardiotoxicity with overdose of venlafaxine.

E. Seizures

Because the convulsive threshold is lowered by TCAs and MAOIs, seizures may occur with overdoses of these agents. Overdoses of maprotiline and the SSRIs have also caused seizures.

CLINICAL USES

A. Major Depressive Disorders

Major depression is the primary clinical indication for antidepressant drugs. Patients typically vary in their responsiveness to

TABLE 30–1 Pharmacodynamic characteristics of selected antidepressants.

Drug	Sedation	Muscarinic Receptor Block	NE Reuptake Block	5-HT Reuptake Block
Tricyclics				
Amitriptyline[a]	+++	+++	+	++
Desipramine	+	+	+++	+
Doxepin[a]	+	++	+++	+
Imipramine	++	++	+	++
Nortriptyline	++	+	++	+
SSRIs				
Citalopram, etc	0	0	0	+++
Heterocyclics—SNRIs				
Duloxetine	0	0	++	+++
Venlafaxine	0	0	+	+++
Heterocyclics—5-HT₂ antagonists				
Nefazodone	++	+	0/+	+
Trazodone	++	0	0	+
Heterocyclics—other				
Amoxapine	++	++	++	+
Bupropion	0	0	0	0
Maprotiline	+	+	++	0
Mirtazapine[b]	++	++	+	0

SNRI, serotonin-norepinephrine reuptake inhibitor.

[a]Significant α_1 antagonism.

[b]Significant H_1 and α_2 antagonism.

0/+, minimal activity; +, mild activity; ++, moderate activity; +++, high activity.

individual agents. Because of more tolerable side effects and safety in overdose (see later discussion), the newer drugs (SSRIs, SNRIs, 5-HT antagonists, and certain heterocyclics) are now the most widely prescribed agents. However, none of the newer antidepressants has been shown to be more effective overall than tricyclic drugs. As alternative agents, tricyclic drugs continue to be most useful in patients with psychomotor retardation, sleep disturbances, poor appetite, and weight loss. MAOIs are thought to be most useful in patients with significant anxiety, phobic features, and hypochondriasis. Selegiline, the MAO type B inhibitor used in parkinsonism (see Chapter 28), is now available in a skin-patch formulation for treatment of depression. SSRIs may decrease appetite; overweight patients often lose weight on these drugs, at least during the first 6–12 months of treatment. Concerns have been expressed that SSRIs, SNRIs, and newer heterocyclics may increase suicide risk in children and adolescents.

B. Other Clinical Uses

TCAs are also used in the treatment of bipolar affective disorders, acute panic attacks, phobic disorders (compare with alprazolam; Chapter 22), enuresis, attention deficit hyperkinetic disorder, and chronic pain states. The SNRIs (eg, duloxetine, venlafaxine) are effective in patients with neuropathic pain and fibromyalgia; duloxetine is also approved for the pain of diabetic neuropathy. Clomipramine and the SSRIs are effective in obsessive-compulsive disorders. SSRIs are approved for patients who suffer from generalized anxiety disorders, panic attacks, social phobias, post-traumatic stress disorder, bulimia, and premenstrual dysphoric disorder, and they may also be useful in the treatment of alcohol dependence. Bupropion is used for management of patients attempting to withdraw from nicotine dependence.

TOXICITY & DRUG INTERACTIONS

A. TCAs

The adverse effects of TCAs are largely predictable from their pharmacodynamic actions. These include (1) excessive sedation, lassitude, fatigue, and, occasionally, confusion; (2) sympathomimetic effects, including tachycardia, agitation, sweating, and insomnia; (3) atropine-like effects; (4) orthostatic hypotension, electrocardiogram (ECG) abnormalities, and cardiomyopathies; (5) tremor and paresthesias; and (6) weight gain. Overdosage with tricyclics is extremely hazardous, and the ingestion of as little as a 2-week supply has been lethal. Manifestations include (1) agitation, delirium, neuromuscular irritability, convulsions, and coma; (2) respiratory depression and circulatory collapse; (3) hyperpyrexia; and (4) cardiac conduction defects and severe arrhythmias. The "3 Cs"—coma, convulsions, and cardiotoxicity—are characteristic.

Tricyclic drug interactions (Table 30–2) include additive depression of the CNS with other central depressants, including ethanol, barbiturates, benzodiazepines, and opioids. Tricyclics may also cause reversal of the antihypertensive action of guanethidine by blocking its transport into sympathetic nerve endings. Less commonly, tricyclics may interfere with the antihypertensive actions of methylnorepinephrine (the active metabolite of methyldopa) and clonidine.

B. SSRI Toxicity

Fluoxetine and the other SSRIs may cause nausea, headache, anxiety, agitation, insomnia, and sexual dysfunction. Jitteriness can be alleviated by starting with low doses or by adjunctive use of benzodiazepines. Extrapyramidal effects early in treatment may include akathisia, dyskinesias, and dystonic reactions. Seizures are a consequence of gross overdosage. Cardiac effects of citalopram overdose include QT prolongation. A withdrawal syndrome has been described for SSRIs, which includes nausea, dizziness, anxiety, tremor, and palpitations.

Certain SSRIs are inhibitors of hepatic cytochrome P450 isozymes, an action that has led to increased activity of other drugs, including TCAs and warfarin (Table 30–2). Fluoxetine inhibits CYP2D6 and to a lesser extent 3A4 isoforms; fluvoxamine inhibits CYP1A2 and paroxetine CYP2D6. Through its inhibition of CYP2D6, fluoxetine can increase plasma levels of several drugs including dextromethorphan, propranolol, tamoxifen, and the TCAs. Citalopram causes fewer drug interactions than other SSRIs.

A **serotonin syndrome** was first described for an interaction between fluoxetine and an MAOI (see later discussion). This life-threatening syndrome includes severe muscle rigidity, myoclonus, hyperthermia, cardiovascular instability, and marked CNS stimulatory effects, including seizures. Drugs implicated include MAOIs, TCAs, dextromethorphan, meperidine, St. John's wort, and possibly illicit recreational drugs such as MDMA ("ecstasy"). Antiseizure drugs, muscle relaxants, and blockers of 5-HT receptors (eg, cyproheptadine) have been used in the management of the syndrome.

C. Toxicity of SNRIs, 5-HT$_2$ Antagonists, and Heterocyclic Drugs

Mirtazapine causes weight gain and is markedly sedating, as is trazodone. Amoxapine, maprotiline, mirtazapine, and trazodone cause some autonomic effects. Amoxapine is also a dopamine receptor blocker and may cause akathisia, parkinsonism, and the amenorrhea-galactorrhea syndrome. Adverse effects of bupropion include anxiety, agitation, dizziness, dry mouth, aggravation of psychosis, and at high doses, seizures. Seizures and cardiotoxicity are prominent features of overdosage with amoxapine and maprotiline. Venlafaxine causes a dose-dependent increase in blood pressure and has CNS stimulant effects similar to those of the SSRIs. Severe withdrawal symptoms can occur, even after missing a single dose of venlafaxine. Both nefazodone and venlafaxine are inhibitors of cytochrome P450 isozymes. Through its inhibitory action on CYP3A4, nefazodone enhances the actions of several drugs including carbamazepine, clozapine, HMG-CoA reductase inhibitors ("statins"), and TCAs. Though rare, nefazodone has caused life-threatening hepatotoxicity requiring liver transplantation. Duloxetine is also reported to cause liver dysfunction.

TABLE 30–2 Drug interactions involving antidepressants.

Antidepressant	Taken With	Consequence
Fluoxetine	Lithium, TCAs, warfarin	Increased blood levels of second drug
Fluvoxamine	Alprazolam, theophylline, TCAs, warfarin	Increased blood levels of second drug
MAO inhibitors	SSRIs, sympathomimetics, tyramine-containing foods	Hypertensive crisis, serotonin syndrome
Nefazodone	Alprazolam, triazolam	Increased blood levels of second drug
Paroxetine	Theophylline, TCAs, warfarin	Increased blood levels of second drug
Sertraline	TCAs, warfarin	Increased effects of second drug
TCAs	Ethanol, sedative hypnotics	Increased CNS depression

MAO, monoamine oxidase; SSRIs, selective serotonin reuptake inhibitors; TCAs, tricyclic antidepressants.

D. MAOI Toxicity

Adverse effects of the traditional MAOIs include hypertensive reactions in response to indirectly acting sympathomimetics, hyperthermia, and CNS stimulation leading to agitation and convulsions. Hypertensive crisis may occur in patients taking MAOIs who consume food that contains high concentrations of the indirect sympathomimetic tyramine. In the absence of indirect sympathomimetics, MAOIs typically *lower* blood pressure; overdosage with these drugs may result in shock, hyperthermia, and seizures. MAOIs administered together with SSRIs have resulted in the **serotonin syndrome.**

QUESTIONS

1. A 36-year-old woman presents with symptoms of major depression that are unrelated to a general medical condition, bereavement, or substance abuse. She is not currently taking any prescription or over-the-counter medications. Drug treatment is to be initiated with paroxetine. In your information to the patient, you would tell her that
   (A) It is preferable that she does not take the drug in the evening
   (B) Muscle cramps and twitches can sometimes occur
   (C) She should tell you if she anticipates using other prescription drugs
   (D) The antidepressant effects of paroxetine may take 2 weeks or more to become effective
   (E) All of the above

2. Concerning the proposed mechanisms of action of antidepressant drugs, which statement is accurate?
   (A) Bupropion inhibits 5-HT reuptake into nerve endings in the CNS
   (B) Chronic treatment with tricyclic antidepressants leads to upregulation of adrenoceptors in the CNS
   (C) Decreased levels of NE and 5-HT in cerebrospinal fluid are characteristic of depressed patients before drug therapy
   (D) Nefazodone blocks 5-HT receptors in the CNS
   (E) Selegiline selectively decreases the metabolism of serotonin

3. A 34-year-old male patient who was prescribed citalopram for depression has decided he wants to stop taking the drug. When questioned, he said that it was affecting his sexual performance. You ascertain that he is also trying to overcome his dependency on tobacco products. If you decide to reinstitute drug therapy in this patient, the best choice would be
   (A) Bupropion
   (B) Fluoxetine
   (C) Imipramine
   (D) Paroxetine
   (E) Venlafaxine

4. Regarding the clinical use of antidepressant drugs, which statement is accurate?
   (A) Chronic use of antidepressants increases the activity of hepatic drug metabolizing enzymes
   (B) In the treatment of major depressive disorders, sertraline is usually more effective than fluoxetine
   (C) Tricyclics are highly effective in depressions with attendant anxiety, phobic features, and hypochondriasis
   (D) Weight gain often occurs during the first few months in patients taking SSRIs
   (E) When selecting an appropriate drug for treatment of depression, the history of patient response to specific drugs is a valuable guide

5. A patient under treatment for a major depressive disorder is brought to the emergency department after ingesting 30 times the normal daily therapeutic dose of amitriptyline. In severe tricyclic antidepressant overdose, it would be of minimal value to
   (A) Administer bicarbonate and potassium chloride (to correct acidosis and hypokalemia)
   (B) Administer lidocaine (to control cardiac arrhythmias)
   (C) Initiate hemodialysis (to hasten drug elimination)
   (D) Maintain heart rhythm by electrical pacing
   (E) Use intravenous diazepam to control seizures

6. This drug, an antagonist at 5-HT_2 receptors, is widely used for the management of insomnia.
   (A) Citalopram
   (B) Doxepin
   (C) Trazodone
   (D) Triazolam
   (E) Zolpidem

7. A recently bereaved 73-year-old female patient was treated with a benzodiazepine for several weeks after the death of her husband, but she did not like the daytime sedation it caused even at low dosage. Living independently, she has no major medical problems but appears rather infirm for her age and has poor eyesight. Because her depressive symptoms are not abating, you decide on a trial of an antidepressant medication. Which of the following drugs would be the most appropriate choice for this patient?
   (A) Amitriptyline
   (B) Mirtazapine
   (C) Phenelzine
   (D) Sertraline
   (E) Trazodone

8. SSRIs are much less effective than tricyclic antidepressants in the management of
   (A) Bulimia
   (B) Chronic pain of neuropathic origin
   (C) Generalized anxiety disorder
   (D) Obsessive-compulsive disorder
   (E) Premenstrual dysphoric disorder

9. Which of the following drugs is most likely to be of value in obsessive-compulsive disorders?
   (A) Amitriptyline
   (B) Clomipramine
   (C) Doxepin
   (D) Nefazodone
   (E) Venlafaxine

10. To be effective in breast cancer, tamoxifen must be converted to an active form by CYP2D6. Cases of inadequate treatment of breast cancer have occurred when tamoxifen was administered to patients who were being treated with

(A) Bupropion
(B) Clomipramine
(C) Fluoxetine
(D) Imipramine
(E) Phenelzine

ANSWERS

1. All the statements are appropriate regarding the initiation of treatment with fluoxetine or other SSRI in a depressed patient. The SSRIs have CNS-stimulating effects and may cause agitation, anxiety, "the jitters," and insomnia, especially early in treatment. Consequently, the evening is not the best time to take SSRI drugs. The answer is **E.**

2. The mechanism of action of bupropion is unknown, but the drug does not inhibit either NE or 5-HT transporters. Levels of NE and 5-HT metabolites in the cerebrospinal fluid of depressed patients before drug treatment are not higher than normal. *Downregulation* of adrenoceptors appears to be a common feature of chronic treatment of depression with tricyclic drugs such as amitriptyline. Selegiline is a selective inhibitor of MAO-B, the enzyme form that metabolizes dopamine (see Chapter 28). Nefazodone is a highly selective antagonist at the 5-HT$_2$ receptor subtype. The answer is **D.**

3. The SSRIs and venlafaxine (an SNRI) can cause sexual dysfunction with decreased libido, erectile dysfunction, and anorgasmia. TCAs may also decrease libido or prevent ejaculation. Bupropion is the least likely antidepressant to affect sexual performance. The drug is also purportedly useful in withdrawal from nicotine dependence, which could be helpful in this patient. The answer is **A.**

4. No antidepressant has been shown to increase hepatic drug metabolism. MAO inhibitors (not TCAs), though now used infrequently, are the drugs most likely to be effective in depression with attendant anxiety, phobic features and hypochondriasis. SSRIs are usually associated with weight loss, at least during the first 6 months of treatment. There is no evidence that any SSRI is more effective than another, or more effective overall than a tricyclic drug, in treatment of major depressive disorder. The answer is **E.**

5. TCA overdose is a medical emergency. The "3 Cs"—coma, convulsions, and cardiac problems—are the most common causes of death. Widening of the QRS complex on the ECG is a major diagnostic feature of cardiac toxicity. Arrhythmias resulting from cardiac toxicity require the use of drugs with the least effect on cardiac conductivity (eg, lidocaine). Hemodialysis does not increase the rate of elimination of tricyclic antidepressants in overdose. The answer is **C.**

6. Triazolam and zolpidem are effective hypnotic drugs, but they do not act via antagonism of serotonin 5-HT$_2$ receptors. Trazodone is an antagonist at 5-HT$_2$ receptors and has wide use as a sleeping aid, especially in patients with symptoms of affective disorder. The answer is **C.**

7. Older patients are more likely to be sensitive to antidepressant drugs that cause sedation, atropine-like adverse effects, or postural hypotension. Tricyclics and MAO inhibitors cause many autonomic side effects; mirtazapine and trazodone are highly sedating. Sertraline (or another SSRI) is often the best choice in such patients. The answer is **D.**

8. The SSRIs are not effective in chronic pain of neuropathic origin. All the other uses of SSRIs are approved indications with clinical effectiveness equivalent or superior to that of tricyclic drugs. In addition to treatment of chronic pain states and depression, the tricyclics are also used to treat enuresis and attention deficit hyperkinetic disorder. The answer is **B.**

9. Clomipramine, a tricyclic agent, is a more selective inhibitor of 5-HT reuptake than other drugs in its class. This activity appears to be important in the treatment of obsessive-compulsive disorder. However, the SSRIs have now become the drugs of choice for this disorder because they are safer in overdose than tricyclics. The answer is **B.**

10. Fluoxetine is an inhibitor of hepatic cytochromes P450 especially CYP2D6, and to a lesser extent CYP3A4. Dosages of several drugs may need to be reduced if given concomitantly with fluoxetine. In the case of tamoxifen, however, its antineoplastic action is dependent on its conversion to an active metabolite by CYP2D6. The answer is **C.**

CHECKLIST

When you complete this chapter, you should be able to:

❑ Describe the probable mechanisms of action and the major characteristics of TCAs, including receptor interactions, adverse effects (from chronic use and in overdose), drug interactions, and clinical uses.

❑ Identify the drugs classified as SSRIs and SNRIs, and describe their characteristics, including clinical uses, adverse effects and toxicity, and potential drug interactions.

❑ Identify drugs thought to act via block of serotonin receptors, and describe their characteristics including clinical uses, adverse effects and toxicity, and potential drug interactions.

❑ Be aware of the limited role of MAO inhibitors in affective disorders.

DRUG SUMMARY TABLE: Antidepressants

Subclass	Mechanism of Action	Clinical Applications	Pharmacokinetics & Drug Interactions	Toxicities
Tricyclic antidepressants				
Amitriptyline, clomipramine, imipramine, etc	Block norepinephrine (NE) and 5-HT transporters	Major depression (backup), chronic pain, obsessive-compulsive disorder (OCD)—clomipramine	CYP substrates: interactions with inducers and inhibitors Long half-lives	α block, M block, sedation, weight gain • overdose: arrhythmias, seizures
Selective serotonin reuptake inhibitors (SSRIs)				
Citalopram, fluoxetine, paroxetine, sertraline, etc	Block 5-HT transporters	Major depression, anxiety disorders, OCD, PMDD, PTSD, bulimia, etc	CYP 2D6 and 3A4 inhibition (fluoxetine, paroxetine) • 1A2 (fluvoxamine) Half-lives: 15+ h	Sexual dysfunction
Serotonin-norepinephrine reuptake inhibitors (SNRIs)				
Venlafaxine Desvenlafaxine Duloxetine	Block NE and 5-HT transporters	Major depression, chronic pain, fibromyalgia, menopausal symptoms	Half-lives: 10+h	Anticholinergic, sedation, hypertension (venlafaxine)
5-HT$_2$ antagonists				
Nefazodone Trazodone	Block 5-HT$_2$ receptors	Major depression, hypnosis (trazodone)	Usually require bid dosing • CYP3A4 inhibition (nefazodone) Short half-lives	Sedation • modest α and H$_1$ blockade (trazodone)
Other heterocyclics				
Amoxapine Bupropion Maprotiline Mirtazepine	Mirtazepine blocks presynaptic α$_2$ receptors • mechanism of action of others uncertain	Major depression, smoking cessation (bupropion), sedation (mirtazepine)	Extensive hepatic metabolism • CYP2D6 inhibition (bupropion)	Lowers seizure threshold (amoxapine, bupropion) • sedation and weight gain (mirtazepine)
Monoamine oxidase inhibitors (MAOIs)				
Isocarboxazid Phenelzine Selegiline	Inhibit MAO-A and MAO-B • selegiline more active vs MAO-B	Major depression unresponsive to other drugs	Hypertension with tyramine and sympathomimetics Serotonin syndrome with SSRIs Very long half-lives	Hypotension, insomnia

MAO-A, monoamine oxidase type A; MAO-B, monoamine oxidase type B; PMDD, premenstrual dysphoric disorder; OD, overdose; PTSD, post-traumatic stress disorder.

Opioid Analgesics & Antagonists

The opioids include natural opiates and semisynthetic alkaloids derived from the opium poppy, pharmacologically similar synthetic surrogates, and endogenous peptides. On the basis of their interaction with opioid receptors, the drugs are classified as agonists, mixed agonist-antagonists, and antagonists.

Opioid peptides released from nerve endings modulate transmission in the brain and spinal cord and in primary afferents via their interaction with specific receptors. Many of the pharmacologic actions of opiates and synthetic opioid drugs are effected via their interactions with endogenous opioid peptide receptors.

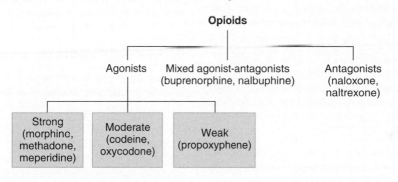

CLASSIFICATION

The opioid analgesics and related drugs are derived from several chemical subgroups and may be classified in several ways.

A. Spectrum of Clinical Uses

Opioid drugs can be subdivided on the basis of their major therapeutic uses (eg, analgesics, antitussives, and antidiarrheal drugs).

B. Strength of Analgesia

On the basis of their relative abilities to relieve pain, the analgesic opioids may be classified as strong, moderate, and weak agonists. Partial agonists are opioids that exert less analgesia than morphine, the prototype of a strong analgesic, or full agonist.

C. Ratio of Agonist to Antagonist Effects

Opioid drugs may be classified as agonists (receptor activators [full or partial]), antagonists (receptor blockers) or mixed agonist-antagonists, which are capable of activating one opioid receptor subtype and blocking another subtype.

PHARMACOKINETICS

A. Absorption and Distribution

Most drugs in this class are well absorbed when taken orally, but morphine, hydromorphone, and oxymorphone undergo extensive first-pass metabolism. In most cases, opioids can be given parenterally, and sustained-release forms of some drugs are now available, including morphine and oxycodone. Opioid drugs are

High-Yield Terms to Learn

Opiate	A drug derived from alkaloids of the opium poppy
Opioid	The class of drugs that includes opiates, opiopeptins, and all synthetic and semisynthetic drugs that mimic the actions of the opiates
Opioid peptides	Endogenous peptides that act on opioid receptors
Opioid agonist	A drug that activates some or all opioid receptor subtypes and does not block any
Partial agonist	A drug that can activate an opioid receptor to effect a submaximal response
Opioid antagonist	A drug that blocks some or all opioid receptor subtypes
Mixed agonist-antagonist	A drug that activates some opioid receptor subtypes and blocks other opioid receptor subtypes

widely distributed to body tissues. They cross the placental barrier and exert effects on the fetus that can result in both respiratory depression and, with continuous exposure, physical dependence in neonates.

B. Metabolism

With few exceptions, the opioids are metabolized by hepatic enzymes, usually to inactive glucuronide conjugates, before their elimination by the kidney. However, morphine-6-glucuronide has analgesic activity equivalent to that of morphine, and morphine-3-glucuronide (the primary metabolite) is neuroexcitatory. Codeine, oxycodone, and hydrocodone are metabolized by cytochrome CYP2D6, an isozyme exhibiting genotypic variability. In the case of codeine, this may be responsible for variability in analgesic response because the drug is demethylated by CYP2D6 to form the active metabolite, morphine. The ingestion of alcohol causes major increases in the peak serum levels of several opioids including hydromorphone and oxymorphone. Meperidine is metabolized to normeperidine, which may cause seizures at high plasma levels. Depending on the specific drug, the duration of their analgesic effects ranges from 1–2 h (eg, fentanyl) to 6–8 h (eg, buprenorphine). However, long-acting formulations of some drugs may provide analgesia for 24 h or more. The elimination half-life of opioids increases in patients with liver disease. Remifentanil, a congener of fentanyl, is metabolized by plasma and tissue esterases and has a very short half-life.

MECHANISMS OF ACTION

A. Receptors

Many of the effects of opioid analgesics have been interpreted in terms of their interactions with specific receptors for endogenous peptides in the CNS and peripheral tissues. Certain opioid receptors are located on primary afferents and spinal cord pain *transmission* neurons (ascending pathways) and on neurons in the midbrain and medulla (descending pathways) that function in pain *modulation* (Figure 31–1). Other opioid receptors that may be involved in altering *reactivity* to pain are located on neurons in the basal ganglia, the hypothalamus, the limbic structures, and the cerebral cortex. Three major opioid receptor subtypes have been extensively characterized pharmacologically: μ, δ, and κ receptors. All 3 receptor subtypes appear to be involved in antinociceptive and analgesic mechanisms at both spinal and supraspinal levels. The μ-receptor activation plays a major role in the respiratory depressant actions of opioids and together with κ-receptor activation slows gastrointestinal transit; κ-receptor activation also appears to be involved in sedative actions; δ-receptor activation may play a role in the development of tolerance.

B. Opioid Peptides

Opioid receptors are thought to be activated by endogenous peptides under physiologic conditions. These peptides, which include endorphins such as β-endorphin, enkephalins, and dynorphins, are synthesized in the soma and are transported to the nerve endings where they accumulate in synaptic vesicles. On release from nerve endings, they bind to opioid receptors and can be displaced from binding by opioid antagonists. Endorphins have highest affinity for μ receptors, enkephalins for δ receptors, and dynorphins for κ receptors. Although it remains unclear whether these peptides function as classic neurotransmitters, they appear to modulate transmission at many sites in the brain and spinal cord and in primary afferents. Opioid peptides are also found in the adrenal medulla and neural plexus of the gut.

C. Ionic Mechanisms

Opioid analgesics *inhibit* synaptic activity partly through direct activation of opioid receptors and partly through release of the endogenous opioid peptides, which are themselves inhibitory to neurons. All 3 major opioid receptors are coupled to their effectors by G proteins and activate phospholipase C or inhibit adenylyl cyclase. At the postsynaptic level, activation of these receptors can open potassium ion channels to cause membrane hyperpolarization (inhibitory postsynaptic potentials). At the presynaptic level, opioid receptor activation can close voltage-gated calcium ion channels to inhibit neurotransmitter release (Figure 31–2). Presynaptic actions result in the inhibition of release of multiple neurotransmitters, including acetylcholine (ACh), norepinephrine, serotonin, glutamate, and substance P.

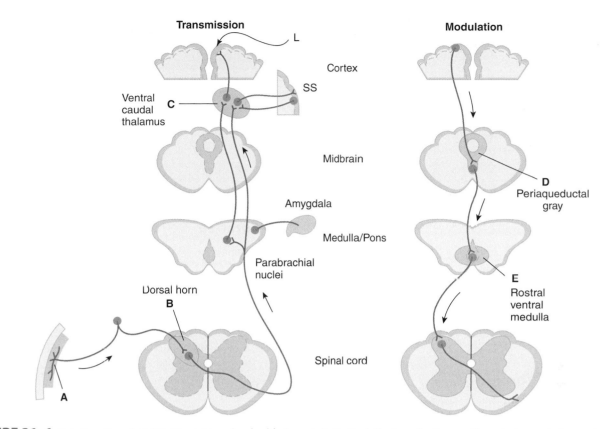

FIGURE 31–1 Putative sites of action of opioid analgesics (*darker color*). On the left, sites of action on the pain transmission pathway from the periphery to the higher centers are shown. **(A)** Direct action of opioids on inflamed or damaged peripheral tissues. **(B)** Inhibition also occurs in the spinal cord. **(C)** Possible sites of action in the thalamus. Different thalamic regions project to somatosensory (SS) or limbic (L) cortex. Parabrachial nuclei (medulla/pons) project to the amygdala. On the right, actions of opioids on pain-modulating neurons in the midbrain **(D)**, rostral ventral medulla **(E)**, and the locus coeruleus indirectly control pain transmission pathways by enhancing descending inhibition to the dorsal horn. (Adapted, with permission, from Katzung BG, editor: *Basic & Clinical Pharmacology*, 10th ed. McGraw-Hill, 2007.)

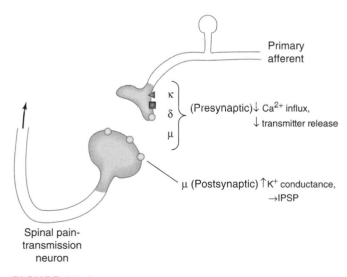

FIGURE 31–2 Spinal sites of opioid action. The μ, κ, and δ agonists reduce excitatory transmitter release from presynaptic terminals of nociceptive primary afferents. The μ agonists also hyperpolarize second-order pain transmission neurons by increasing K^+ conductance, evoking an inhibitory postsynaptic potential (IPSP). (Reproduced, with permission, from Katzung BG, editor: *Basic & Clinical Pharmacology*, 10th ed. McGraw-Hill, 2007.)

ACUTE EFFECTS

A. Analgesia

The opioids are the most powerful drugs available for the relief of pain. They attenuate both emotional and sensory aspects of the pain experience. Strong agonists (ie, those with the highest analgesic efficacy, full agonists) include morphine, methadone, meperidine, fentanyl, levorphanol, and heroin. Drugs with mixed agonist-antagonist actions (eg, buprenorphine, see below) may antagonize the analgesic actions of full agonists and should not be used concomitantly. Codeine, hydrocodone, and oxycodone are partial agonists with mild to moderate analgesic efficacy. They are commonly available in combinations with acetaminophen and nonsteroidal anti-inflammatory drugs (NSAIDs). Propoxyphene, a very weak agonist drug, is also available combined with acetaminophen.

B. Sedation and Euphoria

These effects may occur at doses lower than those required for maximum analgesia. The sedation is additive with other CNS depressants, but there is little amnesia. Some patients experience dysphoric effects from opioid drugs. At higher doses, the drugs may cause mental clouding and result in a stuporous, or even a comatose, state.

C. Respiratory Depression

Opioid actions in the medulla lead to inhibition of the respiratory center, with decreased response to carbon dioxide challenge. With full agonists, respiratory depression may be seen at conventional analgesic doses. Increased PCO_2 may cause cerebrovascular dilation, resulting in increased blood flow and increased intracranial pressure. Opioid analgesics are relatively contraindicated in patients with head injuries.

D. Antitussive Actions

Suppression of the cough reflex by unknown mechanisms is the basis for the clinical use of opioids as antitussives. This action can be obtained with the use of doses lower than those needed for analgesia.

E. Nausea and Vomiting

Nausea and vomiting are caused by activation of the chemoreceptor trigger zone and are increased by ambulation.

F. Gastrointestinal Effects

Constipation occurs through decreased intestinal peristalsis, which is probably mediated by effects on opioid receptors in the enteric nervous system. This powerful action is the basis for the clinical use of these drugs as antidiarrheal agents.

G. Smooth Muscle

Opioids (with the exception of meperidine) cause contraction of biliary tract smooth muscle, which can result in biliary colic or spasm, increased ureteral and bladder sphincter tone, and a reduction in uterine tone, which may contribute to prolongation of labor.

H. Miosis

Pupillary constriction is a characteristic effect of all opioids except meperidine, which has a muscarinic blocking action. Little on no tolerance occurs. Miosis is blocked by the opioid antagonist naloxone and by atropine.

I. Miscellaneous

Opioid analgesics, especially morphine, can cause flushing and pruritus through histamine release. They cause release of antidiuretic hormone (ADH) and prolactin but may inhibit the release of luteinizing hormone (LH). Exaggerated responses to opioid analgesics may occur in patients with adrenal insufficiency or hypothyroidism.

SKILL KEEPER: OPIOID PEPTIDES AND SUBSTANCE P (SEE CHAPTERS 6 AND 17)

These peptides are relevant to understanding the analgesic actions of opioid-analgesic drugs in terms of CNS function. What are the roles of these peptides in peripheral tissues? The Skill Keeper Answers appear at the end of the chapter.

CHRONIC EFFECTS

A. Tolerance

Marked tolerance can develop to the just-mentioned acute pharmacologic effects, with the exception of miosis and constipation. The mechanism of opioid tolerance development may involve receptor "uncoupling." Antagonists of glutamate *N*-methyl-D-aspartate (NMDA) receptors (eg, ketamine), as well as δ-receptor antagonists, are reported to block opioid tolerance. Although there is **cross-tolerance** between different opioid agonists, it is not complete. This provides the basis for "opioid rotation," whereby analgesia is maintained (eg, in cancer patients) by changing from one drug to another.

B. Dependence

Physical dependence is an anticipated physiologic response to chronic therapy with drugs in this group, particularly the strong agonists. Physical dependence is revealed on abrupt discontinuance as an **abstinence syndrome,** which includes rhinorrhea, lacrimation, chills, gooseflesh, muscle aches, diarrhea, yawning, anxiety, and hostility. A more intense state of **precipitated withdrawal** results when an opioid antagonist is administered to a physically dependent individual.

CLINICAL USES

A. Analgesia

Treatment of relatively constant moderate to severe pain is the major indication. Although oral formulations are most commonly used, buccal and suppository forms of some drugs are available. In the acute setting, strong agonists are usually given parenterally. Prolonged analgesia, with some reduction in adverse effects, can be achieved with epidural administration of certain strong agonist drugs (eg, fentanyl and morphine). Fentanyl has also been used by the transdermal route providing analgesia for up to 72 h. For less severe pain and in the chronic setting, moderate agonists are given by the oral route, sometimes in combinations with acetaminophen or NSAIDs.

B. Cough Suppression

Useful oral antitussive drugs include codeine and dextromethorphan. The latter, an over-the-counter drug, has recently been the subject of FDA warnings regarding its abuse potential. Large doses of dextromethorphan may cause hallucinations, confusion, excitation, increased or decreased pupil size, nystagmus, seizures, coma, and decreased breathing.

C. Treatment of Diarrhea

Selective antidiarrheal opioids include diphenoxylate and loperamide. They are given orally.

D. Management of Acute Pulmonary Edema

Morphine (parenteral) may be useful in acute pulmonary edema because of its hemodynamic actions; its calming effects probably also contribute to relief of the pulmonary symptoms.

E. Anesthesia

Opioids are used as preoperative medications and as intraoperative adjunctive agents in balanced anesthesia protocols. High-dose intravenous opioids (eg, morphine, fentanyl) are often the major component of anesthesia for cardiac surgery.

F. Opioid Dependence

Methadone, one of the longer acting opioids, is used in the management of opioid withdrawal states and in maintenance programs for addicts. In withdrawal states, methadone permits a slow tapering of opioid effect that diminishes the intensity of abstinence symptoms. Buprenorphine (see later discussion) has an even longer duration of action and is sometimes used in withdrawal states. In maintenance programs, the prolonged action of methadone blocks the euphoria-inducing effects of doses of shorter acting opioids (eg, heroin, morphine).

TOXICITY

Most of the adverse effects of the opioid analgesics (eg, nausea, constipation, respiratory depression) are predictable extensions of their pharmacologic effects. In addition, overdose and drug interaction toxicities are very important.

A. Overdose

A triad of pupillary constriction, comatose state, and respiratory depression is characteristic; the latter is responsible for most fatalities. Diagnosis of overdosage is confirmed if intravenous injection of naloxone, an antagonist drug, results in prompt signs of recovery. Treatment of overdose involves the use of antagonists such as naloxone and other therapeutic measures, especially ventilatory support.

B. Drug Interactions

The most important drug interactions involving opioid analgesics are additive CNS depression with ethanol, sedative-hypnotics, anesthetics, antipsychotic drugs, tricyclic antidepressants, and antihistamines. Concomitant use of certain opioids (eg, meperidine) with monoamine oxidase inhibitors increases the incidence of hyperpyrexic coma. Meperidine has also been implicated in the serotonin syndrome when used with selective serotonin reuptake inhibitors.

AGONIST-ANTAGONIST DRUGS

A. Analgesic Activity

The analgesic activity of mixed agonist-antagonists varies with the individual drug but is somewhat less than that of strong full agonists like morphine. Buprenorphine, butorphanol, and nalbuphine afford greater analgesia than pentazocine, which is similar to codeine in analgesic efficacy.

B. Receptors

Butorphanol, nalbuphine, and pentazocine are κ agonists, with weak μ-receptor antagonist activity. Butorphanol may act as a partial agonist or antagonist at the μ-receptor.

Buprenorphine is a μ-receptor partial agonist with weak antagonist effects at κ and δ receptors. These characteristics can lead to decreased analgesia, or even precipitate withdrawal symptoms, when such drugs are used in patients taking conventional full μ-receptor agonists. Buprenorphine has a long duration of effect binding strongly to μ receptors. Although prolonged activity of buprenorphine may be clinically useful (eg, to suppress withdrawal signs in dependency states), this property renders its effects resistant to naloxone reversal, since the antagonist drug has a short half-life. In overdose, respiratory depression caused by nalbuphine may also be resistant to naloxone reversal. Naloxone is included in some formulations of these agonist-antagonist drugs to discourage abuse.

C. Effects

The mixed agonist-antagonist drugs often cause sedation at analgesic doses. Dizziness, sweating, and nausea may also occur, and anxiety, hallucinations, and nightmares are possible adverse effects. Respiratory depression may be less intense than with pure agonists but is not predictably reversed by naloxone. Tolerance develops with chronic use but is less than the tolerance that develops to the pure agonists, and there is minimal cross-tolerance. Physical dependence occurs, but the abuse liability of mixed agonist-antagonist drugs is less than that of the full agonists.

D. Miscellaneous

Tramadol is a weak μ-receptor agonist only partially antagonized by naloxone. The analgesic activity of tramadol is mainly based on blockade of serotonin reuptake; it is a weak norepinephrine reuptake blocker. Tramadol is effective in treatment of moderate pain and has been used as an adjunct to opioids in chronic pain syndromes. The drug is relatively contraindicated in patients with a history of seizure disorders, and there is risk of the serotonin syndrome if it is co-administered with SSRIs. No significant effects on cardiovascular functions or respiration have been reported.

Tapentadol is a newer analgesic with strong norepinephrine reuptake-inhibiting activity (its activity is blocked by alpha antagonists) and only modest μ-opioid receptor affinity. It is not as effective as oxycodone in the treatment of moderate to severe pain but causes less gastrointestinal distress and nausea. Tapentadol has been implicated in the serotonin syndrome and should be used with caution in patients with seizure disorders.

OPIOID ANTAGONISTS

Naloxone, nalmefene, and naltrexone are pure opioid receptor antagonists that have few other effects at doses that produce marked antagonism of agonist effects. These drugs have greater affinity for μ receptors than for other opioid receptors. A major clinical use of the opioid antagonists is in the management of acute opioid overdose. Naloxone and nalmefene are given intravenously. Because naloxone has a short duration of action (1–2 h), multiple doses may be required in opioid analgesic overdose. Nalmefene has a duration of action of 8–12 h. Naltrexone has a long elimination half-life, blocking the actions of strong agonists (eg, heroin) for up to 48 h after oral use. Naltrexone decreases the craving for ethanol and is approved for adjunctive use in alcohol dependency programs. Unlike the older drugs, two new antagonists, methylnaltrexone and almivopan, do not cross the blood-brain barrier. These agents block adverse effects of strong opioids on peripheral μ receptors, including those in the gastrointestinal tract responsible for constipation, with minimal effects on analgesic actions and without precipitating an abstinence syndrome.

QUESTIONS

Questions 1 and 2. A 63-year-old man is undergoing radiation treatment as an outpatient for metastatic bone cancer. His pain has been managed with a fixed combination of oxycodone plus acetaminophen taken orally. Despite increasing doses of the analgesic combination, the pain is getting worse.

1. The most appropriate oral medication for his increasing pain is
   (A) Buprenorphine
   (B) Codeine plus aspirin
   (C) Levorphanol
   (D) Pentazocine
   (E) Propoxyphene

2. It is possible that this patient will have to increase the dose of the analgesic as his condition progresses as a result of developing tolerance. However, tolerance will not develop to a significant extent with respect to
   (A) Biliary smooth muscle
   (B) Constipation
   (C) Nausea and vomiting
   (D) Sedation
   (E) Urinary retention

3. You are on your way to take an examination and you suddenly get an attack of diarrhea. If you stop at a nearby drugstore for an over-the-counter opioid with antidiarrheal action, you will be asking for
   (A) Codeine
   (B) Dextromethorphan
   (C) Diphenoxylate
   (D) Loperamide
   (E) Tramadol

4. An emergency department patient with severe pain thought to be of gastrointestinal origin received 80 mg of meperidine. He subsequently developed a severe reaction characterized by tachycardia, hypertension, hyperpyrexia, and seizures. Questioning revealed that the patient had been taking a drug for a psychiatric condition. Which drug is most likely to be responsible for this untoward interaction with meperidine?
   (A) Alprazolam
   (B) Bupropion
   (C) Isocarboxazid
   (D) Lithium
   (E) Mirtazapine

5. Genetic polymorphisms in certain hepatic enzymes involved in drug metabolism are established to be responsible for variations in analgesic response to
   (A) Codeine
   (B) Fentanyl
   (C) Meperidine
   (D) Methadone
   (E) Tramadol

Questions 6 and 7. A young male patient is brought to the emergency department in an anxious and agitated state. He informs the attending physician that he uses "street drugs" and that he gave himself an intravenous "fix" approximately 12 h ago. He now has chills and muscle aches and has also been vomiting. His symptoms include hyperventilation and hyperthermia. The attending physician notes that his pupil size is larger than normal.

6. What is the most likely cause of these signs and symptoms?
   (A) The patient had injected methamphetamine
   (B) The patient has hepatitis B
   (C) The patient has overdosed with an opioid
   (D) The signs and symptoms are those of the opioid abstinence syndrome
   (E) These are early signs of toxicity due to contaminants in "street heroin"

7. Which drug will be most effective in alleviating the symptoms experienced by this patient?
   (A) Acetaminophen
   (B) Codeine
   (C) Diazepam
   (D) Methadone
   (E) Naltrexone

8. Which statement about butorphanol is accurate?
   (A) Activates μ receptors
   (B) Does not cause respiratory depression
   (C) Is a nonsedating opioid
   (D) Pain-relieving action is not superior to that of codeine
   (E) Response to naloxone in overdose may be unreliable

9. Which drug does not activate opioid receptors, has been proposed as a maintenance drug in treatment programs for opioid addicts, and with a single oral dose, will block the effects of injected heroin for up to 48 h?
   (A) Amphetamine
   (B) Buprenorphine
   (C) Naloxone
   (D) Naltrexone
   (E) Propoxyphene

10. Which statement about dextromethorphan is accurate?
    (A) Activates κ receptors
    (B) Analgesia equivalent to pentazocine
    (C) Highly effective antiemetic
    (D) Less constipation than codeine
    (E) No abuse potential

ANSWERS

1. In most situations, pain associated with metastatic carcinoma ultimately necessitates the use of an opioid analgesic that is equivalent in strength to morphine, so hydromorphone, oxymorphone, or levorphanol would be indicated. Pentazocine or the combination of codeine plus salicylate would not be as effective as the original drug combination. Propoxyphene is even less active than codeine alone. Buprenorphine, a mixed agonist-antagonist, is not usually recommended for cancer-associated pain because of its analgesic "ceiling" and because of possible dysphoric and psychotomimetic effects. The answer is **C.**

2. Chronic use of strong opioid analgesics leads to the development of tolerance to their analgesic, euphoric, and sedative actions. Tolerance also develops to their emetic effects and to effects on some smooth muscle, including the biliary and the urethral sphincter muscles. However, tolerance does not develop significantly to the constipating effects or the miotic actions of the opioid analgesics. The answer is **B.**

3. Codeine and possibly nalbuphine could decrease gastrointestinal peristalsis, but not without marked side effects (and a prescription). Dextromethorphan is a cough suppressant. The other 2 drugs listed are opioids with antidiarrheal actions. Diphenoxylate is not available over the counter because it is a constituent of a proprietary combination that includes atropine sulfate (Lomotil). The answer is **D.**

4. Concomitant administration of meperidine and monoamine oxidase inhibitors such as isocarboxazid or phenelzine has resulted in life-threatening hyperpyrexic reactions that may culminate in seizures or coma. Such reactions have occurred even when the MAO inhibitor was administered more than a week after a patient had been treated with meperidine. Note that concomitant use of selective serotonin reuptake inhibitors and meperidine has resulted in the serotonin syndrome, another life-threatening drug interaction (see Chapter 30). The answer is **C.**

5. Codeine, hydrocodone, and oxycodone are metabolized by the cytochrome P450 isoform CYP2D6, and variations in analgesic response to these drugs have been attributed to genotypic polymorphisms in this isozyme. In the case of codeine, this may be especially important since the drug is demethylated by CYP2D6 to form the active metabolite, morphine. The answer is **A.**

6. The signs and symptoms are those of withdrawal in a patient physically dependent on an opioid agonist. They usually start within 6–10 h after the last dose; their intensity depends on the degree of physical dependence, and peak effects usually occur at 36–48 h. Mydriasis is a prominent feature of the abstinence syndrome; other symptoms include rhinorrhea, lacrimation, piloerection, muscle jerks, and yawning. The answer is **D.**

7. Prevention of signs and symptoms of withdrawal after chronic use of a strong opiate like heroin requires replacement with another strong opioid analgesic drug. Methadone is most commonly used, but other strong μ-receptor agonists would also be effective. Acetaminophen and codeine will not be effective. Beneficial effects of diazepam are restricted to relief of anxiety and agitation. The antagonist drug naltrexone may exacerbate withdrawal symptoms. The answer is **D.**

8. Butorphanol and nalbuphine are κ agonists, with weak μ-receptor antagonist activity. They have analgesic efficacy superior to that of codeine, but it is not equivalent to that of strong opioid receptor agonists. Although these mixed agonist-antagonist drugs are less likely to cause respiratory depression than strong μ activators, if depression does occur, reversal with opioid antagonists such as naloxone is unpredictable. Sedation is common. The answer is **E.**

9. The opioid antagonist naltrexone has a much longer half-life than naloxone, and its effects may last 2 d. A high degree of client compliance would be required for naltrexone to be of value in opioid dependence treatment programs. The same reservation is applicable to the use of naltrexone in alcoholism. The answer is **D.**

10. Dextromethorphan, the active component in many over-the-counter cough suppressants, has no appreciable analgesic activity. Compared with codeine, also an effective antitussive, dextromethorphan causes less constipation. When formulated properly and used in small amounts, dextromethoprhan can be safely used as a cough suppressant. However, overdose toxicity in toddlers has raised concern, and abuse of the drug in powdered form has caused disorientation, hallucinations, seizures, and death. The answer is D.

SKILL KEEPER ANSWERS: OPIOID PEPTIDES AND SUBSTANCE P (SEE CHAPTERS 6 AND 17)

1. *Precursor molecules that release opioid peptides are found at various peripheral sites, including the adrenal medulla and the pituitary gland and in some secretomotor neurons and interneurons in the enteric nervous system. In the gut these peptides appear to inhibit the release of ACh, presumably from parasympathetic nerve endings, and thereby inhibit peristalsis. In other tissues, opioid peptides may stimulate the release of transmitters or act as neurohormones.*

2. *Substance P, an undecapeptide, is a member of the tachykinin peptide group. It is an important sensory neuron transmitter in the enteric nervous system and, of course, in primary afferents involved in nociception. Substance P contracts intestinal and bronchiolar smooth muscle but is an arteriolar vasodilator (possibly via nitric oxide release). It may also play a role in renal and salivary gland functions.*

CHECKLIST

When you complete this chapter, you should be able to:

❑ Identify 3 opioid receptor subtypes and describe 2 ionic mechanisms that result from such activation.

❑ Name the major opioid agonists, rank them in terms of analgesic efficacy, and identify specific dynamic or kinetic characteristics.

❑ Describe the cardinal signs and treatment of opioid drug "overdose" and of the "withdrawal" syndrome.

❑ List acute and chronic adverse effects of opioid analgesics.

❑ Identify an opioid receptor antagonist and a mixed agonist-antagonist.

❑ Identify opioids used for antitussive effects and for antidiarrheal effects.

DRUG SUMMARY TABLE: Opioids, Opioid Substitutes, & Opioid Antagonists

Subclass	Mechanism of Action (Receptors)	Clinical Applications	Pharmacokinetics & Interactions	Toxicities
Strong agonists				
Fentanyl Hydromorphone Meperidine Morphine Methadone Oxymorphone	Strong μ agonists • variable δ and κ agonists	Severe pain, anesthesia (adjunctive) • dependence maintenance (methadone)	Hepatic metabolism • duration: 1–4 h (methadone 4–6 h)	Respiratory depression, constipation, addiction liability
Partial agonists				
Codeine Hydrocodone	As above, but lower affinity	Mild-to-moderate pain; cough (codeine) • analgesic combinations with NSAIDs and acetaminophen	Genetic variations in metabolism	As above, but weaker
Mixed agonist-antagonist				
Buprenorphine	Partial μ agonist and κ antagonist	Moderate-to-severe pain • dependence maintenance, reduces craving for alcohol (buprenorphine)	Long duration (buprenorphine) • nalbuphine (parenteral only)	Like strong agonists but can antagonize their effects
Nalbuphine	κ agonist and μ antagonist			
Antagonists				
Naloxone Naltrexone Nalmefene	Antagonists at all receptors	Opioid overdose • dependence maintenance (naltrexone)	Duration: naloxone 2 h • naltrexone and nalmefene >10 h	Rapid antagonism of all opioid actions
Antitussives				
Codeine Dextromethorphan	Mechanism uncertain • partial μ agonists Weak μ agonist • inhibits norepinephrine and 5-HT transporters	Acute debilitating cough	Duration: 0.5–1 h	Reduce cough reflex • toxic in overdose
Tramadol		Moderate pain • adjunctive to opioids in chronic pain states	Duration: 4–6 h	Toxic in overdose (seizures)

NSAIDs, nonsteroidal anti-inflammatory drugs.

Drugs of Abuse

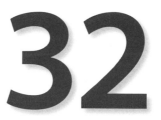

Drug abuse is usually taken to mean the use of an illicit drug or the excessive or nonmedical use of a licit drug. It also denotes the deliberate use of chemicals that generally are not considered drugs by the lay public but may be harmful to the user. A primary motivation for drug abuse appears to be the anticipated feeling of pleasure derived from the CNS effects of the drug. The older term "physical (physiologic) dependence" is now generally denoted as **dependence,** whereas "psychological dependence" is more simply called **addiction**.

THE DOPAMINE HYPOTHESIS OF ADDICTION

Dopamine in the mesolimbic system appears to play a primary role in the expression of "reward," but excessive dopaminergic stimulation may lead to pathologic reinforcement such that behavior may become compulsive and no longer under control—common features of addiction. Though not necessarily the only neurochemical characteristic of drugs of abuse, it appears that most addictive drugs have actions that include facilitation of the effects of dopamine in the CNS.

SEDATIVE-HYPNOTICS

The sedative-hypnotic drugs are responsible for many cases of drug abuse. The group includes **ethanol, barbiturates,** and **benzodiazepines.** Benzodiazepines are commonly prescribed drugs for anxiety and, as Schedule IV drugs, are judged by the US government to have low abuse liability (Table 32–1). Short-acting barbiturates (eg, secobarbital) have high addiction potential. Ethanol is not listed in schedules of controlled substances with abuse liability.

A. Effects

Sedative-hypnotics reduce inhibitions, suppress anxiety, and produce relaxation. All of these actions are thought to encourage repetitive use. Although the primary actions of sedative-hypnotics involve facilitation of the effects of GABA and/or antagonism at ACh-N receptors, these drugs also enhance brain dopaminergic pathways, the latter action possibly related to the development of

addiction. The drugs are CNS depressants, and their depressant effects are enhanced by concomitant use of opioid analgesics, antipsychotic agents, marijuana, and any other drug with sedative properties. Acute overdoses commonly result in death through depression of the medullary respiratory and cardiovascular centers (Table 32–2). Management of overdose includes maintenance of a patent airway plus ventilatory support. Flumazenil can be used to reverse the CNS depressant effects of benzodiazepines, but there is no antidote for barbiturates or ethanol.

Flunitrazepam (Rohypnol), a potent rapid-onset benzodiazepine with marked amnestic properties, has been used in "date rape." Added to alcoholic beverages, **chloral hydrate** or **γ-hydroxybutyrate** (GHB; sodium oxybate) also render the victim incapable of resisting rape. The latter compound, a minor metabolite of GABA, binds to GABA$_B$ receptors in the CNS. When used as a "club drug," GHB causes euphoria, enhanced sensory perception, and amnesia.

B. Withdrawal

Physiologic dependence occurs with continued use of sedative-hypnotics; the signs and symptoms of the withdrawal (abstinence) syndrome are most pronounced with drugs that have a half-life of less than 24 h (eg, ethanol, secobarbital, methaqualone). However, physiologic dependence may occur with any sedative-hypnotic, including the longer acting benzodiazepines. The most important signs of withdrawal derive from excessive *CNS stimulation* and include anxiety, tremor, nausea and vomiting, delirium, and hallucinations (Table 32–2). **Seizures** are not uncommon and may be life-threatening.

Treatment of sedative-hypnotic withdrawal involves administration of a long acting sedative-hypnotic (eg, chlordiazepoxide or diazepam) to suppress the acute withdrawal syndrome, followed by gradual dose reduction. Clonidine or propranolol may also be of value to suppress sympathetic overactivity. The opioid receptor antagonist **naltrexone,** and **acamprosate**, an antagonist at *N*-methyl-D-aspartate (NMDA) glutamate receptors, are both used in the treatment of alcoholism (see Chapter 23).

A syndrome of **therapeutic withdrawal** has occurred on discontinuance of sedative-hypnotics after long-term therapeutic administration. In addition to the symptoms of classic withdrawal presented in Table 32–2, this syndrome includes weight loss, paresthesias, and headache. (See Chapters 22 and 23 for additional details.)

High-Yield Terms to Learn

Abstinence syndrome	A term used to describe the signs and symptoms that occur on withdrawal of a drug in a dependent person
Addiction	Compulsive drug-using behavior in which the person uses the drug for personal satisfaction, often in the face of known risks to health; formerly termed psychological dependence
Controlled substance	A drug deemed to have abuse liability that is listed on governmental Schedules of Controlled Substances.[a] Such schedules categorize illicit drugs, control prescribing practices, and mandate penalties for illegal possession, manufacture, and sale of listed drugs. Controlled substance schedules are presumed to reflect current attitudes toward substance abuse; therefore, which drugs are regulated depends on a social judgment
Dependence	A state characterized by signs and symptoms, frequently the opposite of those *caused* by a drug, when it is withdrawn from chronic use or when the dose is abruptly lowered; formerly termed physical or physiologic dependence
Designer drug	A synthetic derivative of a drug, with slightly modified structure but no major change in pharmacodynamic action. Circumvention of the Schedules of Controlled Drugs is a motivation for the illicit synthesis of designer drugs
Tolerance	A decreased response to a drug, necessitating larger doses to achieve the same effect. This can result from increased disposition of the drug (metabolic tolerance), an ability to compensate for the effects of a drug (behavioral tolerance), or changes in receptor or effector systems involved in drug actions (functional tolerance)

[a]An example of such a schedule promulgated by the US Drug Enforcement Agency is shown in Table 32–1. Note that the criteria given by the agency do not always reflect the actual pharmacologic properties of the drugs.

TABLE 32–1 Schedules of controlled drugs.[a]

Schedule	Criteria	Examples
I	No medical use; high addiction potential	Flunitrazepam, heroin, LSD, mescaline, PCP, MDA, MDMA, STP
II	Medical use; high addiction potential barbiturates, strong opioids	Amphetamines, cocaine, methylphenidate, short acting
III	Medical use; moderate abuse potential moderate opioid agonists	Anabolic steroids, barbiturates, dronabinol, ketamine,
IV	Medical use; low abuse potential	Benzodiazepines, chloral hydrate, mild stimulants (eg, phentermine, sibutramine), most hypnotics (eg, zaleplon, zolpidem), weak opioids

[a]Adapted, with permission, from Katzung BG, editor: *Basic & Clinical Pharmacology*, 11th ed, McGraw-Hill, 2009.

LSD, lysergic acid diethylamide; MDA, methylene dioxyamphetamine; MDMA, methylene dioxymethamphetamine; PCP, phencyclidine; STP (DOM), 2,5-dimethoxy-4-methylamphetamine.

TABLE 32–2 Signs and symptoms of overdose and withdrawal from selected drugs of abuse.

Drug	Overdose Effects	Withdrawal Symptoms
Amphetamines, methylphenidate, cocaine[a]	Agitation, hypertension, tachycardia, delusions, hallucinations, hyperthermia, seizures, death	Apathy, irritability, increased sleep time, disorientation, depression
Barbiturates, benzodiazepines, ethanol[b]	Slurred speech, "drunken" behavior, dilated pupils, weak and rapid pulse, clammy skin, shallow respiration, coma, death	Anxiety, insomnia, delirium, tremors, seizures, death
Heroin, other strong opioids	Constricted pupils, clammy skin, nausea, drowsiness, respiratory depression, coma, death	Nausea, chills, cramps, lacrimation, rhinorrhea, yawning, hyperpnea, tremor

[a]Cardiac arrhythmias, myocardial infarction, and stroke occur more frequently in cocaine overdose.

[b]Ethanol withdrawal includes the excited hallucinatory state of delirium tremens.

OPIOID ANALGESICS

A. Effects

As described in Chapter 31, the primary targets underlying the actions of the opioid analgesics are the μ, κ, and δ receptors. However, the opioids have other actions including disinhibition in dopaminergic pathways in the CNS. The most commonly abused drugs in this group are **heroin, morphine, codeine, oxycodone,** and among health professionals, **meperidine** and **fentanyl.** The effects of intravenous heroin are described by abusers as a "rush" or orgasmic feeling followed by euphoria and then sedation. Intravenous administration of opioids is associated with rapid development of tolerance and psychological and physiologic dependence. Oral administration or smoking of opioids causes milder effects, with a slower onset of tolerance and dependence. Overdose of opioids leads to respiratory depression progressing to coma and death (Table 32–2). Overdose is managed with intravenous naloxone or nalmefene and ventilatory support.

B. Withdrawal

Deprivation of opioids in physiologically dependent individuals leads to an abstinence syndrome that includes lacrimation, rhinorrhea, yawning, sweating, weakness, gooseflesh ("cold turkey"), nausea and vomiting, tremor, muscle jerks ("kicking the habit"), and hyperpnea (Table 32–2). Although extremely unpleasant, withdrawal from opioids is rarely fatal (unlike withdrawal from sedative-hypnotics). Treatment involves replacement of the illicit drug with a pharmacologically equivalent agent (eg, **methadone**), followed by slow dose reduction. **Buprenorphine,** a partial agonist at μ opioid receptors and a longer acting opioid (half-life >40 h), is also used to suppress withdrawal symptoms and as substitution therapy for opioid addicts. The administration of naloxone to a person who is using strong opioids (but not overdosing) may cause more rapid and more intense symptoms of withdrawal (precipitated withdrawal). Neonates born to mothers physiologically dependent on opioids require special management of withdrawal symptoms.

STIMULANTS

A. Caffeine and Nicotine

1. Effects—Caffeine (in beverages) and nicotine (in tobacco products) are legal in most Western cultures even though they have adverse medical effects. In the United States, cigarette smoking is a major preventable cause of death; tobacco use is associated with a high incidence of cardiovascular, respiratory, and neoplastic disease. Addiction (psychological dependence) to caffeine and nicotine has been recognized for some time. More recently, demonstration of abstinence signs and symptoms has provided evidence of dependence.

2. Withdrawal—Withdrawal from caffeine is accompanied by lethargy, irritability, and headache. The anxiety and mental discomfort experienced from discontinuing nicotine are major impediments to quitting the habit. **Varenicline,** a partial agonist at the ACh-N($\alpha_2\beta_2$) subtype nicotinic receptors, which occludes the rewarding effects of nicotine, is used for smoking cessation. **Rimonabant,** an agonist at cannabinoid receptors, approved for use in obesity, is also used off-label in smoking cessation.

3. Toxicity—Acute toxicity from overdosage of caffeine or nicotine includes excessive CNS stimulation with tremor, insomnia, and nervousness; cardiac stimulation and arrhythmias; and, in the case of nicotine, respiratory paralysis (Chapters 6 and 7). Severe toxicity has been reported in small children who ingest discarded nicotine gum or nicotine patches, which are used as substitutes for tobacco products.

B. Amphetamines

1. Effects—Amphetamines inhibit transporters of CNS amines including dopamine, norepinephrine, and serotonin, thus enhancing their actions. They cause a feeling of euphoria and self-confidence that contributes to the rapid development of addiction. Drugs in this class include **dextroamphetamine** and **methamphetamine** ("speed"), a crystal form of which ("ice") can be smoked. Chronic high-dose abuse leads to a psychotic state (with delusions and paranoia) that is difficult to differentiate from schizophrenia. Symptoms of overdose include agitation, restlessness, tachycardia, hyperthermia, hyperreflexia, and possibly seizures (Table 32–2). There is no specific antidote, and supportive measures are directed toward control of body temperature and protection against cardiac arrhythmias and seizures. Chronic abuse of amphetamines is associated with the development of necrotizing arteritis, leading to cerebral hemorrhage and renal failure.

2. Tolerance and withdrawal—Tolerance can be marked, and an abstinence syndrome, characterized by increased appetite, sleepiness, exhaustion, and mental depression, can occur on withdrawal. Antidepressant drugs may be indicated.

3. Congeners of amphetamines—Several chemical congeners of amphetamines have hallucinogenic properties. These include 2,5-dimethoxy-4-methylamphetamine (**DOM [STP]**), methylene dioxyamphetamine (**MDA**), and methylene dioxymethamphetamine (**MDMA; "ecstasy"**). MDMA has a more selective action than amphetamine on the serotonin transporter in the CNS. The drug is purported to facilitate interpersonal communication and act as a sexual enhancer. Positron emission tomography studies of the brains of regular users of MDMA show a depletion of neurons in serotonergic tracts. Overdose toxicity includes hyperthermia, symptoms of the serotonin syndrome (see Chapter 30), and seizures. A withdrawal syndrome with protracted depression has been described in chronic users of MDMA.

C. Cocaine

1. Effects—Cocaine, also an inhibitor of the CNS transporters of dopamine, norepinephrine, and serotonin, has marked amphetamine-like effects ("super-speed"). Its abuse continues to be widespread in the United States partly because of the availability of a free-base form ("crack") that can be smoked. The euphoria, self-confidence, and mental alertness produced by cocaine are short-lasting and positively reinforce its continued use.

Overdoses with cocaine commonly result in fatalities from arrhythmias, seizures, or respiratory depression (see Table 32–2). Cardiac toxicity is partly due to blockade of norepinephrine reuptake by cocaine; its local anesthetic action contributes to the production of seizures. In addition, the powerful vasoconstrictive action of cocaine may lead to severe hypertensive episodes, resulting in myocardial infarcts and strokes. No specific antidote is available. Cocaine abuse during pregnancy is associated with increased fetal morbidity and mortality.

2. Withdrawal—The abstinence syndrome after withdrawal from cocaine is similar to that after amphetamine discontinuance. Severe depression of mood is common and strongly reinforces the compulsion to use the drug. Antidepressant drugs may be indicated. Infants born to mothers who abuse cocaine (or amphetamines) have possible teratogenic abnormalities (cystic cortical lesions) and increased morbidity and mortality and may be cocaine dependent. The signs and symptoms of CNS stimulant overdose and withdrawal are listed in Table 32–2.

HALLUCINOGENS

A. Phencyclidine

The arylcyclohexylamine drugs include **phencyclidine** (PCP; "angel dust") and ketamine ("special K"), which are antagonists at the glutamate NMDA receptor (Chapter 21). Unlike most drugs of abuse, they have no actions on dopaminergic neurons in the CNS. PCP is probably the most dangerous of the hallucinogenic agents. Psychotic reactions are common with PCP, and impaired judgment often leads to reckless behavior. This drug should be classified as a **psychotomimetic.** Effects of overdosage with PCP include both horizontal and vertical nystagmus, marked hypertension, and seizures, which may be fatal. Parenteral benzodiazepines (eg, diazepam, lorazepam) are used to curb excitation and protect against seizures.

B. Miscellaneous Hallucinogenic Agents

Several drugs with hallucinogenic effects have been classified as having abuse liability, including **lysergic acid diethylamide** (LSD), **mescaline,** and **psilocybin.** Hallucinogenic effects may also occur with scopolamine and other antimuscarinic agents. None of these drugs has actions on dopaminergic pathways in the CNS, and interestingly, they do not cause dependence. Terms that have been used to describe the CNS effects of such drugs include "psychedelic" and "mind revealing." The perceptual and psychological effects of such drugs are usually accompanied by marked somatic effects, particularly nausea, weakness, and paresthesias. Panic reactions ("bad trips") may also occur.

MARIJUANA

A. Classification

Marijuana ("grass") is a collective term for the psychoactive constituents in crude extracts of the plant *Cannabis sativa* (hemp), the active principles of which include the cannabinoid compounds **tetrahydrocannabinol (THC),** cannabidiol (CBD), and cannabinol (CBN). **Hashish** is a partially purified material that is more potent.

B. Cannabinoids

Endogenous cannabinoids in the CNS, which include anadamide and 2-arachidonyl glycerol, are released postsynaptically and act as retrograde messengers to inhibit presynaptic release of conventional transmitters including dopamine. The receptors for these compounds are thought to be the "targets" for exogenous cannabinoids present in marijuana.

C. Effects

CNS effects of marijuana include a feeling of being "high," with euphoria, disinhibition, uncontrollable laughter, changes in perception, and achievement of a dream-like state. Mental concentration may be difficult. Vasodilation occurs, and the pulse rate is characteristically increased. Habitual users show a reddened conjunctiva. A mild withdrawal state has been noted only in long-term heavy users of marijuana. The dangers of marijuana use concern its impairment of judgment and reflexes, effects that are potentiated by concomitant use of sedative-hypnotics, including ethanol. Potential therapeutic effects of marijuana include its ability to decrease intraocular pressure and its antiemetic actions. **Dronabinol** (a controlled-substance formulation of THC) is used to combat severe nausea. **Rimonabant,** an agonist at cannabinoid receptors, is approved for use in the treatment of obesity.

INHALANTS

Certain gases or volatile liquids are abused because they provide a feeling of euphoria or disinhibition.

A. Anesthetics

This group includes nitrous oxide, chloroform, and diethylether. Such agents are hazardous because they affect judgment and induce loss of consciousness. Inhalation of nitrous oxide as the pure gas (with no oxygen) has caused asphyxia and death. Ether is highly flammable.

B. Industrial Solvents

Solvents and a wide range of volatile compounds are present in commercial products such as gasoline, paint thinners, aerosol propellants, glues, rubber cements, and shoe polish. Because of their ready availability, these substances are most frequently abused by children in early adolescence. Active ingredients that have been identified include benzene, hexane, methylethylketone, toluene, and trichloroethylene. Many of these are toxic to the liver, kidneys, lungs, bone marrow, and peripheral nerves and cause brain damage in animals.

C. Organic Nitrites

Amyl nitrite, isobutyl nitrite, and other organic nitrites are referred to as "poppers" and are mainly used as sexual intercourse "enhancers." Inhalation of the nitrites causes dizziness, tachycardia, hypotension, and flushing. With the exception of methemoglobinemia, few serious adverse effects have been reported.

STEROIDS

In many countries, including the United States, anabolic steroids are controlled substances based on their potential for abuse. Effects sought by abusers are increases in muscle mass and strength rather than euphoria. However, excessive use can have adverse behavioral, cardiovascular, and musculoskeletal effects. Acne (sometimes severe), premature closure of the epiphyses, and masculinization in females are anticipated androgenic adverse effects. Hepatic dysfunction has been reported, and the anabolic steroids may pose an increased risk of myocardial infarct. Behavioral manifestations include increases in libido and aggression ("roid rage"). A withdrawal syndrome has been described with fatigue and depression of mood.

SKILL KEEPER: DRUG OF ABUSE OVERDOSE SIGNS AND SYMPTOMS (SEE CHAPTERS 22 AND 31)

In an emergency situation, behavioral manifestations of the toxicity of drugs of abuse can be of assistance in diagnosis. What other readily detectable markers will also be helpful? The Skill Keeper Answer appears at the end of the chapter.

QUESTIONS

Questions 1 and 2. A 42-year-old homemaker suffers from anxiety with phobic symptoms and occasional panic attacks. She uses over-the-counter antihistamines for allergic rhinitis and claims that ethanol use is "just 1 or 2 glasses of wine with dinner." Alprazolam is prescribed, and the patient is maintained on the drug for 3 years, with several dose increments over that time period. Her family notices that she does not seem to be improving and that her speech is often slurred in the evenings. She is finally hospitalized with severe withdrawal signs on one weekend while attempting to end her dependence on drugs.

1. Which statement about the use of alprazolam is accurate?
   (A) Additive CNS depression occurs with ethanol
   (B) Abrupt discontinuance of alprazolam after 4 wks of treatment may elicit withdrawal signs
   (C) Alprazolam is a Schedule IV controlled drug judged to have relatively low abuse liability
   (D) Tolerance can occur with chronic use of any benzodiazepine
   (E) All of the above statements are accurate

2. The main reason for hospitalization of this patient was to be able to effectively control
   (A) Cardiac arrhythmias
   (B) Delirium
   (C) Hepatic dysfunction
   (D) Seizures
   (E) None of the above

3. Which drug, a partial agonist at nicotinic acetycholine receptors, is used in smoking cessation programs and heightens the perception of colors?
   (A) Acamprosate
   (B) Buprenorphine
   (C) Nalbuphine
   (D) Rimonabant
   (E) Varenicline

4. Which statement about abuse of the opioid analgesics is false?
   (A) A patient experiencing withdrawal from heroin is free of the symptoms of abstinence in 6–8 d
   (B) Early signs of withdrawal include lacrimation, rhinorrhea, yawning, and sweating
   (C) In withdrawal from opioids, clonidine may be useful in reducing symptoms caused by sympathetic overactivity
   (D) Methadone alleviates most of the symptoms of heroin withdrawal
   (E) Naloxone may precipitate a severe withdrawal state in abusers of opioid analgesics with symptoms starting in less than 15–30 min

5. A young male patient is brought to the emergency department of a hospital suffering from an overdose of cocaine after its intravenous administration. His symptoms are *not* likely to include
   (A) Agitation
   (B) Bradycardia
   (C) Hyperthermia
   (D) Myocardial infarct
   (E) Seizures

6. Which statement about hallucinogens is accurate?
   (A) Dilated pupils and tachycardia are characteristic effects of scopolamine
   (B) LSD is unique among hallucinogens in that animals will self-administer it
   (C) Mescaline and related hallucinogens exert their CNS actions through dopaminergic systems in the brain
   (D) Teratogenic effects occur with the use of phencyclidine during pregnancy
   (E) Withdrawal signs characteristic of dependence occur with abrupt discontinuance of ketamine

7. Which statement about inhalants is accurate?
   (A) Euphoria, numbness, and tingling sensations with visual and auditory disturbances occur in most persons who inhale organic nitrites
   (B) Methemoglobinemia is a common toxicologic problem after repetitive inhalation of industrial solvents
   (C) Nitrous oxide is the most commonly abused drug by medical personnel working in hospitals
   (D) Solvent inhalation is mainly a drug abuse problem in petroleum industry workers
   (E) Isobutyl nitrite is likely to cause headache

8. Which sign or symptom is likely to occur with marijuana?
   (A) Bradycardia
   (B) Conjunctival reddening
   (C) Hypertension
   (D) Increased psychomotor performance
   (E) Mydriasis

Questions 9 and 10. A college student is brought to the emergency department by friends. The physician is informed that the student had taken a drug and then "went crazy." The patient is agitated and delirious. Several persons are required to hold him down. His skin is warm and sweaty, and his pupils are dilated. Bowel sounds are normal. Signs and symptoms include tachycardia, marked hypertension, hyperthermia, increased muscle tone, and both horizontal and vertical nystagmus.

9. The most likely cause of these signs and symptoms is intoxication from
   (A) Cocaine hashish
   (B) LSD
   (C) Methamphetamine
   (D) Phencyclidine
   (E) Scopolamine

10. The management of this patient is likely to include
    (A) Administration of epinephrine
    (B) Alkalinization of the urine to increase drug elimination
    (C) Amitriptyline if psychosis ensues
    (D) Atropine to control hyperthermia
    (E) None of the above

ANSWERS

1. Therapeutic doses of benzodiazepines may lead to dependence with withdrawal symptoms including anxiety and agitation observable on abrupt discontinuance after a few weeks of treatment. Like most sedative-hypnotics, benzodiazepines are schedule-controlled, exhibiting dependence liability and the development of tolerance. Additive depression occurs with ethanol and many other CNS drugs. The answer is **E**.

2. This patient is probably withdrawing from dependence on both alprazolam and alcohol use. In addition to the symptoms described previously, abrupt withdrawal from sedative-hypnotic dependence may include hyperreflexia progressing to seizures, with ensuing coma and possibly death. The risk of a seizure is increased if the patient abruptly withdraws from ethanol use at the same time. Depending on severity of symptoms, initial management may require parenteral diazepam or lorazepam, with the latter drug often favored in hepatic dysfunction. The answer is **D**.

3. Acamprosate is an antagonist of NMDA glutamate receptors used together with counseling in alcohol treatment programs. Varenicline occludes the "rewarding" effects of nicotine and is used in smoking cessation programs. The drug also heightens the awareness of colors. The answer is **E**.

4. Symptoms of opioid withdrawal usually begin within 6–8 h, and the acute course may last 6–8 d. However, a secondary phase of heroin withdrawal, characterized by bradycardia, hypotension, hypothermia, and mydriasis, may last 26–30 wks. Methadone is commonly used in detoxification of the heroin addict because it is a strong agonist, has high oral bioavailability, and has a relatively long half-life. The answer is **A**.

5. Overdoses with amphetamines or cocaine have many signs and symptoms in common. However, the ability of cocaine to block the reuptake of norepinephrine at sympathetic nerve terminals results in greater cardiotoxicity. Tachycardia is the rule, with the possibility of an arrhythmia, infarct, or stroke. The answer is **B**.

6. Psilocybin, mescaline, and LSD have similar central (via serotonergic systems) and peripheral (sympathomimetic) effects, but no actions on dopaminergic receptors in the CNS. None of the hallucinogenic drugs have been shown to have teratogenic potential. Unlike most hallucinogens, PCP (not LSD) acts as a positive reinforcer of self-administration in animals. Emergence reactions can occur after use of ketamine, but they are not signs of withdrawal. Scopolamine blocks muscarinic receptors. The answer is **A**.

7. Male preteens are most likely to "experiment" with solvent inhalation. This can result in central and peripheral neurotoxicity, liver and kidney damage, and pulmonary disease. Opioids, including fentanyl and meperidine, are the most widely abused by medical personnel working in hospitals. Industrial solvents rarely cause methemoglobinemia, but this (and headaches) may occur after excessive use of nitrites. The answer is **E**.

8. Two of the most characteristic signs of marijuana use are increased pulse rate and reddening of the conjunctiva. Decreases in blood pressure and in psychomotor performance occur. Pupil size is *not* changed by marijuana. The answer is **B**.

9. The signs and symptoms point to PCP intoxication. The presence of both horizontal and vertical nystagmus is pathognomonic. The answer is **D**.

10. Management of phencyclidine (PCP) overdose involves ventilatory support and control of seizures (with a benzodiazepine), hypertension, and hyperthermia. Antipsychotic drugs (eg, haloperidol) may also be useful for psychosis. None of the drugs listed are of value. Atropine may cause hyperthermia! Phencyclidine is a weak base, and its renal elimination may be accelerated by urinary *acidification,* not alkalinization! A large percentage of phencyclidine is secreted into the stomach, so removal of the drug may be hastened by activated charcoal or nasogastric suction. The answer is **E**.

SKILL KEEPER ANSWER: DRUG OF ABUSE OVERDOSE SIGNS AND SYMPTOMS (SEE CHAPTERS 22 AND 31)

Readily detectable markers that may assist in diagnosis of the cause of drug overdose toxicity include changes in heart rate, blood pressure, respiration, body temperature, sweating, bowel signs, and pupillary responses. For example, tachycardia, hypertension, increased body temperature, decreased bowel signs, and mydriasis are common characteristics of overdose of CNS stimulants, including amphetamines, cocaine, and most hallucinogens.

Make a brief list of characteristics that would enable you to identify overdose with opioids and with sedative-hypnotics.

CHECKLIST

When you complete this chapter, you should be able to:

❑ Identify the major drugs that are commonly abused.

❑ Describe the signs and symptoms of overdose with, and withdrawal from, CNS stimulants, opioid analgesics, and sedative-hypnotics, including ethanol.

❑ Describe the general principles of the management of overdose of commonly abused drugs.

❑ Identify the most likely causes of death from commonly abused drugs.

DRUG SUMMARY TABLE: Drugs Used to Treat Dependence & Addiction

Subclass	Mechanism of Action	Effects	Clinical Applications	Pharmacokinetics, Toxicities, Interactions
Opioid antagonists				
Naloxone Naltrexone	Antagonists of opioid receptors	Reverse or block effects of opioids	Naloxone: opioid overdose Naltrexone: treatment of alcoholism	Naloxone: Short half-life (1–2 h) Naltrexone: Half-life like morphine (4 h)
Synthetic opioid				
Methadone	Slow-acting agonist at μ opioid receptors	Acute effects like morphine	Substitution therapy for opioid addicts	Variable half-life Toxicity: Like morphine re acute and chronic effects including withdrawal
Partial μ-receptor agonist				
Buprenorphine	Partial agonist at μ opioid receptors	Attenuates acute effects of morphine and other strong opioids	Substitution therapy for opioid addicts	Long half-life (>40 h) • formulated with nalorphine to avoid illicit IV use
N-receptor partial agonist				
Varenicline	Agonist at ACh-N receptor ($\alpha_2\beta_2$) subtype	Blocks "rewarding" effects of nicotine	Smoking cessation	Nausea and vomiting, psychiatric changes, seizures in high dose
Benzodiazepines				
Oxazepam Lorazepam	Modulators of GABA$_A$ receptors	Enhance GABA functions in CNS	Attenuate withdrawal symptoms including seizures from alcohol and other sedative-hypnotics	Half-life 4–15 h; lorazepam kinetics not affected by liver dysfunction
NMDA receptor antagonist				
Acamprosate	Antagonist at glutamate NMDA receptors	May block synaptic plasticity	Treatment of alcoholism (in combination with counseling)	Allergies, arrhythmias, variable BP effects, headaches, and impotence • hallucinations in elderly
Cannabinoid receptor agonist				
Rimonabant	Agonist at CB1 receptors	Decrease GABA and glutamate release in CNS	Treatment of obesity • off-label use for smoking cessation	Major depression • increased suicide risk

ACh, acetylcholine; NMDA, N-methyl-D-aspartate.

CHAPTER

33

Agents Used in Anemias & Hematopoietic Growth Factors

Blood cells play essential roles in oxygenation of tissues, coagulation, protection against infectious agents, and tissue repair. Blood cell deficiency is a relatively common occurrence that can have profound repercussions. The most common cause of erythrocyte deficiency, or anemia, is insufficient supply of iron, vitamin B_{12}, or folic acid, substances required for normal production of erythrocytes. Pharmacologic treatment of these types of anemia usually involves replacement of the missing substance. An alternative therapy for certain types of anemia and for deficiency in other types of blood cells is administration of recombinant hematopoietic growth factors, which stimulate the production of various lineages of blood cells and regulate blood cell function.

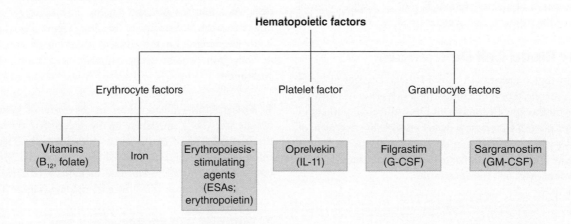

High-Yield Terms to Learn

Cobalamin	Vitamin B_{12}
ESAs	Erythropoiesis-stimulating agents
dTMP synthesis	A set of biochemical reactions that produce deoxythymidylate (dTMP), an essential constituent of DNA synthesis. The cycle depends on the conversion of dihydrofolate to tetrahydrofolate by dihydrofolate reductase (Figure 33–1)
G-CSF	Granulocyte colony-stimulating factor, a hematopoietic growth factor that regulates production and function of neutrophils
GM-CSF	Granulocyte-macrophage colony-stimulating factor, a hematopoietic growth factor that regulates production of granulocytes (basophils, eosinophils, and neutrophils), and other myeloid cells
Hemochromatosis	A condition of chronic excess total body iron caused either by an inherited abnormality of iron absorption or by frequent transfusions to treat certain types of hemolytic disorders (eg, thalassemia major)
Megaloblastic anemia	A deficiency in serum hemoglobin and erythrocytes in which the erythrocytes are abnormally large. Results from either folate or vitamin B_{12} deficiency anemia
Microcytic anemia	A deficiency in serum hemoglobin and erythrocytes in which the erythrocytes are abnormally small. Often caused by iron deficiency
Neutropenia	An abnormally low number of neutrophils in the blood; patients with neutropenia are susceptible to serious infection
Pernicious anemia	A form of megaloblastic anemia resulting from deficiency of intrinsic factor, a protein produced by gastric mucosal cells and required for intestinal absorption of vitamin B_{12}
Thrombocytopenia	An abnormally low number of platelets in the blood; patients with thrombocytopenia are susceptible to hemorrhage

BLOOD CELL DEFICIENCIES

A. Iron and Vitamin Deficiency Anemias

Microcytic hypochromic anemia, caused by iron deficiency, is the most common type of anemia. Megaloblastic anemias are caused by a deficiency of vitamin B_{12} or folic acid, cofactors required for the normal maturation of red blood cells. Pernicious anemia, the most common type of vitamin B_{12} deficiency anemia, is caused by a defect in the synthesis of **intrinsic factor**, a protein required for efficient absorption of dietary vitamin B_{12}, or by surgical removal of that part of the stomach that secretes intrinsic factor.

B. Other Blood Cell Deficiencies

Deficiency in the concentration of the various lineages of blood cells can be a manifestation of a disease or a side effect of radiation or cancer chemotherapy. Recombinant DNA-directed synthesis of hematopoietic growth factors now makes possible the treatment of more patients with deficiencies in erythrocytes, neutrophils, and platelets. Some of these growth factors also play an important role in hematopoietic stem cell transplantation.

IRON

A. Role of Iron

Iron is the essential metallic component of heme, the molecule responsible for the bulk of oxygen transport in the blood. Although most of the iron in the body is contained in hemoglobin, an important fraction is bound to **transferrin,** a transport protein, and **ferritin,** a storage protein. Deficiency of iron occurs most often in women because of menstrual blood loss and in vegetarians or malnourished persons because of inadequate dietary iron intake. Children and pregnant women have increased requirements for iron.

B. Regulation of Iron Stores

Although iron is an essential ion, excessive amounts are highly toxic. As a result, a complex system has evolved for the absorption, transport, and storage of free iron (Figure 33–1). Since there is no mechanism for the efficient excretion of iron, regulation of body iron content occurs through modulation of intestinal absorption.

1. Absorption—Dietary iron in the form of heme and the ferrous ion (Fe^{2+}) are taken up by specialized transporters on the luminal surface of intestinal epithelial cells (Figure 33–1). Intestinal cell iron is either stored as ferritin or the ferrous iron is transported across the basolateral membrane by ferroportin and oxidized to ferric iron (Fe^{3+}) by a ferroxidase (Figure 33–1).

2. Transport and storage—Ferric iron is transported in a complex with transferrin (Figure 33–1). Excess iron is stored in the protein-bound form in gastrointestinal epithelial cells, macrophages, and hepatocytes, and in cases of gross overload, in parenchymal cells of the skin, heart, and other organs.

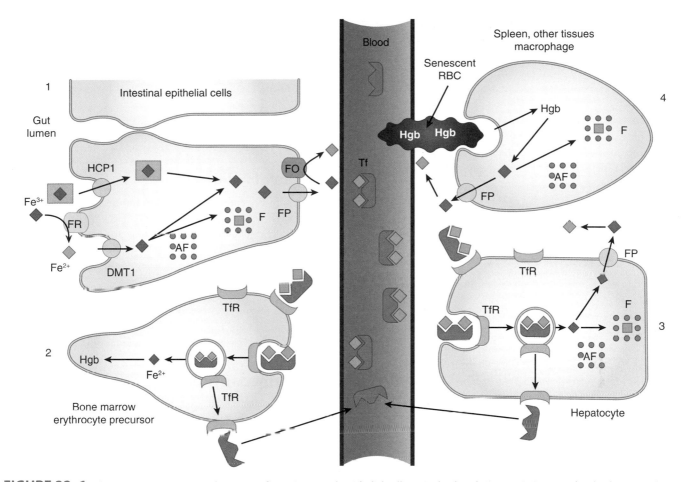

FIGURE 33–1 Absorption, transport, and storage of iron. Intestinal epithelial cells actively absorb inorganic iron via the divalent metal transporter 1 (DMT1) and heme iron via the heme carrier protein 1 (HCP1). Iron that is absorbed or released from absorbed heme iron in the intestine (**section 1**) is actively transported into the blood by ferroportin (FP) or complexed with apoferritin (AF) and stored as ferritin (F). In the blood, iron is transported by transferrin (Tf) to erythroid precursors in the bone marrow for synthesis of hemoglobin (Hgb) (**section 2**) or to hepatocytes for storage as ferritin (**section 3**). The transferrin-iron complex binds to transferrin receptors (TfR) in erythroid precursors and hepatocytes and is internalized. After release of iron, the TfR-Tf complex is recycled to the plasma membrane and Tf is released. Macrophages that phagocytize senescent erythrocytes (RBC) reclaim the iron from the RBC hemoglobin and either export it or store it as ferritin (**section 4**). Hepatocytes use several mechanisms to take up iron and store the iron as ferritin. FO, ferroxidase. (Reproduced, with permission, from Katzung BG, editor: *Basic & Clinical Pharmacology*, 12th ed. McGraw-Hill, 2012: Fig. 33–1.)

3. Elimination—Minimal amounts of iron are lost from the body with sweat and saliva and in exfoliated skin and intestinal mucosal cells.

C. Clinical Use

Prevention or treatment of iron deficiency anemia is the only indication for iron administration. Iron deficiency can be diagnosed from red blood cell changes (microcytic cell size due to diminished hemoglobin content) and from measurements of serum and bone marrow iron stores. The disease is treated by dietary ferrous iron supplementation with **ferrous sulfate, ferrous gluconate,** or **ferrous fumarate.** In special cases, treatment is by parenteral administration of a colloid containing a core of iron oxyhydroxide surrounded by a core of carbohydrate. Parenteral iron preparations include **iron dextran, sodium ferric gluconate complex,** and **iron sucrose.** Iron should *not* be given in hemolytic anemia because iron stores are elevated, not depressed, in this type of anemia.

D. Toxicity of Iron (See Also Chapter 57)

1. Signs and symptoms—Acute iron intoxication is most common in children and usually occurs as a result of accidental ingestion of iron supplementation tablets. Depending on the dose of iron, necrotizing gastroenteritis, shock, metabolic acidosis, coma, and death may result. Chronic iron overload, known as **hemochromatosis,** damages the organs that store excess iron (heart, liver, pancreas). Hemochromatosis occurs most often in individuals with an inherited abnormality of iron absorption and those who receive frequent transfusions for treatment of hemolytic disorders (eg, thalassemia major).

2. Treatment of acute iron intoxication—Immediate treatment is necessary and usually consists of removal of unabsorbed tablets from the gut, correction of acid-base and electrolyte abnormalities, and parenteral administration of **deferoxamine**, which chelates circulating iron.

3. Treatment of chronic iron toxicity—Treatment of the genetic form of hemochromatosis is usually by phlebotomy. Hemochromatosis that is due to frequent transfusions is treated with parenteral deferoxamine or with the newer oral iron chelator **deferasirox**.

VITAMIN B$_{12}$

A. Role of Vitamin B$_{12}$

Vitamin B$_{12}$ (cobalamin), a cobalt-containing molecule, is, along with folic acid, a cofactor in the transfer of 1-carbon units, a step necessary for the synthesis of DNA. Impairment of DNA synthesis affects all cells, but because red blood cells must be produced continuously, deficiency of either vitamin B$_{12}$ or folic acid usually manifests first as anemia. In addition, vitamin B$_{12}$ deficiency can cause neurologic defects, which may become irreversible if not treated promptly.

B. Pharmacokinetics

Vitamin B$_{12}$ is produced only by bacteria; this vitamin cannot be synthesized by multicellular organisms. It is absorbed from the gastrointestinal tract in the presence of **intrinsic factor,** a product of the parietal cells of the stomach. Plasma transport is accomplished by binding to transcobalamin II. Vitamin B$_{12}$ is stored in the liver in large amounts; a normal individual has enough to last 5 yrs. The 2 available forms of vitamin B$_{12}$, cyanocobalamin and hydroxocobalamin, have similar pharmacokinetics, but hydroxocobalamin has a longer circulating half-life.

C. Pharmacodynamics

Vitamin B$_{12}$ is essential in 2 reactions: conversion of methylmalonyl-coenzyme A (CoA) to succinyl-CoA and conversion of homocysteine to methionine. The second reaction is linked to folic acid metabolism and synthesis of deoxythymidylate (dTMP; Figure 33–1, section 2), a precursor required for DNA synthesis. In vitamin B$_{12}$ deficiency, folates accumulate as N^5-methyltetrahydrofolate; the supply of tetrahydrofolate is depleted; and the production of red blood cells slows. Administration of folic acid to patients with vitamin B$_{12}$ deficiency helps refill the tetrahydrofolate pool (Figure 33–1, section 3) and partially or fully corrects the anemia. However, the exogenous folic acid does not correct the neurologic defects of vitamin B$_{12}$ deficiency.

D. Clinical Use and Toxicity

The 2 available forms of vitamin B$_{12}$—hydroxocobalamin and cyanocobalamin—have equivalent effects. The major application is in the treatment of naturally occurring pernicious anemia and anemia caused by gastric resection. Because vitamin B$_{12}$ deficiency anemia is almost always caused by inadequate absorption, therapy should be by replacement of vitamin B$_{12}$, using parenteral therapy. Neither form of vitamin B$_{12}$ has significant toxicity.

FOLIC ACID

A. Role of Folic Acid

Like vitamin B$_{12}$, folic acid is required for normal DNA synthesis, and its deficiency usually presents as megaloblastic anemia. In addition, deficiency of folic acid during pregnancy increases the risk of neural tube defects in the fetus.

B. Pharmacokinetics

Folic acid is readily absorbed from the gastrointestinal tract. Only modest amounts are stored in the body, so a decrease in dietary intake is followed by anemia within a few months.

C. Pharmacodynamics

Folic acid is converted to tetrahydrofolate by the action of dihydrofolate reductase (Figure 33–1, section 3). One important set of reactions involving tetrahydrofolate and dihydrofolate constitutes the dTMP cycle (Figure 33–2, section 2), which supplies the dTMP required for DNA synthesis. Rapidly dividing cells are highly sensitive to folic acid deficiency. For this reason, antifolate drugs are useful in the treatment of various infections and cancers.

D. Clinical Use and Toxicity

Folic acid deficiency is most often caused by dietary insufficiency or malabsorption. Anemia resulting from folic acid deficiency is readily treated by oral folic acid supplementation. Because maternal folic acid deficiency is associated with increased risk of neural tube defects in the fetus, folic acid supplementation is recommended before and during pregnancy. Folic acid supplements correct the anemia but not the neurologic deficits of vitamin B$_{12}$ deficiency. Therefore, vitamin B$_{12}$ deficiency must be ruled out before one selects folic acid as the sole therapeutic agent in the treatment of a patient with megaloblastic anemia. Folic acid has no recognized toxicity.

HEMATOPOIETIC GROWTH FACTORS

More than a dozen glycoprotein hormones that regulate the differentiation and maturation of stem cells within the bone marrow have been identified. Several growth factors, produced by recombinant DNA technology, have FDA approval for the treatment of patients with blood cell deficiencies.

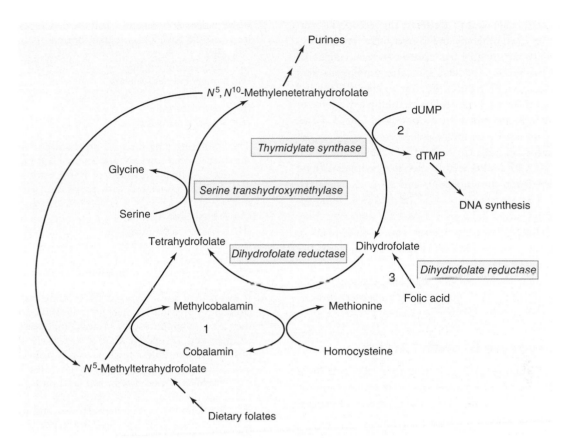

FIGURE 33–2 Enzymatic reactions that use folates. **Section 1** shows the vitamin B_{12}-dependent reaction that allows most dietary folates to enter the tetrahydrofolate cofactor pool and becomes the "folate trap" in vitamin B_{12} deficiency. **Section 2** shows the dTMP cycle. **Section 3** shows the pathway by which folate enters the tetrahydrofolate cofactor pool. Double arrows indicate pathways with more than 1 intermediate step. (Reproduced, with permission, from Katzung BG, editor: *Basic & Clinical Pharmacology*, 12th ed. McGraw-Hill, 2012: Fig. 33–3.)

SKILL KEEPER: ROUTES OF ADMINISTRATION (SEE CHAPTER 1)

All of the recombinant hematopoietic growth factors approved for clinical use are administered by injection. Why can these growth factors not be given orally? Which 3 routes of administration require drug injection? How do these 3 routes compare with regard to onset and duration of drug action and risk of adverse effects? The Skill Keeper Answers appear at the end of the chapter.

A. Erythropoiesis-Stimulating Agents (ESAs)

Erythropoietin is produced by the kidney; reduction in its synthesis underlies the anemia of renal failure. Through activation of receptors on erythroid progenitors in the bone marrow, erythropoietin stimulates the production of red cells and increases their release from the bone marrow.

Erythropoiesis-stimulating agents (ESAs) are routinely used for the anemia associated with renal failure and are sometimes effective for patients with other forms of anemia (eg, primary bone marrow disorders or anemias secondary to cancer chemotherapy or HIV treatment, bone marrow transplantation, AIDS, or cancer). As an alternative to recombinant human erythropoietin (**epoetin alfa**), **darbepoetin alfa**, a glycosylated form of erythropoietin, has a much longer half-life. **Methoxy polyethylene glycol-epoetin beta** is a long-lasting form of erythropoietin that can be administered once or twice a month.

The most common complications of ESA therapy are hypertension and thrombosis. The serum hemoglobin concentration of patients treated with an ESA should not exceed 12 g/dL because hemoglobin concentrations above this target have been linked to an increased rate of mortality and cardiovascular events.

B. Myeloid Growth Factors

Filgrastim (granulocyte colony-stimulating factor; **G-CSF**) and **sargramostim** (granulocyte-macrophage colony-stimulating factor; **GM-CSF**) stimulate the production and function of neutrophils. GM-CSF also stimulates the production of other myeloid and megakaryocyte progenitors. G-CSF and, to a lesser degree, GM-CSF mobilize hematopoietic stem cells (ie, increase their concentration in peripheral blood).

Both growth factors are used to accelerate the recovery of neutrophils after cancer chemotherapy and to treat other forms of secondary and primary neutropenia (eg, aplastic anemia, congenital neutropenia). When given to patients soon after autologous stem cell transplantation, G-CSF reduces the time to engraftment and the duration of neutropenia. In patients with multiple myeloma or non-Hodgkin's lymphoma who respond poorly to G-CSF alone, G-CSF may be combined with the novel hematopoietic stem cell mobilizer **plerixafor,** an inhibitor of the CXC chemokine receptor 4 (CXCR4). G-CSF is also used to mobilize peripheral blood stem cells in preparation for autologous and allogeneic stem cell transplantation. The toxicity of G-CSF is minimal, although the drug sometimes causes bone pain. GM-CSF can cause more severe effects, including fever, arthralgias, and capillary damage with edema. Allergic reactions are rare. **Pegfilgrastim,** a covalent conjugation product of filgrastim and a form of polyethylene glycol, has a much longer serum half-life than recombinant G-CSF. Lenograstim, used widely in Europe, is a glycosylated form of recombinant G-CSF.

C. Megakaryocyte Growth Factors

Oprelvekin (interleukin-11 [**IL-11**]) stimulates the growth of primitive megakaryocytic progenitors and increases the number of peripheral platelets. IL-11 is used for the treatment of patients who have had a prior episode of thrombocytopenia after a cycle of cancer chemotherapy. In such patients, it reduces the need for platelet transfusions. The most common adverse effects of IL-11 are fatigue, headache, dizziness, and fluid retention.

Romiplostim, a thrombopoietin receptor agonist with a novel peptide structure, is used subcutaneously in patients with chronic idiopathic thrombocytopenia who have failed to respond to conventional treatment. **Eltrombopag** is an oral agonist of the thrombopoietin receptor that is also used for patients with chronic idiopathic thrombocytopenia that is refractory to other agents. The risk of hepatotoxicity and hemorrhage has restricted eltrombopag use to registered physicians and patients.

QUESTIONS

Questions 1–4. A 23-year-old pregnant woman is referred by her obstetrician for evaluation of anemia. She is in her fourth month of pregnancy and has no history of anemia; her grandfather had pernicious anemia. Her hemoglobin is 10 g/dL (normal, 12–16 g/dL).

1. If this woman has macrocytic anemia, an increased serum concentration of transferrin, and a normal serum concentration of vitamin B_{12}, the most likely cause of her anemia is deficiency of which of the following?
   (A) Cobalamin
   (B) Erythropoietin
   (C) Folic acid
   (D) Intrinsic factor
   (E) Iron

2. If the patient in Question 1 had the deficiency identified, her infant would have a higher than normal risk of which of the following?
   (A) Cardiac abnormality
   (B) Congenital neutropenia
   (C) Kidney damage
   (D) Limb deformity
   (E) Neural tube defect

3. The laboratory data for your pregnant patient indicate that she does not have macrocytic anemia but rather microcytic anemia. Optimal treatment of normocytic or mild microcytic anemia associated with pregnancy uses which of the following?
   (A) A high-fiber diet
   (B) Erythropoietin injections
   (C) Ferrous sulfate tablets
   (D) Folic acid supplements
   (E) Hydroxocobalamin injections

4. If this patient has a young child at home and is taking iron-containing prenatal supplements, she should be warned that they are a common source of accidental poisoning in young children and advised to make a special effort to keep these pills out of her child's reach. Toxicity associated with acute iron poisoning usually includes which of the following?
   (A) Dizziness, hypertension, and cerebral hemorrhage
   (B) Hyperthermia, delirium, and coma
   (C) Hypotension, cardiac arrhythmias, and seizures
   (D) Necrotizing gastroenteritis, shock, and metabolic acidosis
   (E) Severe hepatic injury, encephalitis, and coma

5. The iron stored in intestinal mucosal cells is complexed to which of the following?
   (A) Apoferritin
   (B) Intrinsic factor
   (C) Oprelvekin
   (D) Transcobalamin II
   (E) Transferrin

6. Which of the following is *most* likely to be required by a 5-year-old boy with chronic renal insufficiency?
   (A) Cyanocobalamin
   (B) Deferoxamine
   (C) Erythropoietin
   (D) Filgrastim (G-CSF)
   (E) Oprelvekin (IL-11)

7. In a patient who requires filgrastim (G-CSF) after being treated with anticancer drugs, the therapeutic objective is to prevent which of the following?
   (A) Allergic reactions
   (B) Cancer recurrence
   (C) Excessive bleeding
   (D) Hypoxia
   (E) Systemic infection

8. The megaloblastic anemia that results from vitamin B_{12} deficiency is due to inadequate supplies of which of the following?
   (A) Cobalamin
   (B) dTMP
   (C) Folic acid
   (D) Homocysteine
   (E) N^5-methyltetrahydrofolate

Questions 9 and 10. After undergoing surgery for breast cancer, a 53-year-old woman is scheduled to receive 4 cycles of cancer chemotherapy. The cycles are to be administered every 3–5 wks. Her first cycle was complicated by severe chemotherapy-induced thrombocytopenia.

9. During the second cycle of chemotherapy, it would be appropriate to consider treating this patient with which of the following?
   (A) Darbepoetin alpha
   (B) Filgrastim (G-CSF)
   (C) Iron dextran
   (D) Oprelvekin (IL-11)
   (E) Vitamin B_{12}

10. Twenty months after finishing her chemotherapy, the woman had a relapse of breast cancer. The cancer was now unresponsive to standard doses of chemotherapy. The decision was made to treat the patient with high-dose chemotherapy followed by autologous stem cell transplantation. Which of the following drugs is most likely to be used to mobilize the peripheral blood stem cells needed for the patient's autologous stem cell transplantation?
    (A) Erythropoietin
    (B) Filgrastim (G-CSF)
    (C) Folic acid
    (D) Intrinsic factor
    (E) Oprelvekin (interleukin-11)

ANSWERS

1. Deficiencies of folic acid or vitamin B_{12} are the most common causes of megaloblastic anemia. If a patient with this type of anemia has a normal serum vitamin B_{12} concentration, folate deficiency is the most likely cause of the anemia. The answer is **C.**

2. Deficiency of folic acid during early pregnancy is associated with increased risk of a neural tube defect in the newborn. In the United States, cereals and grains are supplemented with folic acid in an effort to decrease the incidence of neural tube defects. The answer is **E.**

3. Iron deficiency microcytic anemia is the anemia that is most commonly associated with pregnancy. In this condition, oral iron supplementation is indicated. The answer is **C.**

4. Acute iron poisoning often causes severe gastrointestinal damage resulting from direct corrosive effects, shock from fluid loss in the gastrointestinal tract, and metabolic acidosis from cellular dysfunction. The answer is **D.**

5. The iron stored in intestinal mucosal cells, macrophages, and hepatocytes is in ferritin, a complex of iron and the protein apoferritin. The answer is **A.**

6. The kidney produces erythropoietin; patients with chronic renal insufficiency often require exogenous erythropoietin to avoid chronic anemia. The answer is **C.**

7. Filgrastim (G-CSF) stimulates the production and function of neutrophils, important cellular mediators of the innate immune system that serve as the first line of defense against infection. The answer is **E.**

8. Deficiency of vitamin B_{12} (cobalamin) leads to a deficiency in tetrahydrofolate and subsequently a deficiency of the dTMP required for DNA synthesis. Homocysteine and N^5-methyltetrahydrofolate accumulate. The answer is **B.**

9. Oprelvekin (IL-11) stimulates platelet production and decreases the number of platelet transfusions required by patients undergoing bone marrow suppression therapy for cancer. The answer is **D.**

10. The success of transplantation with peripheral blood stem cells depends on infusion of adequate numbers of hematopoietic stem cells. Administration of G-CSF to the donor (in the case of autologous transplantation, the patient who also will be the recipient of the transplantation) greatly increases the number of hematopoietic stem cells harvested from the donor's blood. The answer is **B.**

SKILL KEEPER ANSWERS: ROUTES OF ADMINISTRATION (SEE CHAPTER 1)

All of the hematopoietic growth factors are proteins with molecular weights greater than 15,000. Like other proteinaceous drugs, the growth factors cannot be administered orally because they have such poor bioavailability. Their peptide bonds are destroyed by stomach acid and digestive enzymes.

Injections are required for intravenous, intramuscular, and subcutaneous administration. The intravenous route offers the fastest onset of drug action and shortest duration of drug action. Because intravenous administration can produce high blood levels, this route of administration has the greatest risk of producing concentration-dependent drug toxicity. Intramuscular injection has a quicker onset of action than subcutaneous injection, and larger volumes of injected fluid can be given. Because protective barriers can be breached by the needle or tubing used for drug injection, all 3 of these routes of administration carry a greater risk of infection than does oral drug administration.

CHECKLIST

When you complete this chapter, you should be able to:

❑ Name the 2 most common types of nutritional anemia, and, for each, describe the most likely biochemical causes.

❑ Diagram the normal pathways of absorption, transport, and storage of iron in the human body.

❑ Name the anemias for which iron supplementation is indicated and those for which it is contraindicated.

❑ List the acute and chronic toxicities of iron.

❑ Sketch the dTMP cycle and show how deficiency of folic acid or deficiency of vitamin B_{12} affects the normal cycle.

❑ Explain the major hazard involved in the use of folic acid as sole therapy for megaloblastic anemia and indicate on a sketch of the dTMP cycle the biochemical basis of the hazard.

❑ Name 3–5 major hematopoietic growth factors that are used clinically and describe the clinical uses and toxicity of each.

❑ Explain the advantage of covalently attaching polyethylene glycol to filgrastim.

DRUG SUMMARY TABLE: Drugs for Anemia & Hematopoietic Growth Factors

Subclass	Mechanism of Action	Clinical Applications	Pharmacokinetics	Toxicities, Interactions
Iron				
Ferrous sulfate	Required for biosynthesis of heme and heme-containing proteins, including hemoglobin	Iron deficiency, which manifests as microcytic anemia	Complicated endogenous system for absorbing, storing, and transporting iron • no mechanism for iron excretion other than cell and blood loss	Acute overdose results in necrotizing gastroenteritis, abdominal pain, bloody diarrhea, shock, lethargy, and dyspnea • chronic iron overload results in hemochromatosis, with damage to the heart, liver, pancreas

Ferrous gluconate and ferrous fumarate: oral iron preparations
Iron dextran, iron sucrose complex, and sodium ferric gluconate complex: parenteral preparations; can cause pain, hypersensitivity reactions

Iron chelators (see also Chapters 57 and 58)				
Deferoxamine	Chelates excess iron	Acute iron poisoning • inherited or acquired hemochromatosis	Preferred route of administration: intramuscular or subcutaneous	Rapid IV administration may cause hypotension • neurotoxicity and increased susceptibility to certain infections has occurred with long-term use

Deferasirox: oral iron chelator for treatment of hemochromatosis

(Continued)

DRUG SUMMARY TABLE: Drugs for Anemia & Hematopoietic Growth Factors (*Continued*)

Subclass	Mechanism of Action	Clinical Applications	Pharmacokinetics	Toxicities, Interactions
Vitamin B$_{12}$				
Cyanocobalamin, hydroxocobalamin	Cofactor required for essential enzymatic reactions that form tetrahydrofolate, convert homocysteine to methionine, and metabolize L-methylmalonyl-CoA	Vitamin B$_{12}$ deficiency, which manifests as megaloblastic anemia and is the basis of pernicious anemia	Parenteral vitamin B$_{12}$ is required for pernicious anemia and other malabsorption syndromes	No toxicity associated with excess vitamin B$_{12}$
Folic acid				
Folacin (pteroylglutamic acid)	Precursor of an essential donor of methyl groups used for synthesis of amino acids, purines, and deoxynucleotides	Folic acid deficiency, which manifests as megaloblastic anemia • prevention of congenital neural tube defects	Oral is well absorbed; need for parenteral administration is rare	Not toxic in overdose, but large amounts can mask vitamin B$_{12}$ deficiency
Erythropoiesis-stimulating agents (ESAs)				
Epoetin alfa	Agonist of erythropoietin receptors expressed by red cell progenitors	Anemia, especially associated with chronic renal failure, HIV infection, cancer, and prematurity • prevention of need for transfusion in patients undergoing certain types of elective surgery	Intravenous or subcutaneous administration 1–3 × per week	Hypertension, thrombotic complications, and, very rarely, pure red cell aplasia • to reduce the risk of serious cardiovascular events, hemoglobin levels should be maintained <12 g/dL

Darbepoetin alfa: long-acting glycosylated form administered weekly
Methoxy polyethylene glycol-epoetin beta: long-acting form administered 1–2 × per month

Myeloid growth factors				
G-CSF (filgrastim)	Stimulates G-CSF receptors expressed on mature neutrophils and their progenitors	Neutropenia associated with congenital neutropenia, cyclic neutropenia, myelodysplasia, and aplastic anemia • secondary prevention of neutropenia in patients undergoing cytotoxic chemotherapy • mobilization of peripheral blood cells in preparation for autologous and allogenic stem cell transplantation	Daily subcutaneous administration	Bone pain • rarely, splenic rupture

Pegfilgrastim: long-acting form of filgrastim that is covalently linked to a type of polyethylene glycol
GM-CSF (sargramostim): myeloid growth factor that acts through a distinct GM-CSF receptor to stimulate proliferation and differentiation of early and late granulocytic progenitor cells, and erythroid and megakaryocyte progenitors. Clinical uses are similar to those of G-CSF, although it is more likely than G-CSF to cause fever, arthralgia, myalgia, and a capillary leak syndrome
Plerixafor: antagonist of CXCR4 receptor used in combination with G-CSF for mobilization of peripheral blood cells prior to autologous transplantation in patients with multiple myeloma or non-Hodgkin's lymphoma who responded suboptimally to G-CSF alone

(*Continued*)

DRUG SUMMARY TABLE: Drugs for Anemia & Hematopoietic Growth Factors (*Continued*)

Subclass	Mechanism of Action	Clinical Applications	Pharmacokinetics	Toxicities, Interactions
Megakaryocyte growth factors				
Oprelvekin (interleukin-11; IL-11)	Recombinant form of an endogenous cytokine • activates IL-11 receptors	Secondary prevention of thrombocytopenia in patients undergoing cytotoxic chemotherapy for nonmyeloid cancers	Daily subcutaneous administration	Fatigue, headache, dizziness, anemia, fluid accumulation in the lungs, and transient atrial arrhythmias

Romiplostim: genetically engineered protein in which the F_c components of a human antibody are fused to multiple copies of a peptide that stimulates the thrombopoietin receptors; approved for treatment of idiopathic thrombocytopenic purpura (ITP)

Eltrombopag: orally active agonist of thrombopoietin receptor; restricted use because of risk of hepatotoxicity and hemorrhage

Drugs Used in Coagulation Disorders

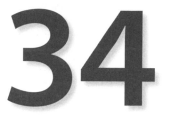

The drugs used in clotting and bleeding disorders fall into 2 major groups: (1) drugs used to decrease clotting or dissolve clots already present in patients at risk for vascular occlusion and (2) drugs used to increase clotting in patients with clotting deficiencies. The first group, the anticlotting drugs, includes some of the most commonly used drugs in the United States. Anticlotting drugs are used in the treatment and prevention of myocardial infarction and other acute coronary syndromes, atrial fibrillation, ischemic stroke, and deep vein thrombosis (DVT). Within the anticlotting group, the anticoagulant and thrombolytic drugs are effective in treatment of both venous and arterial thrombosis, whereas antiplatelet drugs are used primarily for treatment of arterial disease.

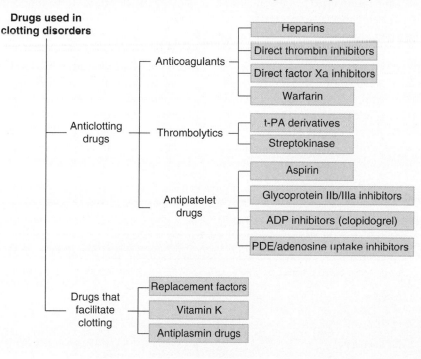

ANTICOAGULANTS

A. Classification

Anticoagulants inhibit the formation of fibrin clots. Three major types of anticoagulants are available: heparin and related products, which must be used parenterally; direct thrombin and factor X inhibitors, which are used parenterally or orally; and the orally active coumarin derivatives (eg, warfarin). Comparative properties of the heparins and warfarin are shown in Table 34–1.

B. Heparin

1. Chemistry—Heparin is a large sulfated polysaccharide polymer obtained from animal sources. Each batch contains molecules of varying size, with an average molecular weight of 15,000–20,000.

High-Yield Terms to Learn

Activated partial thromboplastin time (aPTT) test	Laboratory test used to monitor the anticoagulant effect of unfractionated heparin and direct thrombin inhibitors; prolonged when drug effect is adequate
Antithrombin III	An endogenous anticlotting protein that irreversibly inactivates thrombin and factor Xa. Its enzymatic action is markedly accelerated by the heparins
Clotting cascade	System of serine proteases and substrates in the blood that provides rapid generation of clotting factors in response to blood vessel damage
Glycoprotein IIb/IIIa (GPIIb/IIIa)	A protein complex on the surface of platelets. When activated, it aggregates platelets primarily by binding to fibrin. Endogenous factors including thromboxane A_2, ADP, and serotonin initiate a signaling cascade that activates GPIIb/IIIa
Heparin-induced thrombocytopenia (HIT)	A hypercoagulable state plus thrombocytopenia that occurs in a small number of individuals treated with unfractionated heparin
LMW heparins	Fractionated preparations of heparin of molecular weight 2000—6000. Unfractionated heparin has a molecular weight range of 5000—30,000
Prothrombin time (PT) test	Laboratory test used to monitor the anticoagulant effect of warfarin; prolonged when drug effect is adequate

Heparin is highly acidic and can be neutralized by basic molecules (eg, **protamine**). Heparin is given intravenously or subcutaneously to avoid the risk of hematoma associated with intramuscular injection.

Low-molecular-weight (LMW) fractions of heparin (eg, **enoxaparin**) have molecular weights of 2000–6000. LMW heparins have greater bioavailability and longer durations of action than unfractionated heparin; thus, doses can be given less frequently (eg, once or twice a day). They are given subcutaneously. **Fondaparinux** is a small synthetic drug that contains the biologically active pentasaccharide present in unfractionated

and LMW heparins. It is administered subcutaneously once daily.

2. Mechanism and effects—Unfractionated heparin binds to endogenous **antithrombin III** (ATIII) via a key pentasaccharide sequence. The heparin–ATIII complex combines with and irreversibly inactivates thrombin and several other factors, particularly factor Xa (Figure 34–1). In the presence of heparin, ATIII proteolyzes thrombin and factor Xa approximately 1000-fold faster than in its absence. Because it acts on preformed blood components, heparin provides anticoagulation immediately after administration.

TABLE 34–1 Properties of heparins and warfarin.

Property	Heparins	Warfarin
Structure	Large acidic polysaccharide polymers	Small lipid-soluble molecule
Route of administration	Parenteral	Oral
Site of action	Blood	Liver
Onset of action	Rapid (minutes)	Slow (days); limited by half-lives of preexisting normal factors
Mechanism of action	Activates antithrombin III, which proteolyzes coagulation factors including thrombin and factor Xa	Impairs post-translational modification of factors II, VII, IX and X
Monitoring	aPTT for unfractionated heparin but not LMW heparins	Prothrombin time
Antidote	Protamine for unfractionated heparin; protamine reversal of LMW heparins is incomplete	Vitamin K_1, plasma, prothrombin complex concentrates
Use	Mostly acute, over days	Chronic, over weeks to months
Use in pregnancy	Yes	No

aPTT, activated partial thromboplastin time; LMW, low molecular weight.

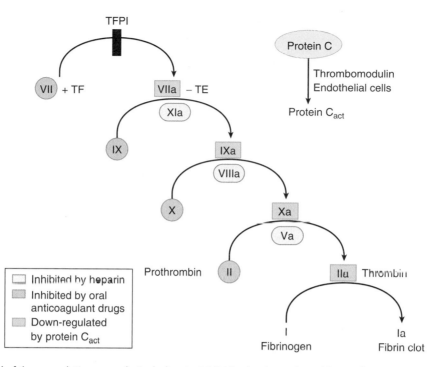

FIGURE 34–1 A model of the coagulation cascade, including its inhibition by the activated form of protein C. Tissue factor (TF) is important in initiating the cascade. Tissue factor pathway inhibitor (TFPI) inhibits the action of the VIIa–TF complex. (Reproduced, with permission, from Katzung BG, editor: *Basic & Clinical Pharmacology*, 11th ed. McGraw-Hill, 2009: Fig. 34–2.)

The action of heparin is monitored with the **activated partial thromboplastin time (aPTT)** laboratory test.

LMW heparins and fondaparinux, like unfractionated heparin, bind ATIII. These complexes have the same inhibitory effect on factor Xa as the unfractionated heparin–ATIII complex. However, the short-chain heparin–ATIII and fondaparinux–ATIII complexes provide a more selective action because they fail to affect thrombin. The aPTT test does not reliably measure the anticoagulant effect of the LMW heparins and fondaparinux; this is a potential problem, especially in renal failure, in which their clearance may be decreased.

3. Clinical use—Because of its rapid effect, heparin is used when anticoagulation is needed immediately (eg, when starting therapy). Common uses include treatment of DVT, pulmonary embolism, and acute myocardial infarction. Heparin is used in combination with thrombolytics for revascularization and in combination with glycoprotein IIb/IIIa inhibitors during angioplasty and placement of coronary stents. Because it does not cross the placental barrier, heparin is the drug of choice when an anticoagulant must be used in pregnancy. LMW heparins and fondaparinux have similar clinical applications.

4. Toxicity—Increased bleeding is the most common adverse effect of heparin and related molecules; the bleeding may result in hemorrhagic stroke. **Protamine** can lessen the risk of serious bleeding that can result from excessive unfractionated heparin. Protamine only partially reverses the effects of LMW heparins and does not affect the action of fondaparinux. Unfractionated heparin causes moderate transient thrombocytopenia in many patients and severe thrombocytopenia and thrombosis (heparin-induced thrombocytopenia or HIT) in a small percentage of patients who produce an antibody that binds to a complex of heparin and platelet factor 4. LMW heparins and fondaparinux are less likely to cause this immune-mediated thrombocytopenia. Prolonged use of unfractionated heparin is associated with osteoporosis.

C. Direct Thrombin Inhibitors

1. Chemistry and pharmacokinetics—Direct thrombin inhibitors are based on proteins made by *Hirudo medicinalis*, the medicinal leech. **Lepirudin** is the recombinant form of the leech protein hirudin, while **desirudin** and **bivalirudin** are modified forms of hirudin. **Argatroban** is a small molecule with a short half-life. All 4 drugs are administered parenterally. **Dabigatran** is an orally active direct thrombin inhibitor.

2. Mechanism and effects—The protein analogs of lepirudin bind simultaneously to the active site of thrombin and to thrombin substrates. Argatroban binds solely to the thrombin-active site. Unlike the heparins, these drugs inhibit both soluble thrombin and the thrombin enmeshed within developing clots. Bivalirudin also inhibits platelet activation.

3. Clinical use—Direct thrombin inhibitors are used as alternatives to heparin primarily in patients with heparin-induced thrombocytopenia. Bivalirudin also is used in combination with aspirin during percutaneous coronary angioplasty. Like unfractionated heparin, the action of these drugs is monitored with the aPTT laboratory test.

4. Toxicity—Like other anticoagulants, the direct thrombin inhibitors can cause bleeding. No reversal agents exist. Prolonged infusion of lepirudin can induce antibodies that form a complex with lepirudin and prolong its action, and it can induce anaphylactic reactions.

D. Direct Oral Factor Xa inhibitors

1. Chemistry and pharmacokinetics—Oral Xa inhibitors, including the small molecules **rivaroxaban** and **apixaban,** have a rapid onset of action and shorter half-lives than warfarin. These drugs are given as fixed oral doses and do not require monitoring. They undergo cytochrome P450-dependent and cytochrome P450-independent elimination.

2. Mechanism and effects—These small molecules directly bind to and inhibit both free factor Xa and factor Xa bound in the clotting complex.

3. Clinical use—Rivaroxaban is approved for prevention of venous thromboembolism following hip or knee surgery and for prevention of stroke in patients with atrial fibrillation.

4. Toxicity—Like other anticoagulants, the factor Xa inhibitors can cause bleeding. No reversal agents exist.

E. Warfarin and Other Coumarin Anticoagulants

1. Chemistry and pharmacokinetics—**Warfarin** and other coumarin anticoagulants are small, lipid-soluble molecules that are readily absorbed after oral administration. Warfarin is highly bound to plasma proteins (>99%), and its elimination depends on metabolism by cytochrome P450 enzymes.

2. Mechanism and effects—Warfarin and other coumarins interfere with the normal post-translational modification of clotting factors in the liver, a process that depends on an adequate supply of reduced vitamin K. The drugs inhibit vitamin K epoxide reductase (VKOR), which normally converts vitamin K epoxide to reduced vitamin K. The vitamin K-dependent factors include thrombin and factors VII, IX, and X (Figure 34–1). Because the clotting factors have half-lives of 8–60 h in the plasma, an anticoagulant effect is observed only after sufficient time has passed for elimination of the normal preformed factors. The action of warfarin can be reversed with vitamin K, but recovery requires the synthesis of new normal clotting factors and is, therefore, slow (6–24 h). More rapid reversal can be achieved by transfusion with fresh or frozen plasma that contains normal clotting factors. The effect of warfarin is monitored by the **prothrombin time (PT)** test.

3. Clinical use—Warfarin is used for chronic anticoagulation in all of the clinical situations described previously for heparin, except in pregnant women.

4. Toxicity—Bleeding is the most important adverse effect of warfarin. Early in therapy, a period of hypercoagulability with subsequent dermal vascular necrosis can occur. This is due to deficiency of protein C, an endogenous vitamin K-dependent anticoagulant with a short half-life. Warfarin can cause bone defects and hemorrhage in the developing fetus and, therefore, is contraindicated in pregnancy.

Because warfarin has a narrow therapeutic window, its involvement in drug interactions is of major concern. Cytochrome P450-inducing drugs (eg, carbamazepine, phenytoin, rifampin, barbiturates) increase warfarin's clearance and reduce the anticoagulant effect of a given dose. Cytochrome P450 inhibitors (eg, amiodarone, selective serotonin reuptake inhibitors, cimetidine) reduce warfarin's clearance and increase the anticoagulant effect of a given dose. Genetic variability in cytochrome P450 2C9 and VKOR affect responses to warfarin. Algorithms to determine initial warfarin dose based on cytochrome P450 2C9 and VKOR, age, body size, and concomitant medications are being tested.

THROMBOLYTIC AGENTS

A. Classification and Prototypes

The thrombolytic drugs used most commonly are either forms of the endogenous **tissue plasminogen activator** (**t-PA**; eg, **alteplase**, tenecteplase, and reteplase) or a protein synthesized by streptococci (**streptokinase**). All are given intravenously.

B. Mechanism of Action

Plasmin is an endogenous fibrinolytic enzyme that degrades clots by splitting fibrin into fragments (Figure 34–2). The thrombolytic enzymes catalyze the conversion of the inactive precursor, **plasminogen**, to plasmin.

1. Tissue plasminogen activator—t-PA is an enzyme that directly converts plasminogen to plasmin (Figure 34–2). It has

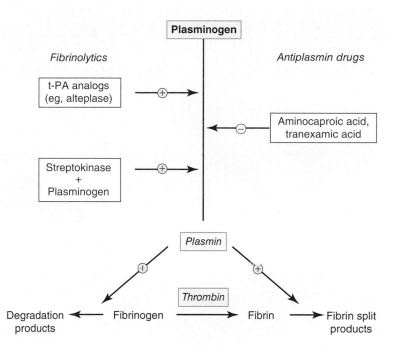

FIGURE 34–2 Diagram of the fibrinolytic system. The useful thrombolytic drugs are shown on the left. These drugs increase the formation of plasmin, the major fibrinolytic enzyme. Antiplasmin drugs are shown on the right. Aminocaproic acid and tranexamic acid inhibit plasmin formation.

little activity unless it is bound to fibrin, which, in theory, should make it selective for the plasminogen that has already bound to fibrin (ie, in a clot) and should result in less danger of widespread production of plasmin and spontaneous bleeding. In fact, t-PA's selectivity appears to be quite limited. **Alteplase** is normal human plasminogen activator. **Reteplase** is a mutated form of human t-PA with similar effects but a slightly faster onset of action and longer duration of action. **Tenecteplase** is another mutated form of t-PA with a longer half-life.

2. Streptokinase—Streptokinase is obtained from bacterial cultures. Although not itself an enzyme, streptokinase forms a complex with endogenous plasminogen; the plasminogen in this complex undergoes a conformational change that allows it to rapidly convert free plasminogen into plasmin. Unlike the forms of t-PA, streptokinase does not show selectivity for fibrin-bound plasminogen.

C. Clinical Use

The major application of the thrombolytic agents is as an alternative to percutaneous coronary angioplasty in the emergency treatment of coronary artery thrombosis. Under ideal conditions (ie, treatment within 6 h), these agents can promptly recanalize the occluded coronary vessel. Very prompt use (ie, within 3 h of the first symptoms) of t-PA in patients with ischemic stroke is associated with a significantly better clinical outcome. Cerebral hemorrhage must be positively ruled out before such use. The thrombolytic agents are also used in cases of severe pulmonary embolism.

D. Toxicity

Bleeding is the most important hazard and has about the same frequency with all the thrombolytic drugs. Cerebral hemorrhage is the most serious manifestation. Streptokinase, a bacterial protein, can evoke the production of antibodies that cause it to lose its effectiveness or induce severe allergic reactions on subsequent therapy. Patients who have had streptococcal infections may have preformed antibodies to the drug. Because they are human proteins, the recombinant forms of t-PA are not subject to this problem. However, they are much more expensive than streptokinase and not much more effective.

ANTIPLATELET DRUGS

Platelet aggregation contributes to the clotting process (Figure 34–3) and is especially important in clots that form in the arterial circulation. Platelets appear to play a central role in pathologic coronary and cerebral artery occlusion. Platelet aggregation is triggered by a variety of endogenous mediators that include the prostaglandin thromboxane, adenosine diphosphate (ADP), thrombin, and fibrin. Substances that increase intracellular cyclic adenosine monophosphate (cAMP; eg, the prostaglandin prostacyclin, adenosine) inhibit platelet aggregation.

A. Classification and Prototypes

Antiplatelet drugs include **aspirin** and other nonsteroidal anti-inflammatory drugs (NSAIDs), glycoprotein IIb/IIIa receptor inhibitors (**abciximab, tirofiban,** and **eptifibatide**), antagonists

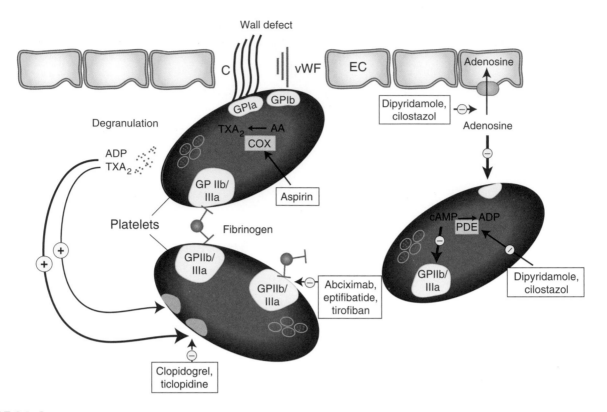

FIGURE 34–3 Thrombus formation at the site of the damaged vascular wall (EC, endothelials cell) and the role of platelets and clotting factors. Platelet membrane receptors include the glycoprotein (GP) la receptor, binding to collagen (C); GP Ib receptor, binding von Willebrand factor (vWF); and GP IIb/IIIa, which binds fibrinogen and other macromolecules. Antiplatelet prostacyclin (PGI$_2$) is released from the endothelium. Aggregating substances released from the degranulating platelet include adenosine diphosphate (ADP), thromboxane A2 (TXA$_2$), and serotonin (5-HT). (Modified and reproduced, with permission, from Katzung BG, editor: *Basic & Clinical Pharmacology*, 12th ed. McGraw-Hill, 2012: Fig. 34–1.)

of ADP receptors (**clopidogrel** and **ticlopidine**), and inhibitors of phosphodiesterase 3 (**dipyridamole** and **cilostazol**).

B. Mechanism of Action

Aspirin and other NSAIDs inhibit thromboxane synthesis by blocking the enzyme cyclooxygenase (COX; Chapter 18). Thromboxane A$_2$ is a potent stimulator of platelet aggregation. Aspirin, an irreversible COX inhibitor, is particularly effective. Because platelets lack the machinery for synthesis of new protein, inhibition by aspirin persists for several days until new platelets are formed. Other NSAIDs, which cause a less persistent antiplatelet effect (hours), are not used as antiplatelet drugs and, in fact, can interfere with the antiplatelet effect of aspirin when used in combination with aspirin.

Abciximab is a monoclonal antibody that reversibly inhibits the binding of fibrin and other ligands to the platelet **glycoprotein IIb/IIIa receptor**, a cell surface protein involved in platelet cross-linking. Eptifibatide and tirofiban also reversibly block the glycoprotein IIb/IIIa receptor.

Clopidogrel, prasugrel, and the older drug ticlopidine are converted in the liver to active metabolites that irreversibly inhibit the platelet ADP receptor and thereby prevent ADP-mediated platelet aggregation.

Dipyridamole and the newer cilostazol appear to have a dual mechanism of action. They prolong the platelet-inhibiting action of intracellular cAMP by inhibiting phosphodiesterase enzymes that degrade cyclic nucleotides, including cAMP, an inhibitor of platelet aggregation, and cyclic guanosine monophosphate (cGMP), a vasodilator (see Chapter 19). They also inhibit the uptake of adenosine by endothelial cells and erythrocytes and thereby increase the plasma concentration of adenosine. Adenosine acts through platelet adenosine A$_2$ receptors to increase platelet cAMP and inhibit aggregation.

C. Clinical Use

Aspirin is used to prevent further infarcts in persons who have had 1 or more myocardial infarcts and may also reduce the incidence of first infarcts. The drug is used extensively to prevent transient ischemic attacks (TIAs), ischemic stroke, and other thrombotic events.

The glycoprotein IIb/IIIa inhibitors prevent restenosis after coronary angioplasty and are used in acute coronary syndromes (eg, unstable angina and non-Q-wave acute myocardial infarction).

Clopidogrel and ticlopidine are effective in preventing TIAs and ischemic strokes, especially in patients who cannot tolerate aspirin.

Clopidogrel is routinely used to prevent thrombosis in patients who have received a coronary artery stent.

Dipyridamole is approved as an adjunct to warfarin in the prevention of thrombosis in those with cardiac valve replacement and has been used in combination with aspirin for secondary prevention of ischemic stroke. Cilostazol is used to treat intermittent claudication, a manifestation of peripheral arterial disease.

D. Toxicity

Aspirin and other NSAIDs cause gastrointestinal and CNS effects (Chapter 36). All antiplatelet drugs significantly enhance the effects of other anticlotting agents. The major toxicities of the glycoprotein IIb/IIIa receptor-blocking drugs are bleeding and, with chronic use, thrombocytopenia. Ticlopidine is used rarely because it causes bleeding in up to 5% of patients, severe neutropenia in about 1%, and very rarely **thrombotic thrombocytopenic purpura (TTP),** a syndrome characterized by the disseminated formation of small thrombi, platelet consumption, and thrombocytopenia. Clopidogrel is less hematotoxic. The most common adverse effects of dipyridamole and cilostazol are headaches and palpitations. Cilostazol is contraindicated in patients with congestive heart failure because of evidence of reduced survival.

DRUGS USED IN BLEEDING DISORDERS

Inadequate blood clotting can result from vitamin K deficiency, genetically determined errors of clotting factor synthesis (eg, hemophilia), a variety of drug-induced conditions, and thrombocytopenia. Treatment involves administration of vitamin K, preformed clotting factors, or antiplasmin drugs. Thrombocytopenia can be treated by administration of platelets or oprelvekin, the recombinant form of the megakaryocyte growth factor interleukin-11 (see Chapter 33).

A. Vitamin K

Deficiency of vitamin K, a fat-soluble vitamin, is most common in older persons with abnormalities of fat absorption and in newborns, who are at risk of vitamin K deficiency bleeding. The deficiency is readily treated with oral or parenteral **phytonadione (vitamin K$_1$).** In the United States, all newborns receive an injection of phytonadione. Large doses of vitamin K$_1$ are used to reverse the anticoagulant effect of excess warfarin.

B. Clotting Factors and Desmopressin

The most important agents used to treat hemophilia are fresh plasma and purified human blood clotting factors, especially **factor VIII** (for hemophilia A) and **factor IX** (for hemophilia B), which are either purified from blood products or produced by recombinant DNA technology. These products are expensive and carry a risk of immunologic reactions and, in the case of factors purified from blood products, infection (although most known blood-borne pathogens are removed by chemical treatment of the plasma extracts.)

The vasopressin V$_2$ receptor agonist **desmopressin acetate** (see Chapter 37) increases the plasma concentration of von Willebrand factor and factor VIII. It is used to prepare patients with mild hemophilia A or von Willebrand disease for elective surgery.

C. Antiplasmin Agents

Antiplasmin agents are valuable for the prevention or management of acute bleeding episodes in patients with hemophilia and others with a high risk of bleeding disorders. **Aminocaproic acid** and **tranexamic acid** are orally active agents that inhibit fibrinolysis by inhibiting plasminogen activation (Figure 34–2). Adverse effects include thrombosis, hypotension, myopathy, and diarrhea.

QUESTIONS

Questions 1–3. A 58-year-old business executive is brought to the emergency department 2 h after the onset of severe chest pain during a vigorous tennis game. She has a history of poorly controlled mild hypertension and elevated blood cholesterol but does not smoke. ECG changes confirm the diagnosis of myocardial infarction. The decision is made to attempt to open her occluded artery.

1. Which of the following drugs accelerates the conversion of plasminogen to plasmin?
   (A) Aminocaproic acid
   (B) Heparin
   (C) Lepirudin
   (D) Reteplase
   (E) Warfarin

2. If a fibrinolytic drug is used for treatment of this woman's acute myocardial infarction, which of the following adverse drug effects is most likely to occur?
   (A) Acute renal failure
   (B) Development of antiplatelet antibodies
   (C) Encephalitis secondary to liver dysfunction
   (D) Hemorrhagic stroke
   (E) Neutropenia

3. If this patient undergoes a percutaneous coronary angiography procedure and placement of a stent in a coronary blood vessel, she may be given eptifibatide. Which of the following most accurately describes the mechanism of eptifibatide anticlotting action?
   (A) Activation of antithrombin III
   (B) Blockade of post-translational modification of clotting factors
   (C) Inhibition of thromboxane production
   (D) Irreversible inhibition of platelet ADP receptors
   (E) Reversible inhibition of glycoprotein IIb/IIIa receptors

4. The graph shows the plasma concentration of free warfarin as a function of time for a patient who was treated with 2 other agents, drugs B and C, on a daily basis at constant dosage starting at the times shown. Which of the following is the most likely explanation for the observed changes in warfarin concentration?
   (A) Drug B displaces warfarin from plasma proteins; drug C displaces warfarin from tissue-binding sites
   (B) Drug B inhibits hepatic metabolism of warfarin; drug C displaces drug B from tissue-binding sites
   (C) Drug B stimulates hepatic metabolism of warfarin; drug C displaces warfarin from plasma protein
   (D) Drug B increases renal clearance of warfarin; drug C inhibits hepatic metabolism of drug B

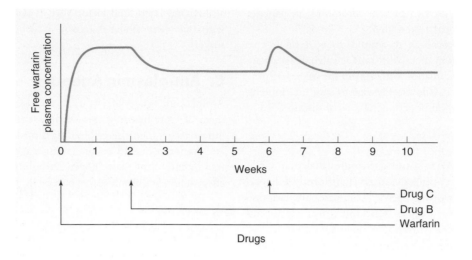

Drugs

Questions 5–7. A 65-year-old man is brought to the emergency department 30 min after the onset of right-sided weakness and aphasia (difficulty speaking). Imaging studies ruled out cerebral hemorrhage as the cause of his acute symptoms of stroke.

5. Prompt administration of which of the following drugs is most likely to improve this patient's clinical outcome?
(A) Abciximab
(B) Alteplase
(C) Factor VIII
(D) Streptokinase
(E) Vitamin K

6. Over the next 2 d, the patient's symptoms resolved completely. To prevent a recurrence of this disease, the patient is most likely to be treated indefinitely with which of the following?
(A) Aminocaproic acid
(B) Aspirin
(C) Enoxaparin
(D) Lepirudin
(E) Warfarin

7. If the patient is unable to tolerate the drug identified in Question 6, he may be treated with clopidogrel. Relative to ticlopidine, clopidogrel
(A) Has a shorter duration of action
(B) Is less likely to cause neutropenia
(C) Is more likely to induce antiplatelet antibodies
(D) Is more likely to precipitate serious bleeding
(E) Will have a greater antiplatelet effect

Questions 8 and 9. A 67-year-old woman presents with pain in her left thigh muscle. Duplex ultrasonography indicates the presence of deep vein thrombosis (DVT) in the affected limb.

8. The decision was made to treat this woman with enoxaparin. Relative to unfractionated heparin, enoxaparin
(A) Can be used without monitoring the patient's aPTT
(B) Has a shorter duration of action
(C) Is less likely to have a teratogenic effect
(D) Is more likely to be given intravenously
(E) Is more likely to cause thrombosis and thrombocytopenia

9. During the next week, the patient was started on warfarin and her heparin was discontinued. Two months later, she returned after a severe nosebleed. Laboratory analysis revealed an INR (international normalized ratio) of 7.0 (INR value in such a warfarin-treated patient should be 2.0–3.0). To prevent severe hemorrhage, the warfarin should be discontinued and this patient should be treated immediately with which of the following?
(A) Aminocaproic acid
(B) Desmopressin
(C) Factor VIII
(D) Protamine
(E) Vitamin K_1

10. A patient develops severe thrombocytopenia in response to treatment with unfractionated heparin and still requires parenteral anticoagulation. The patient is most likely to be treated with which of the following?
(A) Abciximab
(B) Cilostazol
(C) Lepirudin
(D) Plasminogen
(E) Vitamin K_1

ANSWERS

1. Reteplase is the only thrombolytic drug listed. Heparin and warfarin are anticoagulants. Lepirudin is a direct inhibitor of thrombin, and aminocaproic acid is an inhibitor, not an activator, of the conversion of plasminogen to plasmin. The answer is **D.**

2. The most common serious adverse effect of the fibrinolytics is bleeding, especially in the cerebral circulation. The fibrinolytics do not usually have serious effects on the renal, hepatic, or hematologic systems. Unlike heparin, they do not induce antiplatelet antibodies. The answer is **D.**

3. Eptifibatide is a reversible inhibitor of glycoprotein IIb/IIIa, a protein on the surface of platelets that serves as a key role in platelet aggregation. Glycoprotein IIb/IIIa receptor antagonists help prevent platelet-induced occlusion of coronary stents. The answer is **E.**

4. A drug that increases metabolism (clearance) of the anticoagulant lowers the steady-state plasma concentration (both free and bound forms), whereas one that displaces the anticoagulant increases the plasma level of the free form only until elimination of the drug has again lowered it to the steady-state level. The answer is **C**.

5. Alteplase improves the clinical outcome in patients with ischemic stroke if given within 3 h after the onset of symptoms, after ruling out hemorrhagic stroke. Use of streptokinase results in unacceptably high rates of bleeding. Glycoprotein IIb/IIIa receptor inhibitors like abciximab have not been tested in ischemic stroke. The answer is **B**.

6. Aspirin, an irreversible inhibitor of platelet cyclooxygenase, prevents recurrence of TIAs and ischemic stroke. The answer is **B**.

7. Ticlopidine and clopidogrel have similar mechanisms of action and therapeutic efficacy. The key difference between these 2 drugs is that clopidogrel is less likely to cause hematologic adverse effects (neutropenia, TTP) and therefore does not require routine monitoring of blood cell counts during therapy. The answer is **B**.

8. Enoxaparin is an LMW heparin. LMW heparins have a longer half-life than standard heparin and a more consistent relationship between dose and therapeutic effect. Enoxaparin is given subcutaneously, not intravenously. It is less, not more, likely to cause thrombosis and thrombocytopenia. Neither LMW heparins nor standard heparin are teratogenic. The aPTT is not useful for monitoring the effects of LMW heparins. The answer is **A**.

9. The elevated INR indicates excessive anticoagulation with a high risk of hemorrhage. Warfarin should be discontinued and vitamin K_1 administered to accelerate formation of vitamin K-dependent factors. The answer is **E**.

10. Direct thrombin inhibitors such as lepirudin and argatroban provide parenteral anticoagulation similar to that achieved with heparin, but the direct thrombin inhibitors do not induce formation of antiplatelet antibodies. The answer is **C**.

SKILL KEEPER ANSWERS: TREATMENT OF ATRIAL FIBRILLATION (SEE CHAPTERS 13 AND 14)

1. *The β adrenoceptor-blocking drugs (class II; eg, propranolol, acebutolol) and calcium channel-blocking drugs (class IV; eg, verapamil, diltiazem) are useful for atrial fibrillation because they slow atrioventricular (AV) nodal conduction and thereby help control ventricular rate. Though rarely used, digoxin can be effective by increasing the effective refractory period in AV nodal tissue and decreasing AV nodal conduction velocity. If symptoms persist in spite of effective rate control, other class I or class III antiarrhythmic drugs (eg, amiodarone, procainamide, flecainide, sotalol) can be used in an attempt to provide rhythm control.*

2. *With warfarin, one is always concerned about pharmacodynamic and pharmacokinetic drug interactions. A metabolite of amiodarone inhibits the metabolism of warfarin and can increase the anticoagulant effect of warfarin. None of the other antiarrhythmic drugs mentioned appears to have significant interactions with warfarin.*

CHECKLIST

When you complete this chapter, you should be able to:

❏ List the 3 major classes of anticlotting drugs and compare their usefulness in venous and arterial thromboses.

❏ Name 3 types of anticoagulants and describe their mechanisms of action.

❏ Explain why the onset of warfarin's action is relatively slow.

❏ Compare the oral anticoagulants, standard heparin, and LMW heparins with respect to pharmacokinetics, mechanisms, and toxicity.

❏ Give several examples of warfarin's role in pharmacokinetic and pharmacodynamic drug interactions.

❏ Diagram the role of activated platelets at the site of a damaged blood vessel wall and show where the 4 major classes of antiplatelet drugs act.

❏ Compare the pharmacokinetics, clinical uses, and toxicities of the major antiplatelet drugs.

❏ List 3 drugs used to treat disorders of excessive bleeding.

DRUG SUMMARY TABLE: Drugs Used for Anticoagulation & for Bleeding Disorders

Subclass	Mechanism of Action	Clinical Applications	Pharmacokinetics	Toxicities, Drug Interactions
Anticoagulants				
Heparins				
Unfractionated heparin	Complexes with antithrombin III • irreversibly inactivates the coagulation factors thrombin and factor Xa	Venous thrombosis, pulmonary embolism, myocardial infarction, unstable angina, adjuvant to percutaneous coronary intervention (PCI) and thrombolytics	Parenteral administration	Bleeding (monitor with aPTT, protamine is reversal agent) • thrombocytopenia • osteoporosis with chronic use

LMW heparins (enoxaparin, dalteparin, tinzaparin): more selective anti-factor X activity, more reliable pharmacokinetics with renal elimination, protamine reversal only partially effective, less risk of thrombocytopenia
Fondaparinux: effects similar to LMW heparins

Direct factor X inhibitors				
Rivaroxaban	Binds to the active site of factor Xa and inhibits its enzymatic action	Venous thrombosis, pulmonary embolism, prevention of stroke in patients with atrial fibrillation	Oral administration • fixed dose no routine monitoring (factor Xa test)	Bleeding • no specific reversal agent
Direct thrombin inhibitors				
Lepirudin and dabigatran	Binds to thrombin's active site and inhibits its enzymatic action	Anticoagulation in patients with heparin-induced thrombocytopenia (HIT)	Lepirudin: IV administration Dabigatran: oral administration	Both: Bleeding (monitor with aPTT) Lepirudin: anaphylactic reactions
Coumadin anticoagulant				
Warfarin	Inhibits vitamin K poxide reductase and thereby interferes with production of functional vitamin K-dependent clotting and anticlotting factors	Venous thrombosis, pulmonary embolism, prevention of thromboembolic complications of atrial fibrillation or cardiac valve replacement	Oral administration • delayed onset and offset of anticoagulant activity • many drug interactions	Bleeding (monitor with PT, vitamin K_1 is a reversal agent) • thrombosis early in therapy due to protein C deficiency • teratogen
Thrombolytic drugs				
Alteplase, recombinant human tissue plasminogen activator (t-PA)	Converts plasminogen to plasmin, which degrades the fibrin in thrombi	Coronary artery thrombosis, ischemic stroke, pulmonary embolism	Parenteral administration	Bleeding, especially cerebral hemorrhage

Reteplase, tenecteplase: similar to alteplase but with a longer half-life
Streptokinase: bacterial protein that forms a complex with plasminogen that rapidly converts plasminogen to plasmin. Subject to inactivating antibodies and allergic reactions

(Continued)

DRUG SUMMARY TABLE: Drugs Used for Anticoagulation & for Bleeding Disorders (*Continued*)

Subclass	Mechanism of Action	Clinical Applications	Pharmacokinetics	Toxicities, Drug Interactions
Antiplatelet drugs				
COX inhibitor				
Aspirin	Nonselective, irreversible COX inhibitor • reduces platelet production of thromboxane A_2, a potent stimulator of platelet aggregation	Prevention and treatment of arterial thrombosis	Dose required for antithrombotic effect is lower than anti-inflammatory dose (see Chapter 36) • duration of activity is longer than pharmacokinetic half-life due to irreversible action	Gastrointestinal toxicity, nephrotoxicity • hypersensitivity reaction due to increased leukotrienes; tinnitus, hyperventilation metabolic acidosis, hyperthermia, coma in overdose
Glycoprotein IIb/IIIa inhibitor (GP IIb/IIIa)				
Abciximab	Inhibits platelet aggregation by interfering with GPIIb/IIIa binding to fibrinogen and other ligands	Used during PCI to prevent restenosis • acute coronary syndrome	Parenteral administration	Bleeding, thrombocytopenia with prolonged use
Eptifibatide, tirofiban: Reversible GP IIb/IIIa inhibitors of smaller size than abciximab				
ADP receptor antagonists				
Clopidogrel	Prodrug: active metabolite irreversibly inhibits platelet ADP receptor	Acute coronary syndrome, prevention of restenosis after PCI, prevention and treatment of arterial thrombosis	Oral administration	Bleeding, gastrointestinal disturbances, hematologic abnormalities
Ticlopidine: older ADP receptor antagonist with more toxicity, particularly leukopenia and thrombotic thrombocytopenic purpura *Prasugrel:* newer drug, similar to clopidogrel with less variable kinetics				
Dipyridamole				
Dipyridamole	Inhibits adenosine uptake and inhibits phosphodiesterase enzymes that degrade cyclic nucleotides (cAMP, cGMP)	Prevention of thromboembolic complications of cardiac valve replacement • combined with aspirin for secondary prevention of ischemic stroke	Oral administration	Headache, palpitations, contraindicated in congestive heart failure
Cilostazol: similar to dipyridamole				
Drugs used in bleeding disorders				
Reversal agents				
Vitamin K_1 (phytonadione)	Increases supply of reduced vitamin K, which is required for synthesis of functional vitamin K-dependent clotting and anticlotting factors	Vitamin K deficiency, reversal of excessive warfarin anticlotting activity	Oral or parenteral administration	Severe infusion reaction when given IV or IM
Protamine: acidic protein administered parenterally to reverse excessive anticlotting activity of unfractionated heparin				

(Continued)

DRUG SUMMARY TABLE: Drugs Used for Anticoagulation & for Bleeding Disorders (*Continued*)

Subclass	Mechanism of Action	Clinical Applications	Pharmacokinetics	Toxicities, Drug Interactions
Clotting factors				
Factor VIII	Key factor in the clotting cascade	Hemophilia A	Parenteral administration	Infusion reaction, hypersensitivity reaction

Plasma and purified human clotting factors: available to treat other forms of hemophilia
Desmopressin: vasopressin V2 receptor agonist increases concentrations of von Willebrand factor and factor VIII (see Chapter 37)

Subclass	Mechanism of Action	Clinical Applications	Pharmacokinetics	Toxicities, Drug Interactions
Antiplasmin drugs				
Aminocaproic acid	Competitively inhibits plasminogen activation	Excessive fibrinolysis	Oral or parenteral administration	Thrombosis, hypotension, myopathy, diarrhea

Tranexamic acid: analog of aminocaproic acid

aPTT, activated partial thromboplastin time; cAMP, cyclic adenosine monophosphate; cGMP, cyclic guanosine monophosphate; COX, cyclooxygenase; GP, glycoprotein; PCI, percutaneous coronary intervention.

Drugs Used in the Treatment of Hyperlipidemias

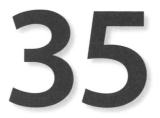

Atherosclerosis is the leading cause of death in the Western world. Drugs discussed in this chapter prevent the sequelae of atherosclerosis (heart attacks, angina, peripheral arterial disease, ischemic stroke) and decrease mortality in patients with a history of cardiovascular disease and hyperlipidemia. Although the drugs are generally safe and effective, they can cause problems, including drug-drug interactions and toxic reactions in skeletal muscle and the liver.

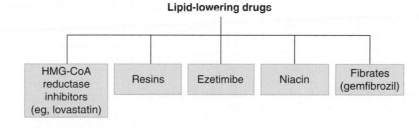

HYPERLIPOPROTEINEMIA

A. Pathogenesis

Premature or accelerated development of atherosclerosis is strongly associated with elevated concentrations of certain plasma lipoproteins, especially the low-density lipoproteins (LDLs) that participate in cholesterol transport. A *depressed* level of high-density lipoproteins (HDLs) is also associated with increased risk of atherosclerosis. In some families, hypertriglyceridemia is similarly correlated with atherosclerosis. Chylomicronemia, the occurrence of chylomicrons in the serum while fasting, is a recessive trait that is correlated with a high incidence of acute pancreatitis and managed by restriction of total fat intake (Table 35–1).

Regulation of plasma lipoprotein levels involves a complex interplay of dietary fat intake, hepatic processing, and utilization in peripheral tissues (Figure 35–1). Primary disturbances in regulation occur in a number of genetic conditions involving mutations in apolipoproteins, their receptors, transport mechanisms, and lipid-metabolizing enzymes. Secondary disturbances are associated with a Western diet, many endocrine conditions, and diseases of the liver or kidneys.

B. Treatment Strategies

1. Diet—Cholesterol and saturated fats are the primary dietary factors that contribute to elevated levels of plasma lipoproteins. Dietary measures designed to reduce the total intake of these substances constitute the first method of management and may be sufficient to reduce lipoprotein levels to a safe range. Because alcohol raises triglyceride and very-low-density lipoprotein (VLDL) levels, it should be avoided by patients with hypertriglyceridemia.

2. Drugs—For an individual patient, the choice of drug treatment is based on the lipid abnormality. The drugs that are most

High-Yield Terms to Learn

Lipoproteins	Macromolecular complexes in the blood that transport lipids
Apolipoproteins	Proteins on the surface of lipoproteins; they play critical roles in the regulation of lipoprotein metabolism and uptake into cells
Low-density lipoprotein (LDL)	Cholesterol-rich lipoprotein whose regulated uptake by hepatocytes and other cells requires functional LDL receptors; an elevated LDL concentration is associated with atherosclerosis
High-density lipoprotein (HDL)	Cholesterol-rich lipoprotein that transports cholesterol from the tissues to the liver; a low concentration is associated with atherosclerosis
Very-low-density lipoprotein (VLDL)	Triglyceride- and cholesterol-rich lipoprotein secreted by the liver that transports triglycerides to the periphery; precursor of LDL
HMG-CoA reductase	3-Hydroxy-3-methylglutaryl-coenzyme A reductase; the enzyme that catalyzes the rate-limiting step in cholesterol biosynthesis
Lipoprotein lipase (LPL)	An enzyme found primarily on the surface of endothelial cells that releases free fatty acids from triglycerides in lipoproteins; the free fatty acids are taken up into cells
Proliferator-activated receptor-alpha (PPAR-α)	Member of a family of nuclear transcription regulators that participate in the regulation of metabolic processes; target of the fibrate drugs and omega-3 fatty acids

effective at lowering LDL cholesterol include the HMG-CoA reductase inhibitors, resins, ezetimibe, and niacin. The fibric acid derivatives (eg, gemfibrozil), niacin and marine omega-3 fatty acids are most effective at lowering triglyceride and VLDL concentrations and raising HDL cholesterol concentrations (Table 35–2).

HMG-CoA REDUCTASE INHIBITORS

A. Mechanism and Effects

The rate-limiting step in hepatic cholesterol synthesis is conversion of hydroxymethylglutaryl coenzyme A (**HMG-CoA**) to

TABLE 35–1 Primary hyperlipoproteinemias and their drug treatment.

Condition/Cause	Manifestations, Cause	Single Drug	Drug Combination
Primary chylomicronemia	Chylomicrons, VLDL increased; deficiency in LPL or apoC-II	Dietary management (omega-3 fatty acids, niacin, or fibrate)	Niacin plus fibrate[a]
Familial hypertriglyceridemia Severe	VLDL, chylomicrons increased; decreased clearance of VLDL	Omega-3 fatty acids, niacin or fibrate	Niacin plus fibrate
Moderate	VLDL increased, chylomicrons may be increased; increased production of VLDL	Omega-3 fatty acids, niacin or fibrate	
Familial combined hyperlipoproteinemia	Increased hepatic apoB and VLDL production		
	VLDL increased	Omega-3 fatty acids, niacin, fibrate, statin	Two or 3 of the individual drugs
	LDL increased	Niacin, statin, ezetimibe	Two or 3 of the individual drugs
	VLDL, LDL increased	Omega-3 fatty acids, niacin, statin	Niacin or fibrate plus statin
Familial dysbetalipoproteinemia	VLDL remnants, chylomicron remnants increased; deficiency in apoE	Omega-3 fatty acids, fibrate, niacin	Fibrate plus niacin, or either plus statin
Familial hypercholesterolemia	LDL increased; defect in LDL receptors		
Heterozygous		Statin, resin, niacin, ezetimibe	Two or 3 of the individual drugs
Homozygous		Niacin, atorvastatin, rosuvastatin, ezetimibe	Niacin plus statin plus ezetimibe

[a]Single-drug therapy with marine omega-3 dietary supplement should be evaluated before drug combinations are used.

Modified and reproduced, with permission, from Katzung BG, editor: *Basic & Clinical Pharmacology,* 12th ed. McGraw-Hill, 2012.

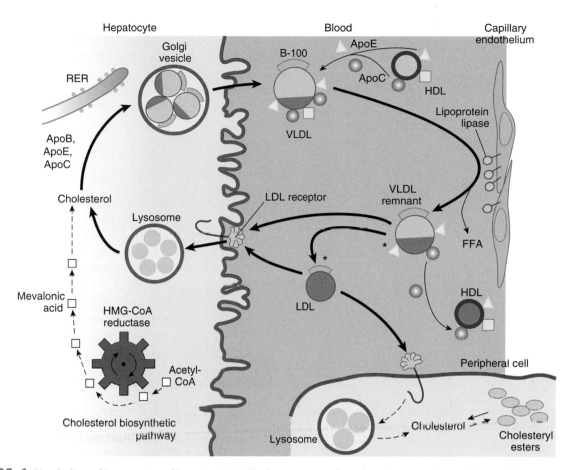

FIGURE 35–1 Metabolism of lipoproteins of hepatic origin. The heavy arrows show the primary pathways. Nascent VLDL are secreted via the Golgi apparatus. They acquire additional apoC lipoproteins and apoE from HDL. VLDL is converted to VLDL remnants by lipolysis via lipoprotein lipase associated with capillaries in peripheral tissue supplies. In the process, C apolipoproteins and a portion of apoE are given back to HDL. Some of the VLDL remnants are converted to LDL by further loss of triglycerides and loss of apoE. A major pathway for LDL degradation involves the endocytosis of LDL by LDL receptors in the liver and the peripheral tissues, for which apoB-100 is the ligand. Dark color denotes cholesteryl esters; light color, triglycerides; the asterisk denotes a functional ligand for LDL receptors; triangles indicate apoE; circles and squares represent C apolipoproteins. FFA, free fatty acid; RER, rough endoplasmic reticulum. (Reproduced, with permission, from Katzung BG, editor: *Basic & Clinical Pharmacology,* 12th ed. McGraw-Hill, 2012: Fig. 35–1.)

TABLE 35–2 Lipid-modifying effects of antihyperlipidemic drugs.

Drug or Drug Group	LDL Cholesterol	HDL Cholesterol	Triglycerides
Statins			
Atorvastatin, rosuvastatin, simvastatin	−25 to −50%	+5 to +15%	↓↓
Lovastatin, pravastatin	−25 to −40%	+5 to +10%	↓
Fluvastatin	−20 to −30%	+5 to +10%	↓
Resins	−15 to −25%	+5 to +10%	±[a]
Ezetimibe	−20%	+5%	±
Niacin	−15 to −25%	+25 to +35%	↓↓
Gemfibrozil	−10 to −15%[b]	+ 15 to +20%	↓↓

LDL, low-density lipoprotein; HDL, high-density lipoprotein; ±, variable, if any.

[a]Resins can increase triglycerides in some patients with combined hyperlipidemia.

[b]Gemfibrozil and other fibrates can increase LDL cholesterol in patients with combined hyperlipidemia.

Modified and reproduced, with permission, from McPhee SJ, Papadakis MA, Tierney LM, editors: *Current Medical Diagnosis & Treatment,* 46th ed. McGraw-Hill, 2006.

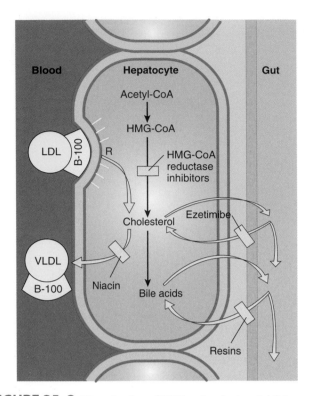

FIGURE 35–2 Sites of action of HMG-coA reductase inhibitors, niacin, ezetimibe, and bile acid-binding resins. Low-density lipoprotein (LDL) receptor synthesis is increased by treatment with drugs that reduce the hepatocyte reserve of cholesterol. (Reproduced, with permission, from Katzung BG, editor: *Basic & Clinical Pharmacology,* 12th ed. McGraw-Hill, 2012: Fig. 35–2)

mevalonate by HMG-CoA reductase. The **statins** are structural analogs of HMG-CoA that competitively inhibit the enzyme (Figure 35–2). Lovastatin and simvastatin are prodrugs, whereas the other HMG-CoA reductase inhibitors (atorvastatin, fluvastatin, pravastatin, and rosuvastatin) are active as given.

Although the inhibition of hepatic cholesterol synthesis contributes a small amount to the total serum cholesterol-lowering effect of these drugs, a much greater effect derives from the response to a reduction in a tightly regulated hepatic pool of cholesterol. The liver compensates by increasing the number of high-affinity LDL receptors, which clear LDL and VLDL remnants from the blood (Figure 35–1). HMG-CoA reductase inhibitors also have direct anti-atherosclerotic effects, and have been shown to prevent bone loss.

B. Clinical Use

Statins can reduce LDL cholesterol levels dramatically (Table 35–2), especially when used in combination with other cholesterol-lowering drugs (Table 35–1). These drugs are used commonly because they are effective and well tolerated. Large clinical trials have shown that they reduce the risk of coronary events and mortality in patients with ischemic heart disease, and they also reduce the risk of ischemic stroke.

Rosuvastatin, atorvastatin, and simvastatin have greater maximal efficacy than the other HMG-CoA reductase inhibitors. These drugs also reduce triglycerides and increase HDL cholesterol in patients with triglycerides levels that are higher than 250 mg/dL and with reduced HDL cholesterol levels. Fluvastatin has less maximal efficacy than the other drugs in this group.

C. Toxicity

Mild elevations of serum aminotransferases are common but are not often associated with hepatic damage. Patients with preexisting liver disease may have more severe reactions. An increase in creatine kinase (released from skeletal muscle) is noted in about 10% of patients; in a few, severe muscle pain and even rhabdomyolysis may occur. HGM-CoA reductase inhibitors are metabolized by the cytochrome P450 system; drugs or foods (eg, grapefruit juice) that inhibit cytochrome P450 activity increase the risk of hepatotoxicity and myopathy. Because of evidence that the HMG-CoA reductase inhibitors are teratogenic, these drugs should be avoided in pregnancy.

SKILL KEEPER: ANGINA (SEE CHAPTER 12)

The antihyperlipidemic drugs, especially the HMG-CoA reductase inhibitors, are commonly used to treat patients with ischemic heart disease. One of the most common manifestations of ischemic heart disease and coronary atherosclerosis is angina.

1. *What are the 3 major forms of angina?*
2. *Name the 3 major drug groups used to treat angina and specify which form of angina each is useful for.*

The Skill Keeper Answers appear at the end of the chapter.

RESINS

A. Mechanism and Effects

Normally, over 90% of bile acids, metabolites of cholesterol, are reabsorbed in the gastrointestinal tract and returned to the liver for reuse. Bile acid-binding resins (**cholestyramine, colestipol, and colesevelam**) are large nonabsorbable polymers that bind bile acids and similar steroids in the intestine and prevent their absorption (Figure 35–2).

By preventing the recycling of bile acids, bile acid-binding resins divert hepatic cholesterol to synthesis of new bile acids, thereby reducing the amount of cholesterol in a tightly regulated pool. A compensatory increase in the synthesis of high-affinity LDL receptors increases the removal of LDL lipoproteins from the blood.

The resins cause a modest reduction in LDL cholesterol (Table 35–2) but have little effect on HDL cholesterol or triglycerides. In some patients with a genetic condition that predisposes them to hypertriglyceridemia and hypercholesterolemia (familial combined hyperlipidemia), resins increase triglycerides and VLDL.

B. Clinical Use

The resins are used in patients with hypercholesterolemia (Table 35–1). They have also been used to reduce pruritus in patients with cholestasis and bile salt accumulation.

C. Toxicity

Adverse effects from resins include bloating, constipation, and an unpleasant gritty taste. Absorption of vitamins (eg, vitamin K, dietary folates) and drugs (eg, thiazide diuretics, warfarin, pravastatin, fluvastatin) is impaired by the resins.

EZETIMIBE

A. Mechanism and Effects

Ezetimibe is a prodrug that is converted in the liver to the active glucuronide form. This active metabolite inhibits a transporter that mediates gastrointestinal uptake of cholesterol and phytosterols (plant sterols that normally enter gastrointestinal epithelial cell but then are immediately transported back into the intestinal lumen.)

By preventing absorption of dietary cholesterol and cholesterol that is excreted in bile, ezetimibe reduces the cholesterol in the tightly regulated hepatic pool. A compensatory increase in the synthesis of high-affinity LDL receptors increases the removal of LDL lipoproteins from the blood.

As monotherapy, ezetimibe reduces LDL cholesterol by about 18% (Table 35–2). When combined with an HMG-CoA reductase inhibitor, it is even more effective.

B. Clinical Use

Ezetimibe is used for treatment of hypercholesterolemia and phytosterolemia, a rare genetic disorder that results from impaired export of phytosterols.

C. Toxicity

Ezetimibe is well tolerated. When combined with HMG-CoA reductase inhibitors, it may increase the risk of hepatic toxicity. Serum concentrations of the glucuronide form are increased by fibrates and reduced by cholestyramine.

NIACIN (NICOTINIC ACID)

A. Mechanism and Effects

Through multiple actions, niacin (but not nicotinamide) reduces LDL cholesterol, triglycerides, and VLDL and also often increases HDL cholesterol. In the liver, niacin reduces VLDL synthesis, which in turn reduces LDL levels (Figures 35–1 and 35–2). In adipose tissue, niacin appears to activate a signaling pathway that reduces hormone-sensitive lipase activity and thus decreases plasma fatty acid and triglyceride levels. Consequently, LDL formation is reduced, and there is a decrease in LDL cholesterol. Increased clearance of VLDL by the lipoprotein lipase associated

with capillary endothelial cells has also been demonstrated and probably accounts for the reduction in plasma triglyceride concentrations. Niacin reduces the catabolic rate for HDL. Finally, niacin decreases circulating fibrinogen and increases tissue plasminogen activator.

B. Clinical Use

Because it lowers serum LDL cholesterol and triglyceride concentrations and increases HDL cholesterol concentrations, niacin has wide clinical usefulness in the treatment of hypercholesterolemia, hypertriglyceridemia, and low levels of HDL cholesterol.

C. Toxicity

Cutaneous flushing is a common adverse effect of niacin. Pretreatment with aspirin or other nonsteroidal anti-inflammatory drugs (NSAIDs) reduces the intensity of this flushing, suggesting that it is mediated by prostaglandin release. Tolerance to the flushing reaction usually develops within a few days. Dose-dependent nausea and abdominal discomfort often occur. Pruritus and other skin conditions are reported. Moderate elevations of liver enzymes and even severe hepatotoxicity may occur. Severe liver dysfunction has been associated with an extended-release preparation, which is not the same as the sustained-release formulation. Hyperuricemia occurs in about 20% of patients, and carbohydrate tolerance may be moderately impaired.

FIBRIC ACID DERIVATIVES

A. Mechanism and Effects

Fibric acid derivatives (eg, **gemfibrozil**, fenofibrate) are ligands for the peroxisome proliferator-activated receptor-alpha (**PPAR-α**) protein, a receptor that regulates transcription of genes involved in lipid metabolism. This interaction with PPAR-α results in increased synthesis by adipose tissue of lipoprotein lipase, which associates with capillary endothelial cells and enhances clearance of triglyceride-rich lipoproteins (Figure 35–1). In the liver, fibrates stimulate fatty acid oxidation, which limits the supply of triglycerides and decreases VLDL synthesis. They also decrease expression of apoC-III, which impedes the clearance of VLDL, and increases the expression of apoA-I and apoA-II, which in turn increases HDL levels. In most patients, fibrates have little or no effect on LDL concentrations. However, fibrates can *increase* LDL cholesterol in patients with a genetic condition called familial combined hyperlipoproteinemia, which is associated with a combined increase in VLDL and LDL.

B. Clinical Use

Gemfibrozil and other fibrates are used to treat hypertriglyceridemia. Because these drugs have only a modest ability to reduce LDL cholesterol and can increase LDL cholesterol in some patients, they often are combined with other cholesterol-lowering drugs for treatment of patients with elevated concentrations of both LDL and VLDL.

C. Toxicity

Nausea is the most common adverse effect with all members of the fibric acid derivatives subgroup. Skin rashes are common with gemfibrozil. A few patients show decreases in white blood count or hematocrit, and these drugs can potentiate the action of anticoagulants. There is an increased risk of cholesterol gallstones; these drugs should be used with caution in patients with a history of cholelithiasis. When used in combination with reductase inhibitors, the fibrates significantly increase the risk of myopathy.

COMBINATION THERAPY

All patients with hyperlipidemia are treated first with dietary modification, but this is often insufficient and drugs must be added. Drug combinations are often required to achieve the maximum lowering possible with minimum toxicity and to achieve the desired effect on the various lipoproteins (LDL, VLDL, and HDL).

Certain drug combinations provide advantages (Table 35–1), whereas others present specific challenges. Because resins interfere with the absorption of certain HMG-CoA reductase inhibitors (pravastatin, cerivastatin, atorvastatin, and fluvastatin), these must be given at least 1 h before or 4 h after the resins. The combination of reductase inhibitors with either fibrates or niacin increases the risk of myopathy.

QUESTIONS

1. Increased serum levels of which of the following is associated with a *decreased* risk of atherosclerosis?
   (A) Cholesterol
   (B) LDL
   (C) HDL
   (D) Triglyceride
   (E) VLDL

2. A 58-year-old man with a history of hyperlipidemia was treated with a drug. The chart below shows the results of the patient's fasting lipid panel before treatment and 6 mo after initiating drug therapy. Normal values are also shown. Which of the following drugs is most likely to be the one that this man received?
   (A) Colestipol
   (B) Ezetimibe
   (C) Gemfibrozil
   (D) Lovastatin
   (E) Niacin

Questions 3–6. A 35-year-old woman appears to have familial combined hyperlipidemia. Her serum concentrations of total cholesterol, LDL cholesterol, and triglyceride are elevated. Her serum concentration of HDL cholesterol is somewhat reduced.

3. Which of the following drugs is most likely to increase this patient's triglyceride and VLDL cholesterol concentrations when used as monotherapy?
   (A) Atorvastatin
   (B) Cholestyramine
   (C) Ezetimibe
   (D) Gemfibrozil
   (E) Niacin

4. If this patient is pregnant, which of the following drugs should be avoided because of a risk of harming the fetus?
   (A) Cholestyramine
   (B) Ezetimibe
   (C) Fenofibrate
   (D) Niacin
   (E) Pravastatin

5. The patient is started on gemfibrozil. Which of the following is a major mechanism of gemfibrozil's action?
   (A) Increased excretion of bile acid salts
   (B) Increased expression of high-affinity LDL receptors
   (C) Increased secretion of VLDL by the liver
   (D) Increased triglyceride hydrolysis by lipoprotein lipase
   (E) Reduced uptake of dietary cholesterol

6. Which of the following is a major toxicity associated with gemfibrozil therapy?
   (A) Bloating and constipation
   (B) Cholelithiasis
   (C) Hyperuricemia
   (D) Liver damage
   (E) Severe cardiac arrhythmia

Questions 7–10. A 43-year-old man has heterozygous familial hypercholesterolemia. His serum concentrations of total cholesterol and LDL are markedly elevated. His serum concentration of HDL cholesterol, VLDL cholesterol, and triglycerides are normal or slightly elevated. The patient's mother and older brother died of myocardial infarctions before the age of 50. This patient recently experienced mild chest pain when walking upstairs and has been diagnosed as having angina of effort. The patient is somewhat overweight. He drinks alcohol most evenings and smokes about 1 pack of cigarettes per week.

7. Consumption of alcohol is associated with which of the following changes in serum lipid concentrations?
   (A) Decreased chylomicrons
   (B) Decreased HDL cholesterol
   (C) Decreased VLDL cholesterol
   (D) Increased LDL cholesterol
   (E) Increased triglyceride

Time of Lipid Measurement	Triglyceride	Total Cholesterol	LDL Cholesterol	VLDL Cholesterol	HDL Cholesterol
Before treatment	1000	640	120	500	20
Six months after starting treatment	300	275	90	150	40
Normal values	<150	<200	<130	<30	>35

8. If the patient has a history of gout, which of the following drugs is most likely to exacerbate this condition?
   (A) Colestipol
   (B) Ezetimibe
   (C) Gemfibrozil
   (D) Niacin
   (E) Simvastatin

9. After being counseled about lifestyle and dietary changes, the patient was started on atorvastatin. During his treatment with atorvastatin, it is important to routinely monitor serum concentrations of which of the following?
   (A) Blood urea nitrogen
   (B) Alanine and aspartate aminotransferase
   (C) Platelets
   (D) Red blood cells
   (E) Uric acid

10. Six months after beginning atorvastatin, the patient's total and LDL cholesterol concentrations remained above normal, and he continued to have anginal attacks despite good adherence to his antianginal medications. His physician decided to add ezetimibe. Which of the following is the most accurate description of ezetimibe's mechanism of an action?
    (A) Decreased lipid synthesis in adipose tissue
    (B) Decreased secretion of VLDL by the liver
    (C) Decreased gastrointestinal absorption of cholesterol
    (D) Increased endocytosis of HDL by the liver
    (E) Increased lipid hydrolysis by lipoprotein lipase

ANSWERS

1. Increased serum concentrations of LDL and total cholesterol are associated with *increased* risk of atherosclerosis. High serum concentration of HDL cholesterol is associated with a decrease in the risk of atherosclerotic disease. The answer is **C**.

2. This patient presents with striking hypertriglyceridemia, elevated VLDL cholesterol, and depressed HDL cholesterol. Six months after drug treatment was initiated, his triglyceride and VLDL cholesterol have dropped dramatically and his HDL cholesterol level has doubled. The drug that is most likely to have achieved all of these desirable changes, particularly the large increase in HDL cholesterol, is niacin. Although gemfibrozil lowers triglyceride and VLDL concentrations, it does not cause such large increases in HDL cholesterol and decreases in LDL cholesterol. The answer is **E**.

3. In some patients with familial combined hyperlipidemia and elevated VLDL, the resins increase VLDL and triglyceride concentrations even though they also lower LDL cholesterol. The answer is **B**.

4. The HMG-CoA reductase inhibitors are contraindicated in pregnancy because of the risk of teratogenic effects. The answer is **E**.

5. A major mechanism recognized for gemfibrozil is increased activity of the lipoprotein lipase associated with capillary endothelial cells. Gemfibrozil and other fibrates decrease VLDL secretion, presumably by stimulating hepatic fatty acid oxidation. The answer is **D**.

6. A major toxicity of the fibrates is increased risk of gallstone formation, which may be due to enhanced biliary excretion of cholesterol. The answer is **B**.

7. Chronic ethanol ingestion can increase serum concentrations of VLDL and triglycerides. This is one of the factors that places patients with alcoholism at risk of pancreatitis. Chronic ethanol ingestion also has the possibly beneficial effect of raising, not decreasing, serum HDL concentrations. The answer is **E**.

8. Niacin can exacerbate both hyperuricemia and glucose intolerance. The answer is **D**.

9. The 2 primary adverse effects of the HMG-CoA reductase inhibitors are hepatotoxicity and myopathy. Patients taking these drugs should have liver function tests performed before starting therapy, and at regular intervals during therapy. Serum concentrations of alanine and aspartate aminotransferase are used as markers of hepatocellular toxicity. The answer is **B**.

10. The major recognized effect of ezetimibe is inhibition of absorption of cholesterol in the intestine. The answer is **C**.

SKILL KEEPER ANSWERS: ANGINA (SEE CHAPTER 12)

1. *The 3 major forms of angina are (1) angina of effort, which is associated with a fixed plaque that partially occludes 1 or more coronary arteries; (2) vasospastic angina, which involves unpredictably timed, reversible coronary spasm; and (3) unstable angina, which often immediately precedes a myocardial infarction and requires emergency treatment.*

2. *The 3 major drug groups used in angina are nitrates, calcium channel blockers, and β blockers. Nitrates are used in all 3 types of angina. Calcium channel blockers are useful for treatment of angina of effort and vasospastic angina. They can be added to β blockers and nitroglycerin in patients with refractory unstable angina. β blockers are not useful in vasospastic angina or for an acute attack of angina of effort. They are primarily used for prophylaxis of angina of effort and also in emergency treatment of acute coronary syndromes.*

CHECKLIST

When you complete this chapter, you should be able to:

❑ Describe the proposed role of lipoproteins in the formation of atherosclerotic plaques.

❑ Describe the dietary management of hyperlipidemia.

❑ List the 5 main classes of drugs used to treat hyperlipidemia. For each, describe the mechanism of action, effects on serum lipid concentrations, and adverse effects.

❑ On the basis of a set of baseline serum lipid values, propose a rational drug treatment regimen.

❑ Argue the merits of combined drug therapy for some diseases, and list 3 rational drug combinations.

DRUG SUMMARY TABLE: Drugs for the Treatment of Hyperlipidemias

Subclass	Mechanism of Action	Clinical Applications	Pharmacokinetics	Toxicities, Drug Interactions
Statins				
Atorvastatin, simvastatin, rosuvastatin	Inhibit HMG-CoA reductase	Atherosclerotic vascular disease (primary and secondary prevention) • acute coronary syndromes	Oral administration • CYP450-dependent metabolism (3A4, 2C9) interacts with CYP inhibitors	Myopathy, hepatic dysfunction, teratogen
Fluvastatin, pravastatin, lovastatin: similar but somewhat less efficacious				
Fibrates				
Gemfibrozil, fenofibrate	PPAR-α agonists[a]	Hypertriglyceridemia, low HDL cholesterol	Oral administration	Myopathy, hepatic dysfunction, cholestasis
Bile acid-binding resins				
Colestipol	Prevents reabsorption of bile acids from the gastrointestinal tract	Elevated LDL cholesterol, pruritus	Oral administration • interferes with absorption of some drugs and vitamins	Constipation, bloating
Cholestyramine, colesevelam: similar to colestipol				
Sterol absorption inhibitor				
Ezetimibe	Reduces intestinal uptake of cholesterol by inhibiting sterol transporter	Elevated LDL cholesterol, phytosterolemia	Oral administration	Rarely, hepatic dysfunction, myositis
Niacin	Decreases VLDL synthesis and LDL cholesterol concentrations • increases HDL cholesterol	Low HDL cholesterol, elevated VLDL and LDL	Oral administration	Gastrointestinal irritation, flushing, hepatic toxicity, hyperuricemia, may reduce glucose tolerance

[a]*PPAR-α, proliferator-activated receptor-alpha. Also responsible for TG-lowering effect of omega-3 fatty acids.*

NSAIDs, Acetaminophen, & Drugs Used in Rheumatoid Arthritis & Gout

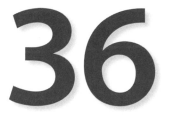

36

Inflammation is a complex response to cell injury that primarily occurs in vascularized connective tissue and often involves the immune response. The mediators of inflammation function to eliminate the cause of cell injury and clear away debris, in preparation for tissue repair. Unfortunately, inflammation also causes pain and, in instances in which the cause of cell injury is not eliminated, can result in a chronic condition of pain and tissue damage such as that seen in rheumatoid arthritis. The nonsteroidal anti-inflammatory drugs (NSAIDs) and

acetaminophen are often effective in controlling inflammatory pain. Other treatment strategies applied to the reduction of inflammation are targeted at immune processes. These include glucocorticoids and disease-modifying antirheumatic drugs (DMARDs). Gout is an inflammatory joint disease caused by precipitation of uric acid crystals. Treatment of acute episodes targets inflammation, whereas treatment of chronic gout targets both inflammatory processes and the production and elimination of uric acid.

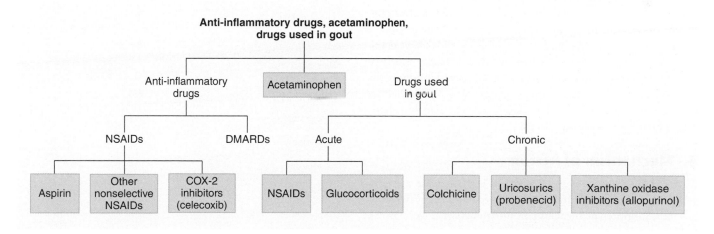

High-Yield Terms to Learn

Antipyretic	A drug that reduces fever (eg, aspirin, NSAIDs, acetaminophen)
Cyclooxygenase (COX)	The enzyme at the head of the enzymatic pathway for prostaglandin synthesis (Figure 36-2)
Cytotoxic drug	Drugs that interfere with essential metabolic processes, especially DNA maintenance and replication and cell division. Such drugs generally kill rapidly dividing cells and are used for cancer chemotherapy and immunosuppression (Chapters 54 and 55)
Disease-modifying antirheumatic drugs (DMARDs)	Diverse group of drugs that modify the inflammatory processes underlying rheumatoid arthritis; they have a slow (weeks to months) onset of clinical effects
Nonsteroidal anti-inflammatory drugs (NSAIDs)	Inhibitors of cyclooxygenase; the term nonsteroidal differentiates them from steroid drugs that mediate anti-inflammatory effects through activation of glucocorticoid receptors (eg, cortisol; Chapter 39)
Reye's syndrome	A rare syndrome of rapid liver degeneration and encephalitis in children treated with aspirin during a viral infection
Tumor necrosis factor-α (TNF-α)	A cytokine that plays a central role in inflammation
Uricosuric agent	A drug that increases the renal excretion of uric acid
Xanthine oxidase	A key enzyme in the purine metabolism pathway that converts hypoxanthine to xanthine and xanthine to uric acid

ASPIRIN & OTHER NONSELECTIVE NSAIDs

A. Classification and Prototypes

Aspirin (acetylsalicylic acid) is the prototype of the salicylates and other NSAIDs (Table 36–1). The other older nonselective NSAIDs (**ibuprofen**, **indomethacin**, many others) vary primarily in their potency, analgesic and anti-inflammatory effectiveness, and duration of action. Ibuprofen and naproxen have moderate effectiveness; indomethacin has greater anti-inflammatory effectiveness; and **ketorolac** has greater analgesic effectiveness. **Celecoxib** was the first member of a newer NSAID subgroup, the cyclooxygenase-2 (COX-2)-selective inhibitors, which were developed in an attempt to lessen the gastrointestinal toxicity associated with COX inhibition while preserving efficacy. Unfortunately, clinical trials involving some of the highly selective COX-2 inhibitors have shown a higher incidence of cardiovascular thrombotic events than the nonselective drugs.

B. Mechanism of Action

As noted in Chapter 18, cyclooxygenase is the enzyme that converts arachidonic acid into the endoperoxide precursors of prostaglandins, important mediators of inflammation (Figure 36–1). Cyclooxygenase has at least 2 isoforms: COX-1 and COX-2. COX-1 is primarily expressed in noninflammatory cells, whereas COX-2 is expressed in activated lymphocytes, polymorphonuclear cells, and other inflammatory cells.

Aspirin and nonselective NSAIDs inhibit both cyclooxygenase isoforms and thereby decrease prostaglandin and thromboxane synthesis throughout the body. Release of prostaglandins necessary for homeostatic function is disrupted, as is release of prostaglandins involved in inflammation. The COX-2-selective inhibitors

TABLE 36–1 Selected NSAIDs.

Drug	Half-life (hours)
Aspirin	0.25
Celecoxib	11
Diclofenac	1.1
Diflunisal	13
Etodolac	6.5
Fenoprofen	2.5
Flurbiprofen	3.8
Ibuprofen	2
Indomethacin	4–5
Ketoprofen	1.8
Ketorolac	4–10
Meloxicam	20
Nabumetone[a]	26
Naproxen	14
Oxaprozin	58
Piroxicam	57
Sulindac	8
Tolmetin	1

[a]Nabumetone is a prodrug; the half-life is for its active metabolite.

(Modified and reproduced, with permission, from Katzung BG, editors: *Basic & Clinical Pharmacology*, 11th ed. McGraw-Hill, 2009.)

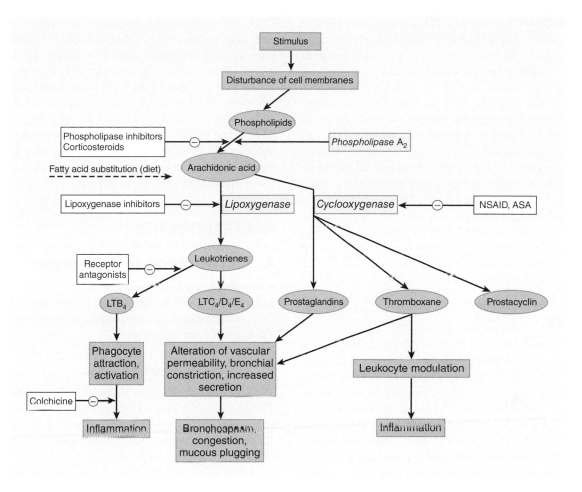

FIGURE 36–1 Prostanoid mediators derived from arachidonic acid and sites of drug action. ASA, acetylsalicylic acid (aspirin); LT, leukotriene; NSAID, nonsteroidal anti-inflammatory drug. (Reproduced, with permission, from Katzung BG, editor: *Basic & Clinical Pharmacology,* 12th ed. McGraw-Hill, 2012: Fig. 36–2.)

have less effect on the prostaglandins involved in homeostatic function, particularly those in the gastrointestinal tract.

The major difference between the mechanisms of action of aspirin and other NSAIDs is that aspirin (but not its active metabolite, salicylate) acetylates and thereby irreversibly inhibits cyclooxygenase, whereas the inhibition produced by other NSAIDs is reversible. The irreversible action of aspirin results in a longer duration of its antiplatelet effect and is the basis for its use as an antiplatelet drug (Chapter 34).

C. Effects

Arachidonic acid derivatives are important mediators of inflammation; cyclooxygenase inhibitors reduce the manifestations of inflammation, although they have no effect on underlying tissue damage or immunologic reactions. These inhibitors also suppress the prostaglandin synthesis in the CNS that is stimulated by pyrogens and thereby reduces fever (antipyretic action). The analgesic mechanism of these agents is less well understood. Activation of peripheral pain sensors may be diminished as a result of reduced production of prostaglandins in injured tissue; in addition, a central mechanism is operative. Cyclooxygenase inhibitors also interfere with the homeostatic function of prostaglandins. Most important, they reduce prostaglandin-mediated cytoprotection in the gastrointestinal tract and autoregulation of renal function.

D. Pharmacokinetics and Clinical Use

1. Aspirin—Aspirin has 3 therapeutic dose ranges: The low range (<300 mg/d) is effective in reducing platelet aggregation; intermediate doses (300–2400 mg/d) have antipyretic and analgesic effects; and high doses (2400–4000 mg/d) are used for an anti-inflammatory effect. Aspirin is readily absorbed and is hydrolyzed in blood and tissues to acetate and salicylic acid. Salicylate is a reversible nonselective inhibitor of cyclooxygenase. Elimination of salicylate is first order at low doses, with a half-life of 3–5 h. At high (anti-inflammatory) doses, half-life increases to 15 h or more and elimination becomes zero order. Excretion is via the kidney.

2. Other NSAIDs—The other NSAIDs are well absorbed after oral administration. Ibuprofen has a half-life of about 2 h, is relatively safe, and is the least expensive of the older, nonselective NSAIDs. Naproxen and piroxicam are noteworthy because of their longer half-lives (Table 36–1), which permit less frequent dosing. These other NSAIDs are used for the treatment of mild to moderate pain, especially the pain of musculoskeletal inflammation such as that seen in arthritis and gout. They are also used to treat many other conditions, including dysmenorrhea, headache, and patent ductus arteriosus in premature infants. Ketorolac is notable as a drug used mainly as a systemic analgesic, not as an anti-inflammatory (although it has typical nonselective NSAID properties). It is the only NSAID available in a parenteral formulation. Nonselective NSAIDs reduce polyp formation in patients with primary familial adenomatous polyposis. Long-term use of NSAIDs reduces the risk of colon cancer.

E. Toxicity

1. Aspirin—The most common adverse effect from therapeutic anti-inflammatory doses of aspirin is gastric upset. Chronic use can result in gastric ulceration, upper gastrointestinal bleeding, and renal effects, including acute failure and interstitial nephritis. Aspirin increases the bleeding time (Chapter 34). When prostaglandin synthesis is inhibited by even small doses of aspirin, persons with aspirin hypersensitivity (especially associated with nasal polyps) can experience asthma from the increased synthesis of leukotrienes. This type of hypersensitivity to aspirin precludes treatment with any NSAID. At higher doses of aspirin, tinnitus, vertigo, hyperventilation, and respiratory alkalosis are observed. At very high doses, the drug causes metabolic acidosis, dehydration, hyperthermia, collapse, coma, and death. Children with viral infections who are treated with aspirin have an increased risk for developing Reye's syndrome, a rare but serious syndrome of rapid liver degeneration and encephalopathy. There is no specific antidote for aspirin.

2. Nonselective NSAIDs—Like aspirin, these agents are associated with significant gastrointestinal disturbance, but the incidence is lower than with aspirin. There is a risk of renal damage with any of the NSAIDs, especially in patients with preexisting renal disease. Because these drugs are cleared by the kidney, renal damage results in higher, more toxic serum concentrations. Use of parenteral ketorolac is generally restricted to 72 h because of the risk of gastrointestinal and renal damage with longer administration. Serious hematologic reactions have been noted with indomethacin.

3. COX-2-selective inhibitors—The COX-2-selective inhibitors (celecoxib, rofecoxib, valdecoxib) have a *reduced* risk of gastrointestinal effects, including gastric ulcers and serious gastrointestinal bleeding. The COX-2 inhibitors carry the same risk of renal damage as nonselective COX inhibitors, presumably because

COX-2 contributes to homeostatic renal effects. Clinical trial data suggest that highly selective COX-2 inhibitors such as rofecoxib and valdecoxib carry an increased risk of myocardial infarction and stroke. The increased risk of arterial thrombosis is believed to be due to the COX-2 inhibitors having a greater inhibitory effect on endothelial prostacyclin (PGI_2) formation than on platelet TXA_2 formation. Prostacyclin promotes vasodilation and inhibits platelet aggregation, whereas TXA_2 has the opposite effects. Several COX-2 inhibitors have been removed from the market, and the others are now labeled with warnings about the increased risk of thrombosis.

ACETAMINOPHEN

A. Classification and Prototype

Acetaminophen is the only over-the-counter non-anti-inflammatory analgesic commonly available in the United States. Phenacetin, a toxic prodrug that is metabolized to acetaminophen, is still available in some other countries.

B. Mechanism of Action

The mechanism of analgesic action of acetaminophen is unclear. The drug is only a weak COX-1 and COX-2 inhibitor in peripheral tissues, which accounts for its lack of anti-inflammatory effect. Evidence suggests that acetaminophen may inhibit a third enzyme, COX-3, in the CNS.

C. Effects

Acetaminophen is an analgesic and antipyretic agent; it lacks anti-inflammatory or antiplatelet effects.

D. Pharmacokinetics and Clinical Use

Acetaminophen is effective for the same indications as intermediate-dose aspirin. Acetaminophen is therefore useful as an aspirin substitute, especially in children with viral infections and in those with any type of aspirin intolerance. Acetaminophen is well absorbed orally and metabolized in the liver. Its half-life, which is 2–3 h in persons with normal hepatic function, is unaffected by renal disease.

E. Toxicity

In therapeutic dosages, acetaminophen has negligible toxicity in most persons. However, when taken in overdose or by patients with severe liver impairment, the drug is a dangerous hepatotoxin. The mechanism of toxicity involves oxidation to cytotoxic intermediates by phase I cytochrome P450 enzymes. This occurs if substrates for phase II conjugation reactions (acetate and glucuronide) are lacking (Chapter 4). Prompt administration of **acetylcysteine**, a sulfhydryl donor, may be lifesaving after an overdose. People who regularly consume 3 or more alcoholic drinks per day are at increased risk of acetaminophen-induced hepatotoxicity (Chapters 4 and 23).

DISEASE-MODIFYING ANTIRHEUMATIC DRUGS (DMARDs)

A. Classification

This heterogeneous group of agents (Table 36–2) has anti-inflammatory actions in several connective tissue diseases. They are called disease-modifying drugs because some evidence shows slowing or even reversal of joint damage, an effect never seen with NSAIDs. They are also called slow-acting antirheumatic drugs because it may take 6 wk to 6 mo for their benefits to become apparent. **Corticosteroids** can be considered anti-inflammatory drugs with an intermediate rate of action (ie, slower than NSAIDs but faster than other DMARDs). However, the corticosteroids are too toxic for routine chronic use (Chapter 39) and are reserved for temporary control of severe exacerbations and long-term use in patients with severe disease not controlled by other agents.

B. Mechanisms of Action and Effects

The mechanisms of action of most DMARDs in treating rheumatoid arthritis are poorly understood. Cytotoxic drugs (eg, **methotrexate**) probably act by reducing the number of immune cells available to maintain the inflammatory response; many of these drugs are also used in the treatment of cancer (Chapter 54). Other drugs appear to interfere with the activity of T lymphocytes (eg, **sulfasalazine, hydroxychloroquine, cyclosporine**, leflunomide, mycophenolate mofetil, abatacept), B lymphocytes (**rituximab**), or macrophages (gold compounds). In recent years, immunoglobulin-based biologic agents that inhibit the action of tumor necrosis factor-α (TNF-α), including **infliximab**, adalimumab, and **etanercept,** have also shown efficacy in rheumatoid arthritis, as has the recombinant human interleukin-1 receptor antagonist anakinra. The immunosuppressant effects of these drugs are discussed in more detail in Chapter 55.

TABLE 36–2 Some disease-modifying antirheumatic drugs (DMARDs).

Drug	Other Clinical Uses	Toxicity When Used for Rheumatoid Arthritis
Abatacept		Infection, exacerbation of COPD, hypersensitivity reactions
Anakinra		Injection-site reaction, infection, neutropenia
Anti-IL-6 drugs (tocilizumab)		Upper respiratory tract infections, headache, hypertension, and elevated liver enzymes
Anti-TNF-α drugs (infliximab, etanercept, adalimumab, golimumab, certolizumab)	Inflammatory bowel disease, other rheumatic disorders	Infection, lymphoma, hepatoxicity, hematologic effects, hypersensitivity reactions, cardiovascular toxicity
Cyclosporine	Tissue transplantation	Nephrotoxicity, hypertension, liver toxicity
Gold compounds		Many adverse effects, including diarrhea, dermatitis, hematologic abnormalities
Hydroxychloroquine, chloroquine	Antimalarial	Rash, gastrointestinal disturbance, myopathy, neuropathy, ocular toxicity
Leflunomide		Teratogen, hepatotoxicity, gastrointestinal disturbance, skin reactions
Methotrexate	Anticancer	Nausea, mucosal ulcers, hematotoxicity, hepatotoxicity, teratogenicity
Penicillamine	Chelating agent	Many adverse effects, including proteinuria, dermatitis, gastrointestinal disturbance, hematologic abnormalities
Rituximab	Non-Hodgkin's lymphoma	Infusion reaction, rash, infection, cardiac toxicity
Sulfasalazine	Inflammatory bowel disease	Rash, gastrointestinal disturbance, dizziness, headache, leukopenia

C. Pharmacokinetics and Clinical Use

Sulfasalazine, hydroxychloroquine, methotrexate, cyclosporine, penicillamine, and leflunomide are given orally. Anti-TNF-α drugs are given by injection. Gold compounds are available for parenteral use (gold sodium thiomalate and aurothioglucose) and for oral administration (auranofin).

Increasingly, DMARDs, particularly low doses of methotrexate, are initiated fairly early in patients with moderate to severe rheumatoid arthritis in an attempt to ameliorate disease progression. Some of these drugs are also used in other rheumatic diseases such as lupus erythematosus, arthritis associated with Sjögren's syndrome, juvenile rheumatoid arthritis, and ankylosing spondylitis, and in other immunologic disorders (Chapter 55).

D. Toxicity

All DMARDs can cause severe or fatal toxicities. Careful monitoring of patients who take these drugs is mandatory. Their major adverse effects are listed in Table 36–2.

DRUGS USED IN GOUT

A. Classification and Prototypes

Gout is associated with increased serum concentrations of uric acid. Acute attacks involve joint inflammation initiated by precipitation of uric acid crystals. Treatment strategies include (1) reducing inflammation during acute attacks (with colchicine, NSAIDs, or glucocorticoids; Figure 36–2); (2) accelerating renal excretion of

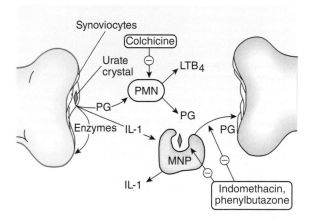

FIGURE 36–2 Sites of action of some anti-inflammatory drugs in a gouty joint. Synoviocytes damaged by uric acid crystals release prostaglandins (PG), interleukins (ILs), and other mediators of inflammation. Polymorphonuclear leukocytes (PMN), macrophages, and other inflammatory cells enter the joint and also release inflammatory substances, including leukotrienes (eg, LTB$_4$), that attract additional inflammatory cells. Colchicine acts on microtubules in the inflammatory cells. NSAIDs act on cyclooxygenase-2 (COX II) and inhibit PG formation in all of the cells of the joint. MNP, mononuclear phagocytes. (Reproduced, with permission, from Katzung BG, editor: *Basic & Clinical Pharmacology*, 12th ed. McGraw-Hill, 2012: Fig. 36–5.)

uric acid with uricosuric drugs (probenecid or sulfinpyrazone); and (3) reducing (with allopurinol or febuxostat) the conversion of purines to uric acid by xanthine oxidase (Figure 36–3).

B. Anti-Inflammatory Drugs Used for Gout

1. Mechanisms—NSAIDs such as **indomethacin** are effective in inhibiting the inflammation of acute gouty arthritis. These agents act through the reduction of prostaglandin formation and the inhibition of crystal phagocytosis by macrophages (Figure 36–2). **Colchicine,** a selective inhibitor of microtubule assembly, reduces leukocyte migration and phagocytosis; the drug may also reduce production of leukotriene B$_4$ and decrease free radical formation.

2. Effects—NSAIDs and glucocorticoids reduce the synthesis of inflammatory mediators in the gouty joint. Because it reacts with tubulin and interferes with microtubule assembly, colchicine is a general mitotic poison. Tubulin is necessary for normal cell division, motility, and many other processes.

3. Pharmacokinetics and clinical use—An NSAID or a glucocorticoid is preferred for the treatment of acute gouty arthritis. Although colchicine can be used for acute attacks, the doses required cause significant gastrointestinal disturbance, particularly diarrhea. Lower doses of colchicine are used to prevent attacks of gout in patients with a history of multiple acute attacks. Colchicine is also of value in the management of familial Mediterranean fever, a disease of unknown cause characterized by fever, hepatitis, peritonitis, pleuritis, arthritis, and, occasionally, amyloidosis. Indomethacin, some glucocorticoids, and colchicine are used orally; parenteral preparations of glucocorticoids and colchicine are also available.

4. Toxicity—NSAIDs can cause renal damage, and indomethacin can additionally cause bone marrow depression. Short courses of glucocorticoids can cause behavioral changes and impaired glucose control. Because colchicine can severely damage the liver and kidney, dosage must be carefully limited and monitored. Overdose is often fatal.

C. Uricosuric Agents

1. Mechanism—Normally, over 90% of the uric acid filtered by the kidney is reabsorbed in the proximal tubules. Uricosuric agents (**probenecid, sulfinpyrazone**) are weak acids that compete with uric acid for reabsorption by the weak acid transport mechanism in the proximal tubules and thereby increase uric acid excretion. At low doses, these agents may also compete with uric acid for **secretion** by the tubule and occasionally can elevate, rather than reduce, serum uric acid concentration. Elevation of uric acid levels by this mechanism occurs with aspirin (another weak acid) over much of its dose range.

2. Effects—Uricosuric drugs inhibit the **secretion** of a large number of other weak acids (eg, penicillin, methotrexate) in addition to inhibiting the reabsorption of uric acid.

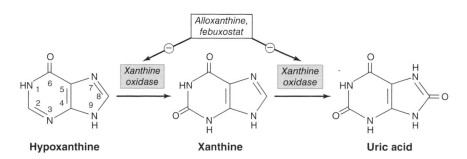

FIGURE 36-3 The action of xanthine oxidase in uric acid synthesis and metabolism of allopurinol. (Modified and reproduced, with permission, from Katzung BG, editor: *Basic & Clinical Pharmacology,* 11th ed. McGraw-Hill, 2012: Fig. 36–7.)

3. Pharmacokinetics and clinical use—Uricosuric drugs are used orally to treat chronic gout. These drugs are of no value in acute episodes.

4. Toxicity—Uricosuric drugs can precipitate an attack of acute gout during the early phase of their action. This can be avoided by simultaneously administering colchicine or indomethacin. Because they are sulfonamides, the uricosuric drugs may share allergenicity with other classes of sulfonamide drugs (diuretics, antimicrobials, oral hypoglycemic drugs).

D. Xanthine Oxidase Inhibitors

1. Mechanism—The production of uric acid can be reduced by inhibition of **xanthine oxidase**, the enzyme that converts hypoxanthine to xanthine and xanthine to uric acid (Figure 36–3). Allopurinol is converted to oxypurinol (alloxanthine) by xanthine oxidase; alloxanthine is an irreversible suicide inhibitor of the enzyme. The newer drug **febuxostat** is a nonpurine inhibitor of xanthine oxidase that is more selective than allopurinol and alloxanthine, which inhibit other enzymes involved in purine and pyrimidine metabolism.

2. Effects—Inhibition of xanthine oxidase increases the concentrations of the more soluble hypoxanthine and xanthine and decreases the concentration of the less soluble uric acid. As a result, there is less likelihood of precipitation of uric acid crystals in joints and tissues. Clinical trials suggest that febuxostat is more effective than allopurinol in lowering serum uric acid.

3. Pharmacokinetics and clinical use—The xanthine oxidase inhibitors are given orally in the management of chronic gout. Like uricosuric agents, these drugs are usually withheld for 1–2 wk after an acute episode of gouty arthritis and are administered in combination with colchicine or an NSAID to avoid an acute attack. Allopurinol is also used as an adjunct to cancer chemotherapy to slow the formation of uric acid from purines released by the death of large numbers of neoplastic cells.

4. Toxicity and drug interactions—Allopurinol causes gastrointestinal upset, rash, and rarely, peripheral neuritis, vasculitis, or bone marrow dysfunction, including aplastic anemia. It inhibits the metabolism of mercaptopurine and azathioprine, drugs that depend on xanthine oxidase for elimination. Febuxostat can cause liver function abnormalities, headache, and gastrointestinal upset.

QUESTIONS

1. Among NSAIDs, aspirin is unique because it
   (A) Irreversibly inhibits its target enzyme
   (B) Prevents episodes of gouty arthritis with long-term use
   (C) Reduces fever
   (D) Reduces the risk of colon cancer
   (E) Selectively inhibits the COX-2 enzyme

2. Which of the following is an analgesic and antipyretic drug that lacks an anti-inflammatory action?
   (A) Acetaminophen
   (B) Celecoxib
   (C) Colchicine
   (D) Indomethacin
   (E) Probenecid

3. A 16-year-old girl comes to the emergency department suffering from the effects of an aspirin overdose. Which of the following syndromes is this patient most likely to exhibit as a result of this drug overdose?
   (A) Bone marrow suppression and possibly aplastic anemia
   (B) Fever, hepatic dysfunction, and encephalopathy
   (C) Hyperthermia, metabolic acidosis, and coma
   (D) Rapid, fulminant hepatic failure
   (E) Rash, interstitial nephritis, and acute renal failure

4. Which of the following drugs is most likely to increase serum concentrations of conventional doses of methotrexate, a weak acid that is primarily cleared in the urine?
   (A) Acetaminophen
   (B) Allopurinol
   (C) Colchicine
   (D) Hydroxychloroquine
   (E) Probenecid

5. The main advantage of ketorolac over aspirin is that ketorolac
(A) Can be combined more safely with an opioid such as codeine
(B) Can be obtained as an over-the-counter agent
(C) Does not prolong the bleeding time
(D) Is available in a parenteral formulation that can be injected intramuscularly or intravenously
(E) Is less likely to cause acute renal failure in patients with some preexisting degree of renal impairment

6. An 18-month-old boy dies from an accidental overdose of acetaminophen. Which of the following is the most likely cause of this patient's death?
(A) Arrhythmia
(B) Hemorrhagic stroke
(C) Liver failure
(D) Noncardiogenic pulmonary edema
(E) Ventilatory failure

Questions 7 and 8. A 52-year-old woman presented with intense pain, warmth, and redness in the first toe on her left foot. Examination of fluid withdrawn from the inflamed joint revealed crystals of uric acid.

7. In the treatment of this woman's acute attack of gout, a high dose of colchicine will reduce the pain and inflammation. However, many physicians prefer to treat acute gout with a corticosteroid or indomethacin because high doses of colchicine are likely to cause
(A) Behavioral changes that include psychosis
(B) High blood pressure
(C) Rash
(D) Severe diarrhea
(E) Sudden gastrointestinal bleeding

8. Over the next 7 mo, the patient had 2 more attacks of acute gout. Her serum concentration of uric acid was elevated. The decision was made to put her on chronic drug therapy to try to prevent subsequent attacks. Which of the following drugs could be used to decrease this woman's rate of production of uric acid?
(A) Allopurinol
(B) Aspirin
(C) Colchicine
(D) Hydroxychloroquine
(E) Probenecid

Questions 9 and 10. A 54-year-old woman presented with signs and symptoms consistent with an early stage of rheumatoid arthritis. The decision was made to initiate NSAID therapy.

9. Which of the following patient characteristics is the most compelling reason for avoiding celecoxib in the treatment of her arthritis?
(A) History of alcohol abuse
(B) History of gout
(C) History of myocardial infarction
(D) History of osteoporosis
(E) History of peptic ulcer disease

10. Although the patient's disease was adequately controlled with an NSAID and methotrexate for some time, her symptoms began to worsen and radiologic studies of her hands indicated progressive destruction in the joints of several fingers. Treatment with another second-line agent for rheumatoid arthritis was considered. Which of the following is a parenterally administered DMARD whose mechanism of anti-inflammatory action is antagonism of tumor necrosis factor?
(A) Cyclosporine
(B) Etanercept
(C) Penicillamine
(D) Phenylbutazone
(E) Sulfasalazine

ANSWERS

1. Aspirin differs from other NSAIDs by **irreversibly** inhibiting cyclooxygenase. The answer is **A.**

2. Acetaminophen is the only drug that fits this description. Indomethacin is a nonselective COX inhibitor and celecoxib is a COX-2 inhibitor; both have analgesic, antipyretic, and anti-inflammatory effects. Colchicine is a drug used for gout that also has an anti-inflammatory action. Probenecid is a uricosuric drug that promotes the excretion of uric acid. The answer is **A.**

3. Salicylate intoxication is associated with metabolic acidosis, dehydration, and hyperthermia. If these problems are not corrected, coma and death ensue. The answer is **C.**

4. Like other weak acids, methotrexate depends on active tubular excretion in the proximal tubule for efficient elimination. Probenecid competes with methotrexate for binding to the proximal tubule transporter and thereby decreases the rate of clearance of methotrexate. The answer is **E.**

5. Ketorolac exerts typical NSAID effects. It prolongs the bleeding time and can impair renal function, especially in a patient with preexisting renal disease. Its primary use is as a parenteral agent for pain management, especially for treatment of postoperative patients. The answer is **D.**

6. In overdose, acetaminophen causes fulminant liver failure as a result of its conversion by hepatic cytochrome P450 enzymes to a highly reactive metabolite. The answer is **C.**

7. At doses needed to treat acute gout, colchicine frequently causes significant diarrhea. Such gastrointestinal effects are less likely with the lower doses used in chronic gout. The answer is **D.**

8. Allopurinol is the only drug listed that decreases production of uric acid. Probenecid increases uric acid excretion. Colchicine and hydroxychloroquine do not affect uric acid metabolism. Aspirin actually slows renal secretion of uric acid and raises uric acid blood levels. It should not be used in gout. The answer is **A.**

9. Celecoxib is a COX-2-selective inhibitor. Although the COX-2 inhibitors have the advantage over nonselective NSAIDs of reduced gastrointestinal toxicity, clinical data suggest that they are more likely to cause arterial thrombotic events. A history of myocardial infarction would be a compelling reason to avoid a COX-2 inhibitor. The answer is **C.**

10. Etanercept is a recombinant protein that binds to tumor necrosis factor and prevents its inflammatory effects. The answer is **B.**

SKILL KEEPER ANSWERS: OPIOIDS (SEE CHAPTER 31)

1. *Morphine is the prototype strong opioid. Fentanyl is a strong agent with a rapid onset that is commonly used in the hospital. Methadone is a strong agonist used in maintenance programs for patients addicted to opioids. Codeine, oxycodone, and hydrocodone are moderate agonists, whereas propoxyphene is a weak agonist.*

2. *Constipation and sedation occur with therapeutic doses; constipation should be managed with stool softeners. In overdose, opioids cause a triad of pinpoint pupils, coma, and respiratory depression.*

3. *Naloxone, a nonselective opioid receptor antagonist, is an antidote for opioid overdose.*

CHECKLIST

When you complete this chapter, you should be able to:

❑ Describe the effects of NSAIDs on prostaglandin synthesis.

❑ Contrast the functions of COX-1 and COX-2.

❑ Compare the actions and toxicity of aspirin, the older nonselective NSAIDs, and the COX-2-selective drugs.

❑ Explain why several of the highly selective COX-2 inhibitors have been withdrawn from the market.

❑ Describe the toxic effects of aspirin.

❑ Describe the effects and the major toxicity of acetaminophen.

❑ Name 5 disease-modifying antirheumatic drugs (DMARDs) and describe their toxicity.

❑ Contrast the pharmacologic treatment of acute and chronic gout.

❑ Describe the mechanisms of action and toxicity of 3 different drug groups used in gout.

DRUG SUMMARY TABLE: NSAIDs, Acetaminophen, & Drugs for Rheumatoid Arthritis & Gout

Subclass	Mechanism of Action	Clinical Applications	Pharmacokinetics	Toxicities, Drug Interactions
Salicylates				
Aspirin	Acetylation of COX-1 and COX-2 results in decreased prostaglandin synthesis	Analgesia, antipyretic, anti-inflammatory, and antithrombotic • prevention of colon cancer	Duration of activity is longer than pharmacokinetic half-life of drug due to irreversible COX inhibition	Gastrointestinal (GI) toxicity, nephrotoxicity, and increased bleeding time at therapeutic levels • hypersensitivity reaction due to increased leukotrienes • tinnitus, hyperventilation metabolic acidosis, hyperthermia, coma in overdose
Nonselective NSAIDs				
Ibuprofen	Reversible inhibition of COX-1 and COX-2 results in decreased prostaglandin synthesis	Analgesia, antipyretic, and anti-inflammatory • closure of patent ductus arteriosus	Rapid metabolism and renal elimination	GI toxicity, nephrotoxicity • hypersensitivity due to increased leukotrienes • interference with aspirin's antithrombotic action
Many nonselective nonsteroidal anti-inflammatory drugs (NSAIDs) available for clinical use. See Table 36-1				
COX-2 inhibitor				
Celecoxib	Selective, reversible inhibition of COX-2 results in decreased prostaglandin synthesis	Analgesia, antipyretic, and anti-inflammatory	Hepatic metabolism	Nephrotoxicity • hypersensitivity due to increased leukotrienes • less risk of GI toxicity than nonselective NSAIDs • greater risk of thrombosis than nonselective NSAIDs
Other analgesic				
Acetaminophen	Mechanism unknown, weak COX inhibitor	Analgesia, antipyretic	Hepatic conjugation	Hepatotoxicity in overdose (antidote is acetylcysteine) • hepatotoxicity more likely with chronic alcohol consumption
Disease-modifying antirheumatic drugs (DMARDs)				
Methotrexate	Cytotoxic to rapidly dividing immune cells due to inhibition of dihydrofolate reductase	Anticancer, rheumatic disorders	Renal elimination	Nausea, mucosal ulcers, hematotoxicity, hepatotoxicity, teratogenicity
Diverse array of DMARDs available for clinical use. See Table 36-2				
Microtubule assembly inhibitor				
Colchicine	Inhibition of microtubule assembly decreases macrophage migration and phagocytosis	Chronic and acute gout, familial Mediterranean fever	Oral drug	Diarrhea, severe liver and kidney damage in overdose
Uricosurics				
Probenecid	Inhibition of renal reuptake of uric acid	Chronic gout, prolongation of antimicrobial drug action	Oral drug	Exacerbation of acute gout, hypersensitivity reactions, inhibits renal tubular secretion of weak acids such as methotrexate
Sulfinpyrazone: similar to probenecid				
Xanthine oxidase inhibitors				
Allopurinol	Active metabolite irreversibly inhibits xanthine oxidase and lowers production of uric acid	Chronic gout, adjunct to cancer chemotherapy	Activated by xanthine oxidase • oral drug	GI upset, hypersensitivity reactions, bone marrow suppression
Febuxostat: reversible inhibitor of xanthine oxidase				

Hypothalamic & Pituitary Hormones

The hormones produced by the hypothalamus and pituitary gland are key regulators of metabolism, growth, and reproduction. Preparations of these hormones, including products made by recombinant DNA technology and drugs that mimic or block their effects, are used in the treatment of a variety of endocrine disorders.

Drugs that mimic or block the effects of hypothalamic and pituitary hormones

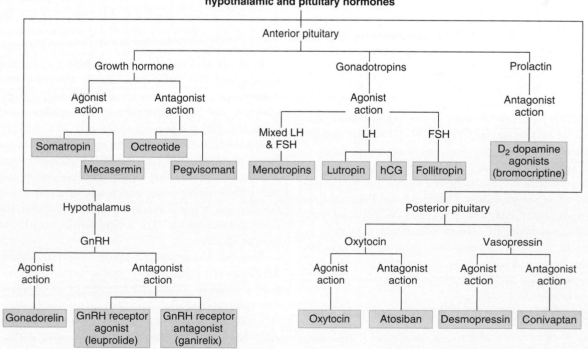

High-Yield Terms to Learn

Acromegaly	A syndrome of growth hormone (GH) excess in adults characterized by abnormal growth of tissues—particularly connective tissue—metabolic abnormalities, and cardiac dysfunction
Central diabetes insipidus	A syndrome of polyuria, polydipsia, and hypernatremia caused by inadequate production of vasopressin
Gigantism	A syndrome of GH excess in children and adolescents with open long bone epiphyses that results in excessive height
Gonadotropins	The 2 anterior pituitary hormones (luteinizing hormone [LH] and follicle-stimulating hormone [FSH]) that regulate reproduction in males and females
Insulin-like growth factor-1 (IGF-1)	A growth factor that is the primary mediator of GH effects
Prolactinoma	Pituitary tumor that secretes excessive amounts of prolactin and is associated with a syndrome of infertility and galactorrhea
Tocolytic	Drug used to inhibit preterm labor (eg, the oxytocin receptor antagonist atosiban; magnesium sulfate; nifedipine; β_2 agonists)

ANTERIOR PITUITARY HORMONES & THEIR HYPOTHALAMIC REGULATORS

The hypothalamic and pituitary hormones and their antagonists are often grouped according to the anatomic site of release of the hormone that they mimic or block—the hypothalamus for gonadotropin-releasing hormone (GnRH); the anterior pituitary for growth hormone (GH), the 2 gonadotropins, luteinizing hormone (LH) and follicle-stimulating hormone (FSH), and prolactin; or the posterior pituitary for oxytocin and vasopressin (antidiuretic hormone [ADH]). This chapter focuses on the agents used commonly; it does not discuss the hypothalamic and pituitary hormones that are either not used clinically or are used solely for specialized diagnostic testing (thyrotropin-releasing hormone [TRH], thyroid-stimulating hormone [TSH], corticotropin-releasing hormone [CRH], adrenocorticotropic hormone [ACTH], and growth hormone-releasing hormone [GHRH]). Hormones of the anterior pituitary are central links in the hypothalamic-pituitary endocrine system (or axis; Figure 37–1). All the anterior pituitary hormones are under the control of a hypothalamic hormone, and with the exception of prolactin, all mediate their ultimate effects by regulating the production by peripheral tissues of other hormones (Table 37–1). Four anterior pituitary hormones (TSH, LH, FSH, and ACTH) and their hypothalamic regulators are subject to feedback regulation by the hormones whose production they control. The complex systems that regulate hormones of the anterior pituitary provide multiple avenues of pharmacologic intervention.

A. Growth Hormone and Mecasermin

1. GH—Growth hormone is required for normal growth during childhood and adolescence and is an important regulator throughout life of lipid and carbohydrate metabolism and lean body mass. Its effects are primarily mediated by regulating the production in peripheral tissues of **insulin-like growth factor 1 (IGF-1)**.

Somatropin, the recombinant form of human GH, is used for GH deficiency in children and adults and in the treatment of children with genetic diseases associated with short stature (eg, Turner syndrome, Noonan syndrome, Prader-Willi syndrome). GH treatment also improves growth in children with failure to thrive due to chronic renal failure or the small-for-gestational-age condition. The most controversial use of GH is for children with idiopathic short stature who are not GH deficient. In this group of children, multiple years of GH therapy at great cost and some risk of toxicity results in a small (1.5-3 inches) average increase in final adult height.

In adults, GH has efficacy in treatment of AIDS-associated wasting and GH deficiency, and it may improve gastrointestinal function in patients who have undergone intestinal resection and have subsequently developed a malabsorption syndrome. GH is a popular component of antiaging programs even though studies in model animal systems have consistently found that analogs of GH and IGF-1 shorten lifespan. GH is also used by athletes for a purported increase in muscle mass and athletic performance and is one of the drugs banned by the Olympic Committee and professional sports associations. Recombinant bovine GH is used in dairy cattle to increase milk production.

Rare but serious adverse effects of GH in children include pseudotumor cerebri, slipped capital femoral epiphysis, progression of scoliosis, edema, and hyperglycemia. Children with GH deficiency should be monitored periodically for concurrent deficiency of other anterior pituitary hormones. Adults generally tolerate GH less well than children. Adverse effects include peripheral edema, myalgia, and arthralgia.

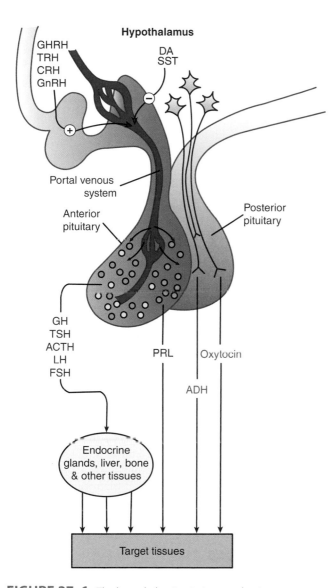

FIGURE 37–1 The hypothalamic-pituitary endocrine system. Except for prolactin, hormones released from the anterior pituitary stimulate the production of hormones by a peripheral endocrine gland, the liver, or other tissues. Prolactin and the hormones released from the posterior pituitary (vasopressin and oxytocin) act directly on target tissues. Hypothalamic factors regulate the release of anterior pituitary hormones. ACTH, adrenocorticotropin; ADH, antidiuretic hormone [vasopressin]; CRH, corticotropin-releasing hormone; DA, dopamine; FSH, follicle-stimulating hormone; GH, growth hormone; GHRH, growth hormone-releasing hormone; GnRH, gonadotropin-releasing hormone; LH, luteinizing hormone; PRL, prolactin; SST, somatostatin; TRH, thyrotropin-releasing hormone; TSH, thyroid-stimulating hormone. (Reproduced, with permission, Katzung BG, editor: *Basic & Clinical Pharmacology*, 12th ed. McGraw-Hill, 2012: Fig. 37–1.)

2. Mecasermin—A small group of children with growth failure unresponsive to GH therapy are deficient in IGF-1. Mecasermin, recombinant human IGF-1, is administered parenterally to children with IGF-1 deficiency. Its most important toxicity is hypoglycemia, which can be prevented by consumption of a snack or meal shortly before mecasermin administration. In some countries, children are treated with mecasermin rinfabate, a combination of recombinant human IGF-1 and human insulin-like growth factor-binding protein-3 (rhIGFBP-3), which increases the half-life of IGF-1.

B. Growth Hormone Antagonists

Growth hormone-secreting pituitary adenomas cause **acromegaly** in adults and, rarely, **gigantism** in children and adolescents who have not completed their growth phase. Pharmacologic treatment of GH excess seeks to inhibit GH secretion or interfere with GH effects.

1. Somatostatin analogs—Somatostatin, a 14-amino-acid peptide, inhibits the release of GH, glucagon, insulin, and gastrin. **Octreotide** and **lanreotide**, long-acting synthetic analogs of somatostatin, are used to treat acromegaly, carcinoid, gastrinoma, glucagonoma, and other endocrine tumors. Regular octreotide must be administered subcutaneously 2–4 times daily, whereas a slow-release intramuscular formulation of octreotide or lanreotide is administered every 4 weeks for long-term therapy. Octreotide and lanreotide cause significant gastrointestinal disturbances, gallstones, and cardiac conduction abnormalities.

2. Dopamine D$_2$ receptor agonists—Dopamine D$_2$ receptor agonists such as **bromocriptine** are more effective at inhibiting prolactin release than inhibiting GH release (see following text). However, high doses of D$_2$ receptor agonists have some efficacy in the treatment of small GH-secreting tumors.

3. Pegvisomant—Pegvisomant is a GH receptor antagonist approved for treatment of acromegaly. Normally, GH, which has 2 distinct receptor binding sites, initiates cellular signaling cascades by dimerizing 2 GH receptors. Pegvisomant is a long-acting derivative of a mutant GH that is able to cross-link GH receptors but is incapable of inducing the conformational changes required for receptor activation.

C. Follicle-Stimulating Hormone (FSH), Luteinizing Hormone, and Their Analogs

In women, FSH directs follicle development, whereas FSH and LH collaborate in the regulation of ovarian steroidogenesis. In men, FSH is the primary regulator of spermatogenesis, whereas LH is the main stimulus for testicular androgen production. The gonadotropins and their analogs are used in combination to stimulate spermatogenesis in infertile men and to induce ovulation in women with anovulation that is not responsive to less complicated treatments (see Chapter 40). In men, the treatment of infertility due to hypogonadism requires months of administration of a mixture of drugs with LH and FSH activity.

Ovulation induction protocols are increasingly complex. They require close monitoring to ensure successful insemination or retrieval of mature oocytes and to prevent the 2 most serious

TABLE 37–1 Links between hypothalamic, anterior pituitary, and target organ hormones or mediators.[a]

Anterior Pituitary Hormone	Hypothalamic Hormone	Target Organ	Primary Target Organ Hormone(s) or Mediator(s)
Growth hormone (GH, somatotropin)	Growth hormone-releasing hormone (GHRH) (+) Somatostatin (−)	Liver, bone, muscle, kidney, and others	Insulin-like growth factor-1 (IGF-1)
Thyroid-stimulating hormone (TSH)	Thyrotropin-releasing hormone (TRH) (+)	Thyroid	Thyroxine, triiodothyronine
Adrenocorticotropin (ACTH)	Corticotropin-releasing hormone (CRH) (+)	Adrenal cortex	Cortisol
Follicle-stimulating hormone (FSH) Luteinizing hormone (LH)	Gonadotropin-releasing hormone (GnRH) (+)[b]	Gonads	Estrogen, progesterone, testosterone
Prolactin (PRL)	Dopamine (−)	Breast	—

(+), stimulant; (−), inhibitor.

[a]All of these hormones act through G protein-coupled receptors except GH and prolactin, which act through JAK/STAT receptors.

[b]Endogenous GnRH, which is released in pulses, stimulates LH and FSH release. When administered continuously as a drug, GnRH and its analogs inhibit LH and FSH release.

Reproduced, with permission, from Katzung BG, editor: *Basic & Clinical Pharmacology*, 12th ed. McGraw-Hill, 2012.

complications of ovulation induction—multiple pregnancies and the ovarian hyperstimulation syndrome, a syndrome of ovarian enlargement, ascites, hypovolemia, and possibly shock. All ovulation induction protocols that use gonadotropins have 3 basic steps. First, endogenous gonadotropin production is inhibited by administration of a GnRH agonist or antagonist (see text that follows). Second, follicle development is driven by daily injections of a preparation with FSH activity (menotropins, FSH, or an FSH analog). Last, the final stage of oocyte maturation is induced with an injection of LH or the LH analog human chorionic gonadotropin (hCG).

A variety of gonadotropin preparations are available. All are administered parenterally.

1. Menotropins—These gonadotropins consist of a mixture of FSH and LH purified from the urine of postmenopausal women (who produce high levels of FSH and LH owing to the disinhibition of pituitary gonadotropin production that results from cessation of ovarian steroidogenesis).

2. FSH and its analogs—Three forms of FSH are available. **Urofollitropin** is a purified preparation extracted from the urine of postmenopausal women. The 2 recombinant forms of human FSH—**follitropin alpha** and follitropin beta—differ in the composition of their carbohydrate side chains.

3. LH and its analogs—**Human chorionic gonadotropin (hCG),** the placental protein that supports the corpus luteum during the early stages of pregnancy, has a structure that is nearly identical to LH and mediates its effects through activation of LH receptors. hCG purified from human urine or recombinant hCG is used commonly for an LH activity. **Lutropin,** a recombinant form of human LH, is also available.

D. Gonadotropin-Releasing Hormone (GnRH) and its Analogs

GnRH is a decapeptide that stimulates gonadotropin release when it is secreted in a pulsatile pattern by the hypothalamus. **Leuprolide** was the first of a set of synthetic peptides with long-acting GnRH agonist activity. Other long-acting GnRH agonists include goserelin, histrelin, nafarelin, and triptorelin.

In men and women, steady dosing with these GnRH agonists inhibits gonadotropin release by downregulating GnRH receptors in the pituitary cells that normally release gonadotropins. Continuous GnRH agonist treatment is used to suppress endogenous gonadotropin secretion in women undergoing ovulation induction with gonadotropins, in women with gynecologic disorders that benefit from ovarian suppression (eg, endometriosis, uterine leiomyomata), in men with advanced prostate cancer, in early pubertal transgender adolescents (to block endogenous puberty prior to treatment with cross-gender gonadal hormones), and in children with central precocious puberty.

In women, continuous treatment with a GnRH agonist causes the typical symptoms of menopause (hot flushes, sweats, headache). Long-term treatment is avoided because of the risk of bone loss and osteoporosis. In men treated continuously with a GnRH agonist, adverse effects include hot flushes, sweats, gynecomastia, reduced libido, decreased hematocrit, and reduced bone density. In men with prostate cancer and children with central precocious puberty, the first few weeks of therapy can temporarily exacerbate the condition.

E. Gonadotropin-Releasing Hormone (GnRH) Antagonists

Ganirelix, cetrorelix, and **degarelix** are GnRH *antagonists*. Ganirelix and cetrorelix can be used during ovulation induction in place of GnRH agonists to suppress endogenous gonadotropin production. Degarelix is approved for the treatment of advanced prostate cancer. The adverse effects of GnRH antagonists are similar to those associated with continuous treatment with a GnRH agonist except that they do not cause a tumor flare when used for treatment of advanced prostate cancer and they may be less likely to cause the ovarian hyperstimulation syndrome when used for ovulation induction.

F. Prolactin Antagonists (Dopamine D₂ Receptor Agonists)

The anterior pituitary hormone prolactin regulates lactation. In women and men, hyperprolactinemia and an associated syndrome of infertility and galactorrhea can result from prolactin-secreting adenomas. Dopamine is the physiologic inhibitor of prolactin release (Figure 37–1). Prolactin-secreting adenomas usually retain their sensitivity to dopamine. In hyperprolactinemia, **bromocriptine** and other orally active D₂ dopamine receptor agonists (eg, cabergoline, pergolide; see Chapter 16) are effective in reducing serum prolactin concentrations and restoring fertility. As previously mentioned, high doses of a dopamine agonist can also be used in the treatment of acromegaly.

> ### SKILL KEEPER: DRUGS THAT CAUSE HYPERPROLACTINEMIA (SEE CHAPTER 29)
>
> *As many as 25% of infertile women have hyperprolactinemia. In women, hyperprolactinemia causes galactorrhea, oligomenorrhea, or amenorrhea as well as infertility (the amenorrhea-galactorrhea syndrome). Although prolactin-secreting tumors are the most common cause of hyperprolactinemia, the condition can also be precipitated by drugs that interfere with the control of prolactin release.*
>
> 1. *What types of pharmacologic actions are most likely to cause hyperprolactinemia?*
> 2. *Name several drugs with this type of pharmacologic action.*
>
> The Skill Keeper Answers appear at the end of the chapter.

POSTERIOR PITUITARY HORMONES

A. Oxytocin

Oxytocin is a nonapeptide synthesized in cell bodies in the paraventricular nuclei of the hypothalamus and transported through the axons of these cells to the posterior pituitary (Figure 37–1). Oxytocin is an effective stimulant of uterine contraction and is used intravenously to induce or reinforce labor. **Atosiban** is an antagonist of the oxytocin receptor that is used in some countries as a **tocolytic**, a drug used to treat preterm labor.

B. Vasopressin (Antidiuretic Hormone [ADH])

Vasopressin is synthesized in neuronal cell bodies in the hypothalamus and released from nerve terminals in the posterior pituitary (Figure 37–1). As discussed in Chapter 15, vasopressin acts through V₂ receptors to increase the insertion of water channels in the apical membranes of collecting duct cells in the kidney and to thereby provide an antidiuretic effect. Extrarenal V₂-like receptors regulate the release of coagulation factor VIII and von Willebrand factor (see Chapter 34). **Desmopressin,** a selective agonist of V₂ receptors, is administered orally, nasally, or parenterally in patients with pituitary diabetes insipidus and in patients with mild hemophilia A or von Willebrand disease.

Vasopressin also contracts vascular smooth muscle by activating V₁ receptors. Because of this vasoconstrictor effect, vasopressin is sometimes used to treat patients with bleeding from esophageal varices or colon diverticula.

Several antagonists of vasopressin receptors (eg, **conivaptan,** tolvaptan) have been developed to offset the fluid retention that results from the excessive production of vasopressin associated with hyponatremia or acute heart failure (see Chapter 15).

QUESTIONS

1. Which of the following is a drug that is purified from the urine of postmenopausal women and used to promote spermatogenesis in infertile men?
   (A) Desmopressin
   (B) Gonadorelin
   (C) Goserelin
   (D) Somatropin
   (E) Urofollitropin

2. A 29-year-old woman in her 41st wk of gestation had been in labor for 12 h. Although her uterine contractions had been strong and regular initially, they had diminished in force during the past hour. Which of the following agents would be used to facilitate this woman's labor and delivery?
   (A) Dopamine
   (B) Leuprolide
   (C) Oxytocin
   (D) Prolactin
   (E) Vasopressin

3. A 3-year-old boy with failure to thrive and metabolic disturbances was found to have an inactivating mutation in the gene that encodes the growth hormone receptor. Which of the following drugs is most likely to improve his metabolic function and promote his growth?
   (A) Atosiban
   (B) Bromocriptine
   (C) Mecasermin
   (D) Octreotide
   (E) Somatropin

4. An important difference between leuprolide and ganirelix is that ganirelix
   (A) Can be administered as an oral formulation
   (B) Can be used alone to restore fertility to hypogonadal men and women
   (C) Immediately reduces gonadotropin secretion
   (D) Initially stimulates pituitary production of LH and FSH
   (E) Must be administered in a pulsatile fashion

5. A 27-year-old woman with amenorrhea, infertility, and galactorrhea was treated with a drug that successfully restored ovulation and menstruation. Before being given the drug, the woman was carefully questioned about previous mental health problems, which she did not have. She was advised to take the drug orally. Which of the following is most likely to be the drug that was used to treat this patient?
   (A) Bromocriptine
   (B) Desmopressin
   (C) Human gonadotropin hormone
   (D) Leuprolide
   (E) Octreotide

6. Who is *least* likely to be treated with somatropin?
   (A) A 3-year-old cow on a dairy farm
   (B) A 4-year-old girl with an XO genetic genotype
   (C) A 4-year-old boy with chronic renal failure and growth deficiency
   (D) A 10-year-old boy with polydipsia and polyuria
   (E) A 37-year-old patient with AIDS-related wasting syndrome

7. A 3-year-old girl presented with hirsutism, breast enlargement, and a height and bone age that was consistent with an age of 9. Diagnostic testing revealed precocious puberty. Which of the following is the most appropriate drug for treatment of this patient's precocious puberty?
   (A) Atosiban
   (B) Follitropin
   (C) Leuprolide
   (D) Octreotide
   (E) Pegvisomant

8. A 47-year-old man exhibited signs and symptoms of acromegaly. Radiologic studies indicated the presence of a large pituitary tumor. Surgical treatment of the tumor was only partially effective in controlling his disease. At this point, which of the following drugs is most likely to be used as pharmacologic therapy?
   (A) Cosyntropin
   (B) Desmopressin
   (C) Leuprolide
   (D) Octreotide
   (E) Somatropin

9. A 37-year-old woman with infertility due to obstructed fallopian tubes was undergoing ovulation induction in preparation for in vitro fertilization. After 10 d of treatment with leuprolide, the next step in the procedure is most likely to involve 10–14 d of treatment with which of the following?
   (A) Bromocriptine
   (B) Follitropin
   (C) Gonadorelin
   (D) hCG
   (E) Pergolide

10. A 7-year-old boy underwent successful chemotherapy and cranial radiation for treatment of acute lymphocytic leukemia. One month after the completion of therapy, the patient presented with excessive thirst and urination plus hypernatremia. Laboratory testing revealed pituitary diabetes insipidus. To correct these problems, this patient is likely to be treated with which of the following?
    (A) Corticotropin
    (B) Desmopressin
    (C) hCG
    (D) Menotropins
    (E) Thyrotropin

ANSWERS

1. Spermatogenesis in males requires the action of FSH and LH. Urofollitropin, which is purified from the urine of postmenopausal women, is used clinically to provide FSH activity. The answer is **E**.

2. Oxytocin is an effective stimulant of uterine contraction that is routinely used to augment labor. The answer is **C**.

3. This child's condition is due to the inability of GH to stimulate the production of insulin-like growth factors, the ultimate mediators of GH effects. Mecasermin, a combination of recombinant IGF-1 and the binding protein that protects IGF-1 from immediate destruction, will help correct the IGF deficiency. Because of the inactive GH receptors, somatropin will not be effective. The answer is **C**.

4. Leuprolide is an agonist of GnRH receptors, whereas ganirelix is an antagonist. Although both drugs can be used to inhibit gonadotropin release, ganirelix does so immediately, whereas leuprolide does so only after about 1 wk of sustained activity. The answer is **C**.

5. Bromocriptine, a dopamine receptor agonist, is used to treat the amenorrhea-galactorrhea syndrome, which is a consequence of hyperprolactinemia. Because of its central dopaminergic effects, the drug should not be used in patients with a history of schizophrenia or other forms of psychotic illness. The answer is **A**.

6. Somatropin, recombinant human GH, promotes growth in children with Turner's syndrome (an XO genetic genotype) or chronic renal failure. It also helps combat the AIDS-associated wasting syndrome. Bovine GH promotes milk production in cows. GH would not be appropriate for the boy with polydipsia and polyuria, which is probably symptomatic of a form of diabetes. The answer is **D**.

7. In precocious puberty, the hypothalamic-pituitary-gonadal axis becomes prematurely active for reasons that are not understood. Treatment involves suppressing gonadotropin secretion with continuous administration of a long-acting GnRH agonist such as leuprolide. The answer is **C**.

8. Octreotide, a somatostatin analog, has some efficacy in reducing the excess GH production that causes acromegaly. The answer is **D**.

9. Once the patient's endogenous gonadotropin production has been inhibited through continuous administration of the GnRH agonist leuprolide, the next step in ovulation induction is the administration of a drug with FSH activity to stimulate follicle maturation. Follitropin is recombinant FSH. The only other drug listed that is used in ovulation induction is hCG, but this is an LH analog. The answer is **B**.

10. Pituitary diabetes insipidus results from deficiency in vasopressin. It is treated with desmopressin, a peptide agonist of vasopressin V_2 receptors. The answer is **B**.

SKILL KEEPER ANSWERS: DRUGS THAT CAUSE HYPERPROLACTINEMIA (SEE CHAPTER 29)

1. *Drugs that block dopamine D_2 receptors cause hyperprolactinemia by blocking the inhibitory effects of endogenous dopamine on the pituitary cells that release prolactin.*

2. *The older antipsychotic drugs (eg, phenothiazines, haloperidol), with their strong dopamine D_2 receptor-blocking activity, are most likely to be the pharmacologic cause of hyperprolactinemia (see Chapter 29). This adverse effect is less likely with atypical antipsychotic drugs (eg, olanzapine). Drugs or drug groups that cause hyperprolactinemia through mechanisms that are not well characterized include methyldopa (an antihypertensive), amphetamines, tricyclic and other types of antidepressants, and opioids.*

CHECKLIST

When you complete this chapter, you should be able to:

❑ Describe the drugs used as substitutes for the natural pituitary hormones, and list their clinical uses.

❑ List the gonadotropin analogs and GnRH agonists and antagonists, and describe their clinical use in treating male and female infertility, endometriosis, and prostate cancer.

❑ Describe the drugs used for treatment of acromegaly and hyperprolactinemia.

DRUG SUMMARY TABLE: Drugs that Mimic or Inhibit Hypothalamic & Pituitary Hormones

Subclass	Mechanism of Action	Clinical Applications	Pharmacokinetics	Toxicities, Interactions
Growth hormone (GH)				
Somatropin	Recombinant human GH • acts through GH receptors to increase the production of IGF-1	Replacement in GH deficiency • increased final adult height in children with certain conditions associated with short stature • wasting in HIV infection • short bowel syndrome	Subcutaneous (SC) injection	In children, pseudotumor cerebri, slipped capital femoral epiphysis, progression of scoliosis, edema, and hyperglycemia • in adults, peripheral edema, myalgia, and arthralgia
IGF-1 agonist				
Mecasermin	Recombinant IGF-1	Replacement in IGF-1 deficiency that is not responsive to exogenous GH	SC injection	Hypoglycemia, intracranial hypertension, increased liver enzymes
Somatostatin analogs				
Octreotide	Somatostatin receptor agonist	Acromegaly and several other hormone-secreting tumors • acute control of bleeding from esophageal varices	SC injection • long-acting formulation injected intramuscularly (IM)	GI disturbances, gallstones, bradycardia, cardiac conduction anomalies
Lanreotide: similar to octreotide; available as a long-acting formulation for acromegaly				
Growth hormone receptor antagonist				
Pegvisomant	Blocks GH receptor signaling	Acromegaly	SC injection	Increased liver enzymes
Gonadotropins: Follicle-stimulating hormone (FSH) analogs				
Follitropin alfa	Follicle-stimulating hormone (FSH) receptor agonist	Controlled ovulation hyperstimulation in women • infertility due to hypogonadotropic hypogonadism in men	SC injection	Ovarian hyperstimulation syndrome and multiple pregnancies in women • gynecomastia in men • headache, depression, edema in both sexes
Follitropin beta: recombinant product with the same peptide sequence as follitropin alfa but differs in its carbohydrate side chains *Urofollitropin:* human FSH purified from the urine of postmenopausal women *Menotropins (hMG):* extract of the urine of postmenopausal women; contains both FSH and LH activity				
Gonadotropins: Luteinizing hormone (LH) analogs				
Human chorionic gonadotropin (hCG)	LH receptor agonist	Initiation of ovulation during controlled ovulation hyperstimulation • ovarian follicle development in women with hypogonadotropic hypogonadism • male hypo-gonadotropic hypogonadism	IM injection	Ovarian hyperstimulation syndrome and multiple pregnancies in women • gynecomastia in men • headache, depression, edema in both sexes
Choriogonadotropin alfa: recombinant form of hCG *Lutropin:* recombinant form of human LH *Menotropins (hMG):* extract of the urine of postmenopausal women; contains both FSH and LH activity				

(Continued)

DRUG SUMMARY TABLE: Drugs that Mimic or Inhibit Hypothalamic & Pituitary Hormones (*Continued*)

Subclass	Mechanism of Action	Clinical Applications	Pharmacokinetics	Toxicities, Interactions
Gonadotropin-Releasing Hormone (GnRH) Analogs				
Leuprolide	GnRH receptor agonist	Ovarian suppression • controlled ovarian hyperstimulation • central precocious puberty • block of endogenous puberty in some transgender early pubertal adolescents • advanced prostate cancer	Administered IV, SC, IM, or intranasally • depot formulations are available	Headache, light-headedness, nausea, injection site reactions • with continuous treatment symptoms of hypogonadism
Gonadorelin: synthetic human GnRH				
Other GnRH analogs: goserelin, histrelin, nafarelin, and triptorelin				
GnRH receptor antagonists				
Ganirelix	Antagonist of GnRH receptors	Prevention of premature LH surges during controlled ovulation hyperstimulation	SC injection	Nausea, headache
Cetrorelix: similar to ganirelix, approved for controlled ovarian hyperstimulation				
Degarelix: approved for advanced prostate cancer				
Dopamine agonists				
Bromocriptine	Dopamine D_2 receptor agonist	Hyperprolactinemia, Parkinson's disease (see Chapter 28)	Administered orally or, for hyperprolactinemia, vaginally	Gastrointestinal disturbances, orthostatic hypotension, headache, psychiatric disturbances, vasospasm and pulmonary infiltrates in high doses
Cabergoline: another ergot derivative with similar effects				
Oxytocin				
Oxytocin	Oxytocin receptor agonist	Induction and augmentation of labor • control of uterine hemorrhage after delivery	IV infusion	Fetal distress, placental abruption, uterine rupture, fluid retention, hypotension
Oxytocin receptor antagonist				
Atosiban	Antagonist of oxytocin receptor	Tocolysis for preterm labor	IV infusion	Concern about rates of infant death • not FDA approved
Vasopressin receptor agonists				
Desmopressin	Agonist of vasopressin V_2 receptors	Pituitary diabetes insipidus • hemophilia A and von Willebrand disease	Oral, IV, SC, or intranasal administration	GI disturbances, headache, hyponatremia, allergic reactions
Vasopressin: treatment of diabetes insipidus and sometimes used to control bleeding from esophageal varices				
Vasopressin receptor antagonist				
Conivaptan	Antagonist of vasopressin V_{1a} and V_2 receptors	Hyponatremia in hospitalized patients	Administered as an IV infusion	Infusion site reactions
Tolvaptan: similar but more selective for vasopressin V_2 receptors; oral administration				

Thyroid & Antithyroid Drugs

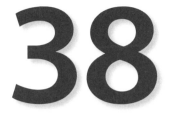

The thyroid secretes 2 types of hormones: iodine-containing amino acids (thyroxine and triiodothyronine) and a peptide (calcitonin). Thyroxine and triiodothyronine have broad effects on growth, development, and metabolism. Calcitonin is important in calcium metabolism and is discussed in Chapter 42. This chapter describes the drugs used in the treatment of hypothyroidism and hyperthyroidism.

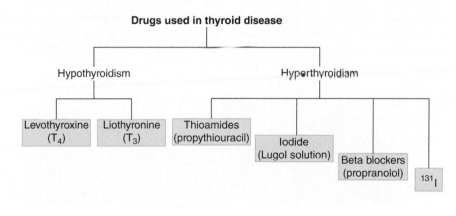

THYROID HORMONES

A. Synthesis and Transport of Thyroid Hormones

The thyroid secretes 2 iodine-containing hormones: thyroxine (T_4) and triiodothyronine (T_3). The iodine necessary for the synthesis of these molecules comes from food or iodide supplements. Iodide ion is actively taken up by and highly concentrated in the thyroid gland, where it is converted to elemental iodine by thyroidal peroxidase (Figure 38–1). The protein **thyroglobulin** serves as a scaffold for thyroid hormone synthesis. Tyrosine residues in thyroglobulin are iodinated to form monoiodotyrosine (MIT) or diiodotyrosine (DIT) in a process known as **iodine organification**. Within thyroglobulin, 2 molecules of DIT combine to form T_4, while 1 molecule each of MIT and DIT combine to form T_3. Proteolysis of thyroglobulin liberates the T_4 and T_3, which are then released from the thyroid. After release from the gland, T_4 and T_3 are transported in the blood by **thyroxine-binding globulin,** a protein synthesized in the liver.

Thyroid function is controlled by the pituitary through the release of thyrotropin (thyroid-stimulating hormone [TSH]) (see Figure 37–1) and by the availability of iodide. Thyrotropin stimulates the uptake of iodide as well as synthesis and release of thyroid hormone. It also has a growth-promoting effect that causes thyroid cell hyperplasia and an enlarged gland (**goiter**). High levels of thyroid hormones inhibit the release of TSH, providing an effective negative feedback control mechanism. In **Graves' disease**, an autoimmune disorder, B lymphocytes produce an antibody that activates the TSH receptor and can cause a syndrome of hyperthyroidism called **thyrotoxicosis**. Because these lymphocytes are not susceptible to negative feedback, patients with Graves' disease can have very high blood concentrations of thyroid hormone at the same time that their blood concentrations of TSH are very low.

High-Yield Terms to Learn

Goiter	Enlargement of the thyroid gland
Graves' disease	Autoimmune disorder that results in hyperthyroidism during the early phase and can progress to hypothyroidism if there is destruction of the gland in later phases
Thyroglobulin	A protein synthesized in the thyroid gland; its tyrosine residues are used to synthesize thyroid hormones
Thyroid-stimulating hormone (TSH)	The anterior pituitary hormone that regulates thyroid gland growth, uptake of iodine and synthesis of thyroid hormone
Thyroid storm	Severe thyrotoxicosis
Thyrotoxicosis	Medical syndrome caused by an excess of thyroid hormone (Table 38–1)
Thyroxine-binding globulin (TBG)	Protein synthesized in the liver that transports thyroid hormone in the blood

B. Mechanisms of Action of T_4 and T_3

T_3 is about 10 times more potent than T_4. Because T_4 is converted to T_3 in target cells, the liver, and the kidneys, most of the effect of circulating T_4 is probably due to T_3. Thyroid hormones bind to intracellular receptors that control the expression of genes responsible for many metabolic processes. The proteins synthesized under T_3 control differ depending on the tissue involved; these proteins include, for example, Na^+/K^+-ATPase, specific contractile proteins in smooth muscle and the heart, enzymes involved in lipid metabolism, and important developmental components in the brain. T_3 may also have a separate membrane receptor-mediated effect in some tissues.

1. Effects of thyroid hormone—The organ-level actions of the thyroid hormones include normal growth and development of the nervous, skeletal, and reproductive systems and control

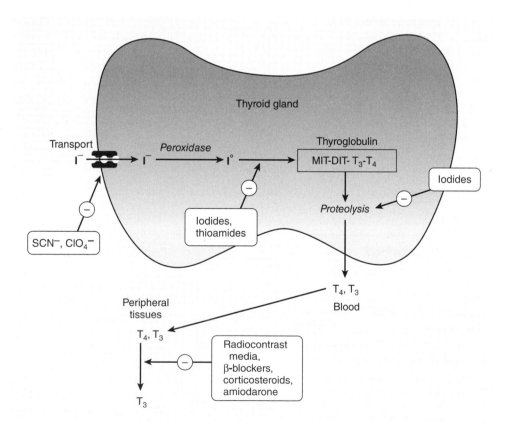

FIGURE 38–1 Sites of action of some antithyroid drugs. I⁻, iodide ion; I°, elemental iodine. Not shown: radioactive iodine (¹³¹I), which destroys the gland through radiation. (Reproduced, with permission, from Katzung BG, editor: *Basic & Clinical Pharmacology,* 12th ed. McGraw-Hill, 2012: Fig. 38–1.)

TABLE 38–1 Key features of thyrotoxicosis and hypothyroidism.

Thyrotoxicosis	Hypothyroidism
Warm, moist skin	Pale, cool, puffy skin
Sweating, heat intolerance	Sensation of being cold
Tachycardia, increased stroke volume, cardiac output, and pulse pressure	Bradycardia, decreased stroke volume, cardiac output, and pulse pressure
Dyspnea	Pleural effusions, hypoventilation, and CO_2 retention
Increased appetite	Reduced appetite
Nervousness, hyperkinesia, tremor	Lethargy, general slowing of mental processes
Weakness, increased deep tendon reflexes	Stiffness, decreased deep tendon reflexes
Menstrual irregularity, decreased fertility	Infertility, decreased libido, impotence, oligospermia
Weight loss	Weight gain
Exophthalmos (Graves' disease)	

of metabolism of fats, carbohydrates, proteins, and vitamins. The key features of excess thyroid activity (thyrotoxicosis) and hypothyroidism are listed in Table 38–1.

2. Clinical use—Thyroid hormone therapy can be accomplished with either T_4 or T_3. Synthetic **levothyroxine** (T_4) is usually the form of choice. T_3 (**liothyronine**) is faster acting but has a shorter half-life and is more expensive.

3. Toxicity—Toxicity is that of thyrotoxicosis (Table 38–1). Older patients, those with cardiovascular disease, and those with longstanding hypothyroidism are highly sensitive to the stimulatory effects of T_4 on the heart. Such patients should receive lower initial doses of T_4.

SKILL KEEPER: THE CYCLIC AMP SECOND-MESSENGER SYSTEM (CHAPTER 2)

Like many neurotransmitters and hormones, TSH mediates its effects in thyroid cells by activating the cAMP (cyclic adenosine monophosphate) second-messenger system. Draw a diagram that shows the key events in this pathway, beginning with the binding of an agonist to its receptor and ending with cellular responses. The Skill Keeper Answer appears at the end of the chapter.

ANTITHYROID DRUGS

A. Thioamides

Methimazole and propylthiouracil (PTU) are small sulfur-containing thioamides that inhibit thyroid hormone synthesis by

blocking peroxidase-catalyzed reactions, iodination of the tyrosine residues of thyroglobulin, and coupling of DIT and MIT (Figure 38–1). Propylthiouracil and, to a much lesser extent, methimazole inhibit peripheral conversion of T_4 to T_3. Because the thioamides do not inhibit the release of preformed thyroid hormone, their onset of activity is usually slow, often requiring 3–4 wk for full effect. The thioamides can be used by the oral route and are effective in young patients with small glands and mild disease. Methimazole is generally preferred because it can be administered once per day. However, PTU is preferred in pregnancy because it is less likely than methimazole to cross the placenta and enter breast milk. Toxic effects include skin rash (common) and severe reactions (rare) such as vasculitis, agranulocytosis, hypoprothrombinemia, and liver dysfunction. These effects are usually reversible.

B. Iodide Salts and Iodine

Iodide salts inhibit iodination of tyrosine and thyroid hormone release (Figure 38–1); these salts also decrease the size and vascularity of the hyperplastic thyroid gland. Because iodide salts inhibit release as well as synthesis of the hormones, their onset of action occurs rapidly, within 2–7 d. However, the effects are transient; the thyroid gland "escapes" from the iodide block after several weeks of treatment. Iodide salts are used in the management of thyroid storm and to prepare patients for surgical resection of a hyperactive thyroid. The usual forms of this drug are Lugol's solution (iodine and potassium iodide) and saturated solution of potassium iodide. Adverse effects include rash, drug fever, metallic taste, bleeding disorders, and, rarely, anaphylactic reactions.

C. Radioactive Iodine

Radioactive iodine (^{131}I) is taken up and concentrated in the thyroid gland so avidly that a dose large enough to severely damage the gland can be given without endangering other tissues.

Unlike the thioamides and iodide salts, an effective dose of ^{131}I can produce a permanent cure of thyrotoxicosis without surgery. ^{131}I should not be used in pregnant or nursing women.

D. Anion Inhibitors

Anions such as thiocyanate (SCN^-) and perchlorate (ClO_4^-) block the uptake of iodide by the thyroid gland through competitive inhibition of the iodide transporter. Their effectiveness is unpredictable and ClO_4^- can cause aplastic anemia, so these drugs are rarely used clinically.

E. Other Drugs

An important class of drugs for the treatment of thyrotoxicosis is the β blockers. These agents are particularly useful in controlling the tachycardia and other cardiac abnormalities of severe thyrotoxicosis. **Propranolol** also inhibits the peripheral conversion of T_4 to T_3.

The iodine-containing antiarrhythmic drug **amiodarone** (Chapter 14) can cause hypothyroidism through its ability to block the peripheral conversion of T_4 to T_3. It also can cause hyperthyroidism either through an iodine-induced mechanism in persons with an underlying thyroid disease such as multinodular goiter or through an inflammatory mechanism that causes leakage of thyroid hormone into the circulation. Amiodarone-associated hypothyroidism is treated with thyroid hormone. Iodine-associated hyperthyroidism caused by amiodarone is treated with thioamides, whereas the inflammatory version is best treated with corticosteroids.

Iodinated radiocontrast media (eg, oral diatrizoate and intravenous iohexol) rapidly suppress the conversion of T_4 to T_3 in the liver, kidney, and other peripheral tissues.

QUESTIONS

Questions 1–3. A 24-year-old woman was found to have mild hyperthyroidism due to Graves' disease. She appears to be in good health otherwise.

1. In Graves' disease, the cause of the hyperthyroidism is the production of an antibody that does which of the following?
   (A) Activates the pituitary thyrotropin-releasing hormone (TRH) receptor and stimulates TSH release
   (B) Activates the thyroid gland TSH receptor and stimulates thyroid hormone synthesis and release
   (C) Activates thyroid hormone receptors in peripheral tissues
   (D) Binds to thyroid gland thyroglobulin and accelerates its proteolysis and the release of its supply of T_4 and T_3
   (E) Binds to thyroid-binding globulin (TBG) and displaces bound T_4 and T_3

2. The decision is made to begin treatment with methimazole. Methimazole reduces serum concentration of T_3 primarily by which of the following mechanisms?
   (A) Accelerating the peripheral metabolism of T_3
   (B) Inhibiting the proteolysis of thyroid-binding globulin
   (C) Inhibiting the secretion of TSH
   (D) Inhibiting the uptake of iodide by cells in the thyroid
   (E) Preventing the addition of iodine to tyrosine residues on thyroglobulin

3. Though rare, a serious toxicity associated with the thioamides is which of the following?
   (A) Agranulocytosis
   (B) Lupus erythematosus-like syndrome
   (C) Myopathy
   (D) Torsades de pointes arrhythmia
   (E) Thrombotic thrombocytic purpura (TTP)

4. A 56-year-old woman presented to the emergency department with tachycardia, shortness of breath, and chest pain. She had had shortness of breath and diarrhea for the last 2 d and was sweating and anxious. A relative reported that the patient had run out of methimazole 2 wk earlier. A TSH measurement revealed a value of <0.01 mIU/L (normal 0.4–4.0 mIU/L). The diagnosis of thyroid storm was made. Which of the following is a drug that is a useful adjuvant in the treatment of thyroid storm?
   (A) Amiodarone
   (B) Betamethasone
   (C) Epinephrine
   (D) Propranolol
   (E) Radioactive iodine

5. A 65-year-old man with multinodular goiter is scheduled for a near-total thyroidectomy. Which of the following drugs will be administered for 10–14 d before surgery to reduce the vascularity of his thyroid gland?
   (A) Levothyroxine
   (B) Liothyronine
   (C) Lugol's solution
   (D) Prednisone
   (E) Radioactive iodine

6. Which of the following is a sign or symptom that would be expected to occur in the event of chronic overdose with exogenous T_4?
   (A) Bradycardia
   (B) Dry, puffy skin
   (C) Large tongue and drooping of the eyelids
   (D) Lethargy, sleepiness
   (E) Weight loss

7. When initiating T_4 therapy for an elderly patient with long-standing hypothyroidism, it is important to begin with small doses to avoid which of the following?
   (A) A flare-up of exophthalmos
   (B) Acute renal failure
   (C) Hemolysis
   (D) Overstimulation of the heart
   (E) Seizures

DIRECTIONS: Questions 8–10. The matching questions in this section consist of a list of 5 lettered options followed by several numbered items. For each numbered item, select the ONE lettered option that is most closely associated with it. Each lettered option may be selected once, more than once, or not at all.

(A) ^{131}I
(B) Amiodarone
(C) Propranolol
(D) Propylthiouracil
(E) Triiodothyronine

8. Hormone produced in the peripheral tissues when T_4 is administered

9. Antiarrhythmic drug that inhibits peripheral conversion of T_4 to T_3

10. Drug that produces a permanent reduction in thyroid activity

ANSWERS

1. The antibodies produced in Graves' disease activate thyroid gland TSH receptors. Their effects mimic those of TSH. The answer is **B.**

2. The thioamides (methimazole and propylthiouracil) act in thyroid cells to prevent conversion of tyrosine residues in thyroglobulin to MIT or DIT. The answer is **E.**

3. Rarely, the thioamides cause severe adverse reactions that include agranulocytosis, vasculitis, hepatic damage, and hypoprothrombinemia. The answer is **A.**

4. In thyroid storm, β blockers such as propranolol are useful in controlling the tachycardia and other cardiac abnormalities, and propranolol also inhibits peripheral conversion of T_4 to T_3. The answer is **D.**

5. Iodides inhibit the synthesis and release of thyroid hormone and decrease the size and vascularity of the hyperplastic gland. Lugol's solution contains a mixture of potassium iodide and iodine. The answer is **C.**

6. In hyperthyroidism, the metabolic rate increases, and even though there is increased appetite, weight loss often occurs. The other choices are symptoms seen in hypothyroidism. The answer is **E.**

7. Patients with longstanding hypothyroidism, especially those who are elderly, are highly sensitive to the stimulatory effects of T_4 on cardiac function. Administration of regular doses can cause overstimulation of the heart and cardiac collapse. The answer is **D.**

8. T_4 is converted into T_3 in the periphery. The answer is **E.**

9. Amiodarone is an iodine-containing antiarrhythmic drug with complex effects on the thyroid gland and thyroid hormones. One of its actions is to inhibit peripheral conversion of T_4 to T_3. The answer is **B.**

10. Radioactive iodine is the only medical therapy that produces a permanent reduction of thyroid activity. The answer is **A.**

SKILL KEEPER ANSWER: THE CYCLIC AMP SECOND-MESSENGER SYSTEM (CHAPTER 2)

Your drawing should show that receptor (Rec) stimulation acts through the G protein G_s to activate the enzyme adenylyl cyclase (AC). Adenylyl cyclase converts ATP to cAMP, which binds to the regulatory subunit (R) of cAMP-dependent protein kinases and thereby frees the catalytic subunit (C) of the kinase so it can transfer phosphate from ATP to substrate proteins (S) that mediate the ultimate cellular responses. These responses are varied and include immediately apparent effects that stem from phosphorylation of substrates such as enzymes and ion channels as well as delayed effects that follow changes in gene transcription. "Brakes" are applied to the pathway by phosphodiesterases (PDE) that hydrolyze cAMP and phosphatases (P'ase) that dephosphorylate substrates.

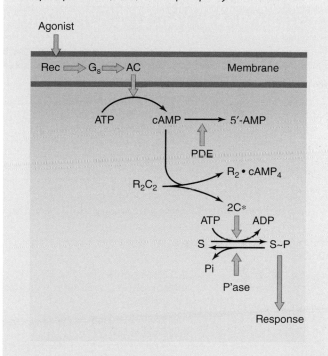

(Reproduced, with permission, from Katzung BG, editor: Basic & Clinical Pharmacology, 11th ed. McGraw-Hill, 2009: Fig. 2–13.)

CHECKLIST

When you complete this chapter, you should be able to:

❑ Sketch the biochemical pathway for thyroid hormone synthesis and release and indicate the sites of action of antithyroid drugs.

❑ List the principal drugs for the treatment of hypothyroidism.

❑ List the principal drugs for the treatment of hyperthyroidism and compare the onset and duration of their action.

❑ Describe the major toxicities of thyroxine and the antithyroid drugs.

DRUG SUMMARY TABLE: Thyroid & Antithyroid Drugs

Subclass	Mechanism of Action	Clinical Applications	Pharmacokinetics	Toxicities, Drug Interactions
Thyroid preparations				
Levothyroxine (T_4) Liothyronine (T_3)	Activation of nuclear receptors results in gene expression with RNA formulation and protein synthesis	Hypothyroidism	T_4 is converted to T_3 in target cells, the liver, and the kidneys • T_3 is 10 × more potent than T_4	See Table 38–1 for symptoms of thyroid excess
Thioamides				
Propylthiouracil (PTU) Methimazole	Inhibit thyroid peroxidase reactions, iodine organification, and peripheral conversion of T_4 to T_3	Hyperthyroidism	Oral administration, delayed onset of activity	Nausea, gastrointestinal disturbances, rash, agranulocytosis, hepatitis, hypothyroidism
Iodides				
Lugol's solution Potassium iodide	Inhibit iodine organification and hormone release • reduce size and vascularity of thyroid gland	Preparation for surgical thyroidectomy	Oral administration, acute onset of activity within 2–7 d	Rare
Radioactive iodine (^{131}I)	Radiation-induced destruction of thyroid parenchyma	Hyperthyroidism	Oral administration	Sore throat, hypothyroidism
Beta blockers				
Propranolol	Inhibition of β receptors; inhibition of conversion of T_4 to T_3	Thyroid storm	Rapid onset of activity	Asthma, AV blockade, hypertension, bradycardia

Corticosteroids & Antagonists

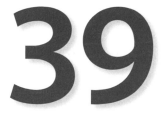

The corticosteroids are steroid hormones produced by the adrenal cortex. They consist of 2 major physiologic and pharmacologic groups: (1) glucocorticoids, which have important effects on intermediary metabolism, catabolism, immune responses, and inflammation; and (2) mineralocorticoids, which regulate sodium and potassium reabsorption in the collecting tubules of the kidney. This chapter reviews the glucocorticoids, the mineralocorticoids, and the adrenocorticosteroid antagonists.

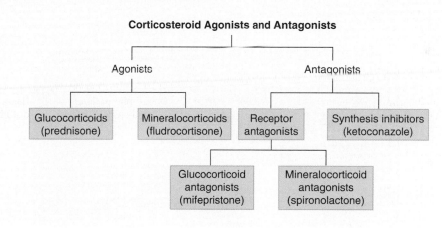

Corticosteroid Agonists and Antagonists

GLUCOCORTICOIDS

A. Mechanism of Action

Corticosteroids enter the cell and bind to cytosolic receptors that transport the steroid into the nucleus. The steroid-receptor complex alters gene expression by binding to glucocorticoid response elements (GREs) or mineralocorticoid-specific elements (Figure 39–1). Tissue-specific responses to steroids are made possible by the presence in each tissue of different protein regulators that control the interaction between the hormone-receptor complex and particular response elements.

B. Organ and Tissue Effects

1. Metabolic effects—Glucocorticoids stimulate gluconeogenesis. As a result, blood glucose rises, muscle protein is catabolized, and insulin secretion is stimulated. Both lipolysis and lipogenesis are stimulated, with a net increase of fat deposition in certain areas (eg, the face and the shoulders and back).

2. Catabolic effects—Glucocorticoids cause muscle protein catabolism. In addition, lymphoid and connective tissue, fat, and skin undergo wasting under the influence of high concentrations of these steroids. Catabolic effects on bone can lead to osteoporosis. In children, growth is inhibited.

3. Immunosuppressive effects—Glucocorticoids inhibit cell-mediated immunologic functions, especially those dependent on lymphocytes. These agents are actively lymphotoxic and, as such, are important in the treatment of hematologic cancers. The drugs do not interfere with the development of normal acquired immunity but delay rejection reactions in patients with organ transplants.

4. Anti-inflammatory effects—Glucocorticoids have a dramatic effect on the distribution and function of leukocytes. These drugs increase neutrophils and decrease lymphocytes, eosinophils, basophils, and monocytes. The migration of leukocytes is also inhibited. The biochemical mechanisms underlying these cellular effects include the induced synthesis of an inhibitor of phospholipase A_2 (Chapter 18), decreased mRNA for cyclooxygenase 2 (COX-2), decreases in interleukin-2 (IL-2) and IL-3, and decreases in platelet activating factor (PAF), an inflammatory cytokine.

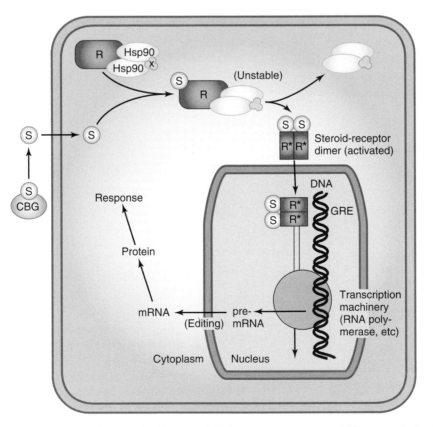

FIGURE 39–1 Mechanism of glucocorticoid action. This figure models the interaction of a steroid (S; eg, cortisol), with its receptor (R) and the subsequent events in a target cell. The steroid is present in the blood bound to corticosteroid-binding globulin (CBG) but enters the cell as the free molecule. The intracellular receptor is bound to stabilizing proteins, including heat shock protein 90 (Hsp90) and several others (X). When the complex binds a molecule of steroid, the Hsp90 and associated molecules are released. The steroid-receptor complex enters the nucleus as a dimer, binds to the glucocorticoid response element (GRE) on the gene, and regulates gene transcription. The resulting mRNA is edited and exported to the cytoplasm for the production of protein that brings about the final hormone response. (Reproduced, with permission, from Katzung BG, editor: *Basic & Clinical Pharmacology*, 12th ed. McGraw-Hill, 2012: Fig. 39–4.)

5. Other effects—Glucocorticoids such as cortisol are required for normal renal excretion of water loads. The glucocorticoids also have effects on the CNS. When given in large doses, these drugs may cause profound behavioral changes. Large doses also stimulate gastric acid secretion and decrease resistance to ulcer formation.

C. Important Glucocorticoids

1. Cortisol—The major natural glucocorticoid is cortisol (hydrocortisone; Figure 39–2). The physiologic secretion of cortisol is regulated by adrenocorticotropin (ACTH) and varies during the day (circadian rhythm); the peak occurs in the morning and the trough occurs about midnight. In the plasma, cortisol is 95% bound to corticosteroid-binding globulin (CBG). Given orally, cortisol is well absorbed from the gastrointestinal tract, is cleared by the liver, and has a short duration of action

compared with its synthetic congeners (Table 39–1). Although it diffuses poorly across normal skin, cortisol is readily absorbed across inflamed skin and mucous membranes.

The cortisol molecule also has a small but significant salt-retaining (mineralocorticoid) effect (Table 39–1). This is an important cause of hypertension in patients with a cortisol-secreting adrenal tumor or a pituitary ACTH-secreting tumor (Cushing's syndrome).

2. Synthetic glucocorticoids—The mechanism of action of these agents is identical with that of cortisol. A large number of synthetic glucocorticoids are available for use; prednisone and its active metabolite, prednisolone, dexamethasone, and triamcinolone are representative. Their properties (compared with cortisol) include longer half-life and duration of action, reduced salt-retaining effect, and better penetration of lipid barriers for topical activity (Table 39–1).

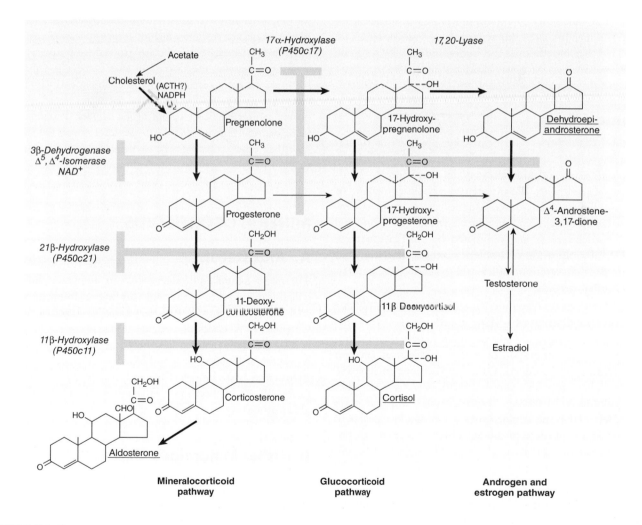

FIGURE 39–2 Outline of major pathways in adrenocortical hormone biosynthesis. The names of major adrenal secretory products are underlined. The enzymes and cofactors for the reactions progressing down each column are shown on the left and across columns at the top of the figure. When a particular enzyme is deficient, hormone production is blocked at points indicated by the shaded bars. (Modified and reproduced, with permission, from Katzung BG, editor: *Basic & Clinical Pharmacology,* 12th ed. McGraw-Hill, 2012: Fig. 39–1.)

TABLE 39–1 Properties of representative corticosteroids.

Agent	Duration of Action (hours)	Anti-inflammatory Potency[a]	Salt-retaining Potency[a]	Topical Activity
Primarily glucocorticoid				
Cortisol	8–12	1	1	0
Prednisone	12–24	4	0.3	(+)
Triamcinolone	15–24	5	0	+++
Dexamethasone	24–36	30	0	+++++
Primarily mineralocorticoid				
Aldosterone	1–2	0.3	3000	0
Fludrocortisone	8–12	10	125–250	0

[a]Relative to cortisol.

Special glucocorticoids have been developed for use in asthma (see Chapter 20) and other conditions in which good surface activity on mucous membranes or skin is needed and systemic effects are to be avoided. **Beclomethasone** and **budesonide** readily penetrate the airway mucosa but have very short half-lives after they enter the blood, so that systemic effects and toxicity are greatly reduced.

D. Clinical Uses

1. Adrenal disorders—Glucocorticoids are essential to preserve life in patients with chronic adrenal cortical insufficiency (Addison's disease) and are necessary in acute adrenal insufficiency associated with life-threatening shock, infection, or trauma. Glucocorticoids are also used in certain types of congenital adrenal hyperplasia, in which synthesis of abnormal forms of corticosteroids are stimulated by ACTH. In these conditions, administration of a potent synthetic glucocorticoid suppresses ACTH secretion sufficiently to reduce the synthesis of the abnormal steroids.

2. Nonadrenal disorders—Many disorders respond to corticosteroid therapy. Some of these are inflammatory or immunologic in nature (eg, asthma, organ transplant rejection, collagen diseases, rheumatic disorders). Other applications include the treatment of hematopoietic cancers, neurologic disorders, chemotherapy-induced vomiting, hypercalcemia, and mountain sickness. Betamethasone, a glucocorticoid with a low degree of protein binding, is given to pregnant women in premature labor to hasten maturation of the fetal lungs. The degree of benefit differs considerably in different disorders, and the toxicity of corticosteroids given chronically limits their use.

E. Toxicity

Most of the toxic effects of the glucocorticoids are predictable from the effects already described. Some are life threatening and include metabolic effects (growth inhibition, diabetes, muscle wasting, osteoporosis), salt retention, and psychosis. Methods for minimizing these toxicities include local application (eg, aerosols for asthma), alternate-day therapy (to reduce pituitary suppression), and tapering the dose soon after achieving a therapeutic response. To avoid adrenal insufficiency in patients who have had long-term therapy, additional "stress doses" may need to be given during serious illness or before major surgery. Patients who are being withdrawn from glucocorticoids after protracted use should have their doses tapered slowly, over the course of several months, to allow recovery of normal adrenal function.

MINERALOCORTICOIDS

A. Aldosterone

The major natural mineralocorticoid in humans is aldosterone, which is discussed in connection with hypertension (see Chapter 11) and with control of its secretion by angiotensin II (see Chapter 17). The secretion of aldosterone is regulated by ACTH and by the renin-angiotensin system and is very important in the regulation of blood volume and blood pressure (see Figure 6–4). Aldosterone has a short half-life and little glucocorticoid activity (Table 39–1). Its mechanism of action is the same as that of the glucocorticoids.

B. Other Mineralocorticoids

Other mineralocorticoids include deoxycorticosterone, the naturally occurring precursor of aldosterone, and **fludrocortisone,** which also has significant glucocorticoid activity. Because of its long duration of action (Table 39–1), fludrocortisone is favored for replacement therapy after adrenalectomy and in other conditions in which mineralocorticoid therapy is needed.

CORTICOSTEROID ANTAGONISTS

A. Receptor Antagonists

Spironolactone and **eplerenone**, antagonists of aldosterone at its receptor, are discussed in connection with the diuretics (see Chapter 15). **Mifepristone (RU-486)** is a competitive inhibitor of glucocorticoid receptors as well as progesterone receptors (see Chapter 40) and has been used in the treatment of Cushing's syndrome.

> ### SKILL KEEPER: ALDOSTERONE ANTAGONISTS AND CONGESTIVE HEART FAILURE (CHAPTERS 13 AND 15)
>
> *Recent clinical trials have shown that the aldosterone receptor antagonists spironolactone and eplerenone decrease morbidity and mortality in patients who are taking other standard therapies.*
>
> 1. *Why is aldosterone elevated in patients with congestive heart failure?*
> 2. *How does the increase in aldosterone contribute to the signs and symptoms of heart failure?*
> 3. *What happens to serum potassium concentrations in patients who are treated with aldosterone antagonists?*
>
> The Skill Keeper Answers appear at the end of the chapter.

B. Synthesis Inhibitors

Several drugs inhibit adrenal steroid synthesis. The most important of these drugs are **ketoconazole, aminoglutethimide,** and **metyrapone. Ketoconazole** (an antifungal drug) inhibits the cytochrome P450 enzymes necessary for the synthesis of all steroids and is used in a number of conditions in which reduced steroid levels are desirable (eg, adrenal carcinoma, hirsutism, breast and prostate cancer). Aminoglutethimide blocks the conversion of cholesterol to pregnenolone (Figure 39–2) and also inhibits synthesis of all hormonally active steroids. It can be used in conjunction with other drugs for treatment of steroid-producing adrenocortical cancer. Metyrapone inhibits the normal synthesis of cortisol but not that of cortisol precursors; the drug can be used in diagnostic tests of adrenal function.

QUESTIONS

1. Which of the following is a pharmacologic effect of exogenous glucocorticoids?
   (A) Increased muscle mass
   (B) Hypoglycemia
   (C) Inhibition of leukotriene synthesis
   (D) Improved wound healing
   (E) Increased excretion of salt and water

2. A 34-year-old woman with ulcerative colitis has required long-term treatment with pharmacologic doses of a glucocorticoid agonist. Which of the following is a toxic effect associated with long-term glucocorticoid treatment?
   (A) A "lupus-like" syndrome
   (B) Adrenal gland neoplasm
   (C) Hepatotoxicity
   (D) Osteoporosis
   (E) Precocious puberty in children

3. A 46-year-old male patient has Cushing's syndrome that is due to the presence of an adrenal tumor. Which of the following drugs would be expected to reduce the signs and symptoms of this man's disease?
   (A) Betamethasone
   (B) Cortisol
   (C) Fludrocortisone
   (D) Ketoconazole
   (E) Triamcinolone

4. A newborn girl exhibited ambiguous genitalia, hyponatremia, hyperkalemia, and hypotension as a result of genetic deficiency of 21β-hydroxylase activity. Treatment consisted of fluid and salt replacement and hydrocortisone administration. In this type of adrenal hyperplasia in which there is excess production of cortisol precursors, which of the following describes the primary therapeutic effect of glucocorticoid administration?
   (A) Increased adrenal estrogen synthesis
   (B) Inhibition of adrenal aldosterone synthesis
   (C) Prevention of hypoglycemia
   (D) Recovery of normal immune function
   (E) Suppression of ACTH secretion

5. Which of the following best describes a glucocorticoid response element?
   (A) A protein regulator that controls the interaction between an activated steroid receptor and DNA
   (B) A short DNA sequence that binds tightly to RNA polymerase
   (C) A small protein that binds to an unoccupied steroid receptor protein and prevents it from becoming denatured
   (D) A specific nucleotide sequence that is recognized by a steroid hormone receptor-hormone complex
   (E) The portion of the steroid receptor that binds to DNA

6. Glucocorticoids have proved useful in the treatment of which of the following medical conditions?
   (A) Chemotherapy-induced vomiting
   (B) Essential hypertension
   (C) Hyperprolactinemia
   (D) Parkinson's disease
   (E) Type II diabetes

7. A 56-year-old woman with systemic lupus erythematosus had been maintained on a moderate daily dose of prednisone for 9 mo. Her disease has finally gone into remission and she now wishes to gradually taper and then discontinue the prednisone. Gradual tapering of a glucocorticoid is required for recovery of which of the following?
   (A) Depressed release of insulin from pancreatic B cells
   (B) Hematopoiesis in the bone marrow
   (C) Normal osteoblast function
   (D) The control by vasopressin of water excretion
   (E) The hypothalamic-pituitary-adrenal system

Questions 8 and 9. A 54-year-old man with advanced tuberculosis has developed signs of severe acute adrenal insufficiency.

8. Which of the following signs or symptoms is this patient most likely to exhibit?
   (A) A moon face
   (B) Dehydration
   (C) Hyperglycemia
   (D) Hypertension
   (E) Hyperthermia

9. The patient should be treated immediately. Which of the following combinations is most rational?
   (A) Aldosterone and fludrocortisone
   (B) Cortisol and fludrocortisone
   (C) Dexamethasone and metyrapone
   (D) Fludrocortisone and metyrapone
   (E) Triamcinolone and dexamethasone

10. Which of the following is a drug that, in high doses, blocks the glucocorticoid receptor?
   (A) Aminoglutethimide
   (B) Beclomethasone
   (C) Ketoconazole
   (D) Mifepristone
   (E) Spironolactone

ANSWERS

1. Glucocorticoids inhibit the production of both leukotrienes and prostaglandins. This is a key component of their anti-inflammatory action. The answer is **C.**

2. One of the adverse metabolic effects of long-term glucocorticoid therapy is a net loss of bone, which can result in osteoporosis. The answer is **D.**

3. Ketoconazole inhibits many types of cytochrome P450 enzymes. It can be used to reduce the unregulated overproduction of corticosteroids by adrenal tumors. The answer is **D.**

4. A 21β-hydroxylase deficiency prevents normal synthesis of cortisol and aldosterone, and causes accumulation of cortisol precursors (Figure 39–2). The hypothalamic-pituitary system responds to the abnormally low levels of cortisol by increasing ACTH release. High levels of ACTH induce adrenal hyperplasia and excess production of adrenal androgens, which can cause virilization of females and prepubertal males. Glucocorticoid is administered to replace the missing mineralocorticoid and glucocorticoid activity and to suppress ACTH release, which removes the stimulus for excess adrenal androgen production. The answer is **E.**

5. Activated steroid hormone receptors mediate their effects on gene expression by binding to hormone response elements, which are short sequences of DNA located near steroid-regulated genes. The answer is **D.**

6. Glucocorticoids are used in combination with other antiemetics to prevent chemotherapy-induced nausea and vomiting, which are commonly associated with anticancer drugs. The answer is **A.**

7. Exogenous glucocorticoids act at the hypothalamus and pituitary to suppress the production of CRF and ACTH.

As a result, adrenal production of endogenous corticosteroids is suppressed. On discontinuance, the recovery of normal hypothalamic-pituitary-adrenal function occurs slowly. Glucocorticoid doses must be tapered slowly, over several months, to prevent adrenal insufficiency. The answer is **E.**

8. In acute adrenal insufficiency, there is loss of salt and water that is primarily due to reduced production of aldosterone. The loss of salt and water can lead to dehydration. The answer is **B.**

9. A rational combination of drugs should include agents with complementary effects (ie, a glucocorticoid and a mineralocorticoid). The combination with these characteristics is cortisol and fludrocortisone. (Note that although fludrocortisone may have sufficient glucocorticoid activity for a patient with mild disease, a patient in severe acute adrenal insufficiency needs a full glucocorticoid such as cortisol.) The answer is **B.**

10. Mifepristone is a competitive antagonist of glucocorticoid and progesterone receptors. Ketoconazole and aminoglutethimide also antagonize corticosteroids; however, they act by inhibiting steroid hormone synthesis. The answer is **D.**

SKILL KEEPER ANSWERS: ALDOSTERONE ANTAGONISTS AND CONGESTIVE HEART FAILURE (CHAPTERS 13 AND 15)

1. *The reduction in cardiac output associated with heart failure decreases the effective arterial blood volume and renal blood flow. Decreased pressure in renal arterioles and increased sympathetic neural activity both stimulate renin release, which increases production of angiotensin II. Angiotensin II is a powerful stimulus of aldosterone secretion.*

2. *Acting through nuclear receptors in the epithelial cells that line renal collecting tubules, aldosterone promotes renal uptake of salt and water. This retention of salt and water exacerbates the peripheral and pulmonary edema associated with congestive heart failure and further overloads the weakened heart. In addition to these renal effects, aldosterone is also implicated in myocardial and vascular fibrosis and baroreceptor dysfunction.*

3. *The aldosterone antagonists are also known as "potassium-sparing diuretics" because, unlike other diuretics, they do not promote renal excretion of potassium. Because the excretion of potassium in the renal tubule is linked to the reuptake of sodium, the reduction in sodium uptake caused by spironolactone and eplerenone results in potassium retention and an increase in serum potassium.*

CHECKLIST

When you complete this chapter, you should be able to:

❏ Describe the major naturally occurring glucocorticosteroid and its actions.

❏ List several synthetic glucocorticoids, and describe differences between these agents and the naturally occurring hormone.

❏ Describe the actions of the naturally occurring mineralocorticoid and 1 synthetic agent in this subgroup.

❏ List the indications for the use of corticosteroids in adrenal and nonadrenal disorders.

❏ Name 3 drugs that interfere with the action or synthesis of corticosteroids, and, for each, describe its mechanism of action.

DRUG SUMMARY TABLE: Corticosteroids & Antagonists

Subclass	Mechanism of Action	Clinical Applications	Pharmacokinetics	Toxicities, Drug Interactions
Glucocorticoid agonists				
Prednisone	Activation of glucocorticoid receptor alters gene transcription	Many inflammatory conditions, organ transplantation, hematologic cancers	Duration of activity is longer than pharmacokinetic half-life of drug owing to gene transcription effects	Adrenal suppression, growth inhibition, muscle wasting, osteoporosis, salt retention, glucose intolerance, behavioral changes
Many other glucocorticoids available for oral and parenteral use (see Table 39–1). Cortisol is the primary endogenous glucocorticoid hormone				
Mineralocorticoid agonist				
Fludrocortisone	Strong agonist of mineralo-corticoid receptors and moderate activation of glucocorticoid receptors	Adrenal insufficiency (Addison's disease)	Long duration of action (see Table 39–1)	Salt and fluid retention, congestive heart failure, signs and symptoms of glucocorticoid excess (see above)
Glucocorticoid receptor antagonist				
Mifepristone	Pharmacologic antagonist of glucocorticoid and progesterone receptors	Medical abortion (see Chapter 40) and very rarely Cushing's syndrome	Oral administration	Vaginal bleeding in females, abdominal pain, gastrointestinal upset, diarrhea, headache
Mineralocorticoid receptor antagonists				
Spironolactone	Pharmacologic antagonist of mineralocorticoid receptor, weak antagonism of androgen receptors	Aldosteronism from any cause, hypokalemia due to other diuretics, post-myocardial infarction	Slow onset and offset of effect Duration: 24–48 h	Hyperkalemia, gynecomastia (spironolactone, not eplerenone), additive interaction with other K-retaining drugs
Eplerenone: similar to spironolactone, more selective for mineralocorticoid receptor				
Synthesis inhibitors				
Ketoconazole	Blocks fungal and mammalian CYP450 enzymes	Inhibits mammalian steroid hormone synthesis and fungal ergosterol synthesis (see Chapter 48)	Oral, topical administration	Hepatic dysfunction, many drug-drug CYP450 interactions
Other adrenal steroid synthesis inhibitors: include aminoglutethimide and metyrapone				

Gonadal Hormones & Inhibitors

The gonadal hormones include the steroids of the ovary (estrogens and progestins) and testis (chiefly testosterone). Because of their importance as contraceptives, many synthetic estrogens and progestins have been produced. These include synthesis inhibitors, receptor antagonists, and some drugs with mixed effects (ie, agonist effects in some tissues and antagonist effects in other tissues). Mixed agonists with estrogenic effects are called selective estrogen receptor modulators (SERMs). Synthetic androgens, including those with anabolic activity, are also available for clinical use. A diverse group of drugs with antiandrogenic effects is used in the treatment of prostate cancer and benign prostatic hyperplasia in men and hyperandrogenism in women.

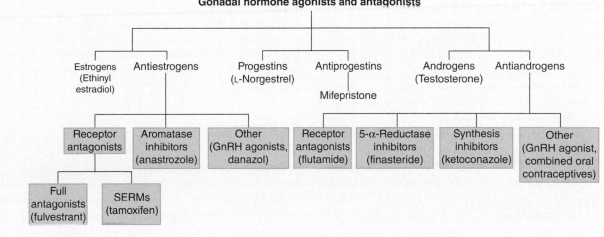

OVARIAN HORMONES

The ovary is the primary source of gonadal hormones in women during the childbearing years (ie, between puberty and menopause). When properly regulated by follicle-stimulating hormone (FSH) and luteinizing hormone (LH) from the pituitary, each menstrual cycle consists of the following events: A follicle in the ovary matures, secretes increasing amounts of estrogen, releases an ovum, and is transformed into a progesterone-secreting corpus luteum. If the ovum is not fertilized and implanted, the corpus luteum degenerates; the uterine endometrium, which has proliferated under the stimulation of estrogen and progesterone, is shed as part of the menstrual flow, and the cycle repeats. The mechanism of action of both estrogen and progesterone involves entry into cells, binding to cytosolic receptors, and translocation of the receptor–hormone complex into the nucleus, where it modulates gene expression (see Figure 39–1).

A. Estrogens

The major ovarian estrogen in women is estradiol. Estradiol has low oral bioavailability but is available in a micronized form

High-Yield Terms to Learn

5α-Reductase	The enzyme that converts testosterone to dihydrotestosterone (DHT); it is inhibited by finasteride, a drug used to treat benign prostatic hyperplasia and prevent male-pattern hair loss in men
Anabolic steroid	Androgen receptor agonists used for anabolic effects (eg, weight gain, increased muscle mass)
Breakthrough bleeding	Vaginal bleeding that occurs outside of the period of regular menstrual bleeding
Combined oral contraceptive (COC or just OC)	Hormonal contraceptive administered orally that contains an estrogen and a progestin
Hirsutism	A male pattern of body hair growth (face, chest, abdomen) in females that results from hyperandrogenism
HRT	Hormone replacement therapy; refers to estrogen replacement for women who have lost ovarian function and nearly always involves combination therapy with estrogen and a progestin
SERM	Selective estrogen receptor modulator such as tamoxifen

for oral use. It can also be administered via transdermal patch, vaginal cream, or intramuscular injection. Long-acting esters of estradiol that are converted in the body to estradiol (eg, estradiol cypionate) can be administered by intramuscular (IM) injection. Mixtures of conjugated estrogens from biologic sources (eg, Premarin) are used orally for hormone replacement therapy (HRT). Synthetic estrogens with high bioavailability (eg, **ethinyl estradiol**, mestranol) are used in hormonal contraceptives.

1. Effects—Estrogen is essential for normal female reproductive development. It is responsible for the growth of the genital structures (vagina, uterus, and uterine tubes) during childhood and for the appearance of secondary sexual characteristics and the growth spurt associated with puberty. Estrogen has many metabolic effects: It modifies serum protein levels and reduces bone resorption. It enhances the coagulability of blood and increases plasma triglyceride levels while reducing low-density lipoprotein (LDL) cholesterol and increasing high-density lipoprotein (HDL) cholesterol. Continuous administration of estrogen, especially in combination with a progestin, inhibits the secretion of gonadotropins from the anterior pituitary (Figure 40–1).

2. Clinical use—Estrogens are used in the treatment of hypogonadism in young females (Table 40–1). Another use is as HRT in women with estrogen deficiency resulting from premature ovarian failure, menopause, or surgical removal of the ovaries. HRT ameliorates hot flushes and atrophic changes in the urogenital tract. It is effective also in preventing bone loss and osteoporosis. The estrogens are components of hormonal contraceptives (see later discussion).

3. Toxicity—In hypogonadal girls, the dosage of estrogen must be adjusted carefully to prevent premature closure of the epiphyses of the long bones and short stature. When used as HRT, estrogen increases the risk of endometrial cancer; this effect is prevented by combining the estrogen with a progestin. Estrogen use by postmenopausal women is associated with a small increase

in the risk of breast cancer and cardiovascular events (myocardial infarction, stroke). Dose-dependent toxicity includes nausea, breast tenderness, increased risk of migraine headache, thromboembolic events (eg, deep vein thrombosis), gallbladder disease, hypertriglyceridemia, and hypertension.

Diethylstilbestrol (DES), a nonsteroidal estrogenic compound, is associated with infertility, ectopic pregnancy, and vaginal adenocarcinoma in the daughters of women who were treated with the drug during pregnancy in a misguided attempt to prevent recurrent spontaneous abortion. These effects appear to be restricted to DES because there is no evidence that the estrogens and progestins in hormonal contraceptives have similar effects or other teratogenic effects.

B. Progestins

Progesterone is the major progestin in humans. A micronized form is used orally for HRT, and progesterone-containing vaginal creams are also available. Synthetic progestins (eg, medroxyprogesterone) have improved oral bioavailability. The 19-nortestosterone compounds differ primarily in their degree of androgenic effects. Older drugs (eg, L-norgestrel and norethindrone) are more androgenic than the newer progestins (eg, norgestimate, desogestrel).

1. Effects—Progesterone induces secretory changes in the endometrium and is required for the maintenance of pregnancy. The other progestins also stabilize the endometrium but do not support pregnancy. Progestins do not significantly affect plasma proteins, but they do affect carbohydrate metabolism and stimulate the deposition of fat. High doses suppress gonadotropin secretion and often cause anovulation in women.

2. Clinical use—Progestins are used as contraceptives, either alone or in combination with an estrogen. They are used in combination with an estrogen in HRT to prevent estrogen-induced endometrial cancer. Progesterone is used in assisted reproductive technology methods to promote and maintain pregnancy.

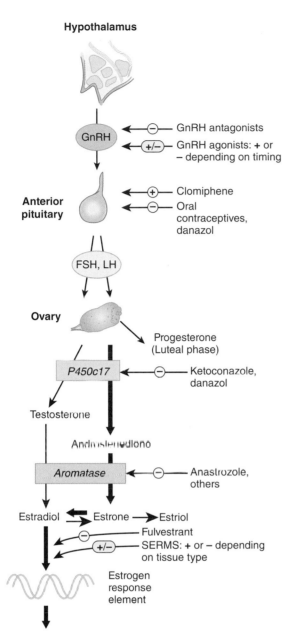

Hypothalamus

GnRH
- ⊖ GnRH antagonists
- +/− GnRH agonists: + or − depending on timing

Anterior pituitary
- ⊕ Clomiphene
- ⊖ Oral contraceptives, danazol

FSH, LH

Ovary

Progesterone (Luteal phase)

P450c17 ← ⊖ Ketoconazole, danazol

Testosterone

Androstenedione

Aromatase ← ⊖ Anastrozole, others

Estradiol ⇄ Estrone → Estriol
- ⊖ Fulvestrant
- +/− SERMS: + or − depending on tissue type

Estrogen response element

Expression in estrogen-responsive cells

FIGURE 40–1 Control of ovarian secretion, the action of its hormones, and some sites of action of antiestrogens. In the follicular phase, the ovary produces mainly estrogens; in the luteal phase it produces estrogens and progesterone. SERMs, selective estrogen receptor modulators. (Reproduced, with permission, from Katzung BG, editor: *Basic & Clinical Pharmacology,* 12th ed. McGraw-Hill, 2012: Fig. 40–5.)

3. Toxicity—The toxicity of progestins is low. However, they may increase blood pressure and decrease HDL. Long-term use of high doses in premenopausal women is associated with a reversible decrease in bone density (a secondary effect of ovarian suppression and decreased ovarian production of estrogen) and delayed resumption of ovulation after termination of therapy.

C. Hormonal Contraceptives

Hormonal contraceptives contain either a combination of an estrogen and a progestin or a progestin alone. Hormonal contraceptives are available in a variety of preparations, including oral pills, long-acting injections, transdermal patches, vaginal rings, and intrauterine devices (IUDs) (Table 40–1). Three types of **oral contraceptives** for women are available in the United States: combination estrogen-progestin tablets that are taken in constant dosage throughout the menstrual cycle (monophasic preparations); combination preparations (biphasic and triphasic) in which the progestin or estrogen dosage, or both, changes during the month (to more closely mimic hormonal changes in a menstrual cycle); and progestin-only preparations.

The **postcoital contraceptives** (also known as "emergency contraception") prevent pregnancy if administered within 72 h after unprotected intercourse. Oral preparations containing a progestin (L-norgestrel) alone, estrogen alone, or the combination of an estrogen and a progestin are effective. The progestin-only preparation causes fewer side effects than the estrogen-containing preparations.

1. Mechanism of action—The combination hormonal contraceptives have several actions, including inhibition of ovulation (the primary action) and effects on the cervical mucus glands, uterine tubes, and endometrium that decrease the likelihood of fertilization and implantation. Progestin-only agents do not always inhibit ovulation and instead act through the other mechanisms listed. The mechanisms of action of postcoital contraceptives are not well understood. When administered before the LH surge, they inhibit ovulation. They also affect cervical mucus, tubal function, and the endometrial lining.

2. Other clinical uses and beneficial effects—Combination hormonal contraceptives are used in young women with primary hypogonadism to prevent estrogen deficiency. Combinations of hormonal contraceptives and progestins are used to treat acne, hirsutism, dysmenorrhea, and endometriosis. Users of combination hormonal contraceptives have reduced risks of ovarian cysts, ovarian and endometrial cancer, benign breast disease, and pelvic inflammatory disease as well as a lower incidence of ectopic pregnancy, iron deficiency anemia, and rheumatoid arthritis.

3. Toxicity—The incidence of dose-dependent toxicity has fallen since the introduction of the low-dose combined oral contraceptives.

a. Thromboembolism—The major toxic effects of the combined hormonal contraceptives relate to the action of the estrogenic component on blood coagulation. There is a well-documented increase in the risk of thromboembolic events (myocardial infarction, stroke, deep vein thrombosis, pulmonary embolism) in older women, smokers, women with a personal or family history of such problems, and women with genetic defects that affect the production or function of clotting factors. However, the risk of thromboembolism incurred by the use of these drugs is usually less than that imposed by pregnancy.

TABLE 40–1 Representative applications for the gonadal hormones and hormone antagonists.

Clinical Application	Drugs
Hypogonadism in girls, women	Conjugated estrogens, ethinyl estradiol, estradiol esters
Hormone replacement therapy	Estrogen component: conjugated estrogens, estradiol, estrone, estriol Progestin component: progesterone, medroxyprogesterone acetate
Oral hormonal contraceptive	Combined: ethinyl estradiol or mestranol plus a progestin Progestin only: norethindrone or norgestrel
Parenteral contraceptive	Medroxyprogesterone as a depot IM injection Ethinyl estradiol and norelgestromin as a weekly patch Ethinyl estradiol and etonogestrel as a monthly vaginal ring L-Norgestrel as an intrauterine device (IUD) Etonogestrel as a subcutaneous implant
Postcoital contraceptive	L-Norgestrel, combined oral contraceptive
Intractable dysmenorrhea or uterine bleeding	Conjugated estrogens, ethinyl estradiol, oral contraceptive, GnRH agonist, depot injection of medroxyprogesterone acetate
Infertility	Clomiphene; hMG and hCG; GnRH analogs; progesterone; bromocriptine
Abortifacient	Mifepristone (RU 486) and misoprostol
Endometriosis	Oral contraceptive, depot injection of medroxyprogesterone acetate, GnRH agonist, danazol
Breast cancer	Tamoxifen, aromatase inhibitors (eg, anastrozole)
Osteoporosis in postmenopausal women	Conjugated estrogens, estradiol, raloxifene (see also Chapter 42)
Hypogonadism in boys, men; replacement therapy	Testosterone enanthate or cypionate; methyltestosterone; fluoxymesterone, testosterone (patch)
Anabolic protein synthesis	Oxandrolone, stanozolol
Prostate hyperplasia (benign)	Finasteride
Prostate carcinoma	GnRH agonist, GnRH receptor antagonist, androgen receptor antagonist (eg, flutamide)
Hirsutism	Combined oral contraceptive, spironolactone, flutamide, GnRH agonist

b. Breast cancer—Evidence suggests that the lifetime risk of breast cancer in women who are current or past users of hormonal contraceptives is not changed, but there may be an earlier onset of breast cancer.

c. Other toxicities—The low-dose combined oral and progestin-only contraceptives cause significant breakthrough bleeding, especially during the first few months of therapy. Other toxicities of the hormonal contraceptives include nausea, breast tenderness, headache, skin pigmentation, and depression. Preparations containing older, more androgenic progestins can cause weight gain, acne, and hirsutism. The high dose of estrogen in estrogen-containing postcoital contraceptives is associated with significant nausea.

ANTIESTROGENS & ANTIPROGESTINS

A. Selective Estrogen Receptor Modulators

Selective estrogen receptor modulators (SERMs) are mixed estrogen agonists that have estrogen agonist effects in some tissues and act as partial agonists or antagonists of estrogen in other tissues.

SKILL KEEPER: CYTOCHROME P450 AND HORMONAL CONTRACEPTIVES (SEE CHAPTERS 4 AND 61)

Hormonal contraceptives usually contain the lowest doses of the estrogen and progestin components that prevent pregnancy. The margin between effective and ineffective serum concentrations of the steroids is narrow, which presents a risk of breakthrough bleeding and also unintended pregnancy resulting from drug–drug interactions. Most steroidal contraceptives are metabolized by cytochrome P450 isozymes.

1. How many drugs can you identify that decrease the efficacy of hormonal contraceptives by increasing their metabolism?

2. When one of these drugs is prescribed for a woman who already is using a combined hormonal contraceptive, what should be done to prevent pregnancy?

The Skill Keeper Answers appear at the end of the chapter.

1. Tamoxifen—Tamoxifen is a SERM that is effective in the treatment of hormone-responsive breast cancer, where it acts as an *antagonist* to prevent receptor activation by endogenous estrogens (Figure 40–2). Prophylactic use of tamoxifen reduces the

incidence of breast cancer in women who are at very high risk. As an *agonist* of endometrial receptors, tamoxifen promotes endometrial hyperplasia and increases the risk of endometrial cancer. The drug also causes hot flushes (an antagonist effect) and increases the risk of venous thrombosis (an agonist effect). Tamoxifen has more agonist than antagonist action on bone and thus prevents osteoporosis in postmenopausal women. **Toremifene** is structurally related to tamoxifen and has similar properties, indications, and toxicity.

2. Raloxifene—Raloxifene, approved for prevention and treatment of osteoporosis in postmenopausal women, has a partial agonist effect on bone. Like tamoxifen, raloxifene has antagonist effects in breast tissue and reduces the incidence of breast cancer in women who are at very high risk. Unlike tamoxifen, the drug has no estrogenic effects on endometrial tissue. Adverse effects include hot flushes (an antagonist effect) and an increased risk of venous thrombosis (an agonist effect).

3. Clomiphene—Clomiphene is a nonsteroidal compound with tissue-selective actions. It is used to induce ovulation in anovulatory women who wish to become pregnant. By selectively blocking estrogen receptors in the pituitary, clomiphene reduces negative feedback and increases FSH and LH output. The increase in gonadotropins stimulates ovulation.

B. Pure Estrogen Receptor Antagonists

Fulvestrant is a pure estrogen receptor antagonist (in all tissues). It is used in the treatment of women with breast cancer that has developed resistance to tamoxifen.

C. Synthesis Inhibitors

1. Aromatase inhibitors—Anastrozole and related compounds (eg, letrozole) are nonsteroidal competitive inhibitors of aromatase, the enzyme required for the last step in estrogen synthesis. **Exemestane** is an irreversible aromatase inhibitor. These drugs are used in the treatment of breast cancer.

2. Danazol—Danazol inhibits several cytochrome P450 enzymes involved in gonadal steroid synthesis and is a weak partial agonist of progestin, androgen, and glucocorticoid receptors. The drug is sometimes used in the treatment of endometriosis and fibrocystic disease of the breast.

D. Gonadotropin-Releasing Hormone Analogs and Antagonists

As discussed in Chapter 37, the continuous administration of gonadotropin-releasing hormone (GnRH) agonists (eg, **leuprolide**) suppresses gonadotropin secretion and thereby inhibits ovarian production of estrogens and progesterone. The GnRH agonists are used in combination with other agents in controlled ovarian hyperstimulation (Chapter 37) and are also used for treatment of precocious puberty in children and short-term (<6 mo) treatment of endometriosis and uterine fibroids in women. Treatment beyond

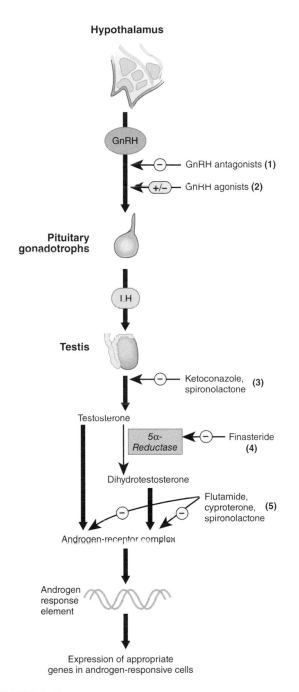

FIGURE 40–2 Control of androgen secretion and activity and some sites of action of antiandrogens: (1) competitive inhibition of GnRH receptors (see Chapter 37); (2) stimulation (+) or inhibition (−) by GnRH agonists; (3) inhibition of testosterone synthesis; (4) inhibition of dihydrotestosterone production by finasteride; (5) inhibition of androgen binding at its receptor by flutamide and other drugs. (Reproduced, with permission, from Katzung BG, editor: *Basic & Clinical Pharmacology*, 12th ed. McGraw-Hill, 2012: Fig. 40–6.)

6 mo in premenopausal women can result in decreased bone density. The GnRH receptor antagonists ganirelix and cetrorelix are used for controlled ovarian hyperstimulation (see Chapter 37).

E. Antiprogestins

Mifepristone (RU 486) is an orally active steroid antagonist of progesterone and glucocorticoids (Chapter 39). Its major use is as an abortifacient in early pregnancy (up to 49 d after the last menstrual period). The combination of mifepristone and the prostaglandin E analog misoprostol (Chapters 18 and 59) achieves a complete abortion in over 95% of early pregnancies. The most common complication is failure to induce a complete abortion. Side effects, which are primarily due to the misoprostol, include nausea, vomiting, and diarrhea plus the vaginal cramping and bleeding associated with passing the pregnancy. Rarely, patients who used mifepristone and misoprostol for medical abortion have experienced serious infection, sepsis, and even death due to unusual infection (eg, *Clostridium sordelli*).

ANDROGENS

Testosterone and related androgens are produced in the testis, the adrenal, and, to a small extent, the ovary. Testosterone is synthesized from progesterone and dehydroepiandrosterone (DHEA). In the plasma, testosterone is partly bound to sex hormone-binding globulin (SHBG), a transport protein. The hormone is converted in several organs (eg, prostate) to **dihydrotestosterone** (DHT), which is the active hormone in those tissues. Because of rapid hepatic metabolism, testosterone given orally has little effect. It may be given by injection in the form of long-acting esters or transdermal patch. Orally active variants are also available (Table 40–1).

Many androgens have been synthesized in an effort to increase the anabolic effect (see Effects, discussed later) without increasing androgenic action. **Oxandrolone** and **stanozolol** are examples of drugs that, in laboratory testing, have an increased ratio of anabolic-androgenic action. However, all the so-called **anabolic steroids** have full androgenic agonist effects when used in humans.

A. Mechanism of Action

Like other steroid hormones, androgens enter cells and bind to cytosolic receptors. The hormone-receptor complex enters the nucleus and modulates the expression of target genes.

B. Effects

Testosterone is necessary for normal development of the male fetus and infant and is responsible for the major changes in the male at puberty (growth of penis, larynx, and skeleton; development of facial, pubic, and axillary hair; darkening of skin; enlargement of muscle mass). After puberty, testosterone acts to maintain secondary sex characteristics, fertility, and libido. It also acts on hair cells to cause male-pattern baldness.

The major effect of androgenic hormones, in addition to development and maintenance of normal male characteristics, is an anabolic action that involves increased muscle size and strength and increased red blood cell production. Excretion of urea nitrogen is reduced, and nitrogen balance becomes more positive. Testosterone also helps maintain normal bone density.

C. Clinical Use

The primary clinical use of the androgens is for replacement therapy in hypogonadism (Table 40–1). Androgens have also been used to stimulate red blood cell production in certain anemias and to promote weight gain in patients with wasting syndromes (eg, AIDS patients). The anabolic effects have been exploited illicitly by athletes to increase muscle bulk and strength and perhaps enhance athletic performance.

D. Toxicity

Use of androgens by females results in virilization (hirsutism, enlarged clitoris, deepened voice) and menstrual irregularity. In women who are pregnant with a female fetus, exogenous androgens can cause virilization of the fetus's external genitalia. Paradoxically, excessive doses in men can result in feminization (gynecomastia, testicular shrinkage, infertility) as a result of feedback inhibition of the pituitary and conversion of the exogenous androgens to estrogens. In both sexes, high doses of anabolic steroids can cause cholestatic jaundice, elevation of liver enzyme levels, and possibly hepatocellular carcinoma.

ANTIANDROGENS

Reduction of androgen effects is an important mode of therapy for both benign and malignant prostate disease, precocious puberty, hair loss, and hirsutism. Drugs are available that act at different sites in the androgen pathway (Figure 40–2).

A. Receptor Inhibitors

Flutamide and related drugs are nonsteroidal competitive antagonists of androgen receptors. These drugs are used to decrease the action of endogenous androgens in patients with prostate carcinoma. **Spironolactone,** a drug used principally as a potassium-sparing diuretic (Chapter 15), also inhibits androgen receptors and is used in the treatment of hirsutism in women.

B. 5α-Reductase Inhibitors

Testosterone is converted to DHT by the enzyme 5α-reductase. Some tissues, most notably prostate cells and hair follicles, depend on DHT rather than testosterone for androgenic stimulation. This enzyme is inhibited by **finasteride,** a drug used to treat benign prostatic hyperplasia and, at a lower dose, to prevent hair loss in men. Because the drug does not interfere with the action of testosterone, it is less likely than other antiandrogens to cause impotence, infertility, and loss of libido. Dutasteride is a newer 5α-reductase inhibitor with a much longer half-life than that of finasteride.

C. Gonadotropin-Releasing Hormone Analogs and Antagonists

Suppression of gonadotropin secretion, especially LH, reduces the production of testosterone. This can be effectively accomplished with long-acting depot preparations of **leuprolide** or similar gonadotropin-releasing hormone (GnRH) agonists (Chapter 37). These analogs are used in prostatic carcinoma. During the first week of therapy, an androgen receptor antagonist (eg, flutamide) is added to prevent the tumor flare that can result from the surge in testosterone synthesis caused by the initial agonistic action of the GnRH agonist. Within several weeks, testosterone production falls to low levels. As discussed in Chapter 37, the GnRH receptor antagonists abarelix and degarelix are approved for advanced prostate cancer.

D. Combined Hormonal Contraceptives

Combined hormonal contraceptives are used in women with androgen-induced hirsutism. The estrogen in the contraceptive acts in the liver to increase the production of sex hormone-binding globulin, which in turn reduces the concentration of the free androgen in the blood that is causing the male-pattern hair growth characteristic of hirsutism.

E. Inhibitors of Steroid Synthesis

Ketoconazole, an antifungal drug (Chapter 48), inhibits gonadal and adrenal steroid synthesis. The drug has been used to suppress adrenal steroid synthesis in patients with steroid-responsive metastatic prostate cancer.

QUESTIONS

1. Which of the following is an estrogen that is used in most combined hormonal contraceptives?
   (A) Clomiphene
   (B) Estrone
   (C) Ethinyl estradiol
   (D) Diethylstilbestrol (DES)
   (E) Norgestrel

2. A 23-year-old woman desires a combined oral contraceptive for pregnancy protection. Which of the following patient factors would lead a health professional to recommend an alternative form of contraception?
   (A) Evidence of hirsutism
   (B) History of gastroesophageal reflux disease and is currently taking omeprazole
   (C) History of pelvic inflammatory disease
   (D) History of migraine headache that is well controlled by sumatriptan
   (E) She plans to use this contraceptive for about 1 yr and will then attempt to become pregnant

3. Men who use large doses of anabolic steroids are at increased risk of which of the following?
   (A) Anemia
   (B) Cholestatic jaundice and elevation of aspartate transaminase levels in the blood
   (C) Hirsutism
   (D) Hyperprolactinemia
   (E) Testicular enlargement

4. A 50-year-old woman with a positive mammogram undergoes lumpectomy and a small carcinoma is removed. Biochemical analysis of the cancer reveals the presence of estrogen and progesterone receptors. After this procedure, she will probably receive which of the following drugs?
   (A) Danazol
   (B) Flutamide
   (C) Leuprolide
   (D) Mifepristone
   (E) Tamoxifen

5. A 60-year-old man is found to have a prostate lump and an elevated prostate-specific antigen (PSA) blood test. Magnetic resonance imaging suggests several enlarged lymph nodes in the lower abdomen, and an x-ray reveals 2 radiolucent lesions in the bony pelvis. This patient is likely to be treated with which of the following drugs?
   (A) Anastrozole
   (B) Desogestrel
   (C) Flutamide
   (D) Methyltestosterone
   (E) Oxandrolone

6. A young woman complains of abdominal pain at the time of menstruation. Careful evaluation indicates the presence of significant endometrial deposits on the pelvic peritoneum. Which of the following is the most appropriate medical therapy for this patient?
   (A) Flutamide, orally
   (B) Medroxyprogesterone acetate by intramuscular injection
   (C) Norgestrel as an IUD
   (D) Oxandrolone by intramuscular injection
   (E) Raloxifene orally

7. Diethylstilbestrol (DES) should never be used in pregnant women because it is associated with which of the following?
   (A) Deep vein thrombosis
   (B) Feminization of the external genitalia of male offspring
   (C) Infertility and development of vaginal cancer in female offspring
   (D) Miscarriages
   (E) Virilization of the external genitalia of female offspring

8. Which of the following is a unique property of SERMs?
   (A) Act as agonists in some tissues and antagonists in other tissues
   (B) Activate a unique plasma membrane-bound receptor
   (C) Have both estrogenic and progestational agonist activity
   (D) Inhibit the aromatase enzyme required for estrogen synthesis
   (E) Produce estrogenic effects without binding to estrogen receptors

9. Finasteride has efficacy in the prevention of male-pattern baldness by virtue of its ability to do which of the following?
   (A) Competitively antagonize androgen receptors
   (B) Decrease the release of gonadotropins
   (C) Increase the serum concentration of sex hormone-binding globulin
   (D) Inhibit the synthesis of testosterone
   (E) Reduce the production of dihydrotestosterone

10. A 52-year-old postmenopausal patient has evidence of low bone mineral density. She and her physician are considering therapy with raloxifene or a combination of conjugated estrogens and medroxyprogesterone acetate. Which of the following patient characteristics is *most* likely to lead them to select raloxifene?

(A) Previous hysterectomy
(B) Recurrent vaginitis
(C) Rheumatoid arthritis
(D) Strong family history of breast cancer
(E) Troublesome hot flushes

ANSWERS

1. Ethinyl estradiol, a synthetic estrogen with good bioavailability, is the estrogenic component of most combined oral contraceptives, the transdermal contraceptive, and the vaginal ring contraceptive. The answer is **C.**

2. Estrogen-containing hormonal contraceptives increase the risk of episodes of migraine headache. The answer is **D.**

3. In men, large doses of anabolic steroids are associated with liver impairment, including cholestasis and elevation of serum concentrations of transaminases. The answer is **B.**

4. Tamoxifen has proved useful in adjunctive therapy of breast cancer; the drug decreases the rate of recurrence of cancer. The answer is **E.**

5. Antiandrogen drugs are used to treat metastatic prostate cancer because they have efficacy, whereas conventional cytotoxic drugs do not. Flutamide is a competitive antagonist of the androgen receptor that is used in combination with a GnRH agonist in the treatment of men with prostate cancer. The answer is **C.**

6. In endometriosis, suppression of ovarian function and production of gonadal steroids are useful. Intramuscular injection of relatively large doses of medroxyprogesterone provides 3 mo of an ovarian suppressive effect because of inhibition of pituitary production of gonadotropins. The answer is **B.**

7. Diethylstilbestrol (DES) is a nonsteroidal estrogen agonist. Several decades ago, misguided use of the drug in pregnant women appears to have resulted in fetal damage that predisposed female offspring to infertility and a rare form of vaginal cancer. For this reason, the drug should be avoided in pregnant women. Other estrogenic drugs do not appear to have these same effects. Although estrogens do increase the risk of deep vein thrombosis, this is not the reason why DES should be avoided. The answer is **C.**

8. SERMs such as tamoxifen and raloxifene exhibit tissue-specific estrogenic and antiestrogenic effects. The answer is **A.**

9. Finasteride inhibits 5α-reductase, the enzyme that converts testosterone to DHT, the principal androgen in androgen-sensitive hair follicles. The answer is **E.**

10. Conjugated estrogens and raloxifene both improve bone mineral density and protect against osteoporosis. The 2 advantages of raloxifene over full estrogen receptor agonists are that raloxifene has antagonist effects in breast tissue and lacks an agonist effect in endometrium. If a patient's uterus was removed by surgery, the difference in the endometrial effect is moot. In patients with a strong family history of breast cancer, raloxifene may be a better choice than a full estrogen agonist because it will not further increase the woman's risk of breast cancer and may even lower her risk. The answer is **D.**

SKILL KEEPER ANSWERS: CYTOCHROME P450 AND HORMONAL CONTRACEPTIVES (SEE CHAPTERS 4 AND 61)

1. *Gonadal steroids and their derivatives are metabolized primarily by the cytochrome P450 3A4 (CYP3A4) family of enzymes. Inducers of CYP3A4 include barbiturates, carbamazepine, corticosteroids, griseofulvin, phenytoin, pioglitazone, rifampin, and rifabutin. The potential reduction in contraceptive efficacy of hormonal contraceptives by carbamazepine and phenytoin are of particular importance because these drugs are known teratogens. St. John's wort, an unregulated herbal product, contains an ingredient that induces CYP3A4 enzymes and can reduce the efficacy of hormonal contraceptives.*

2. *To prevent an unwanted pregnancy, it would be advisable to use a combined hormonal contraceptive pill with a higher dose of estrogen (eg, a formulation containing 50 mcg of ethinyl estradiol). Alternatively, or additionally, women may use a barrier form of contraception or switch to an IUD.*

CHECKLIST

When you complete this chapter, you should be able to:

❏ Describe the hormonal changes that occur during the menstrual cycle.

❏ Name 3 estrogens and 4 progestins. Describe their pharmacologic effects, clinical uses, and toxicity.

❏ List the benefits and hazards of hormonal contraceptives.

❏ List the benefits and hazards of postmenopausal estrogen therapy.

❏ Describe the use of gonadal hormones and their antagonists in the treatment of cancer in women and men.

❏ List or describe the toxic effects of anabolic steroids used to build muscle mass.

❏ Name 2 SERMs and describe their unique properties.

DRUG SUMMARY TABLE: Gonadal Hormones & Inhibitors

Subclass	Mechanism of Action	Clinical Applications	Pharmacokinetics	Toxicities, Drug Interactions
Estrogens				
Ethinyl estradiol	Activation of estrogen receptors leads to changes in the rates of transcription of estrogen-regulated genes	See Table 40–1	Oral, parenteral, or transdermal administration • metabolism relies on cytochrome P450 systems • enterohepatic recirculation occurs	Moderate toxicity: Breakthrough bleeding, nausea, breast tenderness Serious toxicity: Thromboembolism, gallbladder disease, hypertriglyceridemia, migraine headache, hypertension, depression In postmenopausal women: breast cancer, endometrial hyperplasia (unopposed estrogen) Combination with cytochrome P450 inducer can lead to breakthrough bleeding and reduced contraceptive efficacy

Mestranol: a prodrug that is converted to ethinyl estradiol, contained in some contraceptives
Estrogen esters (eg, estradiol cypionate): long-acting estrogens administered IM and used for hypogonadism in young females

Subclass	Mechanism of Action	Clinical Applications	Pharmacokinetics	Toxicities, Drug Interactions
Progestins				
Norgestrel	Activation of progesterone receptors leads to changes in the rates of transcription of progesterone-regulated genes	See Table 40–1	Oral, parenteral, or transdermal administration • metabolism relies on cytochrome P450 systems • enterohepatic recirculation occurs	Weight gain, reversible decrease in bone mineral density (high doses)

Progesterone derivatives: medroxyprogesterone acetate, megestrol acetate
Older 19-nortestosterone derivatives: norethindrone, ethynodiol
Newer 19-nortestosterone derivatives: desogestrel, norelgestromin, norgestimate, etonogestrel
Spironolactone derivative: drospirenone

Subclass	Mechanism of Action	Clinical Applications	Pharmacokinetics	Toxicities, Drug Interactions
Antiestrogens				
SERMS				
Tamoxifen	Estrogen antagonist actions in breast tissue and CNS • estrogen agonist effects in liver and bone	Prevention and adjuvant treatment of hormone-responsive breast cancer	Oral administration	Hot flushes, thromboembolism, endometrial hyperplasia

Toremifene: similar to tamoxifen
Raloxifene: approved for osteoporosis and prevention of breast cancer in selected patients; antagonist effects in breast, CNS, and endometrium and agonist effects in the liver
Clomiphene: used for ovulation induction; antagonist effect in pituitary increases gonadotropin secretion

(Continued)

DRUG SUMMARY TABLE: Gonadal Hormones & Inhibitors (*Continued*)

Subclass	Mechanism of Action	Clinical Applications	Pharmacokinetics	Toxicities, Drug Interactions
Receptor antagonist Fulvestrant	Estrogen receptor antagonist in all tissues	Adjuvant treatment of hormone-responsive breast cancer that is resistant to first-line antiestrogen therapy	Intramuscular administration	Hot flushes, headache, injection site reactions
Aromatase inhibitors Anastrozole	Reduces estrogen synthesis by inhibiting aromatase enzyme	Adjuvant treatment of hormone-responsive breast cancer	Oral administration	Hot flushes, musculoskeletal disorders, reduced bone mineral density Joint symptoms (arthralgia, arthrosis, arthritis, cervical spondylosis, osteoarthritis, and disk herniation)
Letrozole: similar to anastrozole *Exemestane:* irreversible aromatase inhibitor				
GnRH agonist Leuprolide	See Chapter 37			
GnRH receptor antagonist Ganirelix, cetrorelix	See Chapter 37			
Other Danazol	Weak cytochrome P450 inhibitor and partial agonist of progestin and androgen receptors	Endometriosis, fibrocystic breast disease	Oral administration • drug interactions due to cytochrome P450 inhibition	Acne, hirsutism, weight gain, menstrual disturbances, hepatic dysfunction
Antiprogestin				
Mifepristone	Progestin and glucocorticoid receptor antagonist	Used in combination with a prostaglandin (eg, misoprostol) for medical abortion	Oral administration	Gastrointestinal disturbances (mostly due to coadministration of misoprostol) • vaginal bleeding, atypical infection
Androgens				
Testosterone	Androgen receptor agonist	Male hypogonadism • weight gain in patients with wasting syndromes	Transdermal, buccal, subcutaneous implant	In females, virilization In men, high doses can cause gynecomastia, testicular shrinkage, infertility

Fluoxymesterone, methyltestosterone: oral androgens
Testosterone esters (eg, testosterone cypionate): long-acting androgens for parenteral administration
Anabolic steroids (eg, oxandrolone, nandrolone decanoate): increased ratio of anabolic-to-androgenic activity in laboratory animals, cholestatic jaundice, liver toxicity

(*Continued*)

DRUG SUMMARY TABLE: Gonadal Hormones & Inhibitors (*Continued*)

Subclass	Mechanism of Action	Clinical Applications	Pharmacokinetics	Toxicities, Drug Interactions
Antiandrogens				
5α-reductase inhibitors				
Finasteride	Inhibition of 5α-reductase enzyme that converts testosterone to dihydrotestosterone	Benign prostatic hyperplasia (BPH), male-pattern hair loss	Oral administration	Rarely, impotence, gynecomastia
Dutasteride: Similar to finasteride				
Receptor antagonists				
Flutamide	Competitive inhibition of androgen receptor	Advanced prostate cancer	Oral administration	Gynecomastia, hot flushes, impotence, hepatoxicity
Bicalutamide, nilutamide: similar to flutamide but lower risk of hepatotoxicity				
Spironolactone: mineralocorticoid receptor antagonist used mainly as a potassium-sparing diuretic (see Chapter 15); also has androgen-receptor antagonist activity, used for the treatment of hirsutism				
GnRH agonist				
Leuprolide	See Chapter 37			
GnRH receptor antagonist				
Abarelix, degarelix	See Chapter 37			
Synthesis inhibitor				
Ketoconazole (see Chapter 48)	Inhibition of cytochrome P450 enzymes involved in androgen synthesis	Advanced prostate cancer that is resistant to first-line antiandrogen drugs	Oral administration	Interferes with synthesis of other steroids • many drug interactions due to cytochrome P450 inhibition

41

Pancreatic Hormones, Antidiabetic Agents, & Glucagon

In the endocrine pancreas, the islets of Langerhans contain at least 4 types of endocrine cells, including A (alpha, glucagon producing), B (beta, insulin, and amylin producing), D (delta, somatostatin producing), and F (pancreatic polypeptide producing). Of these, the B (insulin-producing) cells are the most numerous.

The most common pancreatic disease requiring pharmacologic therapy is diabetes mellitus, a deficiency of insulin production or effect. Diabetes is treated with several parenteral formulations of insulin and oral or parenteral noninsulin antidiabetic agents. Glucagon, a hormone that affects the liver, cardiovascular system, and gastrointestinal tract, can be used to treat severe hypoglycemia.

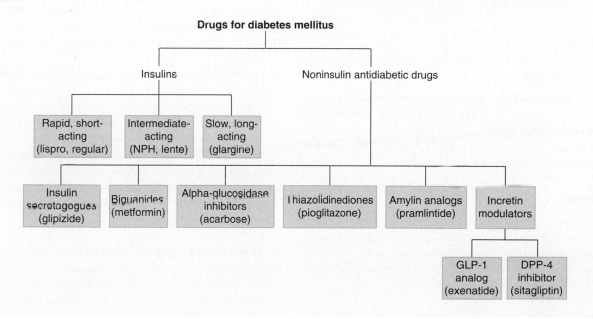

DIABETES MELLITUS

Two major forms of diabetes mellitus have been identified. Type 1 diabetes usually has its onset during childhood and results from autoimmune destruction of pancreatic B cells. Type 2 diabetes is a progressive disorder characterized by increasing insulin resistance and diminishing insulin secretory capacity. Type 2 diabetes is frequently associated with obesity and is much more common than type 1 diabetes. Although type 2 diabetes usually has its onset in adulthood, the incidence in children and adolescents is rising

High-Yield Terms to Learn

α-Glucosidase	An enzyme in the gastrointestinal tract that converts complex starches and oligosaccharides to monosaccharides; inhibited by acarbose and miglitol
Beta (B) cells in the islets of Langerhans	Insulin-producing cells in the endocrine pancreas
Hypoglycemia	Dangerously lowered serum glucose concentration; a toxic effect of high insulin concentrations and the secretagogue class of oral antidiabetic drugs
Lactic acidosis	Acidemia due to excess serum lactic acid; can result from excess production or decreased metabolism of lactic acid
Type 1 diabetes mellitus	A form of chronic hyperglycemia caused by immunologic destruction of pancreatic beta cells
Type 2 diabetes mellitus	A form of chronic hyperglycemia initially caused by resistance to insulin; often progresses to insulin deficiency

dramatically, in parallel with the increase in obesity in children and adolescents.

The clinical history and course of these 2 forms differ considerably, but treatment in both cases requires careful attention to diet, fasting and postprandial blood glucose concentrations, and serum concentrations of hemoglobin A_{1c}, a glycosylated hemoglobin that serves as a marker of glycemia. Type 1 diabetes requires treatment with insulin. The early stages of type 2 diabetes usually can be controlled with noninsulin antidiabetic drugs. However, patients in the later stages of type 2 diabetes often require the addition of insulin to their drug regimen.

INSULIN

A. Physiology

Insulin is synthesized as the prohormone **proinsulin,** an 86-amino-acid single-chain polypeptide. Cleavage of proinsulin and cross-linking result in the 2-chain 51-peptide insulin molecule and a 31-amino-acid residual C-peptide. Neither proinsulin nor C-peptide appears to have any physiologic actions.

B. Effects

Insulin has important effects on almost every tissue of the body. When activated by the hormone, the insulin receptor, a transmembrane tyrosine kinase, phosphorylates itself and a variety of intracellular proteins when activated by the hormone. The major target organs for insulin action include:

1. Liver—Insulin increases the storage of glucose as glycogen in the liver. This involves the insertion of additional GLUT2 glucose transport molecules in cell plasma membranes; increased synthesis of the enzymes pyruvate kinase, phosphofructokinase, and glucokinase; and suppression of several other enzymes. Insulin also decreases protein catabolism.

2. Skeletal muscle—Insulin stimulates glycogen synthesis and protein synthesis. Glucose transport into muscle cells is facilitated by insertion of GLUT4 transporters into cell plasma membranes.

3. Adipose tissue—Insulin facilitates triglyceride storage by activating plasma lipoprotein lipase, increasing glucose transport into cells via GLUT4 transporters, and reducing intracellular lipolysis.

C. Insulin Preparations

Human insulin is manufactured by bacterial recombinant DNA technology. The available forms provide 4 rates of onset and durations of effect that range from rapid-acting to long-acting (Figure 41–1). The goals of insulin therapy are to control both basal and postprandial (after a meal) glucose levels while minimizing the risk of hypoglycemia. Insulin formulations with different rates of onset and effect are often combined to achieve these goals.

1. Rapid-acting—Three insulin analogs (**insulin lispro**, insulin aspart, and insulin glulisine) have rapid onsets and early peaks of activity (Figure 41–1) that permit control of postprandial glucose levels. The 3 rapid-acting insulins have small alterations in their primary amino acid sequences that speed their entry into the circulation without affecting their interaction with the insulin receptor. The rapid-acting insulins are injected immediately before a meal and are the preferred insulin for continuous subcutaneous infusion devices. They also can be used for emergency treatment of uncomplicated diabetic ketoacidosis.

2. Short-acting—**Regular insulin** is used intravenously in emergencies or administered subcutaneously in ordinary maintenance regimens, alone or mixed with intermediate- or long-acting preparations. Before the development of rapid-acting insulins, it was the primary form of insulin used for controlling postprandial glucose concentrations, but it requires administration 1 h or more before a meal.

3. Intermediate-acting—Neutral protamine Hagedorn insulin (**NPH insulin**) is a combination of regular insulin and protamine (a highly basic protein also used to reverse the action of unfractionated heparin, Chapter 34) that exhibits a delayed onset and peak of action (Figure 41–1). NPH insulin is often combined with regular and rapid-acting insulins.

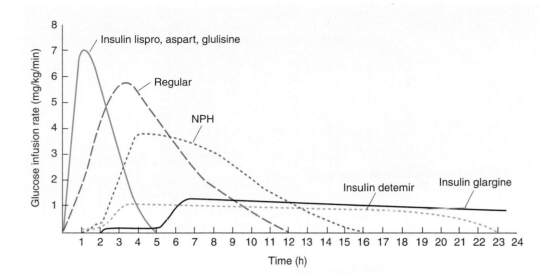

FIGURE 41–1 Extent and duration of action of various types of insulin as indicated by the glucose infusion rates (mg/kg/min) required to maintain a constant glucose concentration. The durations of action shown are typical of an average dose of 0.2–0.3 U/kg; the duration of regular and NPH insulin increases considerably when dosage is increased. (Reproduced, with permission, from Katzung BG, editor: *Basic & Clinical Pharmacology*, 12th ed. McGraw-Hill, 2012: Fig. 41–5.)

4. Long-acting—Insulin glargine and insulin detemir are modified forms of human insulin that provide a peakless basal insulin level lasting more than 20 h, which helps control basal glucose levels without producing hypoglycemia.

5. Insulin delivery systems—The standard mode of insulin therapy is subcutaneous injection with conventional disposable needles and syringes. More convenient means of administration are also available.

Portable pen-sized injectors are used to facilitate subcutaneous injection. Some contain replaceable cartridges, whereas others are disposable.

Continuous subcutaneous insulin infusion devices avoid the need for multiple daily injections and provide flexibility in the scheduling of patients' daily activities. Programmable pumps deliver a constant 24-h basal rate, and manual adjustments in the rate of delivery can be made to accommodate changes in insulin requirements (eg, before meals or exercise).

D. Hazards of Insulin Use

The most common complication is **hypoglycemia**, resulting from excessive insulin effect. To prevent the brain damage that may result from hypoglycemia, prompt administration of glucose (sugar or candy by mouth, glucose by vein) or of glucagon (by intramuscular injection) is essential. Patients with advanced renal disease, the elderly, and children younger than 7 years are most susceptible to the detrimental effects of hypoglycemia.

The most common form of insulin-induced immunologic complication is the formation of antibodies to insulin or non-insulin protein contaminants, which results in resistance to the action of the drug or allergic reactions. With the current use of highly purified human insulins, immunologic complications are uncommon.

NONINSULIN ANTIDIABETIC DRUGS

Four well-established groups of oral antidiabetic drugs are used most commonly to treat type 2 diabetes. These include **insulin secretagogues**, the **biguanide metformin, thiazolidinediones**, and **α-glucosidase inhibitors** (Figure 41–2). Three novel agents—pramlintide, exenatide, and sitagliptin—target endogenous regulators of glucose homeostasis. The durations of action of important members of these groups are listed in Table 41–1

A. Insulin Secretagogues

1. Mechanism and effects—Insulin secretagogues stimulate the release of endogenous insulin by promoting closure of potassium channels in the pancreatic B-cell membrane (Figure 41–2). Channel closure depolarizes the cell and triggers insulin release. Insulin secretagogues are not effective in patients who lack functional pancreatic B cells.

Most insulin secretagogues are in the chemical class known as **sulfonylureas.** The second-generation sulfonylureas (**glyburide, glipizide, glimepiride**) are considerably more potent and used more commonly than the older agents (**tolbutamide, chlorpropamide,** others). **Repaglinide**, a meglitinide, and **nateglinide,** a D-phenylalanine derivative, are also insulin secretagogues. Both have a rapid onset and short duration of action that make them useful for administration just before a meal to control postprandial glucose levels.

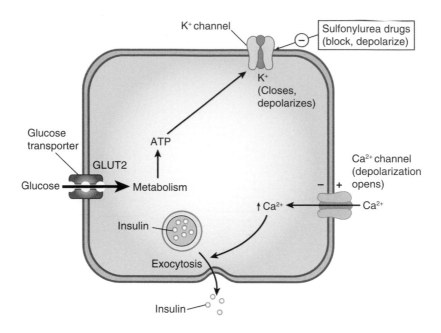

FIGURE 41–2 Control of insulin release from the pancreatic beta cell by glucose and by sulfonylurea drugs. When the extracellular glucose concentration increases, more glucose enters the cell via the GLUT2 glucose transporter and leads, through metabolism, to increased intracellular ATP production with subsequent closure of ATP-dependent K^+ channels, membrane depolarization, opening of voltage-gated Ca^{2+} channels, increased intracellular Ca^{2+}, and insulin secretion. Sulfonylurea and other insulin secretagogues enhance insulin release by blocking ATP-dependent K^+ channels and thereby triggering the events subsequent to reduced K^+ influx. (Reproduced, with permission, from Katzung BG, editor: *Basic & Clinical Pharmacology*, 12th ed. McGraw-Hill, 2012: Fig. 41–2.)

2. Toxicities—The insulin secretagogues, especially those with a high potency (eg, glyburide and glipizide), can precipitate hypoglycemia, although the risk is less than that associated with the insulins. The older sulfonylureas (tolbutamide and chlorpropamide) are extensively bound to serum proteins, and drugs that compete for protein binding may enhance their hypoglycemic effects. Occasionally these drugs cause rash or other allergic reactions. Weight gain is common and is especially undesirable in the large fraction of patients with type 2 diabetes who already are overweight.

B. Biguanides

1. Mechanism and effects—**Metformin**, the primary member of the biguanide group, reduces postprandial and fasting glucose levels. Biguanides inhibit hepatic and renal gluconeogenesis (Figure 41–3). Other effects include stimulation of glucose uptake and glycolysis in peripheral tissues, slowing of glucose absorption from the gastrointestinal tract, and reduction of plasma glucagon levels. The molecular mechanism of biguanide reduction in hepatic glucose production appears to involve activation of an AMP-stimulated protein kinase.

In patients with insulin resistance, metformin reduces endogenous insulin production presumably through enhanced insulin sensitivity. Because of this insulin-sparing effect and because it does not increase weight—unlike insulin, secretagogues, or the thiazolidinediones—metformin is increasingly the drug of first choice in overweight patients with type 2 diabetes. Recent clinical trials suggest that metformin reduces the risk of diabetes in high-risk patients. Metformin is also used to restore fertility in anovulatory women with polycystic ovary disease (PCOD) and evidence of insulin resistance.

TABLE 41–1 Duration of action of representative oral antidiabetic drugs.

Drug	Duration of Action (hours)
Secretagogues	
Chlorpropamide	Up to 60
Tolbutamide	6–12
Glimepiride	12–24
Glipizide	10–24
Glyburide	10–24
Repaglinide	4–5
Nateglinide	4
Biguanides	
Metformin	10–12
Thiazolidinediones	
Pioglitazone	15–24
Rosiglitazone	>24
Alpha-glucosidase inhibitors	
Acarbose	3–4
Miglitol	3–4
Incretin modifiers	
Sitagliptin	8–14

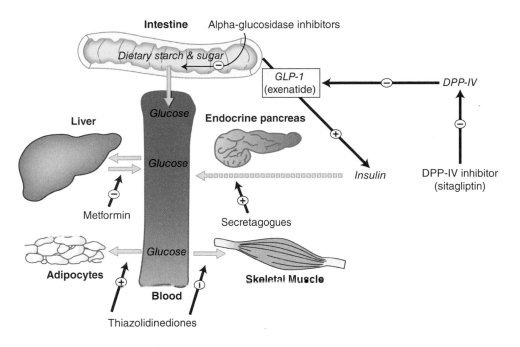

FIGURE 41–3 Major actions of the principal oral antidiabetic drugs used to treat type 2 diabetes.

2. Toxicities—Unlike the sulfonylureas, the biguanides do not cause hypoglycemia. Their most common toxicity is gastrointestinal distress (nausea, diarrhea), and they can cause lactic acidosis, especially in patients with renal or liver disease, alcoholism, or conditions that predispose to tissue anoxia and lactic acid production (eg, chronic cardiopulmonary dysfunction).

C. Thiazolidinediones

1. Mechanism and effects—The thiazolidinediones, **rosiglitazone** and **pioglitazone**, increase target tissue sensitivity to insulin by activating the peroxisome proliferator-activated receptor-gamma nuclear receptor (**PPAR-γ receptor**). This nuclear receptor regulates the transcription of genes encoding proteins involved in carbohydrate and lipid metabolism. A primary effect of the thiazolidinediones is increasing glucose uptake in muscle and adipose tissue (Figure 41–3). They also inhibit hepatic gluconeogenesis and have effects on lipid metabolism and the distribution of body fat. Thiazolidinediones reduce both fasting and postprandial hyperglycemia. They are used as monotherapy or in combination with insulin or other oral antidiabetic drugs. Like metformin, the thiazolidinediones have been shown to reduce the risk of diabetes in high-risk patients.

2. Toxicities—When these drugs are used alone, hypoglycemia is extremely rare. Thiazolidinediones can cause fluid retention, which presents as mild anemia and edema and may increase the risk of heart failure. Recent data have linked rosiglitazone to increased risk of myocardial infarction. The original thiazolidinedione (troglitazone) was removed from the market in several countries because of hepatotoxicity. Rosiglitazone and pioglitazone have not been linked to serious liver dysfunction but still require routine monitoring of liver function. Female patients taking thiazolidinediones appear to have an increased risk of bone fractures. Pioglitazone and troglitazone induce cytochrome P450 activity (especially the 3A4 isozyme) and can reduce the serum concentrations of drugs that are metabolized by these enzymes (eg, oral contraceptives, cyclosporine).

D. α-Glucosidase Inhibitors

1. Mechanism and effects—**Acarbose** and miglitol are carbohydrate analogs that act within the intestine to inhibit α-glucosidase, an enzyme necessary for the conversion of complex starches, oligosaccharides, and disaccharides to the monosaccharides that can be transported out of the intestinal lumen and into the bloodstream. As a result of slowed absorption, postprandial hyperglycemia is reduced. These drugs lack an effect on fasting blood sugar. Both drugs can be used as monotherapy or in combination with other antidiabetic drugs. They are taken just before a meal. Like metformin and the thiazolidinediones, the α-glucosidase inhibitors have been shown to prevent type 2 diabetes in prediabetic persons.

2. Toxicities—The primary adverse effects of the α-glucosidase inhibitors include flatulence, diarrhea, and abdominal pain resulting from increased fermentation of unabsorbed carbohydrate by bacteria in the colon. Patients taking an α-glucosidase inhibitor who experience hypoglycemia should be treated with oral glucose (dextrose) and not sucrose, because the absorption of sucrose will be delayed.

E. Pramlintide

Pramlintide is an injectable synthetic analog of **amylin**, a 37-amino acid hormone produced by pancreatic B cells. Amylin contributes to glycemic control by activating high-affinity receptors that are a complex of the calcitonin receptor and a receptor-activity modifying receptor (RANK). Pramlintide suppresses glucagon release, slows gastric emptying, and works in the CNS to reduce appetite. After subcutaneous injection, it is rapidly absorbed and has a short duration of action. It is used in combination with insulin to control postprandial glucose levels. The major adverse effects associated with pramlintide are hypoglycemia and gastrointestinal disturbances.

F. Exenatide

Glucagon-like peptide-1 (**GLP-1**) is a member of the **incretin** family of peptide hormones, which are released from endocrine cells in the epithelium of the bowel in response to food. The incretins augment glucose-stimulated insulin release from pancreatic B cells, retard gastric emptying, inhibit glucagon secretion, and produce a feeling of satiety. The GLP-1 receptor is a G protein-coupled receptor (GPCR) that increases cAMP and also increases the free intracellular concentration of calcium.

Exenatide, a long-acting injectable peptide analog of GLP-1, is used in combination with metformin or a sulfonylurea for treatment of type 2 diabetes. The major adverse effects are gastrointestinal disturbances, particularly nausea during initial therapy, and hypoglycemia when exenatide is combined with a sulfonylurea. The drug has also caused serious and sometimes fatal acute pancreatitis.

G. Sitagliptin

Sitagliptin is an oral inhibitor of dipeptidyl peptidase-4 (DPP-4), the enzyme that degrades GLP-1 and other incretins. It is approved for use in type 2 diabetes as monotherapy or in combination with metformin or a thiazolidinedione. Like exenatide, sitagliptin promotes insulin release, inhibits glucagon secretion, and has an anorexic effect. The most common adverse effects associated with sitagliptin are headache, nasopharyngitis, and upper respiratory tract infection.

TREATMENT OF DIABETES MELLITUS

A. Type 1 Diabetes

Therapy for type 1 diabetes involves dietary instruction, parenteral insulin (a mixture of shorter and longer acting forms to maintain control of basal and postprandial glucose levels) and possibly pramlintide for improved control of postprandial glucose levels, plus careful attention by the patient to factors that change insulin requirements: exercise, infections, other forms of stress, and deviations from the regular diet. Large clinical studies indicate that **tight control** of blood sugar, by frequent blood sugar testing and insulin injections, reduces the incidence of vascular complications, including renal and retinal damage. The risk of hypoglycemic reactions is increased in tight control regimens but not enough to obviate the benefits of better control.

B. Type 2 Diabetes

Because type 2 diabetes is usually a progressive disease, therapy for an individual patient generally escalates over time. It begins with weight reduction and dietary control. Initial drug therapy usually is oral monotherapy with metformin. Although initial responses to monotherapy usually are good, secondary failure within 5 yr is common. Increasingly, noninsulin antidiabetic agents are being used in combination with each other or with insulin to achieve better glycemic control and minimize toxicity. Because type 2 diabetes involves both insulin resistance and inadequate insulin production, it makes sense to combine an agent that augments insulin's action (metformin, a thiazolidinedione, or an α-glucosidase inhibitor) with one that augments the insulin supplies (insulin secretagogue or insulin). Long-acting drugs (sulfonylureas, metformin, thiazolidinediones, exenatide, sitagliptin, some insulin formulations) help control both fasting and postprandial blood glucose levels, whereas short-acting drugs (α-glucosidase inhibitors, repaglinide, pramlintide, rapid-acting insulins) primarily target postprandial levels. As is the case for type 1 diabetes, clinical trials have shown that tight control of blood glucose in patients with type 2 diabetes reduces the risk of vascular complications.

SKILL KEEPER: DIABETES AND HYPERTENSION (SEE CHAPTER 11)

Diabetes is linked to hypertension in several important ways. Obesity predisposes patients to hypertension as well as to type 2 diabetes, so many patients suffer from both diseases. Both diseases damage the kidney and predispose patients to coronary artery disease. A large clinical trial of patients with type 2 diabetes suggests that poorly controlled hypertension exacerbates the microvascular disease caused by long-standing diabetes. Because of these links, it is important to consider the treatment of hypertension in diabetic patients.

1. *Identify the major drug groups used for chronic treatment of essential hypertension.*

2. *Which of these drug groups have special implications for the treatment of patients with diabetes?*

The Skill Keeper Answers appear at the end of the chapter.

HYPERGLYCEMIC DRUGS: GLUCAGON

A. Glucagon

1. Chemistry, mechanism, and effects—Glucagon is a protein hormone secreted by the A cells of the endocrine pancreas. Acting through G protein-coupled receptors in heart, smooth muscle, and liver, glucagon increases heart rate and force of contraction, increases hepatic glycogenolysis and gluconeo-genesis, and relaxes smooth muscle. The smooth muscle effect is particularly marked in the gut.

2. Clinical uses—Glucagon is used to treat severe hypogly-cemia in diabetics, but its hyperglycemic action requires intact hepatic glycogen stores. The drug is given intramuscularly or intravenously. In the management of severe β-blocker overdose, glucagon may be the most effective method for stimulating the depressed heart because it increases cardiac cAMP without requir-ing access to β receptors (Chapter 59).

QUESTIONS

Questions 1 and 2. A 13-year-old boy with type 1 diabetes is brought to the hospital complaining of dizziness. Laboratory findings include severe hyperglycemia, ketoacidosis, and a blood pH of 7.15.

1. Which of the following agents should be administered to achieve rapid control of the severe ketoacidosis in this diabetic boy?
   (A) Crystalline zinc insulin
   (B) Glyburide
   (C) Insulin glargine
   (D) NPH insulin
   (E) Tolbutamide

2. Which of the following is the most likely complication of insulin therapy in this patient?
   (A) Dilutional hyponatremia
   (B) Hypoglycemia
   (C) Increased bleeding tendency
   (D) Pancreatitis
   (E) Severe hypertension

3. A 24-year-old woman with type 1 diabetes wishes to try tight control of her diabetes to improve her long-term prognosis. Which of the following regimens is *most* appropriate?
   (A) Morning injections of mixed insulin lispro and insulin aspart
   (B) Evening injections of mixed regular insulin and insulin glargine
   (C) Morning and evening injections of regular insulin, supplemented by small amounts of NPH insulin at mealtimes
   (D) Morning injections of insulin glargine, supplemented by small amounts of insulin lispro at mealtimes
   (E) Morning injection of NPH insulin and evening injection of regular insulin

4. Which one of the following drugs promotes the release of endogenous insulin?
   (A) Acarbose
   (B) Glipizide
   (C) Metformin
   (D) Miglitol
   (E) Pioglitazone

5. Which of the following is an important effect of insulin?
   (A) Increased conversion of amino acids into glucose
   (B) Increased gluconeogenesis
   (C) Increased glucose transport into cells
   (D) Inhibition of lipoprotein lipase
   (E) Stimulation of glycogenolysis

6. A 54-year-old obese patient with type 2 diabetes has a history of alcoholism. In this patient, metformin should either be avoided or used with extreme caution because the combina-tion of metformin and ethanol increases the risk of which of the following?
   (A) A disulfiram-like reaction
   (B) Excessive weight gain
   (C) Hypoglycemia
   (D) Lactic acidosis
   (E) Serious hepatotoxicity

7. Which of the following drugs is taken during the first part of a meal for the purpose of delaying the absorption of dietary carbohydrates?
   (A) Acarbose
   (B) Exenatide
   (C) Glipizide
   (D) Pioglitazone
   (E) Repaglinide

8. The PPAR-γ receptor that is activated by thiazolidinediones increases tissue sensitivity to insulin by which of the following mechanisms?
   (A) Activating adenylyl cyclase and increasing the intracel-lular concentration of cAMP
   (B) Inactivating a cellular inhibitor of the GLUT2 glucose transporter
   (C) Inhibiting acid glucosidase, a key enzyme in glycogen breakdown pathways
   (D) Regulating transcription of genes involved in glucose utilization
   (E) Stimulating the activity of a tyrosine kinase that phosphorylates the insulin receptor

9. Which of the following drugs is *most* likely to cause hypogly-cemia when used as monotherapy in the treatment of type 2 diabetes?
   (A) Acarbose
   (B) Glyburide
   (C) Metformin
   (D) Miglitol
   (E) Rosiglitazone

10. Which of the following patients is *most* likely to be treated with intravenous glucagon?
    (A) An 18-year-old woman who took an overdose of cocaine and now has a blood pressure of 190/110 mm Hg
    (B) A 27-year-old woman with severe diarrhea caused by a flare in her inflammatory bowel disease
    (C) A 57-year-old woman with type 2 diabetes who has not taken her glyburide for the last 3 d
    (D) A 62-year-old man with severe bradycardia and hypoten-sion resulting from ingestion of an overdose of atenolol
    (E) A 74-year-old man with lactic acidosis as a complication of severe infection and shock

ANSWERS

1. Oral antidiabetic agents (listed in Table 41–1) are inappropriate in this patient because he has insulin-dependent diabetes. He needs a rapid-acting insulin preparation that can be given intravenously (see Figure 41–1). The answer is **A.**

2. Because of the risk of brain damage, the most important complication of insulin therapy is hypoglycemia. The other choices are not common effects of insulin. The answer is **B.**

3. Insulin regimens for tight control usually take the form of establishing a basal level of insulin with a small amount of a long-acting preparation (eg, insulin glargine) and supplementing the insulin levels, when called for by food intake, with short-acting insulin lispro. Less tight control may be achieved with 2 injections of intermediate-acting insulin per day. Because intake of glucose is mainly during the day, long-acting insulins are usually given in the morning, not at night. The answer is **D.**

4. Glipizide is a second-generation sulfonylurea that promotes insulin release by closing potassium channels in pancreatic B cells. The answer is **B.**

5. Insulin lowers serum glucose concentration in part by driving glucose into cells, particularly into muscle cells. The answer is **C.**

6. Biguanides, especially the older drug phenformin, have been associated with lactic acidosis. Thus, metformin should be avoided or used with extreme caution in patients with conditions that increase the risk of lactic acidosis, including acute ethanol ingestion. The answer is **D.**

7. To be absorbed, carbohydrates must be converted into monosaccharides by the action of α-glucosidase enzymes in the gastrointestinal tract. Acarbose inhibits α-glucosidase and, when present during digestion, delays the uptake of carbohydrates. The answer is **A.**

8. The PPAR-γ receptor belongs to a family of nuclear receptors. When activated, these receptors translocate to the nucleus, where they regulate the transcription of genes encoding proteins involved in the metabolism of carbohydrate and lipids. The answer is **D.**

9. The insulin secretagogues, including the sulfonylurea glyburide, can cause hypoglycemia as a result of their ability to increase serum insulin levels. The biguanides, thiazolidinediones, and α-glucosidase inhibitors are euglycemics that are unlikely to cause hypoglycemia when used alone. The answer is **B.**

10. Glucagon acts through cardiac glucagon receptors to stimulate the rate and force of contraction of the heart. Because this bypasses cardiac β adrenoceptors, glucagon is useful in the treatment of β-blocker-induced cardiac depression. The answer is **D.**

SKILL KEEPER ANSWERS: DIABETES AND HYPERTENSION (CHAPTER 11)

1. *The major antihypertensive drug groups are (a) β-adrenoceptor blockers; (b) α_1-selective adrenoceptor blockers (eg, prazosin); (c) centrally acting sympathoplegics (eg, clonidine or methyldopa); (d) calcium channel blockers (eg, diltiazem, nifedipine, verapamil); (e) angiotensin-converting enzyme (ACE) inhibitors (eg, captopril); (f) angiotensin receptor antagonists (eg, losartan); and (g) thiazide diuretics.*

2. *ACE inhibitors slow the progression of diabetic nephropathy and help stabilize renal function. Angiotensin receptor antagonists may have similar protective effects in patients with diabetes. Beta-adrenoceptor blockers can, in theory, mask the symptoms of hypoglycemia in diabetic patients; however, many patients with diabetes and cardiovascular disease are successfully treated with these drugs. A large clinical trial showed that control of hypertension decreases diabetes-associated microvascular disease. This trial included many patients being maintained on β-adrenoceptor blockers. Thiazide diuretics impair the release of insulin and tissue utilization of glucose, so they should be used with caution for patients with diabetes.*

CHECKLIST

When you complete this chapter, you should be able to:

❑ Describe the effects of insulin on hepatocytes, muscle, and adipose tissue.

❑ List the types of insulin preparations and their durations of action.

❑ Describe the major hazards of insulin therapy.

❑ List the prototypes and describe the mechanisms of action, key pharmacokinetic features, and toxicities of the major classes of agents used to treat type 2 diabetes.

❑ Give 3 examples of rational drug combinations for treatment of type 2 diabetes mellitus.

❑ Describe the clinical uses of glucagon.

DRUG SUMMARY TABLE: Antidiabetic Agents

Subclass	Mechanism of Action	Clinical Applications	Pharmacokinetics	Toxicities, Drug Interactions
Insulins				
Regular insulin	Activate insulin receptor	Type 1 and type 2 diabetes	Parenteral administration, short-acting	Hypoglycemia, weight gain
Rapid-acting: lispro, aspart, glulisine *Intermediate-acting: NPH Long-acting:* detemir, glargine				
Biguanides				
Metformin	Decreased endogenous glucose production	Type 2 diabetes	Oral administration	Gastrointestinal (GI) disturbances, lactic acidosis (rare)
Insulin secretagogues				
Glipizide	Increases insulin secretion from pancreatic beta cells by closing ATP-sensitive K⁺ channels	Type 2 diabetes	Oral administration	Hypoglycemia, weight gain
Glyburide, glimepiride: like glipizide, sulfonylurea drugs with intermediate duration of action *Repaglinide, nateglinide:* fast-acting insulin secretagogues *Chlorpropamide, tolbutamide:* older sulfonylurea drugs, lower potency, greater toxicity; rarely used				
Alpha-glucosidase inhibitors				
Acarbose	Inhibit intestinal α-glucosidases	Type 2 diabetes	Oral administration	GI disturbances
Miglitol: Similar to acarbose				
Thiazolidinediones				
Rosiglitazone	Regulates gene expression by binding to PPAR-γ	Type 2 diabetes	Oral administration	Fluid retention, edema, anemia, weight gain, bone fractures in women, may worsen heart disease and increase risk of myocardial infarction
Pioglitazone: Similar to rosiglitazone possibly less cardiovascular adverse effects				
Incretin-based drugs				
Exenatide	Analog of glucagon-like peptide-1 (GLP-1) activates GLP-1 receptors	Type 2 diabetes	Parenteral administration	GI disturbances, headache, pancreatitis
Sitagliptin	Inhibitor of the dipeptidyl peptidase-4 (DPP-4) that degrades GLP-1 and other incretins	Type 2 diabetes	Oral administration	Rhinitis, upper respiratory infections, rare allergic reactions
Amylin analog				
Pramlintide	Analog of amylin activates amylin receptors	Type 1 and type 2 diabetes	Parenteral administration	GI disturbances, hypoglycemia, headache
Glucagon				
Glucagon	Activates glucagon receptors	Severe hypoglycemia, β-blocker overdose	Parenteral administration	GI disturbances, hypotension

PPAR-γ, peroxisome proliferator-activated receptor-gamma.

Drugs That Affect Bone Mineral Homeostasis

CHAPTER

42

Calcium and phosphorus, the 2 major elements of bone, are crucial not only for the mechanical strength of the skeleton but also for the normal function of many other cells in the body. Accordingly, a complex regulatory mechanism has evolved to tightly regulate calcium and phosphate homeostasis. Parathyroid hormone (PTH) and vitamin D are primary regulators (Figure 42–1), whereas calcitonin, glucocorticoids, and estrogens play secondary roles. These hormones or drugs that mimic or suppress their actions are used in the treatment of bone mineral disorders (eg, osteoporosis, rickets, osteomalacia, Paget's disease), as are several nonhormonal agents.

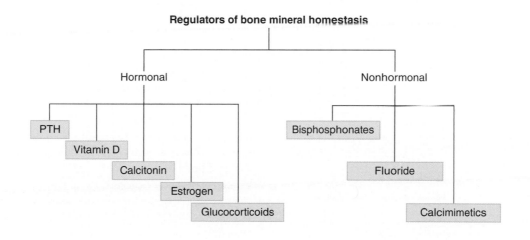

HORMONAL REGULATORS OF BONE MINERAL HOMEOSTASIS

A. Parathyroid Hormone

Parathyroid hormone (PTH), an 84-amino-acid peptide, acts on membrane G protein-coupled receptors to increase cyclic adenosine monophosphate (cAMP) in bone and renal tubular cells. In the kidney, PTH inhibits calcium excretion, promotes phosphate excretion, and stimulates the production of active vitamin D metabolites (Figure 42–1, Table 42–1). In bone, PTH promotes bone turnover by increasing the activity of both osteoblasts and osteoclasts (Figure 42–2B). Osteoclast activation is not a direct effect and instead results from PTH stimulation of osteoblast formation of RANK ligand (RANKL), a member of the tumor necrosis factor (TNF) cytokine family that stimulates the activity of mature osteoclasts and the differentiation of osteoclast precursors.

At the continuous high concentrations seen in hyperparathyroidism, the net effect of elevated PTH is increased bone resorption, hypercalcemia, and hyperphosphatemia. However, low intermittent doses of PTH produce a net increase in bone formation; this is the basis of the use of **teriparatide**, a recombinant truncated form of PTH, for parenteral treatment of osteoporosis.

High-Yield Terms to Learn

Hyperparathyroidism	A condition of PTH excess characterized by hypercalcemia, bone pain, cognitive abnormalities, and renal stones. Primary disease results from parathyroid gland dysfunction. Secondary disease most commonly results from chronic kidney disease
Osteoblast	Bone cell that promotes bone *formation*
Osteoclast	Bone cell that promotes bone *resorption*
Osteomalacia	A condition of abnormal mineralization of adult bone secondary to nutritional deficiency of vitamin D or inherited defects in the formation or action of active vitamin D metabolites
Osteoporosis	Abnormal loss of bone with increased risk of fractures, spinal deformities, and loss of stature; remaining bone is histologically normal
Paget's disease	A bone disorder, of unknown origin, characterized by excessive bone destruction and disorganized repair. Complications include skeletal deformity, musculoskeletal pain, kidney stones, and organ dysfunction secondary to pressure from bony overgrowth
Rickets	The same as osteomalacia, but it occurs in the growing skeleton
RANK ligand	An osteoblast-derived growth factor that stimulates osteoclast activity and osteoclast precursor differentiation

The synthesis and secretion of PTH is primarily regulated by the serum concentration of free ionized calcium; a drop in free ionized calcium stimulates PTH release. Active metabolites of vitamin D play a secondary role in regulating PTH secretion by inhibiting PTH synthesis (Figure 42–2A).

B. Vitamin D

Vitamin D, a fat-soluble vitamin (Figure 42–3), can be synthesized in the skin from 7-dehydrocholesterol under the influence of ultraviolet light or absorbed from the diet in the natural form (vitamin D_3, **cholecalciferol**) or the plant form (vitamin D_2, **ergocalciferol**). Active metabolites are formed in the liver (25-hydroxyvitamin D or calcifediol) and kidney (1,25-dihydroxyvitamin D or **calcitriol** plus other metabolites). Renal synthesis of active vitamin D metabolites is stimulated by PTH and by fibroblast growth factor 23 (FGF23), a factor produced by osteoblasts and osteoclasts. Renal synthesis of 1,25-dihydroxyvitamin D_2 is inhibited by phosphate and vitamin D metabolites (Figure 41–2). The action of vitamin D metabolites is mediated by activation of 1 or possibly a family of nuclear receptors that regulate gene expression.

Active vitamin D metabolites cause a net increase in serum concentrations of calcium and phosphate by increasing intestinal absorption and bone resorption and decreasing renal excretion (Figure 42–1, Table 42–1). Because their effect in the gastrointestinal (GI) tract and bone is greater than their effect in the kidney, they also increase urinary calcium. Active vitamin D metabolites are required for normal mineralization of bone; deficiencies cause rickets in growing children and adolescents and osteomalacia in adults. Vitamin D metabolites inhibit PTH secretion directly and indirectly, by increasing serum calcium.

Vitamin D, vitamin D metabolites, and synthetic derivatives are used to treat deficiency states, including nutritional deficiency, intestinal osteodystrophy, chronic kidney or liver disease, hypoparathyroidism, and nephrotic syndrome. They are also used, in combination with calcium supplementation, to prevent and treat osteoporosis in older women and men. Topical formulations are

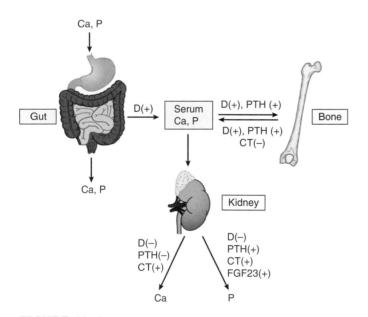

FIGURE 42–1 Effects of active metabolites of vitamin D (D), parathyroid hormone (PTH), calcitonin (CT), and fibroblast growth factor 23 (FGF23) on calcium and phosphorus homeostasis. Active metabolites of vitamin D increase absorption of calcium from both gut and bone, whereas PTH increases reabsorption from bone. Vitamin D metabolites and PTH both reduce urinary excretion of calcium. In animals with vitamin D deficiency, active metabolites of vitamin D produce a net increase in bone mineralization by increasing the availability of serum calcium and phosphate. (Reproduced, with permission, from Katzung BG, editor: *Basic & Clinical Pharmacology*, 12th ed. McGraw-Hill, 2012: Fig. 42–1.)

TABLE 42–1 Actions of PTH and active vitamin D metabolites on intestine, kidney, and bone.

Organ	PTH	Active Vitamin D Metabolites
Intestine	Indirectly increases calcium and phosphate absorption by increasing vitamin D metabolites	Increased calcium and phosphate absorption
Kidney	Decreased calcium excretion, increased phosphate excretion	Increased resorption of calcium and phosphate but usually net increase in urinary calcium due to effects in GI tract and bone
Bone	Calcium and phosphate resorption increased by continuous high concentrations. Low intermittent doses increase bone formation	Direct effect is increased calcium and phosphate resorption; indirect effect is promoting mineralization by increasing the availability of calcium and phosphate
Net effect on serum levels	Serum calcium increased, serum phosphate decreased	Serum calcium and phosphate both increased

Reproduced and modified, with permission, from Katzung BG, editor: *Basic & Clinical Pharmacology,* 12th ed. McGraw-Hill, 2012.

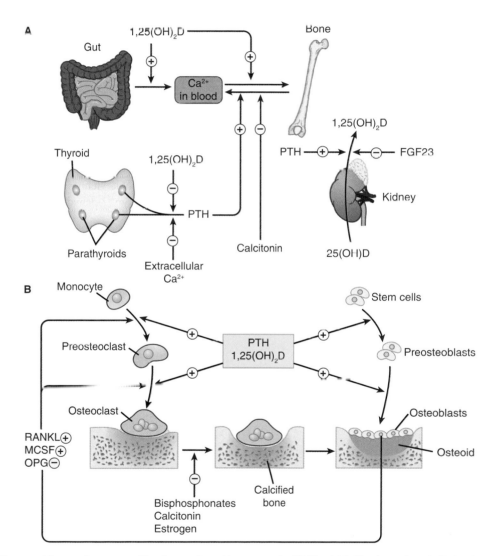

FIGURE 42–2 Hormonal interactions controlling bone mineral homeostasis. (**A**) The 1,25-dihydroxyvitamin D that is produced by the kidney under control of parathyroid hormone (PTH) and fibroblast growth hormone 23 (FGF23) stimulates intestinal uptake of calcium and phosphate, and, in those with vitamin D deficiency, promotes bone formation. Calcitonin inhibits resorption from bone, whereas PTH stimulates bone resorption. Extracellular calcium and 1,25-dihydroxyvitamin D inhibit PTH production. (**B**) Both PTH and 1,25-dihydroxyvitamin D regulate bone formation and resorption. This is accomplished by their activation of precursor differentiation and by stimulation of osteoblast production of signaling factors, including RANK ligand (RANKL), macrophage colony-stimulating factor (MCSF), and osteoprotegerin. (Reproduced and modified, with permission, from Katzung BG, editor: *Basic & Clinical Pharmacology,* 12th ed. McGraw-Hill, 2012: Fig. 42–2.)

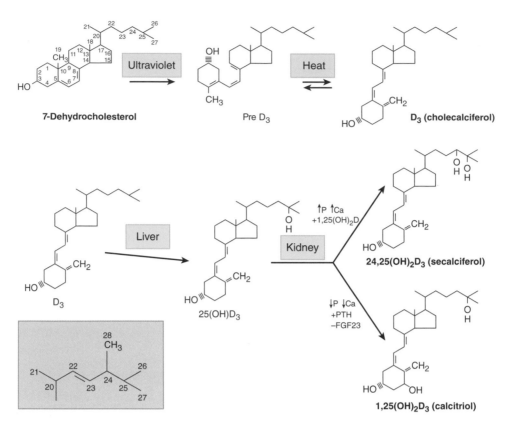

FIGURE 42–3 Conversion of 7-dehydroxycholesterol to vitamin D$_3$ and metabolism of vitamin D$_3$ to 1,25-dihydroxyvitamin D$_3$ (1,25(OH)$_2$D$_3$) and to 24,25-dihydroxyvitamin D$_3$ (24,25(OH)$_2$D$_3$). The inset shows the side chain for ergosterol. Ergosterol undergoes similar transformation to vitamin D$_2$ (ergocalciferol), which, in turn is metabolized to 1,25-dihydroxyvitamin D$_2$ and 24,25-dihydroxyvitamin D$_2$. In humans, corresponding D$_2$ and D$_3$ have equivalent effects and potency. They are therefore referred to in the text without a subscript. (Reproduced, with permission, from Katzung BG, editor: *Basic & Clinical Pharmacology*, 12th ed. McGraw-Hill, 2012: Fig. 42–3.)

used in psoriasis, a hyperproliferative skin disorder. The 2 forms of vitamin D—cholecalciferol and ergocalciferol—are available as oral supplements and are commonly added to dairy products and other foods. In patients with conditions that impair vitamin D activation (chronic kidney disease, liver disease, hypoparathyroidism), an active form of vitamin D such as calcitriol is required. In the treatment of secondary hyperparathyroidism associated with chronic kidney disease, calcitriol reduces PTH levels, corrects hypocalcemia, and improves bone disease, but it can also result in hypercalcemia and hypercalciuria through direct effects on intestinal, bone, and renal handling of calcium and phosphate. Several forms of active vitamin D that selectively inhibit PTH formation while posing less risk of hypercalcemia have been developed. 1α-Hydroxyvitamin D$_2$ (**doxercalciferol**) is a prodrug that is converted in the liver to 1,25-dihyroxyvitamin D, whereas 19-nor-1,25-dihydroxyvitamin D$_2$ (**paricalcitol**) and **calcipotriene** (calcipotriol) are analogs of calcitriol. All cause less hypercalcemia and, in patients with normal renal function, less hypercalciuria than calcitriol. Oral and parenteral doxercalciferol and oral paricalcitol are approved for treatment of secondary hyperparathyroidism in patients with chronic kidney disease. Calcipotriene (calcipotriol) is approved for topical treatment of psoriasis. These and other analogs are being investigated for use in various malignancies and inflammatory disorders.

The primary toxicity caused by chronic overdose with vitamin D or its active metabolites is hypercalcemia, hyperphosphatemia, and hypercalciuria.

C. Calcitonin

Calcitonin, a peptide hormone secreted by the thyroid gland, decreases serum calcium and phosphate by inhibiting bone resorption and inhibiting renal excretion of these minerals (Figure 42–1). Bone formation is not impaired initially, but ultimately it is reduced. The hormone has been used in conditions in which an acute reduction of serum calcium is needed (eg, Paget's disease and hypercalcemia). Calcitonin is approved for treatment of osteoporosis and has been shown to increase bone mass and to reduce spine fractures. However, it is not as effective as teriparatide or bisphosphonates. Although human calcitonin is available, salmon calcitonin is most often selected for clinical use because of its longer half-life and greater potency. Calcitonin is administered by injection or as a nasal spray.

D. Estrogens

Estrogens and selective estrogen receptor modulators (SERMs; eg, **raloxifene**) can prevent or delay bone loss in postmenopausal women (see Chapter 40). Their action involves the inhibition of PTH-stimulated bone resorption (Figure 42–2B).

E. Glucocorticoids

The glucocorticoids (Chapter 39) inhibit bone mineral maintenance. As a result, chronic systemic use of these drugs is a common cause of osteoporosis in adults. However, these hormones are useful in the intermediate-term treatment of hypercalcemia.

SKILL KEEPER: DIURETICS AND CALCIUM (SEE CHAPTER 15)

The kidney is a key regulator of serum calcium concentrations. Several diuretics affect the kidney's handling of filtered calcium.

1. *Which 2 classes of diuretics have opposite effects on calcium elimination?*
2. *What mechanisms are responsible for their opposing effects?*
3. *What is the clinical importance of these effects?*

The Skill Keeper Answers appear at the end of the chapter.

NONHORMONAL AGENTS

A. Bisphosphonates

The bisphosphonates (**alendronate, etidronate, ibandronate, pamidronate, risedronate, tiludronate,** and **zoledronic acid**) are short-chain organic polyphosphate compounds that reduce both the resorption and the formation of bone by an action on the basic hydroxyapatite crystal structure. The bisphosphonates have other complex cellular effects, including effects on vitamin D production and calcium absorption from the GI tract, and direct effects on osteoclasts, including inhibition of farnesyl pyrophosphate synthase, an enzyme that appears to play a critical role in osteoclast survival. Bisphosphonates are used to manage the hypercalcemia associated with some malignancies and to treat Paget's disease. Chronic bisphosphonate therapy is used commonly to prevent and treat all forms of osteoporosis. It has been shown to increase bone density and reduce fractures.

Pamidronate, zoledronic acid, or etidronate are available for parenteral treatment of hypercalcemia associated with Paget's disease and malignancies. Etidronate and the other bisphosphonates listed above are available as oral medications. Oral bioavailability of bisphosphonates is low (<10%), and food impairs their absorption. Bisphosphonate treatment of osteoporosis is accomplished with daily oral dosing (alendronate, risedronate, ibandronate); weekly oral dosing (alendronate, risedronate); monthly oral dosing (ibandronate); quarterly injection dosing (ibandronate); or annual infusions (zoledronate). The primary toxicity of the low oral bisphosphonate doses used for osteoporosis is gastric and esophageal irritation. To reduce esophageal irritation, patients are advised to take the drugs with large quantities of water and avoid situations that permit esophageal reflux. The higher doses of bisphosphonates used to treat hypercalcemia have been associated with renal impairment and osteonecrosis of the jaw.

B. Rank Ligand (RANKL) Inhibitor

Denosumab is a human monoclonal antibody that binds to and prevents the action of RANKL. Denosumab inhibits osteoclast formation and activity. It is at least as effective as the potent bisphosphonates in inhibiting bone resorption and can be used for treatment of postmenopausal osteoporosis.

Denosumab is administered subcutaneously every 6 mo, which avoids gastrointestinal side effects. The drug appears to be well tolerated, but there could be an increased risk of infection due to RANKL's role in the immune response.

C. Calcimimetics

Cinacalcet lowers PTH by activating the calcium-sensing receptor in the parathyroid gland. It is used for oral treatment of secondary hyperparathyroidism in chronic kidney disease and for the treatment of hypercalcemia in patients with parathyroid carcinoma. Its toxicities include hypocalcemia and adynamic bone disease, a condition of profoundly decreased bone cell activity.

D. Fluoride

Appropriate concentrations of fluoride ion in drinking water or as an additive in toothpaste have a well-documented ability to reduce dental caries. Chronic exposure to the ion, especially in high concentrations, may increase new bone synthesis. It is not clear, however, whether this new bone is normal in strength. Clinical trials of fluoride in patients with osteoporosis have not demonstrated a reduction in fractures. Acute toxicity of fluoride (usually caused by ingestion of rat poison) is manifested by gastrointestinal and neurologic symptoms.

E. Other Drugs with Effects on Serum Calcium and Phosphate

Strontium ranelate, an organic ion bound to 2 atoms of strontium, promotes osteoclast apoptosis and increases concentrations of bone formation markers; it is used in Europe for treatment of osteoporosis. **Gallium nitrate** is effective in managing the hypercalcemia associated with some malignancies and possibly Paget's disease. It acts by inhibiting bone resorption. To prevent nephrotoxicity, patients need to be well hydrated and to have good renal output. The antibiotic **plicamycin (mithramycin)** has been used to reduce serum calcium and bone resorption in Paget's disease and hypercalcemia. Because of the risk of serious toxicity (eg, thrombocytopenia, hemorrhage, hepatic and renal damage), plicamycin is mainly restricted to short-term treatment of serious hypercalcemia. Several diuretics, most notably **thiazide diuretics** and **furosemide,** can affect serum and urinary calcium levels (see this chapter's Skill Keeper). The phosphate-binding gel **sevelamer** is used in combination with calcium supplements and dietary phosphate restriction to treat hyperphosphatemia, a common complication of renal failure, hypoparathyroidism, and vitamin D intoxication.

QUESTIONS

1. Which of the following drugs is routinely added to calcium supplements and milk for the purpose of preventing rickets in children and osteomalacia in adults?
   (A) Cholecalciferol
   (B) Calcitriol
   (C) Gallium nitrate
   (D) Sevelamer
   (E) Plicamycin

2. Which of the following drugs is *most* useful for the treatment of hypercalcemia in Paget's disease?
   (A) Fluoride
   (B) Hydrochlorothiazide
   (C) Pamidronate
   (D) Raloxifene
   (E) Teriparatide

3. The active metabolites of vitamin D act through a nuclear receptor to produce which of the following effects?
   (A) Decrease the absorption of calcium from bone
   (B) Increase PTH formation
   (C) Increase renal production of erythropoietin
   (D) Increase the absorption of calcium from the gastrointestinal tract
   (E) Lower the serum phosphate concentration

4. Which of the following conditions is an indication for the use of raloxifene?
   (A) Chronic kidney failure
   (B) Hypoparathyroidism
   (C) Intestinal osteodystrophy
   (D) Postmenopausal osteoporosis
   (E) Rickets

Questions 5–7. A 58-year-old postmenopausal woman was sent for dual-energy x-ray absorptiometry to evaluate the bone mineral density of her lumbar spine, femoral neck, and total hip. The test results revealed significantly low bone mineral density in all sites.

5. Chronic use of which of the following medications is *most* likely to have contributed to this woman's osteoporosis?
   (A) Lovastatin
   (B) Metformin
   (C) Prednisone
   (D) Propranolol
   (E) Thiazide diuretic

6. If this patient began oral therapy with alendronate, she would be advised to drink large quantities of water with the tablets and remain in an upright position for at least 30 min and until eating the first meal of the day. These instructions would be given to decrease the risk of which of the following?
   (A) Cholelithiasis
   (B) Diarrhea
   (C) Constipation
   (D) Erosive esophagitis
   (E) Pernicious anemia

7. The patient's condition was not sufficiently controlled with alendronate, so she began therapy with a nasal spray containing a protein that inhibits bone resorption. The drug contained in the nasal spray was which of the following?
   (A) Calcitonin
   (B) Calcitriol
   (C) Cinacalcet
   (D) Cortisol
   (E) Teriparatide

Questions 8–10. A 67-year-old man with chronic kidney disease was found to have an elevated serum PTH concentration and a low serum concentration of 25-hydroxyvitamin D. He was successfully treated with ergocalciferol. Unfortunately, his kidney disease progressed so that he required dialysis and his serum PTH concentration became markedly elevated.

8. Which of the following drugs is *most* likely to lower this patient's serum PTH concentration?
   (A) Calcitriol
   (B) Cholecalciferol
   (C) Furosemide
   (D) Gallium nitrate
   (E) Risedronate

9. Although the drug therapy was effective at lowering serum PTH concentrations, the patient experienced several episodes of hypercalcemia. He was switched to a vitamin D analog that suppresses PTH with less risk of hypercalcemia. Which drug was the patient switched to?
   (A) Calcitriol
   (B) Cholecalciferol
   (C) Furosemide
   (D) Paricalcitol
   (E) Risedronate

10. In the treatment of patients like this with secondary hyperparathyroidism due to chronic kidney disease, cinacalcet is an alternative to vitamin D-based drugs. Cinacalcet lowers PTH by which of the following mechanisms?
    (A) Activating a steroid receptor that inhibits expression of the PTH gene
    (B) Activating the calcium-sensing receptor in parathyroid cells
    (C) Activating transporters in the GI tract that are involved in calcium absorption
    (D) Inducing the liver enzyme that converts vitamin D_3 to 25-hydroxyvitamin D_3
    (E) Inhibiting the farnesyl pyrophosphate synthase found in osteoclasts

ANSWERS

1. The 2 forms of vitamin D—cholecalciferol and ergocalciferol—are commonly added to calcium supplements and dairy products. Calcitriol, the active 1,25-dihydroxyvitamin D_3 metabolite, would prevent vitamin D deficiency and is available as an oral formulation. However, because it is not subject to the complex mechanisms that regulate endogenous production of active vitamin D metabolites, it is not suitable for widespread use. The answer is **A.**

2. Paget's disease is characterized by excessive bone resorption, poorly organized bone formation, and hypercalcemia.

Bisphosphonates and calcitonin are first-line treatments. Pamidronate is a powerful bisphosphonate used parenterally to treat hypercalcemia. The answer is **C**.

3. The active metabolites of vitamin D increase serum calcium and phosphate by promoting calcium and phosphate uptake from the gastrointestinal tract, increasing bone resorption, and decreasing renal excretion of both electrolytes. They inhibit, rather than stimulate, PTH formation. The answer is **D**.

4. Raloxifene, a SERM, is approved for use in postmenopausal women with osteoporosis. The answer is **D**.

5. Long-term therapy with glucocorticoids such as prednisone is associated with a reduction in bone mineral density and an increased risk of fractures. The other drugs are not known to have significant effects on bone or serum calcium. The answer is **C**.

6. Oral bisphosphonates such as alendronate can irritate the esophagus and stomach. The risk of this toxicity is reduced by drinking water and by remaining in an upright position for 30 min after taking the medication. The answer is **D**.

7. Calcitonin is a peptide hormone that prevents bone resorption. Salmon calcitonin is available as a nasal spray or a parenteral form for injection. The answer is **A**.

8. In patients with chronic kidney disease that requires dialysis, the impaired production of active vitamin D metabolites compounded with elevated serum phosphate due to renal impairment leads to secondary hyperparathyroidism. Administration of the active vitamin D metabolite calcitriol acts directly on the parathyroid to inhibit PTH production. Cholecalciferol, a form of vitamin D, is not effective in patients with advanced renal disease who cannot form adequate amounts of active vitamin D metabolites. The answer is **A**.

9. Paricalcitol is an analog of 1,25-dihydroxyvitamin D_3 (calcitriol) that lowers serum PTH at doses that only rarely precipitate hypercalcemia. The molecular basis of this selective action is poorly understood but is of value in the management of hyperparathyroidism and psoriasis. The answer is **D**.

10. Cinacalcet is a member of a novel class of drugs that activate the calcium-sensing receptor in parathyroid cells. When this receptor is activated by cinacalcet or free ionized calcium, it activates a signaling pathway that suppresses PTH synthesis and release. The answer is **B**.

CHECKLIST

When you complete this chapter, you should be able to:

❑ Identify the major and minor endogenous regulators of bone mineral homeostasis.

❑ Sketch the pathway and sites of formation of 1,25-dihydroxyvitamin D.

❑ Compare and contrast the clinical uses and effects of the major forms of vitamin D and its active metabolites.

❑ Describe the major effects of PTH and vitamin D derivatives on the intestine, the kidney, and bone.

❑ Describe the agents used in the treatment of hypercalcemia and the agents used in the treatment of osteoporosis.

❑ Recall the effects of adrenal and gonadal steroids on bone structure and the actions of diuretics on serum calcium levels.

DRUG SUMMARY TABLE: Drugs Affecting Bone Mineral Metabolism

Subclass	Mechanism of Action	Clinical Applications	Pharmacokinetics	Toxicities, Drug Interactions
Vitamin D, metabolites, analogs				
Cholecalciferol, ergocalciferol	Regulates gene transcription via the vitamin D receptor to produce the effects detailed in Table 42–1	Vitamin D deficiency	Oral administration Requires metabolism in liver or kidney to active forms	Hypercalcemia, hyperphosphatemia, hypercalciuria

Calcitriol: used for management of secondary hyperparathyroidism in patients with chronic kidney disease and for management of hypocalcemia in patients with hypoparathyroidism. Note that drug is active form, does not require metabolism
Doxercalciferol (1-hydroxyvitamin D₃): used for management of secondary hyperparathyroidism in patients with chronic kidney disease
Paricalcitol: an analog of calcitriol used for management of secondary hyperparathyroidism in patients with chronic kidney disease
Calcipotriene: an analog of calcitriol approved for psoriasis

Subclass	Mechanism of Action	Clinical Applications	Pharmacokinetics	Toxicities, Drug Interactions
Bisphosphonates				
Alendronate	Suppresses the activity of osteoclasts and inhibits bone resorption	Osteoporosis, Paget's disease	Oral administration daily or weekly	Adynamic bone, esophageal irritation, osteonecrosis of the jaw (rare)

Risedronate, ibandronate, pamidronate, zoledronate: similar to alendronate

Subclass	Mechanism of Action	Clinical Applications	Pharmacokinetics	Toxicities, Drug Interactions
Parathyroid hormone (PTH) analog				
Teriparatide	Acts through PTH receptors to produce a net increase in bone formation	Osteoporosis	Subcutaneous injection	Hypercalcemia, hypercalciuria • osteosarcoma in experimental animals
Calcitonin				
Calcitonin	Acts through calcitonin receptors to inhibit bone resorption	Osteoporosis	Subcutaneous injection or intranasal	Rhinitis with the nasal spray
Selective estrogen-receptor modulator (see Chapter 40)				
Raloxifene	Estrogen agonist effect in bone • estrogen antagonist effects in breast and endometrium	Osteoporosis in postmenopausal women	Oral administration	Hot flushes, thromboembolism
Rank Ligand (RANKL) Inhibitor				
Denosumab	Binds to RANKL and prevents it from stimulating osteoclast differentiation and function	Osteoporosis	Subcutaneously every 6 mo	May increase risk of infections
Calcimimetic				
Cinacalcet	Activates the calcium-sensing receptor	Hyperparathyroidism	Oral administration	Nausea, hypocalcemia, adynamic bone

PART VIII CHEMOTHERAPEUTIC DRUGS

The emergence of **microbial resistance** poses a constant challenge to the use of antimicrobial drugs. Mechanisms underlying microbial resistance to cell wall synthesis inhibitors include the production of antibiotic-inactivating enzymes, changes in the structure of target receptors, increased efflux via drug transporters, and decreases in the permeability of microbes' cellular membranes to antibiotics. Strategies designed to combat microbial resistance include the use of adjunctive agents that can protect against antibiotic inactivation, the use of antibiotic combinations, the introduction of new (and often expensive) chemical derivatives of established antibiotics, and efforts to avoid the indiscriminate use or misuse of antibiotics.

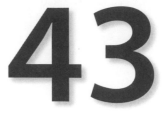

Beta-Lactam Antibiotics & Other Cell Wall Synthesis Inhibitors

Penicillins and cephalosporins are the major antibiotics that inhibit bacterial cell wall synthesis. They are called beta-lactams because of the unusual 4-member ring that is common to all their members. The beta-lactams include some of the most effective, widely used, and well-tolerated agents available for the treatment of microbial infections. Vancomycin, fosfomycin, and bacitracin also inhibit cell wall synthesis but are not nearly as important as the beta-lactam drugs. The selective toxicity of the drugs discussed in this chapter is mainly due to specific actions on the synthesis of a cellular structure that is unique to the microorganism. More than 50 antibiotics that act as cell wall synthesis inhibitors are currently available, with individual spectra of activity that afford a wide range of clinical applications.

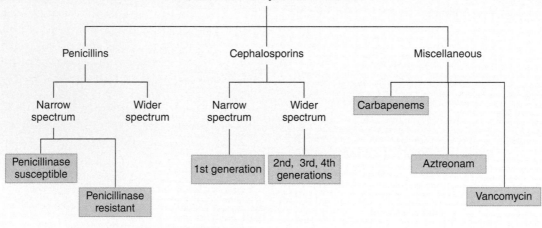

PENICILLINS

A. Classification

All penicillins are derivatives of 6-aminopenicillanic acid and contain a beta-lactam ring structure that is essential for antibacterial activity. Penicillin subclasses have additional chemical substituents that confer differences in antimicrobial activity, susceptibility to acid and enzymatic hydrolysis, and biodisposition.

B. Pharmacokinetics

Penicillins vary in their resistance to gastric acid and therefore vary in their oral bioavailability. Parenteral formulations of ampicillin, piperacillin, and ticarcillin are available for injection. Penicillins are polar compounds and are not metabolized extensively. They are usually excreted unchanged in the urine via glomerular filtration and tubular secretion; the latter process is inhibited by probenecid. Nafcillin is excreted mainly in the bile and ampicillin

High-Yield Terms to Learn

Bactericidal	An antimicrobial drug that can eradicate an infection in the absence of host defense mechanisms; kills bacteria
Bacteriostatic	An antimicrobial drug that inhibits antimicrobial growth but requires host defense mechanisms to eradicate the infection; does not kill bacteria
Beta-lactam antibiotics	Drugs with structures containing a beta-lactam ring: includes the penicillins, cephalosporins and carbapenems. This ring must be intact for antimicrobial action
Beta-lactamases	Bacterial enzymes (penicillinases, cephalosporinases) that hydrolyze the beta-lactam ring of certain penicillins and cephalosporins
Beta-lactam inhibitors	Potent inhibitors of some bacterial beta-lactamases used in combinations to protect hydrolyzable penicillins from inactivation
Minimal inhibitory concentration (MIC)	Lowest concentration of antimicrobial drug capable of inhibiting growth of an organism in a defined growth medium
Penicillin-binding proteins (PBPs)	Bacterial cytoplasmic membrane proteins that act as the initial receptors for penicillins and other beta-lactam antibiotics
Peptidoglycan	Chains of polysaccharides and polypeptides that are cross-linked to form the bacterial cell wall
Selective toxicity	More toxic to the invader than to the host; a property of useful antimicrobial drugs
Transpeptidases	Bacterial enzymes involved in the cross-linking of linear peptidoglycan chains, the final step in cell wall synthesis

undergoes enterohepatic cycling. The plasma half-lives of most penicillins vary from 30 min to 1 h. Procaine and benzathine forms of penicillin G are administered intramuscularly and have long plasma half-lives because the active drug is released very slowly into the bloodstream. Most penicillins cross the blood-brain barrier only when the meninges are inflamed.

C. Mechanisms of Action and Resistance

Beta-lactam antibiotics are **bactericidal** drugs. They act to inhibit cell wall synthesis by the following steps (Figure 43–1): (1) binding of the drug to specific enzymes (**penicillin-binding proteins [PBPs]**) located in the bacterial cytoplasmic membrane; (2) inhibition of the **transpeptidation reaction** that cross-links the linear peptidoglycan chain constituents of the cell wall; and (3) activation of **autolytic** enzymes that cause lesions in the bacterial cell wall.

Enzymatic hydrolysis of the beta-lactam ring results in loss of antibacterial activity. The formation of **beta-lactamases (penicillinases)** by most staphylococci and many gram-negative organisms is a major mechanism of bacterial resistance. Inhibitors of these bacterial enzymes (eg, clavulanic acid, sulbactam, tazobactam) are often used in combination with penicillins to prevent their inactivation. Structural change in target PBPs is another mechanism of resistance and is responsible for methicillin resistance in staphylococci and for resistance to penicillin G in pneumococci (eg, PRSP, penicillin resistant *Streptococcus pneumoniae*) and enterococci. In some gram-negative rods (eg, *Pseudomonas aeruginosa*), changes in the porin structures in the outer cell wall membrane may contribute to resistance by impeding access of penicillins to PBPs.

D. Clinical Uses

1. Narrow-spectrum penicillinase-susceptible agents—
Penicillin G is the prototype of a subclass of penicillins that have a limited spectrum of antibacterial activity and are susceptible to beta-lactamases. Clinical uses include therapy of infections caused by common streptococci, meningococci, gram-positive bacilli, and spirochetes. Many strains of pneumococci are now resistant to penicillins (penicillin-resistant *Streptococcus pneumoniae* [PRSP] strains). Most strains of *Staphylococcus aureus* and a significant number of strains of *Neisseria gonorrhoeae* are resistant via production of beta-lactamases. Although no longer suitable for treatment of gonorrhea, penicillin G remains the drug of choice for syphilis. Activity against enterococci is enhanced by aminoglycoside antibiotics. **Penicillin V** is an oral drug used mainly in oropharyngeal infections.

2. Very-narrow-spectrum penicillinase-resistant drugs—
This subclass of penicillins includes **methicillin** (the prototype, but rarely used owing to its nephrotoxic potential), **nafcillin**, and **oxacillin**. Their primary use is in the treatment of known or suspected staphylococcal infections. Methicillin-resistant (MR) staphylococci (*S aureus* [MRSA] and *S epidermidis* [MRSE]) are resistant to all penicillins and are often resistant to multiple antimicrobial drugs.

3. Wider-spectrum penicillinase-susceptible drugs
a. Ampicillin and amoxicillin—These drugs make up a penicillin subgroup that has a wider spectrum of antibacterial activity than penicillin G but remains susceptible to penicillinases. Their clinical uses include indications similar to penicillin G

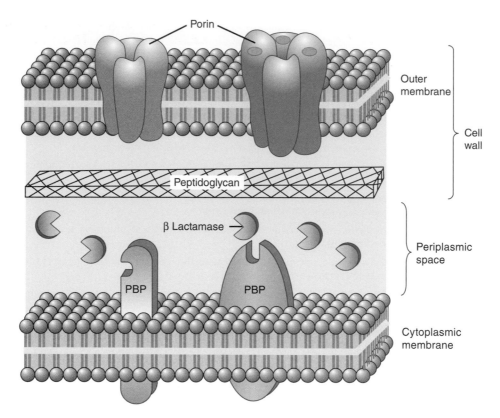

FIGURE 43–1 Beta-lactams and bacterial cell wall synthesis. The outer membrane shown in this simplified diagram is present only in gram-negative organisms. It is penetrated by proteins (porins) that are permeable to hydrophilic substances such as beta-lactam antibiotics. The peptidoglycan chains (mureins) are cross-linked by transpeptidases located in the cytoplasmic membrane, closely associated with penicillin-binding proteins (PBPs). Beta-lactam antibiotics bind to PBPs and inhibit transpeptidation, the final step in cell wall synthesis. They also activate autolytic enzymes that cause lesions in the cell wall. Beta-lactamases, which inactivate beta-lactam antibiotics, may be present in the periplasmic space or on the outer surface of the cytoplasmic membrane. (Reproduced, with permission, from Katzung BG, editor: *Basic & Clinical Pharmacology*, 12th ed. McGraw-Hill, 2012: Fig. 43–3.)

as well as infections resulting from enterococci, *Listeria monocytogenes, Escherichia coli, Proteus mirabilis, Haemophilus influenzae,* and *Moraxella catarrhalis,* although resistant strains occur. When used in combination with inhibitors of penicillinases (eg, clavulanic acid), their antibacterial activity is often enhanced. In enterococcal and listerial infections, ampicillin is synergistic with aminoglycosides.

b. Piperacillin and ticarcillin—These drugs have activity against several gram-negative rods, including *Pseudomonas, Enterobacter,* and in some cases *Klebsiella* species. Most drugs in this subgroup have synergistic actions when used with aminoglycosides against such organisms. Piperacillin and ticarcillin are susceptible to penicillinases and are often used in combination with penicillinase inhibitors (eg, tazobactam and clavulanic acid) to enhance their activity.

E. Toxicity

1. Allergy—Allergic reactions include urticaria, severe pruritus, fever, joint swelling, hemolytic anemia, nephritis, and anaphylaxis. About 5–10% of persons with a history of penicillin reaction have an allergic response when given a penicillin again. Methicillin causes interstitial nephritis, and nafcillin is associated

with neutropenia. Antigenic determinants include degradation products of penicillins such as penicilloic acid. Complete **cross-allergenicity** between different penicillins should be assumed. Ampicillin frequently causes maculopapular skin rash that does not appear to be an allergic reaction.

2. Gastrointestinal disturbances—Nausea and diarrhea may occur with oral penicillins, especially with ampicillin. Gastrointestinal upsets may be caused by direct irritation or by overgrowth of gram-positive organisms or yeasts. Ampicillin has been implicated in pseudomembranous colitis.

CEPHALOSPORINS

A. Classification

The cephalosporins are derivatives of 7-aminocephalosporanic acid and contain the beta-lactam ring structure. Many members of this group are in clinical use. They vary in their antibacterial activity and are designated first-, second-, third-, or fourth-generation drugs according to the order of their introduction into clinical use.

B. Pharmacokinetics

Several cephalosporins are available for oral use, but most are administered parenterally. Cephalosporins with side chains may undergo hepatic metabolism, but the major elimination mechanism for drugs in this class is renal excretion via active tubular secretion. Cefoperazone and ceftriaxone are excreted mainly in the bile. Most first- and second-generation cephalosporins do not enter the cerebrospinal fluid even when the meninges are inflamed.

C. Mechanisms of Action and Resistance

Cephalosporins bind to PBPs on bacterial cell membranes to inhibit bacterial cell wall synthesis by mechanisms similar to those of the penicillins. Cephalosporins are bactericidal against susceptible organisms.

Structural differences from penicillins render cephalosporins less susceptible to penicillinases produced by staphylococci, but many bacteria are resistant through the production of other beta-lactamases that can inactivate cephalosporins. Resistance can also result from decreases in membrane permeability to cephalosporins and from changes in PBPs. Methicillin-resistant staphylococci are also resistant to cephalosporins.

D. Clinical Uses

1. First-generation drugs—Cefazolin (parenteral) and cephalexin (oral) are examples of this subgroup. They are active against gram-positive cocci, including staphylococci and common streptococci. Many strains of *E coli* and *K pneumoniae* are also sensitive. Clinical uses include treatment of infections caused by these organisms and surgical prophylaxis in selected conditions. These drugs have minimal activity against gram-negative cocci, enterococci, methicillin-resistant staphylococci, and most gram-negative rods.

2. Second-generation drugs—Drugs in this subgroup usually have slightly less activity against gram-positive organisms than the first-generation drugs but have an extended gram-negative coverage. Marked differences in activity occur among the drugs in this subgroup. Examples of clinical uses include infections caused by the anaerobe *Bacteroides fragilis* (**cefotetan, cefoxitin**) and sinus, ear, and respiratory infections caused by *H influenzae* or *M catarrhalis* (**cefamandole, cefuroxime, cefaclor**).

3. Third-generation drugs—Characteristic features of third-generation drugs (eg, **ceftazidime, cefoperazone, cefotaxime**) include increased activity against gram-negative organisms resistant to other beta-lactam drugs and ability to penetrate the blood-brain barrier (except cefoperazone and cefixime). Most are active against *Providencia, Serratia marcescens,* and beta-lactamase-producing strains of *H influenzae* and *Neisseria*; they are less active against *Enterobacter* strains that produce extended-spectrum beta-lactamases. Ceftriaxone and cefotaxime are currently the most active cephalosporins against penicillin-resistant pneumococci (PRSP strains), but resistance is reported. Individual drugs also have activity against *Pseudomonas* (**cefoperazone, ceftazidime**) and *B fragilis* (**ceftizoxime**). Drugs in this subclass should usually be reserved for treatment of serious infections. **Ceftriaxone** (parenteral) and **cefixime** (oral), currently drugs of choice in gonorrhea, are exceptions. Likewise, in acute otitis media, a single injection of ceftriaxone is usually as effective as a 10-day course of treatment with amoxicillin.

4. Fourth-generation drugs—**Cefepime** is more resistant to beta-lactamases produced by gram-negative organisms, including *Enterobacter, Haemophilus, Neisseria,* and some penicillin-resistant pneumococci. Cefepime combines the gram-positive activity of first-generation agents with the wider gram-negative spectrum of third-generation cephalosporins. **Ceftaroline** is a newly introduced agent with activity against methicillin-resistant staphylococci.

E. Toxicity

1. Allergy—Cephalosporins cause a range of allergic reactions from skin rashes to anaphylactic shock. These reactions occur less frequently with cephalosporins than with penicillins. Complete cross-hypersensitivity between different cephalosporins should be assumed. Cross-reactivity between penicillins and cephalosporins is incomplete (5–10%), so penicillin-allergic patients are sometimes treated successfully with a cephalosporin. However, patients with a history of *anaphylaxis* to penicillins should not be treated with a cephalosporin.

2. Other adverse effects—Cephalosporins may cause pain at intramuscular injection sites and phlebitis after intravenous administration. They may increase the nephrotoxicity of aminoglycosides when the two are administered together. Drugs containing a methylthiotetrazole group (eg, cefamandole, cefoperazone, cefotetan) may cause hypoprothrombinemia and disulfiram-like reactions with ethanol.

OTHER BETA-LACTAM DRUGS

A. Aztreonam

Aztreonam is a **monobactam** that is resistant to beta-lactamases produced by certain gram-negative rods, including *Klebsiella, Pseudomonas,* and *Serratia.* The drug has no activity against gram-positive bacteria or anaerobes. It is an inhibitor of cell wall synthesis, preferentially binding to a specific penicillin-binding protein (PBP3), and is synergistic with aminoglycosides.

Aztreonam is administered intravenously and is eliminated via renal tubular secretion. Its half-life is prolonged in renal failure. Adverse effects include gastrointestinal upset with possible superinfection, vertigo and headache, and rarely hepatotoxicity. Although skin rash may occur, there is no cross-allergenicity with penicillins.

B. Imipenem, Doripenem, Meropenem, and Ertapenem

These drugs are **carbapenems** (chemically different from penicillins but retaining the beta-lactam ring structure) with low susceptibility to beta-lactamases. They have wide activity against gram-positive cocci (including some penicillin-resistant pneumococci), gram-negative rods, and anaerobes. With the exception of ertapenem, the carbapenems are active against *P aeruginosa* and *Acinetobacter* species. For pseudomonal infections, they are often used in combination with an aminoglycoside. The carbapenems are administered parenterally and are useful for infections caused by organisms resistant to other antibiotics. However, MRSA strains of staphylococci are resistant. Carbapenems are currently co-drugs of choice for infections caused by *Enterobacter, Citrobacter,* and *Serratia* species. Imipenem is rapidly inactivated by renal dehydropeptidase I and is administered in fixed combination with cilastatin, an inhibitor of this enzyme. Cilastatin increases the plasma half-life of imipenem and inhibits the formation of a potentially nephrotoxic metabolite. The other carbapenems are not significantly degraded by the kidney.

Adverse effects of imipenem-cilastatin include gastrointestinal distress, skin rash, and, at very high plasma levels, CNS toxicity (confusion, encephalopathy, seizures). There is partial cross-allergenicity with the penicillins. **Meropenem** is similar to imipenem except that it is not metabolized by renal dehydropeptidases and is less likely to cause seizures. **Ertapenem** has a long half-life but is less active against enterococci and *Pseudomonas,* and its intramuscular injection causes pain and irritation.

C. Beta-Lactamase Inhibitors

Clavulanic acid, sulbactam, and **tazobactam** are used in fixed combinations with certain hydrolyzable penicillins. They are most active against plasmid-encoded beta-lactamases such as those produced by gonococci, streptococci, *E coli,* and *H influenzae.* They are not good inhibitors of inducible chromosomal beta-lactamases formed by *Enterobacter, Pseudomonas,* and *Serratia.*

OTHER CELL WALL OR MEMBRANE-ACTIVE AGENTS

A. Vancomycin

Vancomycin is a bactericidal glycoprotein that binds to the D-Ala-D-Ala terminal of the nascent peptidoglycan pentapeptide side chain and inhibits transglycosylation. This action prevents elongation of the peptidoglycan chain and interferes with cross-linking. Resistance in strains of enterococci (vancomycin-resistant enterococci [VRE]) and staphylococci (vancomycin-resistant *S aureus* [VRSA]) involves a decreased affinity of vancomycin for the binding site because of the replacement of the terminal D-Ala by D-lactate. Vancomycin has a narrow spectrum of activity and is used for serious infections caused by drug-resistant gram-positive organisms, including methicillin-resistant staphylococci (MRSA), and in combination with a third-generation cephalosporin such as ceftriaxone for treatment of infections due to penicillin-resistant pneumococci (PRSP). Vancomycin is also a backup drug for treatment of infections caused by *Clostridium difficile.* **Teicoplanin** and **telavancin,** other glycopeptide derivatives, have similar characteristics.

Vancomycin-resistant enterococci are increasing and pose a potentially serious clinical problem because such organisms usually exhibit multiple-drug resistance. Vancomycin-intermediate strains of *S aureus* resulting in treatment failures have also been reported. Vancomycin is not absorbed from the gastrointestinal tract and may be given orally for bacterial enterocolitis. When given parenterally, vancomycin penetrates most tissues and is eliminated unchanged in the urine. Dosage modification is mandatory in patients with renal impairment. Toxic effects of vancomycin include chills, fever, phlebitis, ototoxicity, and nephrotoxicity. Rapid intravenous infusion may cause diffuse flushing ("red man syndrome") from histamine release.

B. Fosfomycin

Fosfomycin is an antimetabolite inhibitor of cytosolic enolpyruvate transferase. This action prevents the formation of *N*-acetylmuramic acid, an essential precursor molecule for peptidoglycan chain formation. Resistance to fosfomycin occurs via decreased intracellular accumulation of the drug.

Fosfomycin is excreted by the kidney, with urinary levels exceeding the **minimal inhibitory concentrations (MICs)** for many urinary tract pathogens. In a single dose, the drug is less effective than a 7-day course of treatment with fluoroquinolones. With multiple dosing, resistance emerges rapidly and diarrhea is common. Fosfomycin may be synergistic with beta-lactam and quinolone antibiotics in specific infections.

C. Bacitracin

Bacitracin is a peptide antibiotic that interferes with a late stage in cell wall synthesis in gram-positive organisms. Because of its marked nephrotoxicity, the drug is limited to topical use.

D. Cycloserine

Cycloserine is an antimetabolite that blocks the incorporation of D-Ala into the pentapeptide side chain of the peptidoglycan. Because of its potential neurotoxicity (tremors, seizures, psychosis), cycloserine is only used to treat tuberculosis caused by organisms resistant to first-line antituberculous drugs.

E. Daptomycin

Daptomycin is a novel cyclic lipopeptide with spectrum similar to vancomycin but active against vancomycin-resistant strains of enterococci and staphylococci. The drug is eliminated via the kidney. Creatine phosphokinase should be monitored since daptomycin may cause myopathy.

QUESTIONS

1. The primary mechanism of antibacterial action of the penicillins involves inhibition of
   (A) Beta-lactamases
   (B) *N*-acetylmuramic acid synthesis
   (C) Peptidoglycan cross-linking
   (D) Synthesis of cell membranes
   (E) Transglycosylation

Questions 2 and 3. A 33-year-old man was seen in a clinic with a complaint of dysuria and urethral discharge of yellow pus. He had a painless clean-based ulcer on the penis and nontender enlargement of the regional lymph nodes. Gram stain of the urethral exudate showed gram-negative diplococci within polymorphonucleocytes. The patient informed the clinic staff that he was unemployed and had not eaten a meal for 2 days.

2. The most appropriate treatment of gonorrhea in this patient is
   (A) Ampicillin orally for 7 d
   (B) Ceftriaxone intramuscularly as a single dose
   (C) Procaine penicillin G intramuscularly as a single dose plus oral probenecid
   (D) Tetracycline orally for 5 d
   (E) Vancomycin intramuscularly as a single dose

3. Immunofluorescent microscopic examination of fluid expressed from the penile chancre of this patient revealed treponemes. Because he appears to be infected with *Treponema pallidum*, the best course of action would be to
   (A) Administer a single oral dose of fosfomycin
   (B) Give no other antibiotics because drug treatment of gonorrhea provides coverage for incubating syphilis
   (C) Inject intramuscular benzathine penicillin G
   (D) Treat with oral tetracycline for 7 d
   (E) Treat with vancomycin

4. Which statement about imipenem is accurate?
   (A) Active against methicillin-resistant staphylococci
   (B) Has a narrow spectrum of antibacterial action
   (C) In renal dysfunction, dosage reduction is necessary to avoid seizures
   (D) Is highly susceptible to beta-lactamases produced by *Enterobacter* species
   (E) Is used in fixed combination with sulbactam

5. A 36-year-old woman recently treated for leukemia is admitted to the hospital with malaise, chills, and high fever. Gram stain of blood reveals the presence of gram-negative bacilli. The initial diagnosis is bacteremia, and parenteral antibiotics are indicated. The records of the patient reveal that she had a severe urticarial rash, hypotension, and respiratory difficulty after oral penicillin V about 6 mo ago. The most appropriate drug regimen for empiric treatment is
   (A) Aztreonam
   (B) Cefazolin
   (C) Imipenem
   (D) Nafcillin
   (E) Ticarcillin plus clavulanic acid

Questions 6–8. A 52-year-old man (weight 70 kg) is brought to the hospital emergency department in a confused and delirious state. He has had an elevated temperature for more than 24 h, during which time he had complained of a severe headache and had suffered from nausea and vomiting. Lumbar puncture reveals an elevated opening pressure, and cerebrospinal fluid findings include elevated protein, decreased glucose, and increased neutrophils. Gram stain of a smear of cerebrospinal fluid reveals gram-positive diplococci, and a preliminary diagnosis is made of purulent meningitis. The microbiology report informs you that for approximately 15% of *S pneumoniae* isolates in the community, the minimal inhibitory concentration for penicillin G is 20 mcg/mL.

6. Treatment of this patient should be initiated immediately with intravenous administration of
   (A) Ampicillin-sulbactam
   (B) Cefazolin
   (C) Cefotaxime plus vancomycin
   (D) Nafcillin
   (E) Ticarcillin

7. Resistance of pneumococci to penicillin G is due to
   (A) Beta-lactamase production
   (B) Changes in chemical structure of target penicillin-binding proteins
   (C) Changes in porin structure
   (D) Changes in the D-Ala-D-Ala building block of peptidoglycan precursor
   (E) Decreased intracellular accumulation of penicillin G

8. If this patient had been 82 years old and the Gram stain of the smear of cerebrospinal fluid had revealed gram-positive rods resembling diphtheroids, the antibiotic regimen for empiric treatment would include
   (A) Ampicillin
   (B) Aztreonam
   (C) Cefazolin
   (D) Fosfomycin
   (E) Meropenem

9. A patient needs antibiotic treatment for native valve, culture-positive infective enterococcal endocarditis. His medical history includes a severe anaphylactic reaction to penicillin G during the last year. The best approach would be treatment with
   (A) Amoxicillin-clavulanate
   (B) Aztreonam
   (C) Cefazolin plus gentamicin
   (D) Meropenem
   (E) Vancomycin

10. Which statement about vancomycin is accurate?
    (A) Active against methicillin-resistant staphylococci
    (B) Bacteriostatic
    (C) Binds to penicillin-binding proteins (PBPs)
    (D) Hepatic metabolism
    (E) Oral bioavailability

ANSWERS

1. Penicillins (and cephalosporins) bind to PBPs acting at the transpeptidation stage of cell wall synthesis (the final step) to inhibit peptidoglycan cross-linking. The beta-lactam antibiotics also activate autolysins, which break down the bacterial cell wall. Synthesis of *N*-acetylmuramic acid is inhibited by fosfomycin. Vancomycin inhibits transglycolase preventing elongation of peptidoglycan chains. The answer is **C.**

2. The treatments of choice for gonorrhea include a single dose of ceftriaxone (intramuscularly). Because of the high incidence of beta-lactamase-producing gonococci, the use of penicillin G or amoxicillin is no longer appropriate for gonorrhea. Similarly, many strains of gonococci are resistant to tetracyclines. Alternative drugs (not listed) for gonorrhea include cefixime, azithromycin (see Chapter 44) or spectinomycin (see Chapter 45). The answer is **B.**

3. This patient with gonorrhea also has primary syphilis. The penile chancre, the enlarged nontender lymph nodes, and the microscopic identification of treponemes in fluid expressed from the lesion are essentials of diagnosis. Although a single dose of ceftriaxone may cure incubating syphilis, it cannot be relied on for treating primary syphilis. The most appropriate course of action in this patient is to administer a single intramuscular injection of 2.4 million units of benzathine penicillin G. For penicillin-allergic patients, oral doxycycline or tetracycline for 15 d (not 7 d) is effective in most cases (see Chapter 44). However, lack of compliance may be a problem with oral therapy. Fosfomycin and vancomycin have no significant activity against spirochetes. The answer is **C.**

4. Like other carbapenems, imipenem has a wide spectrum of activity that includes anaerobes and many beta-lactamase-producing gram-negative rods, including *Enterobacter*. However, the carbapenems are not active against MRSA strains. Imipenem is rapidly hydrolyzed by renal dehydropeptidases and is given in combination with **cilastatin,** an inhibitor of this enzyme. Severe CNS toxicity, including seizures, will occur if the dose of imipenem is not reduced in patients with renal impairment. The answer is **C.**

5. Each of the drugs listed has activity against some gram-negative bacilli. All penicillins should be avoided in patients with a history of allergic reactions to any individual penicillin drug. Cephalosporins should also be avoided in patients who have had anaphylaxis or other severe hypersensitivity reactions after use of a penicillin. There is partial cross-reactivity between penicillins and the carbapenems such as imipenem and meropenem, but no cross-reactivity between the penicillins and aztreonam. The answer is **A.**

6. Pneumococcal isolates with a minimal inhibitory concentration for penicillin G of greater than 2 mcg/mL are highly resistant. Such strains are not killed by the concentrations of penicillin G or ampicillin that can be achieved in the cerebrospinal fluid. Nafcillin has minimal activity against penicillin-resistant pneumococci, and ticarcillin is used mainly for infections caused by gram-negative rods. Cefotaxime and ceftriaxone are the most active cephalosporins against penicillin-resistant pneumococci, and the addition of vancomycin is recommended in the case of highly resistant strains. The answer is **C.**

7. Pneumococcal resistance to penicillins is due to changes in the chemical structures of the target penicillin-binding proteins located in the bacterial cytoplasmic membrane. A similar mechanism underlies the resistance of staphylococci to methicillin (MRSA strains). A structural alteration in the D-Ala-D-Ala component of the pentapeptide side chains of peptidoglycans is the basis for a mechanism of resistance to vancomycin. The answer is **B.**

8. Diphtheroid-like gram-positive rods in the cerebrospinal fluid smear of an elderly patient are indicative of *L monocytogenes*. *Listeria* infections are more common in neonates, elderly patients, and those who have been treated with immunosuppressive agents. Treatment consists of ampicillin with or without an aminoglycoside such as gentamicin. Trimethoprim-sulfamethoxazole can also be used (see Chapter 46). The answer is **A.**

9. In patients who have had a severe reaction to a penicillin, it is inadvisable to administer a cephalosporin or a carbapenem such as meropenem. Aztreonam has no significant activity against gram-positive cocci, so the logical treatment in this case is vancomycin, often with an aminoglycoside (eg, gentamicin) for synergistic activity against enterococci. The answer is **E.**

10. Vancomycin is a bactericidal glycoprotein. It inhibits cell wall synthesis but does not bind to PBPs and is not susceptible to beta-lactamases. Vancomycin is not absorbed after oral administration and is used by this route in the treatment of colitis caused by *C difficile* and staphylococci. It undergoes renal elimination. Vancomycin is commonly considered the drug of first choice for parenteral use against methicillin-resistant staphylococci. The answer is **A.**

CHECKLIST

When you complete this chapter, you should be able to:

❑ Describe the mechanism of antibacterial action of beta-lactam antibiotics.

❑ Describe 3 mechanisms underlying the resistance of bacteria to beta-lactam antibiotics.

❑ Identify the prototype drugs in each subclass of penicillins, and describe their antibacterial activity and clinical uses.

❑ Identify the 4 subclasses of cephalosporins, and describe their antibacterial activities and clinical uses.

❑ List the major adverse effects of the penicillins and the cephalosporins.

❑ Identify the important features of aztreonam, imipenem, and meropenem.

❑ Describe the clinical uses and toxicities of vancomycin.

DRUG SUMMARY TABLE: Beta-Lactam & Other Cell Wall Membrane-Active Antibiotics[a]

Subclass	Activity Spectrum & Clinical Uses	Pharmacokinetics & Interactions	Toxicities
Penicillins			
Narrow spectrum			
Penase-susceptible Penicillin G Penicillin V	Streptococcal and meningococcal infections • syphilis	Rapid renal elimination; short half-lives necessitate frequent dosing • some biliary clearance of nafcillin and oxacillin	Hypersensitivity reactions (~5–6% incidence) • assume complete cross-reactivity; GI distress and maculopapular rash (ampicillin)
Penase–resistant Nafcillin Oxacillin	Staphylococcal infections		
Wider spectrum (+/–) penicillinase inhibitor Ampicillin Amoxicillin Piperacillin Ticarcillin	Greater activity vs gram-negative bacteria All penicillins (and cephalosporins) are bactericidal		
Cephalosporins			
First generation Cephalexin, others	Skin, soft tissue UT infections	Oral use for older drugs Mostly IV for newer drugs • renal elimination Short half-lives Third-generation drugs enter CNS	Hypersensitivity reactions (~2% incidence) • assume complete cross-reactivity between cephalosporins • partial with penicillins • GI distress
Second generation Cefotetan Cefoxitin Cefuroxime	More active vs *S pneumoniae* and *H inflenzae*; *B fragilis* (cefotetan)		
Third generation Ceftriaxone Cefotaxime Ceftazidime	Many uses including pneumonia, meningitis, and gonorrhea		
Fourth generation Cefipime	Broad activity, beta-lactamase-stable		
Carbapenems			
Imipenem-cilastatin Doripenem Meropenem Ertapenem	Broad spectrum includes some PRSP strains (not MRSA), gram-negative rods, and *Pseudomonas* sp	Parenteral; cilastatin inhibits renal metabolism of imipenem • renal elimination	Partial cross-reactivity with penicillins • CNS effects include confusion and seizures

(Continued)

DRUG SUMMARY TABLE: Beta-Lactam & Other Cell Wall Membrane-Active Antibiotics[a] (*Continued*)

Subclass	Activity Spectrum & Clinical Uses	Pharmacokinetics & Interactions	Toxicities
Monobactams			
Aztreonam	Active only vs gram-negative bacteria: *Klebsiella, Pseudomonas*, and *Serratia* spp	Parenteral use • renal elimination	GI upsets, headache, vertigo • no cross-allergenicity with beta-lactams
Glycopeptides			
Vancomycin Teicoplanin	Gram-positive activity includes MRSA and PRSP strains Teicoplanin as for vancomycin	Parenteral (oral for *C difficile* colitis) • renal elimination IV only, long half-life	"Red-man" syndrome, rare nephrotoxicity
Lipopeptide			
Daptomycin	Gram-positive activity; used in endocarditis and sepsis	Renal elimination	Myopathy • monitor CPK weekly

[a]*All the drugs listed are bactericidal cell wall synthesis inhibitors except daptomycin, which destabilizes bacterial cell membranes. CPK, creatine phosphokinase; MRSA, methicillin-resistant Staphyloccus aureus; PRSP, penicillin-resistant Streptococcus pneumoniae; UT, urinary tract.*

Chloramphenicol, Tetracyclines, Macrolides, Clindamycin, Streptogramins, & Linezolid

---

The antimicrobial drugs reviewed in this chapter selectively inhibit bacterial protein synthesis. The mechanisms of protein synthesis in microorganisms are not identical to those of mammalian cells. Bacteria have 70S ribosomes, whereas mammalian cells have 80S ribosomes. Differences exist in ribosomal subunits and in the chemical composition and functional specificities of component nucleic acids and proteins. Such differences form the basis for the selective toxicity of these drugs against microorganisms without causing major effects on protein synthesis in mammalian cells.

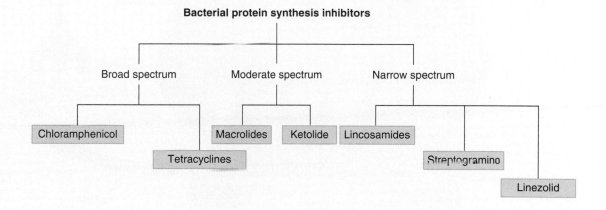

Bacterial protein synthesis inhibitors

INHIBITORS OF MICROBIAL PROTEIN SYNTHESIS

Drugs that inhibit protein synthesis vary considerably in terms of chemical structures and their spectrum of antimicrobial activity. Chloramphenicol, tetracyclines, and the aminoglycosides (see Chapter 45) were the first inhibitors of bacterial protein synthesis to be discovered. Because they had a broad spectrum of antibacterial activity and were thought to have low toxicities, they were overused. Many once highly susceptible bacterial species have become resistant, and most of these drugs are now used for more selected targets. Erythromycin, an older macrolide antibiotic, has a narrower spectrum of action but continues to be active against several important pathogens. Azithromycin and clarithromycin, semisynthetic macrolides, have some distinctive properties compared with erythromycin, as does clindamycin. Newer inhibitors of microbial protein synthesis, which include streptogramins, linezolid, telithromycin, and tigecycline (a tetracycline analog), have activity against certain bacteria that have developed resistance to older antibiotics.

MECHANISMS OF ACTION

Most of the antibiotics reviewed in this chapter are bacteriostatic inhibitors of protein synthesis acting at the ribosomal level (Figure 44–1). With the exception of tetracyclines, the binding sites for these antibiotics are on the 50S ribosomal subunit. Chloramphenicol inhibits transpeptidation (catalyzed by peptidyl transferase) by blocking the binding of the aminoacyl moiety of the charged transfer RNA (tRNA) molecule to the acceptor site on the ribosome-messenger (mRNA) complex. Thus, the peptide at the donor site cannot be transferred to its amino acid acceptor. Macrolides, telithromycin, and clindamycin, which share a common binding site on the 50S ribosome, also block transpeptidation. Tetracyclines bind to the 30S ribosomal subunit preventing binding of amino acid-charged tRNA to the acceptor site of the ribosome-mRNA complex.

Streptogramins are bactericidal for most susceptible organisms. They bind to the 50S ribosomal subunit, constricting the exit channel on the ribosome through which nascent polypeptides are extruded. In addition, tRNA synthetase activity is inhibited, leading to a decrease in free tRNA within the cell. Linezolid is mainly bacteriostatic. The drug binds to a unique site on the 50S ribosome, inhibiting initiation by blocking formation of the tRNA-ribosome-mRNA ternary complex.

Selective toxicity of these protein synthesis inhibitors against microorganisms may be explained by target differences. Chloramphenicol does not bind to the 80S ribosomal RNA of mammalian cells, although it can inhibit the functions of *mitochondrial* ribosomes, which contain 70S ribosomal RNA. Tetracyclines have little effect on mammalian protein synthesis because an active efflux mechanism prevents their intracellular accumulation.

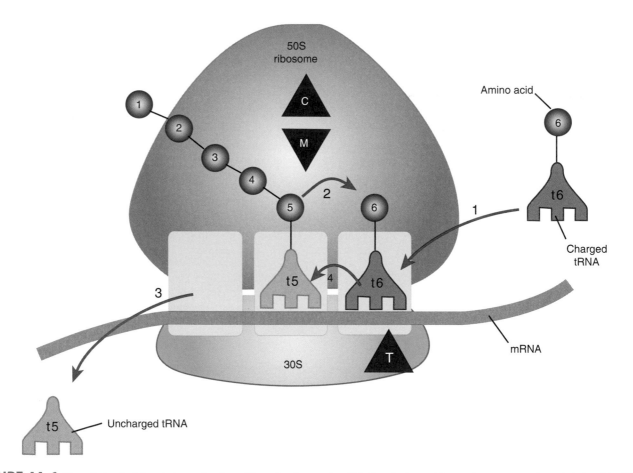

FIGURE 44–1 Steps in bacterial protein synthesis and targets of several antibiotics. Amino acids are shown as numbered circles. The 70S ribosomal mRNA complex is shown with its 50S and 30S subunits. In step 1, the charged tRNA unit carrying amino acid 6 binds to the acceptor site on the 70S ribosome. The peptidyl tRNA at the donor site, with amino acids 1 through 5, then binds the growing amino acid chain to amino acid 6 (transpeptidation, step 2). The uncharged tRNA left at the donor site is released (step 3), and the new 6-amino acid chain with its tRNA shifts to the peptidyl site (translocation, step 4). The antibiotic-binding sites are shown schematically as triangles. Chloramphenicol (C) and macrolides (M) bind to the 50S subunit and block transpeptidation (step 2). The tetracyclines (T) bind to the 30S subunit and prevent binding of the incoming charged tRNA unit (step 1). (Reproduced, with permission, from Katzung BG, editor: *Basic & Clinical Pharmacology,* 12th ed. McGraw-Hill, 2012: Fig. 44–1.)

CHLORAMPHENICOL

A. Classification and Pharmacokinetics

Chloramphenicol has a simple and distinctive structure, and no other antimicrobials have been discovered in this chemical class. It is effective orally as well as parenterally and is widely distributed readily crossing the placental and blood-brain barriers. Chloramphenicol undergoes enterohepatic cycling, and a small fraction of the dose is excreted in the urine unchanged. Most of the drug is inactivated by a hepatic glucuronosyltransferase.

B. Antimicrobial Activity

Chloramphenicol has a wide spectrum of antimicrobial activity and is usually bacteriostatic. Some strains of *Haemophilus influenzae, Neisseria meningitidis,* and *Bacteroides* are highly susceptible, and for these organisms chloramphenicol may be bactericidal. It is not active against *Chlamydia* species. Resistance to chloramphenicol, which is plasmid-mediated, occurs through the formation of acetyltransferases that inactivate the drug.

C. Clinical Uses

Because of its toxicity, chloramphenicol has very few uses as a systemic drug. It is a backup drug for severe infections caused by *Salmonella* species and for the treatment of pneumococcal and meningococcal meningitis in beta-lactam–sensitive persons. Chloramphenicol is sometimes used for rickettsial diseases and for infections caused by anaerobes such as *Bacteroides fragilis.* The drug is commonly used as a topical antimicrobial agent.

D. Toxicity

1. Gastrointestinal disturbances—These conditions may occur from direct irritation and from superinfections, especially candidiasis.

2. Bone marrow—Inhibition of red cell maturation leads to a decrease in circulating erythrocytes. This action is dose-dependent and reversible. Aplastic anemia is a rare idiosyncratic reaction (approximately 1 case in 25,000–40,000 patients treated). It is usually irreversible and may be fatal.

3. Gray baby syndrome—This syndrome occurs in infants and is characterized by decreased red blood cells, cyanosis, and cardiovascular collapse. Neonates, especially those who are premature, are deficient in hepatic glucuronosyltransferase and are sensitive to doses of chloramphenicol, which would be tolerated in older infants.

4. Drug interactions—Chloramphenicol inhibits hepatic drug-metabolizing enzymes, thus increasing the elimination half-lives of drug including phenytoin, tolbutamide and warfarin.

TETRACYCLINES

A. Classification

Drugs in this class are broad-spectrum bacteriostatic antibiotics that have only minor differences in their activities against specific organisms.

B. Pharmacokinetics

Oral absorption is variable, especially for the older drugs, and may be impaired by foods and multivalent cations (calcium, iron, aluminum). Tetracyclines have a wide tissue distribution and cross the placental barrier. All the tetracyclines undergo enterohepatic cycling. Doxycycline is excreted mainly in feces; the other drugs are eliminated primarily in the urine. The half-lives of doxycycline and minocycline are longer than those of other tetracyclines. Tigecycline, formulated only for IV use, is eliminated in the bile and has a half-life of 30–36 h.

C. Antibacterial Activity

Tetracyclines are broad-spectrum antibiotics with activity against gram-positive and gram-negative bacteria, species of *Rickettsia, Chlamydia, Mycoplasma,* and some protozoa.

However, resistance to most tetracyclines is widespread. Resistance mechanisms include the development of mechanisms (efflux pumps) for active extrusion of tetracyclines and the formation of ribosomal protection proteins that interfere with tetracycline binding. These mechanisms do not confer resistance to tigecycline in most organisms, with the exception of the multidrug efflux pumps of *Proteus* and *Pseudomonas* species.

D. Clinical Uses

1. Primary uses—Tetracyclines are recommended in the treatment of infections caused by *Mycoplasma pneumoniae* (in adults), chlamydiae, rickettsiae, vibrios, and some spirochetes. Doxycycline is currently an alternative to macrolides in the initial treatment of community-acquired pneumonia.

2. Secondary uses—Tetracyclines are alternative drugs in the treatment of syphilis. They are also used in the treatment of respiratory infections caused by susceptible organisms, for prophylaxis against infection in chronic bronchitis, in the treatment of leptospirosis, and in the treatment of acne.

3. Selective uses—Specific tetracyclines are used in the treatment of gastrointestinal ulcers caused by *Helicobacter pylori* (tetracycline), in Lyme disease (doxycycline), and in the meningococcal carrier state (minocycline). Doxycycline is also used for the prevention of malaria and in the treatment of amebiasis (Chapter 52). Demeclocycline inhibits the renal actions of antidiuretic hormone (ADH) and is used in the management of patients with ADH-secreting tumors (Chapter 15).

4. Tigecycline—Unique features of this glycylcycline derivative of minocycline include a broad spectrum of action that includes organisms resistant to standard tetracyclines. The antimicrobial activity of tigecycline includes gram-positive cocci resistant to methicillin (MRSA strains) and vancomycin (VRE strains), beta-lactamase–producing gram-negative bacteria, anaerobes, chlamydiae, and mycobacteria. The drug is formulated only for intravenous use.

E. Toxicity

1. Gastrointestinal disturbances—Effects on the gastrointestinal system range from mild nausea and diarrhea to severe, possibly life-threatening enterocolitis. Disturbances in the normal flora may lead to candidiasis (oral and vaginal) and, more rarely, to bacterial superinfections with *S aureus* or *Clostridium difficile*.

2. Bony structures and teeth—Fetal exposure to tetracyclines may lead to tooth enamel dysplasia and irregularities in bone growth. Although usually contraindicated in pregnancy, there may be situations in which the benefit of tetracyclines outweigh the risk. Treatment of younger children may cause enamel dysplasia and crown deformation when permanent teeth appear.

3. Hepatic toxicity—High doses of tetracyclines, especially in pregnant patients and those with preexisting hepatic disease, may impair liver function and lead to hepatic necrosis.

4. Renal toxicity—One form of renal tubular acidosis, Fanconi's syndrome, has been attributed to the use of outdated tetracyclines. Though not directly nephrotoxic, tetracyclines may exacerbate preexisting renal dysfunction.

5. Photosensitivity—Tetracyclines, especially demeclocycline, may cause enhanced skin sensitivity to ultraviolet light.

6. Vestibular toxicity—Dose-dependent reversible dizziness and vertigo have been reported with doxycycline and minocycline.

MACROLIDES

A. Classification and Pharmacokinetics

The macrolide antibiotics (**erythromycin, azithromycin,** and **clarithromycin**) are large cyclic lactone ring structures with attached sugars. The drugs have good oral bioavailability, but azithromycin absorption is impeded by food. Macrolides distribute to most body tissues, but azithromycin is unique in that the levels achieved in tissues and in phagocytes are considerably higher than those in the plasma. The elimination of erythromycin (via biliary excretion) and clarithromycin (via hepatic metabolism and urinary excretion of intact drug) is fairly rapid (half-lives of 2 and 6 h, respectively). Azithromycin is eliminated slowly (half-life 2–4 days), mainly in the urine as unchanged drug.

B. Antibacterial Activity

Erythromycin has activity against many species of *Campylobacter, Chlamydia, Mycoplasma, Legionella,* gram-positive cocci, and some gram-negative organisms. The spectra of activity of azithromycin and clarithromycin are similar but include greater activity against species of *Chlamydia, Mycobacterium avium* complex, and *Toxoplasma*.

Azithromycin is also effective in gonorrhea, as an alternative to ceftriaxone and in syphilis, as an alternative to penicillin G. Resistance to the macrolides in gram-positive organisms involves efflux pump mechanisms and the production of a methylase that adds a methyl group to the ribosomal binding site. Cross-resistance between individual macrolides is complete. In the case of methylase-producing microbial strains, there is partial cross-resistance with other drugs that bind to the same ribosomal site as macrolides, including clindamycin and streptogramins. Resistance in *Enterobacteriaceae* is the result of formation of drug-metabolizing esterases.

C. Clinical Uses

Erythromycin is effective in the treatment of infections caused by *M pneumoniae, Corynebacterium, Campylobacter jejuni, Chlamydia trachomatis, Chlamydophila pneumoniae, Legionella pneumophila, Ureaplasma urealyticum,* and *Bordetella pertussis*. The drug is also active against gram-positive cocci (but not penicillin-resistant *Streptococcus pneumoniae* [PRSP] strains) and beta-lactamase–producing staphylococci (but not methicillin-resistant *S aureus* [MRSA] strains).

Azithromycin has a similar spectrum of activity but is more active against *H influenzae, Moraxella catarrhalis,* and *Neisseria*. Because of its long half-life, a single dose of azithromycin is effective in the treatment of urogenital infections caused by *C trachomatis,* and a 4-day course of treatment has been effective in community-acquired pneumonia.

Clarithromycin has almost the same spectrum of antimicrobial activity and clinical uses as erythromycin. The drug is also used for prophylaxis against and treatment of *M avium* complex and as a component of drug regimens for ulcers caused by *H pylori*.

Fidaxomicin is a narrow-spectrum macrolide antibiotic that inhibits bacterial protein synthesis and is selectively active against gram-positive aerobes and anaerobes. Given orally, systemic absorption is minimal. Fidaxomicin has proved to be as effective as vancomycin for the treatment of *C difficile* colitis, possibly with a lower relapse rate.

D. Toxicity

Adverse effects, especially with erythromycin, include gastrointestinal irritation (common) via stimulation of motolin receptors, skin rashes, and eosinophilia. A hypersensitivity-based acute cholestatic hepatitis may occur with erythromycin estolate. Hepatitis is rare in children, but there is an increased risk with erythromycin estolate in the pregnant patient. Erythromycin inhibits several forms of hepatic cytochrome P450 and can increase the plasma levels of many drugs, including anticoagulants, carbamazepine, cisapride, digoxin, and theophylline. Similar drug interactions have also occurred with clarithromycin. The lactone ring structure of azithromycin is slightly different from that of other macrolides, and drug interactions are uncommon because azithromycin does not inhibit hepatic cytochrome P450.

TELITHROMYCIN

Telithromycin is a ketolide structurally related to macrolides. The drug has the same mechanism of action as erythromycin and a similar spectrum of antimicrobial activity. However, some macrolide-resistant strains are susceptible to telithromycin because it binds more tightly to ribosomes and is a poor substrate for bacterial efflux pumps that mediate resistance. The drug can be used in community-acquired pneumonia including infections caused by multidrug-resistant organisms. Telithromycin is given orally once daily and is eliminated in the bile and the urine. The adverse effects of telithromycin include hepatic dysfunction and prolongation of the QTc interval. The drug is an inhibitor of the CYP3A4 drug-metabolizing system.

CLINDAMYCIN

A. Classification and Pharmacokinetics

Clindamycin inhibits bacterial protein synthesis via a mechanism similar to that of the macrolides, although it is not chemically related. Mechanisms of resistance include methylation of the binding site on the 50S ribosomal subunit and enzymatic inactivation. Gram-negative aerobes are intrinsically resistant because of poor penetration of clindamycin through the outer membrane. Cross-resistance between clindamycin and macrolides is common. Good tissue penetration occurs after oral absorption. Clindamycin undergoes hepatic metabolism, and both intact drug and metabolites are eliminated by biliary and renal excretion.

B. Clinical Use and Toxicity

The main use of clindamycin is in the treatment of severe infections caused by certain anaerobes such as *Bacteroides*. Clindamycin has been used as a backup drug against gram-positive cocci (it is active against community-acquired strains of methicillin-resistant *S aureus*) and is recommended for prophylaxis of endocarditis in valvular disease patients who are allergic to penicillin. The drug is also active against *Pneumocystis jiroveci* and is used in combination with pyrimethamine for AIDS-related toxoplasmosis. The toxicity of clindamycin includes gastrointestinal irritation, skin rashes, neutropenia, hepatic dysfunction, and possible superinfections such as *C difficile* pseudomembranous colitis.

STREPTOGRAMINS

Quinupristin-dalfopristin, a combination of 2 streptogramins, is bactericidal (see prior discussion of mechanism of action) and has a duration of antibacterial activity longer than the half-lives of the 2 compounds (postantibiotic effects). Antibacterial activity includes penicillin-resistant pneumococci, methicillin-resistant (MRSA) and vancomycin-resistant staphylococci (VRSA), and

resistant *E faecium*; *E faecalis* is intrinsically resistant via an efflux transport system. Administered intravenously, the combination product may cause pain and an arthralgia-myalgia syndrome. Streptogramins are potent inhibitors of CYP3A4 and increase plasma levels of many drugs, including astemizole, cisapride, cyclosporine, diazepam, nonnucleoside reverse transcriptase inhibitors, and warfarin.

LINEZOLID

The first of a novel class of antibiotics (oxazolidinones), linezolid is active against drug-resistant gram-positive cocci, including strains resistant to penicillins (eg, MRSA, PRSP) and vancomycin (eg, VRE). The drug is also active against *L monocytogenes* and corynebacteria. Linezolid binds to a unique site located on the 23S ribosomal RNA of the 50S ribosomal subunit, and there is currently no cross-resistance with other protein synthesis inhibitors. Resistance (rare to date) involves a decreased affinity of linezolid for its binding site. Linezolid is available in both oral and parenteral formulations and should be reserved for treatment of infections caused by multidrug-resistant gram-positive bacteria. The drug is metabolized by the liver and has an elimination half-life of 4–6 h. Thrombocytopenia and neutropenia occur, most commonly in immunosuppressed patients. Linezolid has been implicated in the serotonin syndrome when used in patients taking selective serotonin reuptake inhibitors (SSRIs).

QUESTIONS

1. A 2-year-old child is brought to the hospital after ingesting pills that a parent had used for bacterial dysentery when traveling outside the United States. The child has been vomiting for more than 24 h and has had diarrhea with green stools. He is now lethargic with an ashen color. Other signs and symptoms include hypothermia, hypotension, and abdominal distention. The drug most likely to be the cause of this problem is
   (A) Ampicillin
   (B) Chloramphenicol
   (C) Clindamycin
   (D) Doxycycline
   (E) Erythromycin

2. The mechanism of antibacterial action of doxycycline involves
   (A) Antagonism of bacterial translocase activity
   (B) Binding to a component of the 50S ribosomal subunit
   (C) Inhibition of DNA-dependent RNA polymerase
   (D) Interference with binding of aminoacyl-tRNA to bacterial ribosomes
   (E) Selective inhibition of ribosomal peptidyl transferases

3. Clarithromycin and erythromycin have very similar spectra of antimicrobial activity. The major advantage of clarithromycin is that it
   (A) Does not inhibit hepatic drug-metabolizing enzymes
   (B) Eradicates mycoplasmal infections in a single dose
   (C) Has greater activity against *M avium-intracellulare* complex
   (D) Is active against methicillin-resistant strains of staphylococci
   (E) Is active against strains of streptococci that are resistant to erythromycin

4. The primary mechanism of resistance of gram-positive organisms to erythromycin is
(A) Decreased activity of uptake mechanisms
(B) Decreased drug permeability of the cytoplasmic membrane
(C) Formation of drug-inactivating acetyltransferases
(D) Formation of esterases that hydrolyze the lactone ring
(E) Methylation of binding sites on the 50S ribosomal subunit

5. A 26-year-old woman was treated for a suspected chlamydial infection at a neighborhood clinic. She was given a prescription for oral doxycycline to be taken for 10 d. Three weeks later, she returned to the clinic with a mucopurulent cervicitis. On questioning she admitted not having the prescription filled. The best course of action at this point would be to
(A) Delay drug treatment until the infecting organism is identified
(B) Rewrite the original prescription for oral doxycycline
(C) Treat her in the clinic with a single oral dose of cefixime
(D) Treat her in the clinic with a single oral dose of azithromycin
(E) Write a prescription for oral erythromycin for 10 d

6. A 55-year-old patient with a prosthetic heart valve is to undergo a periodontal procedure involving scaling and root planing. Several years ago, the patient had a severe allergic reaction to procaine penicillin G. Regarding prophylaxis against bacterial endocarditis, which one of the following drugs taken orally is most appropriate?
(A) Amoxicillin 10 min before the procedure
(B) Clindamycin 1 h before the procedure
(C) Erythromycin 1 h before the procedure and 4 h after the procedure
(D) Vancomycin 15 min before the procedure
(E) No prophylaxis is needed because this patient is in the negligible risk category

Questions 7–9. A 24-year-old woman comes to a clinic with complaints of dry cough, headache, fever, and malaise, which have lasted 3 or 4 d. She appears to have some respiratory difficulty, and chest examination reveals rales but no other obvious signs of pulmonary involvement. However, extensive patchy infiltrates are seen on chest x-ray film. Gram stain of expectorated sputum fails to reveal any bacterial pathogens. The patient mentions that a colleague at work has similar symptoms to those she is experiencing. The patient has no history of serious medical problems. She takes loratadine for allergies and supplementary iron tablets, and she drinks at least 6 cups of caffeinated coffee per day. The physician makes an initial diagnosis of community-acquired pneumonia.

7. Regarding the treatment of this patient, which of the following drugs is most suitable?
(A) Amoxicillin
(B) Clindamycin
(C) Doxycycline
(D) Linezolid
(E) Vancomycin

8. If this patient were to be treated with the macrolide erythromycin, she should
(A) Avoid exposure to sunlight
(B) Avoid taking supplementary iron tablets
(C) Decrease her intake of caffeinated beverages
(D) Discontinue loratadine temporarily
(E) Have her plasma urea nitrogen or creatinine checked before treatment

9. A 5-d course of treatment for community-acquired pneumonia would be effective in this patient with little risk of drug interactions if the drug prescribed were
(A) Ampicillin
(B) Azithromycin
(C) Clindamycin
(D) Erythromycin
(E) Vancomycin

10. Concerning quinupristin-dalfopristin, which statement is accurate?
(A) Active in treatment of infections caused by *E faecalis*
(B) Bacteriostatic
(C) Hepatotoxicity has led to FDA drug alerts
(D) Induce formation of hepatic drug-metabolizing enzymes
(E) Used in management of infections caused by multidrug-resistant streptococci

ANSWERS

1. Chloramphenicol is commonly used outside the United States for treatment of bacillary dysentery. The drug causes a dose-dependent (reversible) suppression of erythropoiesis. Although the gray baby syndrome was initially described in neonates, a similar syndrome has occurred with overdosage of chloramphenicol in older children and adults, especially those with hepatic dysfunction. The answer is **B**.

2. Doxycycline and other tetracyclines inhibit bacterial protein synthesis by interfering with the binding of aminoacyl-tRNA molecules to bacterial ribosomes. Peptidyl transferase is inhibited by chloramphenicol. The answer is **D**.

3. Clarithromycin can be administered less frequently than erythromycin, but it is not effective in single doses against susceptible organisms. Organisms resistant to erythromycin, including pneumococci and methicillin-resistant staphylococci, are also resistant to other macrolides. Drug interactions have occurred with clarithromycin through its ability to inhibit cytochrome P450. Clarithromycin is more active than erythromycin against *M avium* complex, *T gondii,* and *H pylori*. The answer is **C**.

4. Methylase production and methylation of the receptor site are established mechanisms of resistance of gram-positive organisms to macrolide antibiotics. Such enzymes may be inducible by macrolides or constitutive; in the latter case, cross-resistance occurs between macrolides and clindamycin. Increased expression of efflux pumps is also a mechanism of macrolide resistance. Esterase formation is a mechanism of macrolide resistance seen in coliforms. The answer is **E**.

5. Cervicitis or urethritis is often caused by *C trachomatis*. Such infections may develop slowly because of the long incubation period of chlamydial infection. Treatment with oral doxycycline for 14 d (as originally prescribed) would have eradicated *C trachomatis* and most other organisms commonly associated with nongonococcal cervicitis or urethritis. Given the limited compliance of this patient, the best course of action would be the administration (in the clinic) of a single oral dose of azithromycin. The answer is **D**.

6. This patient is in the high-risk category for bacterial endocarditis and should receive prophylactic antibiotics before many dental procedures. The American Heart Association recommends that clindamycin be used in patients allergic to penicillins. Oral erythromycin is not recommended because it is no more effective than clindamycin and causes more gastrointestinal side effects. Intravenous vancomycin (not oral), sometimes with gentamicin, is recommended for prophylaxis in high-risk penicillin-allergic patients undergoing genitourinary and lower gastrointestinal surgical procedures. Complete cross-allergenicity must be assumed between individual penicillins. The answer is **B.**

7. It is often difficult to establish a definite cause of community-acquired pneumonia (CAP). Approximately 86% of cases are caused by typical pathogens such as *S pneumoniae, H influenzae,* or *M catarrhalis,* and 15% are due to the nonzoonotic atypical pathogens such as *Legionella* species, *Mycoplasma* species, or *C pneumoniae.* Currently, monotherapy coverage of both typical and atypical pathogens in CAP is preferred to double-drug therapy. Preferred initial therapy includes a macrolide, doxycycline, or a quinolone active against respiratory pathogens (Chapter 46). Amoxicillin, clindamycin, and vancomycin have low activity against atypical pathogens in CAP. The answer is **C.**

8. The inhibition of liver cytochrome P450 by erythromycin has led to serious drug interactions. Although erythromycin does not inhibit loratadine metabolism, it does inhibit the CYP1A2 form of cytochrome P450, which metabolizes methylxanthines. Consequently, cardiac and/or CNS toxicity may occur with excessive ingestion of caffeine. Unlike the tetracyclines, the oral absorption of erythromycin is not affected by cations and the drug does not cause photosensitivity. Because erythromycin undergoes biliary excretion, there is little reason to assess renal function before treatment. The answer is **C.**

9. Azithromycin has a half-life of more than 70 h, which allows for once-daily dosing and a 5-d course of treatment for community-acquired pneumonia. Unlike other macrolides, azithromycin does not inhibit cytochrome P450 enzymes involved in drug metabolism. The answer is B.

10. Quinupristin-dalfopristin is bactericidal against many drug-resistant gram-positive cocci, including multidrug-resistant streptococci, MRSA, and vancomycin-resistant enterococci. The streptogramins have activity against *E faecium* (not *E fecalis*). The drugs are potent *inhibitors* of CYP3A4 and interfere with the metabolism of many other drugs. The streptogramins are not hepatotoxic. The answer is **E.**

CHECKLIST

When you complete this chapter, you should be able to:

❏ Explain (1 sentence per drug class) how these agents inhibit bacterial protein synthesis.

❏ Identify the primary mechanisms of resistance to each of these drug classes.

❏ Name the most important agents in each drug class, and list 3 clinical uses of each.

❏ Recall distinctive pharmacokinetic features of the major drugs.

❏ List the characteristic toxic effects of the major drugs in each class.

DRUG SUMMARY TABLE: Tetracyclines, Macrolides, & Other Protein Synthesis Inhibitors

Subclass	Mechanism of Action	Activity & Clinical Uses	Pharmacokinetics & Interactions	Toxicities
Tetracyclines				
Tetracycline Doxycycline Minocycline Tigecycline	Bind to 30S ribosomal subunit • bacteriostatic; tigecycline has broadest spectrum and resistance is less common	Infections due to chlamydiae, mycoplasma, rickettsiae, spirochetes, and *H pylori*; treatment of acne (low dose)	Oral, IV • renal and biliary clearance Doxycycline mainly gastrointestinal (GI) elimination and long half-life	GI upsets, deposition in developing bones and teeth, photosensitivity, superinfection
Macrolides				
Erythromycin Azithromycin Clarithromycin Telithromycin Fidaxomicin	Bind to 50S ribosomal subunit • bacteriostatic • least resistance to telithromycin	Community-acquired pneumonia, pertussis, corynebacteria, and chlamydial infections	Oral • IV for erythromycin, azithromycin Hepatic clearance, azithromycin long half-life (>40 h)	GI upsets, hepatic dysfunction • QT elongation • CYP450 inhibition (*not* azithromycin)
Lincosamide				
Clindamycin	Bind to 50S ribosomal subunit • bacteriostatic	Skin, soft tissue, and anaerobic infections	Oral, IV • hepatic clearance	GI upsets • *C difficile* colitis
Streptogramins				
Quinupristin-dalfopristin	Binds to 50S ribosomal subunit • bactericidal	Staphylococcal infections, vancomycin-resistant *E faecium*	IV • renal clearance	Infusion-related arthralgia and myalgia • CYP450 inhibition
Chloramphenicol	Binds to 50S ribosomal subunit • bacteriostatic	Wide spectrum, but mainly backup	Oral, IV; hepatic clearance, short half-life	Dose-related anemia • gray baby syndrome
Oxazolidinone				
Linezolid	Binds to 23S RNA of 50S subunit • bacteriostatic	Activity includes MRSA, PRSP, and VRE strains	Oral, IV; hepatic clearance	Dose-related anemia, neuropathy, optic neuritis • serotonin syndrome with SSRIs

MRSA, methicillin-resistant staphylococci; PRSP, penicillin-resistant pneumococci; SSRIs, selective serotonin reuptake inhibitors; VRE, vancomycin-resistant enterococci.

Aminoglycosides

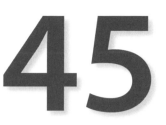
MODES OF ANTIBACTERIAL ACTION

In the treatment of microbial infections with antibiotics, multiple daily dosage regimens traditionally have been designed to maintain serum concentrations above the minimal inhibitory concentration (MIC) for as long as possible. However, the in vivo effectiveness of some antibiotics, including aminoglycosides, results from a **concentration-dependent** killing action. As the plasma level is increased above the MIC, aminoglycosides kill an increasing proportion of bacteria and do so at a more rapid rate. Many antibiotics, including penicillins and cephalosporins, cause **time-dependent** killing of microorganisms, wherein their in vivo efficacy is directly related to time above MIC and becomes independent of concentration once the MIC has been reached.

Aminoglycosides are also capable of exerting a **postantibiotic effect** such that their killing action continues when their plasma levels have declined below measurable levels. Consequently, aminoglycosides have greater efficacy when administered as a single large dose than when given as multiple smaller doses. The toxicity (in contrast to the antibacterial efficacy) of aminoglycosides depends both on a critical plasma concentration and on the time that such a level is exceeded. The time above such a threshold is shorter with administration of a single large dose of an aminoglycoside than when multiple smaller doses are given. These concepts form the basis for once-daily aminoglycoside dosing protocols, which can be more effective and less toxic than traditional dosing regimens.

PHARMACOKINETICS

Aminoglycosides are structurally related amino sugars attached by glycosidic linkages. They are polar compounds, not absorbed after oral administration, and must be given intramuscularly or intravenously for systemic effect. They have limited tissue penetration and do not readily cross the blood-brain barrier. Glomerular filtration is the major mode of excretion, and plasma levels of these drugs are greatly affected by changes in renal function. Excretion of aminoglycosides is directly proportional to creatinine clearance. With normal renal function, the elimination half-life of aminoglycosides is 2–3 h. Dosage adjustments must be made in renal insufficiency to prevent toxic accumulation. Monitoring of plasma levels of aminoglycosides is important for safe and effective dosage selection and adjustment. For traditional dosing regimens (2 or 3 times daily), peak serum levels are measured 30–60 min after administration and trough levels just before the next dose. With once-daily dosing, peak levels are less important since they will naturally be high.

MECHANISM OF ACTION

Aminoglycosides are bactericidal inhibitors of protein synthesis. Their penetration through the bacterial cell envelope is partly dependent on oxygen-dependent active transport, and they have minimal activity against strict anaerobes. Aminoglycoside transport can be enhanced by cell wall synthesis inhibitors, which may be the basis of antimicrobial synergism. Inside the cell, aminoglycosides bind to the 30S ribosomal subunit and interfere with protein synthesis in at least 3 ways: (1) they block formation of the initiation complex; (2) they cause misreading of the code on the mRNA template; and (3) they inhibit translocation (Figure 45–1). Aminoglycosides may also disrupt polysomal structure, resulting in nonfunctional monosomes.

MECHANISMS OF RESISTANCE

Streptococci, including *Streptococcus pneumoniae,* and enterococci are relatively resistant to gentamicin and most other aminoglycosides owing to failure of the drugs to penetrate into the cell. However, the primary mechanism of resistance to aminoglycosides, especially in gram-negative bacteria, involves the plasmid-mediated formation of inactivating enzymes. These enzymes are **group transferases** that catalyze the acetylation of amine functions and the transfer of phosphoryl or adenylyl groups to the oxygen atoms of hydroxyl groups on the aminoglycoside. Individual aminoglycosides have varying susceptibilities to such enzymes. For example, transferases produced by enterococci can inactivate amikacin, gentamicin, and tobramycin but not streptomycin. However, amikacin is often resistant to many enzymes that inactivate gentamicin and tobramycin. In addition, resistance to streptomycin, which is common, appears to be due to changes in the ribosomal binding site.

CLINICAL USES

The main differences among the individual aminoglycosides lie in their activities against specific organisms, particularly gram-negative rods. **Gentamicin, tobramycin,** and **amikacin** are

Normal bacterial cell

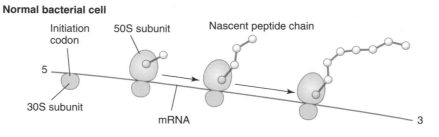

Aminoglycoside-treated bacterial cell

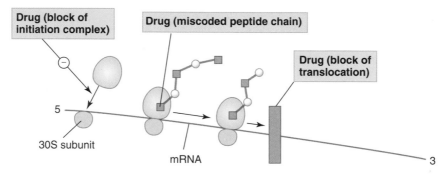

FIGURE 45–1 Putative mechanisms of action of the aminoglycosides. Normal protein synthesis is shown in the top panel. At least 3 aminoglycoside effects have been described, as shown in the bottom panel: block of formation of the initiation complex; miscoding of amino acids in the emerging peptide chain due to misreading of the mRNA; and block of translocation on mRNA. Block of movement of the ribosome may occur after the formation of a single initiation complex, resulting in an mRNA chain with only a single ribosome on it, a so-called monosome.

important drugs for the treatment of serious infections caused by aerobic gram-negative bacteria, including *Escherichia coli* and *Enterobacter, Klebsiella, Proteus, Providencia, Pseudomonas,* and *Serratia* species. These aminoglycosides also have activity against strains of *Haemophilus influenzae, Moraxella catarrhalis,* and *Shigella* species, although they are not drugs of choice for infections caused by these organisms. In most cases, aminoglycosides are used in combination with a beta-lactam antibiotic. When used alone, aminoglycosides are not reliably effective in the treatment of infections caused by gram-positive cocci. Antibacterial synergy may occur when aminoglycosides are used in combination with cell wall synthesis inhibitors. Examples include their combined use with penicillins in the treatment of pseudomonal, listerial, and enterococcal infections.

Streptomycin in combination with penicillins is often more effective in enterococcal carditis than regimens that include other aminoglycosides. This combination is also used in the treatment of tuberculosis, plague, and tularemia. Other aminoglycosides are usually effective in these conditions. Multidrug-resistant strains of *Mycobacterium tuberculosis* that are resistant to streptomycin may be susceptible to amikacin. Because of the risk of ototoxicity, streptomycin should not be used when other drugs will serve. Owing to their toxic potential, **neomycin and kanamycin** are usually restricted to topical or oral use (eg, to eliminate bowel flora). Gentamicin is also available for topical use.

Netilmicin has been used for treatment of serious infections caused by organisms resistant to the other aminoglycosides. Netilmicin is no longer available in the United States.

Spectinomycin is an aminocyclitol related to the aminoglycosides. Its sole use is as a backup drug, administered intramuscularly as a single dose for the treatment of gonorrhea, most commonly in patients allergic to beta-lactams. There is no cross-resistance with other drugs used in gonorrhea. Spectinomycin may cause pain at the injection site.

TOXICITY

A. Ototoxicity

Auditory or vestibular damage (or both) may occur with any aminoglycoside and may be irreversible. Auditory impairment is more likely with amikacin and kanamycin; vestibular dysfunction is more likely with gentamicin and tobramycin. Ototoxicity risk is proportional to the plasma levels and thus is especially high if dosage is not appropriately modified in a patient with renal dysfunction. Ototoxicity may be increased by the use of loop diuretics. Because ototoxicity has been reported after fetal exposure, the aminoglycosides are contraindicated in pregnancy unless their potential benefits are judged to outweigh risk.

B. Nephrotoxicity

Renal toxicity usually takes the form of acute tubular necrosis. This adverse effect, which is often reversible, is more common in elderly patients and in those concurrently receiving amphotericin B, cephalosporins, or vancomycin. Gentamicin and tobramycin are the most nephrotoxic.

C. Neuromuscular Blockade

Though rare, a curare-like block may occur at high doses of aminoglycosides and may result in respiratory paralysis. It is usually reversible by treatment with calcium and neostigmine, but ventilatory support may be required.

D. Skin Reactions

Allergic skin reactions may occur in patients, and contact dermatitis may occur in personnel handling the drug. Neomycin is the agent most likely to cause this adverse effect.

SKILL KEEPER: NEPHROTOXICITY

One of the characteristics of aminoglycoside antibiotics is their nephrotoxic potential. What other drugs can you identify that are known to have adverse effects on renal function? The Skill Keeper Answer appears at the end of the chapter.

QUESTIONS

1. Regarding the mechanism of action of aminoglycosides, the drugs
   (A) Are bacteriostatic
   (B) Bind to the 50S ribosomal subunit
   (C) Cause misreading of the code on the mRNA template
   (D) Inhibit peptidyl transferase
   (E) Stabilize polysomes

2. A 50-kg patient with creatinine clearance of 80 mL/min has a gram-negative infection. Amikacin is administered intramuscularly at a dose of 5 mg/kg every 8 h, and the patient begins to respond. After 2 d, creatinine clearance declines to 40 mL/min. Assuming that no information is available about amikacin plasma levels, what would be the most reasonable approach to management of the patient at this point?
   (A) Administer 5 mg/kg every 12 h
   (B) Decrease the dosage to a daily total of 200 mg
   (C) Decrease the dosage to 125 mg every 8 h
   (D) Discontinue amikacin and switch to gentamicin
   (E) Maintain the patient on the present dosage and test auditory function

3. All of the following statements about the clinical uses of the aminoglycosides are accurate EXCEPT
   (A) Effective in the treatment of infections caused by *Bacteroides fragilis*
   (B) Gentamicin is used with ampicillin for synergistic effects in the treatment of enterococcal endocarditis
   (C) Netilmicin is more likely to be effective than streptomycin in the treatment of a hospital-acquired infection caused by *Serratia marcescens*
   (D) Often used in combination with cephalosporins in the empiric treatment of life-threatening bacterial infections
   (E) Owing to their polar nature, aminoglycosides are not absorbed after oral administration

4. Which statement is accurate regarding the antibacterial action of gentamicin?
   (A) Antibacterial activity is often reduced by the presence of an inhibitor of cell wall synthesis
   (B) Antibacterial action is not concentration-dependent
   (C) Antibacterial action is time-dependent
   (D) Efficacy is directly proportional to the duration of time that the plasma level is greater than the minimal inhibitory concentration
   (E) Gentamicin continues to exert antibacterial effects even after plasma levels decrease below detectable levels

5. An adult patient (weight 60 kg) has bacteremia suspected to be due to a gram-negative rod. Tobramycin is to be administered using a once-daily dosing regimen, and the loading dose must be calculated to achieve a peak plasma level of 20 mg/L. Assume that the patient has normal renal function. Pharmacokinetic parameters of tobramycin in this patient are as follows: $V_d = 20$ L; $t_{1/2} = 3$ h; $CL = 80$ mL/min. What loading dose should be given?
   (A) 100 mg
   (B) 200 mg
   (C) 400 mg
   (D) 600 mg
   (E) 800 mg

6. A 67-year-old man is seen in a hospital emergency department complaining of pain in and behind the right ear. Physical examination shows edema of the external otic canal with purulent exudate and weakness of the muscles on the right side of the face. The patient informs the physician that he is a diabetic. Gram stain of the exudate from the ear shows many polymorphonucleocytes and gram-negative rods, and samples are sent to the microbiology laboratory for culture and drug susceptibility testing. A preliminary diagnosis is made of external otitis. At this point, which of the following is most appropriate?
   (A) Amikacin should be administered by intramuscular injection, and the patient should be sent home
   (B) Analgesics should be prescribed for pain, but antibiotics should be withheld pending the results of cultures
   (C) Oral cefaclor should be prescribed together with analgesics, and the patient should be sent home
   (D) The patient should be hospitalized and treatment started with gentamicin plus ticarcillin
   (E) The patient should be hospitalized and treatment started with intravenous imipenem-cilastatin

7. Regarding the toxicity of aminoglycosides, which statement is accurate?
   (A) Gentamicin and tobramycin are the least likely to cause renal damage
   (B) Ototoxicity due to amikacin and gentamicin includes vestibular dysfunction that is often irreversible
   (C) Ototoxicity is reduced if loop diuretics are used to facilitate aminoglycoside renal excretion
   (D) Skin reactions are rare with use of topical neomycin
   (E) With traditional dosage regimens, the earliest sign of nephrotoxicity is a reduced blood creatinine

8. This drug has characteristics almost identical to those of gentamicin but has much weaker activity in combination with penicillin against enterococci.
   (A) Amikacin
   (B) Erythromycin
   (C) Netilmicin
   (D) Spectinomycin
   (E) Tobramycin

9. Your 23-year-old female patient is pregnant and has gonorrhea. The medical history includes anaphylaxis following exposure to amoxicillin. The most appropriate drug to use is
   (A) Azithromycin
   (B) Cefixime
   (C) Ceftriaxone
   (D) Ciprofloxacin
   (E) Doxycycline

10. Which statement about "once-daily" dosing with aminoglycosides is *not* accurate?
    (A) Convenient for outpatient therapy
    (B) Dosage adjustment is less important in renal insufficiency
    (C) Less nursing time is required for drug administration
    (D) Often less toxic than conventional (multiple) dosing regimens
    (E) Underdosing is less of a problem

ANSWERS

1. Aminoglycosides are bactericidal inhibitors of protein synthesis binding to specific components of the 30S ribosomal subunit. Their actions include block of the formation of the initiation complex, miscoding, and polysomal breakup. Peptidyl transferase is inhibited by chloramphenicol, not aminoglycosides. The answer is **C.**

2. Monitoring plasma drug levels is important when aminoglycosides are used. In this case, the patient seems to be improving, so a decrease of the amikacin dose in proportion to decreased creatinine clearance is most appropriate. Because creatinine clearance is only one half of the starting value, a dose reduction should be made to one half of that given initially. The answer is **C.**

3. Aminoglycoside antibiotics act at the ribosomal level and their intracellular accumulation by bacteria is oxygen dependent. Anaerobic bacteria including *B fragilis* are innately resistant. The answer is **A.**

4. The antibacterial action of aminoglycosides is concentration dependent rather than time dependent. The activity of gentamicin continues to increase as its plasma level rises above the minimal inhibitory concentration (MIC). When the plasma level falls below the MIC, gentamicin continues to exert antibacterial effects for several hours, exerting a post-antibiotic effect. Inhibitors of bacterial cell wall synthesis often exert synergistic effects with aminoglycosides, possibly by increasing the intracellular accumulation of the aminoglycoside. The answer is **E.**

5. The loading dose of any drug is calculated by multiplying the desired plasma concentration (mg/L) by the volume of distribution (L). The answer is **C.**

6. The diabetic patient with external otitis is at special risk because of the danger of spread to the middle ear and possibly the meninges, so hospitalization is advisable, especially in the elderly. Likely pathogens include *E coli* and *Pseudomonas aeruginosa,* and coverage must be provided for these and possibly other gram-negative rods. The combination of an aminoglycoside plus a wider spectrum penicillin is most suitable in this case and is synergistic against many pseudomonas strains. Imipenem-cilastatin is also possible, but resistant strains of *P aeruginosa* have emerged during treatment. Cefaclor lacks antipseudomonal activity. The answer is **D.**

7. Gentamicin and tobramycin are the most likely aminoglycosides to cause nephrotoxicity. The incidence of nephrotoxic effects with gentamicin is 2 to 3 times greater than the incidence of ototoxicity. With traditional dosage regimens, the first indication of potential nephrotoxicity is an increase in trough serum levels of aminoglycosides, which is followed by an *increase* in blood creatinine. Although ototoxicity resulting from aminoglycosides such as gentamicin and tobramycin usually involves irreversible effects on vestibular function, hearing loss can also occur. Ototoxicity is *enhanced* by loop diuretics. Skin reactions are common with topical use of neomycin. The answer is **B.**

8. Tobramycin is almost identical to gentamicin in both its pharmacodynamic and pharmacokinetic properties. However, it is much less active than either gentamicin or streptomycin when used in combination with a penicillin in the treatment of enterococcal endocarditis. The answer is **E.**

9. All of the listed drugs have been used for treatment of gonorrhea. Cephalosporins should be avoided in patients with a history of severe hypersensitivity to penicillins, and fluoroquinolones (see Chapter 46) should be avoided in pregnancy. Tetracyclines including doxycycline have been used in the past for gonorrhea, but not as single doses, and they too should be avoided in pregnancy. The answer is **A.**

10. In "once-daily dosing" with aminoglycosides, the selection of an appropriate dose is particularly critical in patients with renal insufficiency. The aminoglycosides are eliminated by the kidney in proportion to creatinine clearance. Knowledge of the degree of insufficiency, based on plasma creatinine (or BUN), is essential for estimation of the appropriate single daily dose of an aminoglycoside. The answer is **B.**

SKILL KEEPER ANSWER: NEPHROTOXICITY

Drugs with nephrotoxic potential include ACE inhibitors, acetazolamide, aminoglycosides, aspirin, amphotericin B, cyclosporine, furosemide, gold salts, lithium, methicillin, methoxyflurane, NSAIDs, pentamidine, sulfonamides, tetracyclines (degraded), thiazides, and triamterene.

CHECKLIST

When you complete this chapter, you should be able to:

❑ Describe 3 actions of aminoglycosides on protein synthesis and 2 mechanisms of resistance to this class of drugs.

❑ List the major clinical applications of aminoglycosides and identify their 2 main toxicities.

❑ Describe aminoglycoside pharmacokinetic characteristics with reference to their renal clearance and potential toxicity.

❑ Understand time-dependent and concentration-dependent killing actions of antibiotics and what is meant by "postantibiotic effect."

DRUG SUMMARY TABLE: Aminoglycosides & Spectinomycin

Drugs	Mechanism of Action	Activity & Clinical Uses	Pharmacokinetics & Interactions	Toxicities
Gentamicin Tobramycin Amikacin Streptomycin Neomycin Spectinomycin	Bactericidal • inhibit protein synthesis via binding to 30S ribosomal subunit • amikacin least resistance • concentration-dependent action; also exert postantibiotic effects	Aerobic gram-negative bacteria, *H influenzae, M catarrhalis, and Shigella* species • often used in combinations with beta-lactams Gonorrhea (spectinomycin, IM) • tuberculosis (streptomycin, IM)	IV • renal clearance with half-lives 2–4 h • once-daily dosing effective with less toxicity • oral and topical (neomycin, gentamicin)	Nephrotoxicity (reversible), ototoxicity (irreversible), neuromuscular blockade

46

Sulfonamides, Trimethoprim, & Fluoroquinolones

Sulfonamides and trimethoprim are antimetabolites selectively toxic to microorganisms because they interfere with folic acid synthesis. Sulfonamides continue to be used selectively as individual antimicrobial agents, although resistance is common. The combination of a sulfonamide with trimethoprim causes a sequential blockade of folic acid synthesis. This results in a synergistic action against a wide spectrum of microorganisms; resistance occurs but has been relatively slow in development.

Fluoroquinolones, which selectively inhibit microbial nucleic acid metabolism, also have a broad spectrum of antimicrobial activity that includes many common pathogens. Resistance has emerged to the older antibiotics in this class but has been offset to some extent by the introduction of newer fluoroquinolones with expanded activity against common pathogenic organisms.

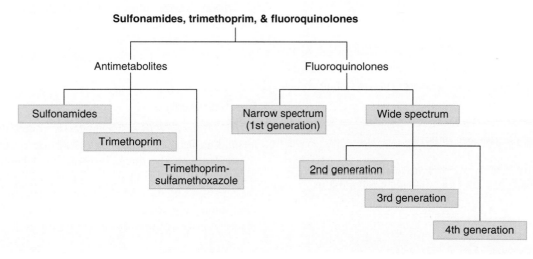

ANTIFOLATE DRUGS

A. Classification and Pharmacokinetics

The antifolate drugs used in the treatment of infectious diseases are the sulfonamides, which inhibit microbial enzymes involved in folic acid synthesis, and trimethoprim, a selective inhibitor of dihydrofolate reductase.

1. Sulfonamides—The sulfonamides are weakly acidic compounds that have a common chemical nucleus resembling *p*-aminobenzoic acid (PABA). Members of this group differ mainly in their pharmacokinetic properties and clinical uses. Pharmacokinetic features include modest tissue penetration, hepatic metabolism, and excretion of both intact drug and acetylated metabolites in the urine. Solubility may be decreased in acidic urine, resulting in precipitation of the drug or its metabolites. Because of the solubility limitation, a combination of 3 separate sulfonamides (**triple sulfa**) has been used to reduce the likelihood that any one drug will precipitate. The sulfonamides may be classified as short-acting (eg, sulfisoxazole), intermediate-acting (eg, sulfamethoxazole), and long-acting (eg, sulfadoxine). Sulfonamides bind to plasma proteins at sites shared by bilirubin and by other drugs.

2. Trimethoprim—This drug is structurally similar to folic acid. It is a weak base and is trapped in acidic environments, reaching high concentrations in prostatic and vaginal fluids. A large percentage of trimethoprim is excreted unchanged in the urine. The half-life of this drug is similar to that of sulfamethoxazole (10–12 h).

B. Mechanisms of Action

1. Sulfonamides—The sulfonamides are bacteriostatic inhibitors of folic acid synthesis. As antimetabolites of PABA, they are competitive inhibitors of dihydropteroate synthase (Figure 46–1).

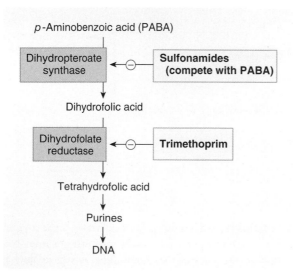

FIGURE 46–1 Inhibitory effects of sulfonamides and trimethoprim on folic acid synthesis. Inhibition of 2 successive steps in the formation of tetrahydrofolic acid constitutes sequential blockade and results in antibacterial synergy.

They can also act as substrates for this enzyme, resulting in the synthesis of nonfunctional forms of folic acid. The selective toxicity of sulfonamides results from the inability of mammalian cells to synthesize folic acid; they must use preformed folic acid that is present in the diet.

2. Trimethoprim—Trimethoprim is a selective inhibitor of bacterial dihydrofolate reductase that prevents formation of the active tetrahydro form of folic acid (Figure 46–1). Bacterial dihydrofolate reductase is 4–5 orders of magnitude more sensitive to inhibition by trimethoprim than the human enzyme.

3. Trimethoprim plus sulfamethoxazole—When the 2 drugs are used in combination, antimicrobial synergy results from the **sequential blockade** of folate synthesis (Figure 46–1). The drug combination is bactericidal against susceptible organisms.

C. Resistance

Bacterial resistance to sulfonamides is common and may be plasmid-mediated. It can result from decreased intracellular accumulation of the drugs, increased production of PABA by bacteria, or a decrease in the sensitivity of dihydropteroate synthase to the sulfonamides. Clinical resistance to trimethoprim most commonly results from the production of dihydrofolate reductase that has a reduced affinity for the drug.

D. Clinical Use

1. Sulfonamides—The sulfonamides are active against gram-positive and gram-negative organisms, *Chlamydia*, and *Nocardia*. Specific members of the sulfonamide group are used by the following routes for the conditions indicated:

a. Simple urinary tract infections—Oral (eg, triple sulfa, sulfisoxazole).

b. Ocular infections—Topical (eg, sulfacetamide).

c. Burn infections—Topical (eg, mafenide, silver sulfadiazine).

d. Ulcerative colitis, rheumatoid arthritis—Oral (eg, sulfasalazine).

e. Toxoplasmosis—Oral sulfadiazine plus pyrimethamine (a dihydrofolate reductase inhibitor) plus folinic acid.

2. Trimethoprim-sulfamethoxazole (TMP-SMZ)—This drug combination is effective orally in the treatment of urinary tract infections and in respiratory, ear, and sinus infections caused by *Haemophilus influenzae* and *Moraxella catarrhalis*. In the immunocompromised patient, TMP-SMZ is used for infections due to *Aeromonas hydrophila* and is the drug of choice for prevention and treatment of pneumocystis pneumonia. An intravenous formulation is available for patients unable to take the drug by mouth and is used for treatment of severe pneumocystis pneumonia and for gram-negative sepsis. TMP-SMZ is also the drug of choice in nocardiosis, a possible backup drug for cholera, typhoid fever, and shigellosis, and has been used in the treatment of infections caused by methicillin-resistant staphylococci and *Listeria monocytogenes*.

E. Toxicity of Sulfonamides

1. Hypersensitivity—Allergic reactions, including skin rashes and fever, occur commonly. Cross-allergenicity between the individual sulfonamides should be assumed and may also occur with chemically related drugs (eg, oral hypoglycemics, thiazides). Exfoliative dermatitis, polyarteritis nodosa, and Stevens-Johnson syndrome have occurred rarely.

2. Gastrointestinal—Nausea, vomiting, and diarrhea occur commonly. Mild hepatic dysfunction can occur, but hepatitis is uncommon.

3. Hematotoxicity—Although such effects are rare, sulfonamides can cause granulocytopenia, thrombocytopenia, and aplastic anemia. Acute hemolysis may occur in persons with glucose-6-phosphate dehydrogenase deficiency.

4. Nephrotoxicity—Sulfonamides may precipitate in the urine at acidic pH, causing crystalluria and hematuria.

5. Drug interactions—Competition with warfarin and methotrexate for plasma protein binding transiently increases the plasma levels of these drugs. Sulfonamides can displace bilirubin from plasma proteins, with the risk of kernicterus in the neonate if used in the third trimester of pregnancy.

F. Toxicity of Trimethoprim

Trimethoprim may cause the predictable adverse effects of an antifolate drug, including megaloblastic anemia, leukopenia, and granulocytopenia. These effects are usually ameliorated by supplementary folinic acid. The combination of TMP-SMZ may cause any of the adverse effects associated with the sulfonamides. AIDS patients given TMP-SMZ have a high incidence of adverse effects, including fever, rashes, leukopenia, and diarrhea.

FLUOROQUINOLONES

A. Classification

Fluoroquinolines are classified by "generation" based on their antimicrobial spectrum of activity. **Norfloxacin,** a first-generation fluoroquinolone derived from nalidixic acid, has activity against the common pathogens that cause urinary tract infections. **Ciprofloxacin** and **ofloxacin** (second-generation fluoroquinolones) have greater activity against gram-negative bacteria and are also active against the gonococcus, many gram-positive cocci, mycobacteria, and agents of atypical pneumonia (*Mycoplasma pneumoniae, Chlamydophila pneumoniae*). Third-generation fluoroquinolones (**levofloxacin, gemifloxacin,** and **moxifloxacin**) are slightly less active than ciprofloxacin and ofloxacin against gram-negative bacteria but have greater activity against gram-positive cocci, including *S pneumoniae* and some strains of enterococci and methicillin-resistant *Staphylococcus aureus* (MRSA). Third-generation drugs are commonly referred to as "respiratory fluoroquinolones." The most recently introduced drugs (eg, **gemifloxacin, moxifloxacin**) are the broadest-spectrum fluoroquinolones introduced to date, with enhanced activity against anaerobes.

B. Pharmacokinetics

All the fluoroquinolones have good oral bioavailability (antacids containing multivalent cations may interfere) and penetrate most body tissues. However, norfloxacin does not achieve adequate plasma levels for use in most systemic infections. Elimination of most fluoroquinolones is through the kidneys via active tubular secretion, which can be blocked by probenecid. Dosage reductions are usually needed in renal dysfunction except for moxifloxacin which is eliminated partly by hepatic metabolism and also by biliary excretion. Use of moxifloxacin in urinary tract infections is not recommended. Half-lives of fluoroquinolones are usually in the range of 3–8 h.

C. Mechanism of Action

The fluoroquinolones interfere with bacterial DNA synthesis by inhibiting topoisomerase II (DNA gyrase), especially in gram-negative organisms and topoisomerase IV, especially in gram-positive organisms. They block the relaxation of supercoiled DNA that is catalyzed by DNA gyrase, a step required for normal transcription and duplication. Inhibition of topoisomerase IV by fluoroquinolones interferes with the separation of replicated chromosomal DNA during cell division. Fluoroquinolones are usually bactericidal against susceptible organisms. Like aminoglycosides, the fluoroquinolones exhibit postantibiotic effects, whereby bacterial growth continues to be inhibited even after the plasma concentration of the drug has fallen below the minimum inhibitory concentration of the bacterium (see Chapter 45).

D. Resistance

Fluoroquinolone resistance has emerged rapidly in the case of second-generation fluoroquinolones, especially in *Campylobacter jejuni* and gonococci, but also in gram-positive cocci (eg, MRSA), *Pseudomonas aeruginosa* and *Serratia* species. Mechanisms of resistance include decreased intracellular accumulation of the drug via the production of efflux pumps or changes in porin structure (in gram-negative bacteria). Efflux mechanisms appear to be responsible for resistance in strains of *M tuberculosis, S aureus,* and *S pneumoniae.* Changes in the sensitivity of the target enzymes via point mutations in the antibiotic binding regions are also established to confer resistance against specific fluoroquinolones. Mutations in the quinolone resistance-determining region of the *gyrA* gene that encodes DNA gyrase is responsible for resistance in gonococci.

E. Clinical Use

Fluoroquinolones are effective in the treatment of infections of the urogenital and gastrointestinal tracts caused by gram-negative organisms, including gonococci, *E coli, Klebsiella pneumoniae, Campylobacter jejuni, Enterobacter, Pseudomonas aeruginosa, Salmonella,* and *Shigella* species. They have been used widely for respiratory tract, skin, and soft tissue infections, but their effectiveness is now variable because of the emergence of resistance. Ciprofloxacin and ofloxacin in single oral doses have been used as alternatives to ceftriaxone or cefixime in gonorrhea, but they are not currently recommended because resistance is now common. Ofloxacin eradicates *Chlamydia trachomatis,* but a 7-d course of treatment is required. Levofloxacin has activity against most organisms associated with community-acquired pneumonia, including chlamydiae, mycoplasma, and legionella species. Gemifloxacin and moxifloxacin have the widest spectrum of activity, which includes both gram-positive and gram-negative organisms, atypical pneumonia agents, and some anaerobic bacteria. Fluoroquinolones have also been used in the meningococcal carrier state, in the treatment of tuberculosis, and in prophylactic management of neutropenic patients.

F. Toxicity

Gastrointestinal distress is the most common adverse effect. The fluoroquinolones may cause skin rashes, headache, dizziness, insomnia, abnormal liver function tests, phototoxicity, and both tendinitis and tendon rupture. Opportunistic infections caused by *C albicans* and streptococci have occurred. The fluoroquinolones are not recommended for children or pregnant women because they may damage growing cartilage and cause arthropathy. Fluoroquinolones may increase the plasma levels of theophylline and other methylxanthines, enhancing their toxicity. Newer fluoroquinolones (gemifloxacin, levofloxacin, moxifloxacin) prolong the QTc interval. They should be avoided in patients with known QTc prolongation and those on certain antiarrhythmic drugs (Chapter 14) or other drugs that increase the QTc interval.

QUESTIONS

1. Trimethoprim-sulfamethoxazole is established to be effective against which of the following opportunistic infections in the AIDS patient?
   (A) Cryptococcal meningitis
   (B) Disseminated herpes simplex
   (C) Oral candidiasis
   (D) Toxoplasmosis
   (E) Tuberculosis

2. A 24-year-old woman has returned from a vacation abroad suffering from traveler's diarrhea, and her problem has not responded to antidiarrheal drugs. A pathogenic gram-negative bacillus is suspected. Which drug is most likely to be effective in the treatment of this patient?
   (A) Amoxicillin
   (B) Ciprofloxacin
   (C) Sulfacetamide
   (D) Trimethoprim
   (E) Vancomycin

3. Which statement about the clinical use of sulfonamides is false?
   (A) Active against *C trachomatis* and can be used topically for the treatment of chlamydial infections of the eye
   (B) Are not effective as sole agents in the treatment of prostatitis
   (C) Effective in Rocky Mountain spotted fever in patients allergic to tetracyclines
   (D) Resistance can occur in some strains of bacteria because of increased production of PABA
   (E) Some resistant bacterial strains exhibit decreased intracellular accumulation of sulfonamides

4. A 31-year-old man has gonorrhea. He has no drug allergies, but a few years ago acute hemolysis followed use of an antimalarial drug. The physician is concerned that the patient has an accompanying urethritis caused by *C trachomatis,* although no cultures or enzyme tests have been performed. Which of the following drugs will be reliably effective against both gonococci and *C trachomatis* and safe to use in this patient?
   (A) Cefixime
   (B) Ciprofloxacin
   (C) Spectinomycin
   (D) Sulfamethoxazole-trimethoprim
   (E) None of the above

5. Which statement about the fluoroquinolones is accurate?
   (A) A fluoroquinolone is the drug of choice for treatment of an uncomplicated urinary tract infection in a 7-year-old girl
   (B) Antacids increase the oral bioavailability of fluoroquinolones
   (C) Gonococcal resistance to fluoroquinolones may involve changes in DNA gyrase
   (D) Modification of moxifloxacin dosage is required in patients when creatinine clearance is less than 50 mL/min
   (E) The fluoroquinolones are contraindicated in patients with hepatic dysfunction

6. A 55-year-old man complains of periodic bouts of diarrhea with lower abdominal cramping and intermittent rectal bleeding. Seen in the clinic, he appears well nourished, with blood pressure in the normal range. Examination reveals moderate abdominal pain and tenderness. His current medications are limited to loperamide for his diarrhea. Sigmoidoscopy reveals mucosal edema, friability, and some pus. Laboratory findings include mild anemia and decreased serum albumin. Microbiologic examination via stool cultures and mucosal biopsies do not reveal any evidence for bacterial, amebic, or cytomegalovirus involvement. The most appropriate drug to use in this patient is
   (A) Amoxicillin
   (B) Ciprofloxacin
   (C) Doxycycline
   (D) Sulfasalazine
   (E) Trimethoprim-sulfamethoxazole

7. Which adverse effect is most likely to occur with sulfonamides?
   (A) Fanconi's aminoaciduria syndrome
   (B) Hematuria
   (C) Kernicterus in the newborn
   (D) Neurologic dysfunction
   (E) Skin reactions

8. Which drug is effective in the treatment of nocardiosis and, in combination with pyrimethamine, is prophylactic against *Pneumocystis jiroveci* infections in AIDS patients?
   (A) Amoxicillin
   (B) Ciprofloxacin
   (C) Clindamycin
   (D) Sulfadiazine
   (E) Trimethoprim

9. Which statement about ciprofloxacin is accurate?
   (A) Active against most MRSA strains of staphylococci
   (B) Antagonism occurs if it is used with inhibitors of dihydrofolate reductase
   (C) During treatment, tendinitis and even tendon rupture may occur
   (D) Most "first-time" urinary tract infections are resistant to ciprofloxacin
   (E) Organisms associated with middle ear infections are highly resistant

10. Supplementary folinic acid may prevent anemia in folate-deficient persons who use this drug; it is a weak base achieving tissue levels similar to those in plasma
   (A) Ciprofloxacin
   (B) Moxifloxacin
   (C) Sulfacetamide
   (D) Sulfamethoxazole
   (E) Trimethoprim

ANSWERS

1. Trimethoprim-sulfamethoxazole is not effective in the treatment of infections caused by viruses, fungi, or mycobacteria. However, the drug combination is active against certain protozoans, including *Toxoplasma,* and can be used for both prevention and treatment of toxoplasmosis in the AIDS patient. The answer is **D.**

2. The second-generation fluoroquinolones are very effective in diarrhea caused by bacterial gram-negative pathogens, including *E coli, Shigella,* and *Salmonella.* None of the other drugs listed would be appropriate. Many coliforms are now resistant to amoxicillin and ampicillin. Sulfacetamide is a topical agent used for bacterial conjunctivitis. Although trimethoprim is available as a single drug, resistance emerges rapidly during treatment unless it is used for urinary tract infections, in which high concentrations can be achieved. Vancomycin has no activity against gram-negative bacilli. The answer is **B.**

3. Sulfonamides have minimal therapeutic actions in rickettsial infections. Chloramphenicol may be used for Rocky Mountain spotted fever in patients with established allergy or other contraindication to tetracyclines. All of the other statements about sulfonamide antimicrobial drugs are accurate. The answer is **C.**

4. Although cefixime in a single oral dose is effective in gonorrhea (Chapter 43), it has no activity against organisms causing nongonococcal urethritis. Spectinomycin (Chapter 45) is active against most gonococci, but does not eradicate a urogenital chlamydial infection. Although ciprofloxacin might be effective in both gonorrhea and chlamydial urethritis, it is no longer recommended for treatment of gonorrhea in the United States, since resistance is now common. This patient could be treated by *single* oral doses of cefixime plus azithromycin (not listed). Sulfamethoxazole or TMP-SMZ would not be useful and may cause acute hemolysis in this patient. The answer is **E.**

5. Antacids can *decrease* oral bioavailability of fluoroquinolones. Neither hepatic or renal dysfunction is a *contraindication* to the use of fluoroquinolones. Most fluoroquinolones undergo renal elimination and dosage should be modified with creatinine clearance < 50 mL/min. Moxifloxacin elimination occurs mainly via the liver. The fluoroquinolones should not be used to treat uncomplicated first-time urinary tract infections in children because of possible effects on cartilage development. Uncomplicated urinary tract infections in children are usually due to a strain of *E coli* that is sensitive to many other drugs, including beta-lactam antibiotics. The answer is **C.**

6. In the absence of any evidence pointing toward a definite microbial cause for the colitis in this patient, a drug that decreases inflammation is indicated. Sulfasalazine has significant anti-inflammatory action, and its oral use results in symptomatic improvement in 50–75% of patients suffering from ulcerative colitis. The drug is also used for its anti-inflammatory effects in rheumatoid arthritis. The answer is **D.**

7. The most common adverse effect of the sulfonamides is a skin rash caused by hypersensitivity. Neurologic dysfunction and hematuria occur less frequently. Sulfonamides are usually avoided in the third trimester of pregnancy or in neonates, so kernicterus is rare. Fanconi's syndrome is associated with the use of outdated tetracyclines. The answer is **E.**

8. Sulfadiazine and TMP-SMZ are drugs of choice in nocardiosis. In combination with pyrimethamine (an effective dihydrofolate reductase inhibitor in protozoa), sulfadiazine is effective in toxoplasmosis and is prophylactic against pneumocystis pneumonia in the AIDS patient. However, TMP-SMZ is more commonly used for the latter purpose. The answer is **D.**

9. Ciprofloxacin is commonly used for the treatment of urinary tract infections and is active against most strains of common causative agents of otitis media, including *H influenzae* and pneumococci. However, up to 50% of strains of MRSA are now resistant to ciprofloxacin. No clinical antagonism has been reported between fluoroquinolones and inhibitors of folic acid synthesis. Fluoroquinolones are not recommended for use in pregnancy or for children younger than 10 years because they may damage growing cartilage. The answer is **C.**

10. Trimethoprim is the only weak base listed (fluoroquinolones and sulfonamides are acidic compounds), and its high lipid solubility at blood pH allows penetration of the drug into prostatic and vaginal fluid to reach levels similar to those in plasma. Leukopenia and thrombocytopenia may occur in folate deficiency when the drug is used alone or in combination with sulfamethoxazole. Fluoroquinolones do not exacerbate symptoms of folic acid deficiency. The answer is **E.**

SKILL KEEPER ANSWER: PROLONGATION OF THE QT INTERVAL (SEE CHAPTER 14)

The most important drugs that prolong the QT interval are antiarrhythmics. These include drugs from class IA and class III, including amiodarone, bretylium, disopyramide, procainamide, quinidine, and sotalol. You may recall that although group IA drugs are classified as Na^+ channel blockers, they also block K^+ channels and prolong the duration of the ventricular action potential. Other drugs implicated in QT prolongation include erythromycin, mefloquine, pentamidine, thioridazine and possibly other tricyclic antidepressants, and ziprasidone.

CHECKLIST

When you complete this chapter, you should be able to:

❑ Describe how sulfonamides and trimethoprim affect bacterial folic acid synthesis and how resistance to the antifolate drugs occurs.

❑ Identify major clinical uses of sulfonamides and trimethoprim, singly and in combination, and describe their characteristic pharmacokinetic properties and toxic effects.

❑ Describe how fluoroquinolones inhibit nucleic acid synthesis and identify mechanisms involved in bacterial resistance to these agents.

❑ List the major clinical uses of fluoroquinolones and describe their characteristic pharmacokinetic properties and toxic effects.

DRUG SUMMARY TABLE: Sulfonamides, Trimethoprim, & Fluoroquinolones

Subclass	Mechanism of Action	Activity & Clinical Uses	Pharmacokinetics & Interactions	Toxicities
Trimethoprim-sulfamethoxazole	Synergistic inhibition of folic acid synthesis • the combination is bactericidal–"sequential blockade"	Urinary tract, respiratory, ear, and sinus infections • *P jiroveci* pneumonia • toxoplasmosis • nocardiosis	Oral, IV • renal clearance, half-life ~8 h	Rash, fever, bone marrow suppression, hyperkalemia • high incidence of adverse effects in AIDS
Other folate antagonists				
Sulfisoxazole Sulfadiazine (+/– pyrimethamine) Trimethoprim Pyrimethamine (+/– sulfadoxine)	Sulfonamides inhibit dihydropteroate synthase Trimethoprim and pyrimethamine inhibit dihydrofolate reductase	Simple urinary tract infections (oral) and topical in burn or eye infections (sulfonamides) • toxoplasmosis (sulfadiazine + pyrimethamine) • malaria (sulfadoxine + pyrimethamine)	Hepatic and renal clearance and extensive plasma protein binding of sulfonamides (displace bilirubin, methotrexate, and warfarin)	Common—oral doses of sulfonamides cause GI upsets, acute hemolysis in G6PDH deficiency, possible crystalluria and rash (assume cross-hypersensitivity
Ciprofloxacin	Inhibits DNA replication via binding to DNA gyrase (gram-negative organisms) and topoisomerase IV (gram-positive organisms) • bactericidal Resistance: see below	Effective in urogenital, GI tracts, and some respiratory infections • activity versus gonococci rapidly declining • limited use in tuberculosis	Oral, IV • mostly renal clearance, half-life 4 h Oral absorption impaired by cations	GI upsets, CNS effects (dizziness, headache) • tendinitis due to effects on cartilage (try to avoid in young children and pregnancy)
Other fluoroquinolones				
Norfloxacin Ofloxacin Levofloxacin Moxifloxacin Gemifloxacin	Mechanism identical to that of ciprofloxacin; bactericidal Resistance via changes in target enzymes (eg DNA gyrase) and possibly formation of inactivating enzymes	Norfloxacin and ofloxacin used mainly for urinary tract infections • levofloxacin and moxifloxacin are "respiratory" fluoroquinolones with enhanced activity against gram-positive cocci and atypicals (chlamydia, mycoplasma)	Oral and IV forms of levofloxacin and moxifloxacin • mostly renal clearance (not moxifloxacin—hepatic) Long half-lives of gemifloxacin and moxifloxacin permit once-daily dosing	Like ciprofloxacin (see above) QTc prolongation (levofloxacin, gemifloxacin, and moxifloxacin) Caution with use of class IA and III antiarrhythmics

G6PDH, glucose-6-phosphate dehydrogenase.

Antimycobacterial Drugs

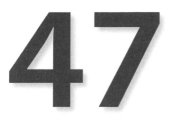

47

The chemotherapy of infections caused by *Mycobacterium tuberculosis, M leprae,* and *M avium-intracellulare* is complicated by numerous factors, including (1) limited information about the mechanisms of antimycobacterial drug actions; (2) the development of resistance; (3) the intracellular location of mycobacteria; (4) the chronic nature of mycobacterial disease, which requires protracted drug treatment and is associated with drug toxicities; and (5) patient compliance. Chemotherapy of mycobacterial infections almost always involves the use of drug combinations to delay the emergence of resistance and to enhance antimycobacterial efficacy.

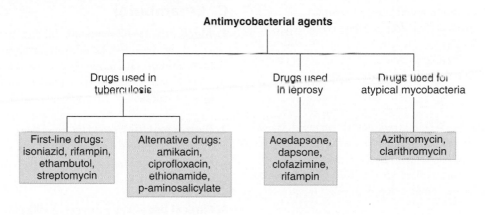

DRUGS FOR TUBERCULOSIS

The major drugs used in tuberculosis are **isoniazid (INH), rifampin, ethambutol, pyrazinamide,** and **streptomycin.** Actions of these agents on *M tuberculosis* are bactericidal or bacteriostatic depending on drug concentration and strain susceptibility. Appropriate drug treatment involves antibiotic susceptibility testing of mycobacterial isolates. Initiation of treatment of pulmonary tuberculosis usually involves a 3- or 4-drug combination regimen depending on the known or anticipated rate of resistance to isoniazid (INH). Directly observed therapy (DOT) regimens are recommended in noncompliant patients and in drug-resistant tuberculosis.

A. Isoniazid

1. Mechanisms—Isoniazid (INH) is a structural congener of pyridoxine. Its mechanism of action involves inhibition of mycolic acids, characteristic components of mycobacterial cell walls. Resistance can emerge rapidly if the drug is used alone. High-level resistance is associated with deletion in the *katG* gene that codes for a catalase-peroxidase involved in the bioactivation of INH. Low-level resistance occurs via deletions in the *inhA* gene that encodes the "target enzyme," an acyl carrier protein reductase. INH is bactericidal for actively growing tubercle bacilli but is less effective against dormant organisms.

2. Pharmacokinetics—INH is well absorbed orally and penetrates cells to act on intracellular mycobacteria. The liver metabolism of INH is by acetylation and is under genetic control. Patients may be fast or slow inactivators of the drug. INH half-life in "fast acetylators" is 60–90 min; in "slow acetylators" it may be 3–4 h. The proportion of fast acetylators is higher among people of Asian origin (including Native Americans) than those of European or African origin. Fast acetylators may require higher dosage than slow acetylators for equivalent therapeutic effects.

3. Clinical use—INH is the single most important drug used in tuberculosis and is a component of most drug combination regimens. In the treatment of latent infection (formerly known as "prophylaxis") including skin test converters and for close contacts of patients with active disease, INH is given as the sole drug.

4. Toxicity and interactions—Neurotoxic effects are common and include peripheral neuritis, restlessness, muscle twitching, and insomnia. These effects can be alleviated by administration of pyridoxine (25–50 mg/d orally). INH is hepatotoxic and may cause abnormal liver function tests, jaundice, and hepatitis. Fortunately, hepatotoxicity is rare in children. INH may inhibit the hepatic metabolism of drugs (eg, carbamazepine, phenytoin, warfarin). Hemolysis has occurred in patients with glucose-6-phosphate dehydrogenase (G6PDH) deficiency. A lupus-like syndrome has been reported.

B. Rifampin

1. Mechanisms—Rifampin, a derivative of rifamycin, is bactericidal against *M tuberculosis*. The drug inhibits DNA-dependent RNA polymerase (encoded by the *rpo* gene) in *M tuberculosis* and many other microorganisms. Resistance via changes in drug sensitivity of the polymerase often emerges rapidly if the drug is used alone.

2. Pharmacokinetics—When given orally, rifampin is well absorbed and is distributed to most body tissues, including the central nervous system (CNS). The drug undergoes enterohepatic cycling and is partially metabolized in the liver. Both free drug and metabolites, which are orange-colored, are eliminated mainly in the feces.

3. Clinical uses—In the treatment of tuberculosis, rifampin is almost always used in combination with other drugs. However, rifampin can be used as the sole drug in treatment of latent tuberculosis in INH-intolerant patients or in close contacts of patients with INH-resistant strains of the organism. In leprosy, rifampin given monthly delays the emergence of resistance to dapsone. Rifampin may be used with vancomycin for infections due to resistant staphylococci (methicillin-resistant *Staphylococcus aureus* [MRSA] strains) or pneumococci (penicillin-resistant *Streptococcus pneumoniae* [PRSP] strains). Other uses of rifampin include the meningococcal and staphylococcal carrier states.

4. Toxicity and interactions—Rifampin commonly causes light-chain proteinuria and may impair antibody responses. Occasional adverse effects include skin rashes, thrombocytopenia, nephritis, and liver dysfunction. If given less often than twice weekly, rifampin may cause a flu-like syndrome and anemia. Rifampin strongly induces liver drug-metabolizing enzymes and enhances the elimination rate of many drugs, including anticonvulsants, contraceptive steroids, cyclosporine, ketoconazole, methadone, terbinafine, and warfarin.

5. Other rifamycins—**Rifabutin** is equally effective as an antimycobacterial agent and is less likely to cause drug interactions than rifampin. It is usually preferred over rifampin in the treatment of tuberculosis or other mycobacterial infections in AIDS patients, especially those treated with cytochrome P450 substrates including protease inhibitors or efavirenz. **Rifamixin**, a rifampin derivative that is not absorbed from the gastrointestinal tract, has been used in traveler's diarrhea.

C. Ethambutol

1. Mechanisms—Ethambutol inhibits arabinosyl transferases (encoded by the *embCAB* operon) involved in the synthesis of arabinogalactan, a component of mycobacterial cell walls. Resistance occurs rapidly via mutations in the *emb* gene if the drug is used alone.

2. Pharmacokinetics—The drug is well absorbed orally and distributed to most tissues, including the CNS. A large fraction is eliminated unchanged in the urine. Dose reduction is necessary in renal impairment.

3. Clinical use—The main use of ethambutol is in tuberculosis, and it is always given in combination with other drugs.

4. Toxicity—The most common adverse effects are dose-dependent visual disturbances, including decreased visual acuity, red-green color blindness, optic neuritis, and possible retinal damage (from prolonged use at high doses). Most of these effects regress when the drug is stopped. Other adverse effects include headache, confusion, hyperuricemia and peripheral neuritis.

D. Pyrazinamide

1. Mechanisms—The mechanism of action of pyrazinamide is not known; however, its bacteriostatic action appears to require metabolic conversion via pyrazinamidases (encoded by the *pncA* gene) present in *M tuberculosis*. Resistance occurs via mutations in the gene that encodes enzymes involved in the bioactivation of pyrazinamide and by increased expression of drug efflux systems. This develops rapidly when the drug is used alone, but there is minimal cross-resistance with other antimycobacterial drugs.

2. Pharmacokinetics—Pyrazinamide is well absorbed orally and penetrates most body tissues, including the CNS. The drug is partly metabolized to pyrazinoic acid, and both parent molecule and metabolite are excreted in the urine. The plasma half-life of pyrazinamide is increased in hepatic or renal failure.

3. Clinical use—The combined use of pyrazinamide with other antituberculous drugs is an important factor in the success of short-course treatment regimens.

4. Toxicity—Approximately 40% of patients develop nongouty polyarthralgia. Hyperuricemia occurs commonly but is usually asymptomatic. Other adverse effects are myalgia, gastrointestinal irritation, maculopapular rash, hepatic dysfunction, porphyria, and photosensitivity reactions. Pyrazinamide should be avoided in pregnancy.

E. Streptomycin

This aminoglycoside is now used more frequently than before because of the growing prevalence of drug-resistant strains of *M tuberculosis*. Streptomycin is used principally in drug combinations for the treatment of life-threatening tuberculous disease, including meningitis, miliary dissemination, and severe organ tuberculosis. The pharmacodynamic and pharmacokinetic properties of streptomycin are similar to those of other aminoglycosides (see Chapter 45).

F. Alternative Drugs

Several drugs with antimycobacterial activity are used in cases that are resistant to first-line agents; they are considered second-line drugs because they are no more effective, and their toxicities are often more serious than those of the major drugs.

Amikacin is indicated for the treatment of tuberculosis suspected to be caused by streptomycin-resistant or multidrug-resistant mycobacterial strains. To avoid emergence of resistance, amikacin should always be used in combination drug regimens.

Ciprofloxacin and **ofloxacin** are often active against strains of *M tuberculosis* resistant to first-line agents. The fluoroquinolones should always be used in combination regimens with two or more other active agents.

Ethionamide is a congener of INH, but cross-resistance does not occur. The major disadvantage of ethionamide is severe gastrointestinal irritation and adverse neurologic effects at doses needed to achieve effective plasma levels.

p-**Aminosalicylic acid (PAS)** is rarely used because primary resistance is common. In addition, its toxicity includes gastrointestinal irritation, peptic ulceration, hypersensitivity reactions, and effects on kidney, liver, and thyroid function.

Other drugs of limited use because of their toxicity include **capreomycin** (ototoxicity, renal dysfunction) and **cycloserine** (peripheral neuropathy, CNS dysfunction).

G. Antitubercular Drug Regimens

1. Standard regimens—For empiric treatment of pulmonary TB (in most areas of <4% INH resistance), an initial 3-drug regimen of INH, rifampin, and pyrazinamide is recommended. If the

organisms are fully susceptible (and the patient is HIV-negative), pyrazinamide can be discontinued after 2 mo and treatment continued for a further 4 mo with a 2-drug regimen.

2. Alternative regimens—Alternative regimens in cases of fully susceptible organisms include INH + rifampin for 9 mo, or INH + ETB for 18 mo. Intermittent (2 or 3 × weekly) high-dose 4-drug regimens are also effective.

3. Resistance—If resistance to INH is higher than 4%, the initial drug regimen should include ethambutol or streptomycin. Tuberculosis resistant only to INH (the most common form of resistance) can be treated for 6 mo with a regimen of RIF + pyrazinamide + ethambutol or streptomycin. Multidrug-resistant organisms (resistant to both INH and rifampin) should be treated with 3 or more drugs to which the organism is susceptible for a period of more than 18 mo, including 12 mo after sputum cultures become negative.

DRUGS FOR LEPROSY

A. Sulfones

Dapsone (diaminodiphenylsulfone) remains the most active drug against *M leprae*. The mechanism of action of sulfones may involve inhibition of folic acid synthesis. Because of increasing reports of resistance, it is recommended that the drug be used in combinations with rifampin and/or clofazimine (see below). Dapsone can be given orally, penetrates tissues well, undergoes enterohepatic cycling, and is eliminated in the urine, partly as acetylated metabolites. Common adverse effects include gastrointestinal irritation, fever, skin rashes, and methemoglobinemia. Hemolysis may occur, especially in patients with G6PDH deficiency.

Acedapsone is a repository form of dapsone that provides inhibitory plasma concentrations for several months. In addition to its use in leprosy, dapsone is an alternative drug for the treatment of *Pneumocystis jiroveci* pneumonia in AIDS patients.

B. Other Agents

Drug regimens usually include combinations of dapsone with rifampin (or rifabutin, see prior discussion) plus or minus **clofazimine.** Clofazimine, a phenazine dye that may interact with DNA, causes gastrointestinal irritation and skin discoloration ranging from red-brown to nearly black.

DRUGS FOR ATYPICAL MYCOBACTERIAL INFECTIONS

Mycobacterium avium complex (MAC) is a cause of disseminated infections in AIDS patients. Currently, clarithromycin or azithromycin with or without rifabutin is recommended for primary prophylaxis in patients with CD4 counts less than 50/μL. Treatment of MAC infections requires a combination of drugs, one favored regimen consisting of azithromycin or clarithromycin with ethambutol and rifabutin. Infections resulting from other atypical mycobacteria (eg, *M marinum, M ulcerans*), though sometimes asymptomatic, may be treated with the described antimycobacterial drugs (eg, ethambutol, INH, rifampin) or other antibiotics (eg, amikacin, cephalosporins, fluoroquinolones, macrolides, or tetracyclines).

QUESTIONS

1. The primary reason for the use of drug combinations in the treatment of tuberculosis is to
   (A) Delay or prevent the emergence of resistance
   (B) Ensure patient compliance with the drug regimen
   (C) Increase antimycobacterial activity synergistically
   (D) Provide prophylaxis against other bacterial infections
   (E) Reduce the incidence of adverse effects

Questions 2–5. A 21-year-old woman from Southeast Asia has been staying with family members in the United States for the last 3 mo and is looking after her sister's preschool children during the day. Because she has difficulty with the English language, her sister escorts her to the emergency department of a local hospital. She tells the staff that her sister has been feeling very tired for the last month, has a poor appetite, and has lost weight. The patient has been feeling somewhat better lately except for a cough that produces a greenish sputum, sometimes specked with blood. With the exception of rales in the left upper lobe, the physical examination is unremarkable and she does not seem to be acutely ill. Laboratory values show a white count of 12,000/μL and a hematocrit of 33%. Chest x-ray film reveals an infiltrate in the left upper lobe with a possible cavity. A Gram-stained smear of the sputum shows mixed flora with no dominance. An acid-fast stain reveals many thin rods of pinkish hue. A preliminary diagnosis is made of pulmonary tuberculosis. Sputum is sent to the laboratory for culture.

2. At this point, the most appropriate course of action is to
   (A) Hospitalize the patient and start treatment with isoniazid plus rifampin
   (B) Hospitalize the patient and start treatment with 4 antimycobacterial drugs
   (C) Prescribe isoniazid for prophylaxis and send the patient home to await culture results
   (D) Prescribe no drugs and send the patient home to await culture results
   (E) Treat the patient with isoniazid plus rifampin

3. Which drug regimen should be initiated in this patient when treatment is started?
   (A) Amikacin, isoniazid, pyrazinamide, streptomycin
   (B) Ciprofloxacin, cycloserine, isoniazid, PAS
   (C) Ethambutol, isoniazid, ofloxacin, streptomycin
   (D) Ethionamide, pyrazinamide, rifampin, streptomycin
   (E) Isoniazid, rifampin, pyrazinamide, ethambutol

4. Which statement concerning the possible use of isoniazid (INH) in this patient is false?
   (A) A lower maintenance dose than usual is required in a patient from Southeast Asia
   (B) Flushing, sweating, dyspnea, and palpitations may occur after ingestion of tyramine-containing foods
   (C) Peripheral neuritis may occur during treatment
   (D) The patient should take pyridoxine daily
   (E) The risk of the patient developing hepatitis from INH is less than 2%

5. On her release from the hospital, the patient is advised not to rely solely on oral contraceptives to prevent pregnancy because they may be less effective while she is being maintained on antimycobacterial drugs. The agent most likely to interfere with the action of oral contraceptives is
   (A) Amikacin
   (B) Ethambutol
   (C) Isoniazid
   (D) Pyrazinamide
   (E) Rifampin

6. A patient with AIDS and a CD4 cell count of 100/μL has persistent fever and weight loss associated with invasive pulmonary disease due to *M avium* complex (MAC). Optimal management of this patient is to
   (A) Select an antibiotic based on drug susceptibility of the cultured organism
   (B) Start treatment with INH and pyrazinamide
   (C) Treat with rifabutin because it prevents the development of MAC bacteremia
   (D) Treat with the combination of clarithromycin, ethambutol, and rifabutin
   (E) Treat with trimethoprim-sulfamethoxazole

7. A 10-year-old boy has uncomplicated pulmonary tuberculosis. After initial hospitalization, he is now being treated at home with isoniazid, rifampin, and ethambutol. Which statement about this case is accurate?
   (A) A baseline auditory function test is essential before drug treatment is initiated
   (B) His mother, who takes care of him, does not need INH prophylaxis
   (C) His 3-year-old sibling should receive INH prophylaxis
   (D) The patient may develop symptoms of polyarthralgia caused by rifampin
   (E) The potential nephrotoxicity of the prescribed drugs warrants periodic assessment of renal function

8. Which statement about antitubercular drugs is accurate?
   (A) Antimycobacterial actions of streptomycin involve inhibition of arabinosyl transferases
   (B) Cross-resistance of *M tuberculosis* to isoniazid and pyrazinamide is common
   (C) Ocular toxicity of ethambutol is prevented by thiamine
   (D) Pyrazinamide treatment should be discontinued immediately if hyperuricemia occurs
   (E) Resistance to ethambutol involves mutations in the *emb* gene

9. Once weekly administration of which of the following antibiotics has prophylactic activity against bacteremia caused by *M avium* complex in AIDS patients?
   (A) Azithromycin
   (B) Clarithromycin
   (C) Ethambutol
   (D) Kanamycin
   (E) Rifabutin

10. Risk factors for multidrug-resistant tuberculosis include
    (A) A history of treatment of tuberculosis without rifampin
    (B) Recent immigration from Asia and living in an area of over 4% isoniazid resistance
    (C) Recent immigration from Latin America
    (D) Residence in regions where isoniazid resistance is known to exceed 4%
    (E) All of the above

ANSWERS

1. Although it is sometimes possible to achieve synergistic effects against mycobacteria with drug combinations, the primary reason for their use is to delay the emergence of resistance. The answer is **A.**

2. Despite the fact that this patient does not appear to be acutely ill, she would in most cases be treated with 4 drugs that have activity against *M tuberculosis*. This is because organisms infecting patients from Southeast Asia are commonly INH-resistant, and coverage must be provided with 3 other antituberculosis drugs in addition to isoniazid. This patient should be hospitalized for several reasons, including potential difficulties with compliance regarding the drug regimen and the fact that young children are in the home where she is living. The answer is **B.**

3. Sputum cultures will not be available for several weeks, and no information is available regarding drug susceptibility of the organism at this stage. For optimum coverage, the initial regimen should include INH, rifampin, pyrazinamide, and ethambutol. INH-resistant organisms are usually sensitive to both rifampin and pyrazinamide. Streptomycin is usually reserved for use in severe forms of tuberculosis or for infections known to be resistant to first-line drugs. Likewise, amikacin and ciprofloxacin are possible agents for treatment of multidrug-resistant strains of *M tuberculosis*. Cycloserine, PAS, and rifabutin are alternative second-line drugs that may be used in cases of failed response to more conventional agents. The answer is **E.**

4. Patients from Pacific Rim countries do not require lower doses of INH. Fast acetylators, including Native Americans, may require higher doses of the drug than others. Peripheral neuropathy caused by INH is due to pyridoxine deficiency. It is more common in the diabetic, malnourished, or AIDS patient and can be prevented by a daily dose of 25–50 mg of pyridoxine. INH can inhibit monoamine oxidase type A and has caused tyramine reactions. Hepatotoxicity is age-dependent, with an incidence of 0.3% in patients aged 21–35 yr and greater than 2% in patients older than 50 yr. The answer is **A.**

5. Rifampin induces the formation of several microsomal drug-metabolizing enzymes, including cytochrome P450 isoforms. This action increases the rate of elimination of a number of drugs, including anticoagulants, ketoconazole, methadone, and steroids that are present in oral contraceptives. The pharmacologic activity of these drugs can be reduced markedly in patients taking rifampin. The answer is **E.**

6. Combinations of antibiotics are essential for suppression of disease caused by *M avium* complex in the AIDS patient, and treatment should be started before culture results are available. Although rifabutin is prophylactic against MAC bacteremia when it is used as sole therapy in active disease, resistant strains of the organism emerge rapidly. MAC is much less susceptible than *M tuberculosis* to conventional antimycobacterial drugs. Currently, the optimum regimen consists of clarithromycin (or azithromycin) with ethambutol and rifabutin. The answer is **D.**

7. A baseline test of ocular (not auditory) function may be useful before starting ethambutol. None of the drugs prescribed is associated with nephrotoxicity. Polyarthralgia is a common adverse effect of pyrazinamide that was not prescribed in this case. Periodic tests of liver function may be advisable in younger patients who are treated with INH plus rifampin,

especially if higher doses of these drugs are used. Prophylaxis with INH is advisable for all household members and very close contacts of patients with active tuberculosis, *especially* young children. The answer is **C.**

8. Ethambutol inhibits arabinosyl transferases. Ocular toxicity due to ethambutol is dose-dependent and is usually reversible when the drug is discontinued. Thiamine is not protective. There is minimal cross-resistance between pyrazinamide and other antimycobacterial drugs. Pyrazinamide uniformly causes hyperuricemia, but this is not a reason to halt therapy even though the drug may provoke gouty arthritis in susceptible persons. The answer is **E.**

9. Because of its long elimination half-life (3–4 d), weekly administration of azithromycin has proved to be equivalent to daily administration of clarithromycin when used for prophylaxis against *M avium* complex in AIDS patients. The answer is **A.**

10. Multidrug-resistant tuberculosis (MDR-TB) is defined as resistance to 2 or more drugs. All the risk factors are relevent. In the case of resistance to both INH and rifampin, initial regimens still include both drugs plus ethambutol, pyrazinamide, streptomycin (or other aminoglycoside), and a fluoroquinolone. Continuation therapy should include at least 3 drugs shown to be active in vitro against the infecting strain. The appropriate duration of therapy has not been established. The answer is **E.**

SKILL KEEPER ANSWERS: GENOTYPIC VARIATIONS IN DRUG METABOLISM (SEE CHAPTER 4)

Examples of genotypic variations in drug metabolism include succinylcholine (pseudocholinesterase) and isoniazid (N-acetyltransferase). Genetic polymorphisms also occur in isoforms of cytochrome P450 and contribute to variability in the rates of metabolism of phenformin, dextromethorphan, and metoprolol. Variants in the CYP2D6 isoform have been implicated in excessive responses to codeine and nortriptyline, and variants in CYP2C9 may be responsible for unusual sensitivity to the anticoagulant effects of warfarin.

Enzyme	Drugs	Clinical Consequences
Aldehyde dehydrogenase	Ethanol	Facial flushing, emesis, and cardiovascular symptoms in Asians with low enzyme activity
N-acetyltransferase	Isoniazid	Increased dose requirement in fast acetylators
	Hydralazine	Increased risk of lupus-like syndrome in slow acetylators
	Procainamide	Increased cardiotoxicity in fast acetylators
Pseudocholinesterase	Succinylcholine	Deficiences may lead to prolonged apnea

CHECKLIST

When you complete this chapter, you should be able to:

❑ List 5 special problems associated with chemotherapy of mycobacterial infections.

❑ Identify the characteristic pharmacodynamic and pharmacokinetic properties of isoniazid and rifampin.

❑ List the typical adverse effects of ethambutol, pyrazinamide, and streptomycin.

❑ Describe the standard protocols for drug management of latent tuberculosis, pulmonary tuberculosis, and multidrug-resistant tuberculosis.

❑ Identify the drugs used in leprosy and in the prophylaxis and treatment of *M avium-intracellulare* complex disease.

DRUG SUMMARY TABLE: First-Line Antimycobacterial Drugs[a]

Drugs	Mechanism of Action	Activity & Clinical Uses	Pharmacokinetics & Interactions	Toxicities
Isoniazid (INH)	Requires bioactivation; inhibits mycolic acid synthesis • resistance via expression of *katG* and *inhA* genes	Bactericidal • primary drug for LTBI and a primary drug for use in combinations	Oral and IV forms • hepatic clearance (fast and slow acetylators) • inhibits metabolism of carbamazepine, phenytoin and warfarin	Hepatotoxicity, peripheral neuropathy (use pyridoxine) • hemolysis in G6PDH deficiency
Rifamycins Rifampin(RIF)[b] Rifabutin Rifapentine	Inhibit DNA-dependent RNA polymerase • resistance emerges rapidly when drug is used alone	Bactericidal • RIF is an optional drug for LTBI, a primary drug used in combinations for active TB	Rifampin (oral, IV) • others oral • enterohepatic cycling with some metabolism • induced formation of CYP450 by RIF leads to decreased efficacy of many drugs (rifabutin less)	Rash, nephritis, cholestasis, thrombocytopenia • flu-like syndrome with intermittent dosing
Ethambutol (ETB)	Inhibits formation of arabinoglycan, a component of mycobacterial cell wall • resistance emerges rapidly if drug is used alone	Bacteriostatic • component of many drug combination regimens for active TB	Oral • renal elimination with large fraction unchanged • reduce dose in renal dysfunction	Dose-dependent visual disturbances, reversible on discontinuance • headache, confusion, hyperuricemia, and peripheral neuritis
Pyrazinamide (PYR)	Uncertain, but requires bioactivation via hydrolytic enzymes to form pyrazoic acid (active)	Bacteriostatic • component of many drug combination regimens for active TB	Oral • both hepatic and renal elimination (reduce dose in dysfunction)	Polyarthralgia (40% incidence), hyperuricemia, myalgia, maculopapular rash, porphyria, and photosensitivity • avoid in pregnancy
Streptomycin (SM)	Binds to S12 ribosomal subunit inhibiting protein synthesis	Bactericidal • used in TB when injectable drug needed, or in treatment of drug-resistant strains	Parenteral • renal elimination	Ototoxicity, nephrotoxicity

[a]*Backup drugs include amikacin, aminosalicylic acid, ciprofloxacin, cycloserine, ethionamide, and levofloxacin.*
[b]*Rifampin is also used for eradication of staphylococci and meningococci in carriers.*
G6PDH, glucose-6-phosphate dehydrogenase; LTBI, latent tuberculosis infection.

Antifungal Agents

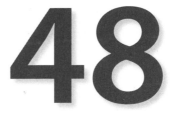

Fungal infections are difficult to treat, particularly in the immunocompromised or neutropenic patient. Most fungi are resistant to conventional antimicrobial agents, and relatively few drugs are available for the treatment of systemic fungal diseases. Amphotericin B and the azoles (fluconazole, itraconazole, ketoconazole, and voriconazole) are the primary drugs used in systemic infections. They are selectively toxic to fungi because they interact with or inhibit the synthesis of ergosterol, a sterol unique to fungal cell membranes.

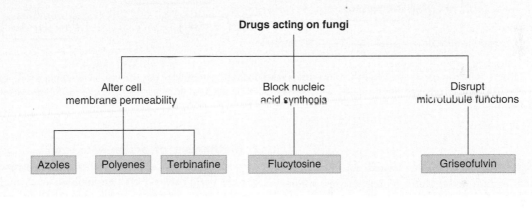

DRUGS FOR SYSTEMIC FUNGAL INFECTIONS

A. Amphotericin B

Amphotericin B continues to be an important drug for the treatment of systemic fungal infections. However, several azoles and echinocandins are proving to be just as effective in some systemic mycoses with less risk of toxic effects.

1. Classification and pharmacokinetics—Amphotericin B is a polyene antibiotic related to nystatin. Amphotericin is poorly absorbed from the gastrointestinal tract and is usually administered intravenously as a nonlipid colloidal suspension, as a lipid complex, or in a liposomal formulation. The drug is widely distributed to all tissues except the central nervous system (CNS). Elimination is mainly via slow hepatic metabolism; the half-life is approximately 2 wk. A small fraction of the drug is excreted in the urine; dosage modification is necessary only in extreme renal dysfunction. Amphotericin B is not dialyzable.

2. Mechanism of action—The fungicidal action of amphotericin B is due to its effects on the permeability and transport properties of fungal membranes. Polyenes are molecules with both hydrophilic and lipophilic characteristics (ie, they are amphipathic). They bind to **ergosterol,** a sterol specific to fungal cell membranes, and cause the formation of artificial pores (Figure 48–1). Resistance, though uncommon, can occur via a decreased level of or a structural change in membrane ergosterol.

3. Clinical uses—Amphotericin B is one of the most important drugs available for the treatment of systemic mycoses and is often used for initial induction regimens before follow-up treatment with an azole. It has the widest antifungal spectrum of any agent and remains the drug of choice, or codrug of choice, for most systemic infections caused by *Aspergillus, Blastomyces, Candida albicans, Cryptococcus, Histoplasma,* and *Mucor.* Amphotericin B is usually given by slow intravenous infusion, but in fungal meningitis intrathecal administration, though dangerous, has been used. Local administration of the drug, with minimal toxicity, has been used in treatment of mycotic corneal ulcers and keratitis.

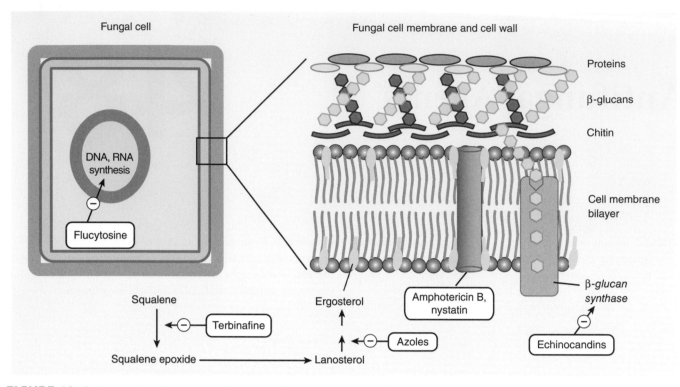

FIGURE 48–1 Targets of antifungal drugs. Except for flucytosine (and possibly griseofulvin, not shown), all available antifungal drugs target the fungal cell membrane or cell wall. (Reproduced, with permission, from Katzung BG, editor: *Basic & Clinical Pharmacology*, 12th ed. McGraw-Hill, 2012: Fig. 48–1.)

4. Toxicity

a. Infusion related—Adverse effects related to intravenous infusion commonly include fever, chills, muscle spasms, vomiting, and a shock-like fall in blood pressure. These effects may be attenuated by a slow infusion rate and by premedication with antihistamines, antipyretics, meperidine, or glucocorticoids.

b. Dose limiting—Amphotericin B decreases the glomerular filtration rate and causes renal tubular acidosis with magnesium and potassium wasting. Anemia may result from decreases in the renal formation of erythropoietin. Although concomitant saline infusion may reduce renal damage, the nephrotoxic effects of the drug are dose-limiting. Dose reduction (with lowered toxicity) is possible in some infections when amphotericin B is used with flucytosine. Liposomal formulations of amphotericin B have reduced nephrotoxic effects, possibly because of decreased binding of the drug to renal cells.

c. Neurotoxicity—Intrathecal administration of amphotericin B may cause seizures and neurologic damage.

B. Flucytosine (5-Fluorocytosine [5-FC])

1. Classification and pharmacokinetics—5-FC is a pyrimidine antimetabolite related to the anticancer drug 5-fluorouracil (5-FU). It is effective orally and is distributed to most body tissues, including the CNS. The drug is eliminated intact in the urine, and the dose must be reduced in patients with renal impairment.

2. Mechanism of action—Flucytosine is accumulated in fungal cells by the action of a membrane permease and converted by cytosine deaminase to 5-FU, an inhibitor of thymidylate synthase (Figure 48–1). Selective toxicity occurs because mammalian cells have low levels of permease and deaminase. Resistance can occur rapidly if flucytosine is used alone and involves decreased activity of the fungal permeases or deaminases. When 5-FC is given with amphotericin B, or triazoles such as itraconazole, emergence of resistance is decreased and synergistic antifungal effects may occur.

3. Clinical uses—The antifungal spectrum of 5-FC is narrow; its clinical use is limited to the treatment, in combination with amphotericin B or a triazole, of infections resulting from *Cryptococcus neoformans,* possibly systemic candidal infections and chromoblastomycosis caused by molds.

4. Toxicity—Prolonged high plasma levels of flucytosine cause reversible bone marrow depression, alopecia, and liver dysfunction.

C. Azole Antifungal Agents

1. Classification and pharmacokinetics—The azoles used for systemic mycoses include **ketoconazole,** an imidazole, and the triazoles **fluconazole, itraconazole,** and **voriconazole.** Oral bioavailability is variable (normal gastric acidity is required). Fluconazole and voriconazole are more reliably absorbed via the oral route than the other azoles. The triazoles are available in both oral and intravenous formulations. The drugs are distributed to most body tissues, but with the exception of fluconazole, drug levels achieved in the CNS are very low. Liver metabolism is responsible for the elimination of ketoconazole, itraconazole, and voriconazole. Inducers of drug-metabolizing enzymes (eg, rifampin) decrease the bioavailability of itraconazole. Fluconazole is eliminated by the kidneys, largely in unchanged form.

2. Mechanism of action—The azoles interfere with fungal cell membrane permeability by inhibiting the synthesis of ergosterol. These drugs act at the step of 14α-demethylation of lanosterol, which is catalyzed by a fungal cytochrome P450 isozyme. With increasing use of azole antifungals, especially for long-term prophylaxis in immunocompromised and neutropenic patients, resistance is occurring, possibly via changes in the sensitivity of the target enzymes.

3. Clinical uses

a. Ketoconazole—Because it has a narrow antifungal spectrum and causes more adverse effects than other azoles, ketoconazole is now rarely used for systemic mycoses. The drug is not available in parenteral form. However, ketoconazole continues to be used for chronic mucocutaneous candidiasis and is also effective against dermatophytes.

b. Fluconazole—Fluconazole is a drug of choice in esophageal and oropharyngeal candidiasis and for most infections caused by *Coccidioides*. A single oral dose usually eradicates vaginal candidiasis. Fluconazole is the drug of choice for treatment and secondary prophylaxis against cryptococcal meningitis and is an alternative drug of choice (with amphotericin B) in treatment of active disease due to *Cryptococcus neoformans*. The drug is also equivalent to amphotericin B in candidemia.

c. Itraconazole—This azole is currently the drug of choice for systemic infections caused by *Blastomyces* and *Sporothrix* and for subcutaneous chromoblastomycosis. Itraconazole is an alternative agent in the treatment of infections caused by *Aspergillus, Coccidioides, Cryptococcus,* and *Histoplasma*. In esophageal candidiasis, the drug is active against some strains resistant to fluconazole. Itraconazole is also used extensively in the treatment of dermatophytoses, especially onychomycosis.

d. Voriconazole—Voriconazole has an even wider spectrum of fungal activity than itraconazole. It is a codrug of choice for treatment of invasive aspergillosis; some studies report greater efficacy than amphotericin B. Voriconzole is an alternative drug in candidemia with activity against some fluconazole-resistant organisms and in AIDS patients has been used in the treatment of candidial esophagitis and stomatitis.

e. Posaconazole—The broadest-spectrum triazole, posaconazole has activity against most species of *Candida* and *Aspergillus*. It is the only azole with activity against *Rhizopus*, one of the agents of mucormycosis, and is used for prophylaxis of fungal infections during cancer chemotherapy and in salvage therapy in invasive aspergillosis.

4. Toxicity—Adverse effects of the azoles include vomiting, diarrhea, rash, and sometimes hepatotoxicity, especially in patients with preexisting liver dysfunction. Ketoconazole is a notorious inhibitor of hepatic cytochrome P450 isozymes and may increase the plasma levels of many other drugs, including cyclosporine, oral hypoglycemics, phenytoin, and warfarin. Inhibition of cytochrome P450 isoforms by ketoconazole interferes with the synthesis of adrenal and gonadal steroids and may lead to gynecomastia, menstrual irregularities, and infertility. The other azoles are more selective inhibitors of fungal cytochrome P450. Although they are less likely than ketoconazole to cause endocrine dysfunction, their inhibitory effects on liver drug-metabolizing enzymes have resulted in drug interactions. Voriconazole causes immediate but transient visual disturbances including blurring of vision of unknown cause in more than 30% of patients. Based on animal studies, voriconazole is a class D drug in terms of pregnancy risk. Visual dysfunction has not been reported with posaconazole, but the drug is an inhibitor of CYP3A4, increasing the levels of cyclosporine and tacrolimus.

> ### SKILL KEEPER: INHIBITORS OF CYTOCHROMES P450 (SEE CHAPTERS 4 AND 61)
>
> Ketoconazole has the unenviable reputation of association with multiple drug interactions because of its inhibition of cytochromes P450 involved in drug metabolism.
>
> 1. How many drugs can you identify that have their metabolism via such enzymes inhibited by ketoconazole?
> 2. How many other drugs that inhibit hepatic cytochromes P450 can you recall?
>
> The Skill Keeper Answers appear at the end of the chapter.

D. Echinocandins

1. Classification and pharmacokinetics—Caspofungin is an echinocandin, the first of a novel class of antifungal agents. Other echinocandins include anidulafungin and micafungin. Used intravenously, the drugs distribute widely to the tissues and are eliminated largely via hepatic metabolism. Caspofungin has a half-life of 9–12 h. The half-life of micafungin is slightly longer, and that of anidulafungin is 24–48 h.

2. Mechanism of action—The echinocandins have a unique fungicidal action, inhibiting the synthesis of β(1-2)glycan, a critical component of fungal cell walls.

3. Clinical uses—Caspofungin is used for disseminated and mucocutaneous *Candida* infections in patients who fail to respond to amphotericin B and in the treatment of mucormycosis. Anidulafungin is used for esophageal and invasive candidiasis. Micofungin is used for mucocutaneous candidiasis and for prophylaxis of *Candida* infections in bone marrow transplant patients.

4. Toxicity—Infusion-related effects of caspofungin include headache, gastrointestinal distress, fever, rash, and flushing (histamine release). Micafungin also causes histamine release and elevates blood levels of the immunosuppressant drugs cyclosporine and sirolimus. Combined use of echinocandins with cyclosporine may elevate liver transaminases.

SYSTEMIC DRUGS FOR SUPERFICIAL FUNGAL INFECTIONS

Drugs used orally in the treatment of dermatophytoses include griseofulvin, terbinafine, and several azole antifungals.

A. Griseofulvin

1. Pharmacokinetics—Oral absorption of griseofulvin depends on the physical state of the drug—ultra-micro-size formulations, which have finer crystals or particles, are more effectively absorbed—and is aided by high-fat foods. The drug is distributed to the stratum corneum, where it binds to keratin. Biliary excretion is responsible for its elimination.

2. Mechanism of action—Griseofulvin interferes with microtubule function in dermatophytes (Figure 48–1) and may also inhibit the synthesis and polymerization of nucleic acids. Sensitive dermatophytes take up the drug by an energy-dependent mechanism, and resistance can occur via decrease in this transport. Griseofulvin is fungistatic.

3. Clinical uses and toxicity—Griseofulvin is not active topically. The oral formulation of the drug is indicated for dermatophytoses of the skin and hair, but has been largely replaced by terbinafine and the azoles. Adverse effects include headaches, mental confusion, gastrointestinal irritation, photosensitivity, and changes in liver function. Griseofulvin should not be used in patients with porphyria. Griseofulvin decreases the bioavailability of warfarin, resulting in decreased anticoagulant effect, and it also causes disulfiram-like reactions with ethanol.

B. Terbinafine

1. Mechanism of action—Terbinafine inhibits a fungal enzyme, squalene epoxidase. It causes accumulation of toxic levels of squalene, which can interfere with ergosterol synthesis. Terbinafine is fungicidal.

2. Clinical uses and toxicity—Terbinafine is available in both oral and topical forms. Like griseofulvin, terbinafine accumulates in keratin, but it is much more effective than griseofulvin in onychomycosis. Adverse effects include gastrointestinal upsets, rash, headache, and taste disturbances. Terbinafine does not inhibit cytochrome P450.

C. Azoles

The azoles other than voriconazole and posaconazole are commonly used orally for the treatment of dermatophytoses. Pulse or intermittent dosing with itraconazole is as effective in onychomycoses as continuous dosing because the drug persists in the nails for several months. Typically, treatment for 1 wk is followed by 3 wk without drug. Advantages of pulse dosing include a lower incidence of adverse effects and major cost savings. Topical forms of various azoles are also available for use in dermatophytoses.

TOPICAL DRUGS FOR SUPERFICIAL FUNGAL INFECTIONS

A number of antifungal drugs are used topically for superficial infections caused by *C albicans* and dermatophytes. **Nystatin** is a polyene antibiotic (toxicity precludes systemic use) that disrupts fungal membranes by binding to ergosterol. Nystatin is commonly used topically to suppress local *Candida* infections and has been used orally to eradicate gastrointestinal fungi in patients with impaired defense mechanisms. Other topical antifungal agents that are widely used include the azole compounds **miconazole, clotrimazole,** and several others.

QUESTIONS

1. Interactions between this drug and cell membrane components can result in the formation of pores lined by hydrophilic groups present in the drug molecule.
   (A) Amphotericin B
   (B) Flucytosine
   (C) Griseofulvin
   (D) Itraconazole
   (E) Terbinafine

2. Which statement about fluconazole is accurate?
   (A) Does not penetrate the blood-brain barrier
   (B) Has the least effect of all azoles on hepatic drug metabolism
   (C) Is an inducer of hepatic drug-metabolizing enzymes
   (D) Is highly effective in the treatment of aspergillosis
   (E) Oral bioavailability is less than that of ketoconazole

Questions 3–5. A 37-year-old woman with leukemia was undergoing chemotherapy with intravenous antineoplastic drugs. During treatment, she developed a systemic infection from an opportunistic pathogen. There was no erythema or edema at the catheter insertion site. A white vaginal discharge was observed. After appropriate specimens were obtained for culture, empiric antibiotic therapy was started with gentamicin, nafcillin, and ticarcillin intravenously. This regimen was maintained for 72 h, during which time the patient's condition did not improve significantly. Her throat was sore, and white plaques had appeared in her pharynx. On day 4, none of the cultures had shown any bacterial growth, but both the blood and urine cultures grew out *Candida albicans*.

3. At this point, the best course of action is to
   (A) Continue current antibiotics and start amphotericin B
   (B) Continue current antibiotics and start flucytosine
   (C) Stop current antibiotics and start amphotericin B
   (D) Stop current antibiotics and start ketoconazole
   (E) Stop current antibiotics and start terbinafine

4. If amphotericin B is administered, the patient should be pre-medicated with
   (A) Diphenhydramine
   (B) Ibuprofen
   (C) Prednisone
   (D) Any or all of the above
   (E) None of the above

5. *Candida* is a major cause of nosocomial bloodstream infection. The opportunistic fungal infection in this patient could have been prevented by administration of
   (A) Caspofungin
   (B) Fluconazole
   (C) Nystatin
   (D) Posaconazole
   (E) None of the above

Questions 6 and 7. A 28-year-old man living on the East Coast was transferred by his employer to central California for several months. On his return, he complains of having influenza-like symptoms with fever and a cough. He also has red, tender nodules on his shins. His physician suspects that these symptoms are due to coccidioidomycosis contracted during his stay in California.

6. This patient should be treated immediately with
   (A) Amphotericin B
   (B) Caspofungin
   (C) Terbinafine
   (D) Voriconazole
   (E) None of these drugs

7. Which is the drug of choice if this patient is suffering from persistent lung lesions or disseminated disease caused by *Coccidioides immitis*?
   (A) Amphotericin B
   (B) Fluconazole
   (C) Ketoconazole
   (D) Micofungin
   (E) Terbinafine

8. Which drug is *least* likely to be effective in the treatment of esophageal candidiasis if it is used by the oral route?
   (A) Clotrimazole
   (B) Fluconazole
   (C) Griseofulvin
   (D) Itraconazole
   (E) Nystatin

9. Serious cardiac effects have occurred when this drug was taken by patients using the antihistamines astemizole or terfenadine
   (A) Amphotericin B
   (B) Fluconazole
   (C) Griseofulvin
   (D) Ketoconazole
   (E) Terbinafine

10. Regarding the clinical use of liposomal formulations of amphotericin B, which statement is accurate?
    (A) Amphotericin B affinity for these lipids is greater than affinity for ergosterol
    (B) Less expensive to use than conventional amphotericin B
    (C) More effective in fungal infections because they increase tissue uptake of amphotericin B
    (D) They decrease the nephrotoxicity of amphotericin B
    (E) They have a wider spectrum of antifungal activity than conventional formulations of amphotericin B

ANSWERS

1. The polyene antifungal drugs are amphipathic molecules that can interact with ergosterol in fungal cell membranes to form artificial pores. In these structures, the lipophilic groups on the drug molecule are arranged on the outside of the pore, and the hydrophilic regions are located on the inside. The fungicidal action of amphotericin B and nystatin derives from this interaction, which results in leakage of intracellular constituents. The answer is **A**.

2. The azoles with activity against *Aspergillus* are itraconazole and voriconazole. Fluconazole is the best absorbed member of the azole group by the oral route and the only one that readily penetrates into cerebrospinal fluid. Although fluconazole may inhibit the metabolism of some drugs, it has the least effect of all azoles on hepatic microsomal drug-metabolizing enzymes. The answer is **B**.

3. The antibiotic regimen should be stopped, since the condition of the patient did not improve after 3 d of such treatment, the cultures were negative for bacteria, and the clinical picture suggested that the patient had a fungal infection. This was subsequently confirmed by blood culture. The answer is **C**.

4. Infusion-related adverse effects of amphotericin B include chills and fevers (the "shake and bake" syndrome), muscle spasms, nausea, headache, and hypotension. Antipyretics, antihistamines, and glucocorticoids all have been shown to be helpful. The administration of a 1-mg test dose of amphotericin B is sometimes useful in predicting the severity of infusion-related toxicity. The answer is **D**.

5. In the case of opportunistic candidal infections in the immunocompromised patient, no prophylactic drugs have been shown to be clinically effective. Prophylaxis against other fungi may be effective in some instances, including suppression of cryptococcal meningitis in AIDS patients with fluconazole. However, prophylactic use of azoles may contribute to the development of fungal resistance. The answer is **E**.

6. A travel history can be important in the diagnosis of fungal disease. If this patient has a fungal infection of the lungs, it is probably due to *C immitis*, which is endemic in dry regions of the western United States. Pulmonary symptoms of coccidioidomycosis are usually self-limiting, and drug therapy is not commonly required in an otherwise healthy patient. Tender red nodules on extensor surfaces constitute a good prognostic sign. Erythema nodosum is a delayed hypersensitivity response to fungal antigens. No organisms are present in the lesions, and it is not a sign of disseminated disease. The answer is **E**.

7. In progressive or disseminated forms of coccidioidomycosis, systemic antifungal drug treatment is needed. Until recently, amphotericin B was the recommended therapy, but fluconazole or itraconazole are now generally preferred. Note that the risk of dissemination is much greater in African Americans (10% incidence) and in pregnant women during the third trimester. The answer is **B**.

8. Griseofulvin has no activity against *C albicans* and is not effective in the treatment of systemic or superficial infections caused by such organisms. "Swish and swallow" formulations of clotrimazole and nystatin have been used commonly. Most of the azoles are effective in esophageal candidiasis. The answer is **C**.

9. Ketoconazole was the first oral azole introduced into clinical use, but it has a greater propensity to inhibit human cytochrome P450 enzymes than other azoles and is no longer widely used in the United States. Cardiotoxicity may occur when ketoconazole is used by patients taking astemizole or terfenadine as a result of the ability of ketoconazole to inhibit their metabolism via hepatic cytochromes P450. The answer is **D.**

10. Liposomal formulations of amphotericin B result in decreased accumulation of the drug in tissues, including the kidney. As a result, nephrotoxicity is decreased. With some lipid formulations, infusion-related toxicity may also be reduced. Lipid formulations do not have a wider antifungal spectrum; their daily cost ranges from 10 to 40 times more than the conventional formulation of amphotericin B. The answer is **D.**

SKILL KEEPER ANSWERS: INHIBITORS OF CYTOCHROMES P450 (SEE CHAPTERS 4 AND 61)

1. *A sampling of commonly used drugs with cytochrome P450-mediated metabolism inhibited by ketoconazole (and to a much lesser extent by other azoles) includes chlordiazepoxide, cisapride, cyclosporine, didanosine, fluoxetine, loratadine, lovastatin, methadone, nifedipine, phenytoin, quinidine, tacrolimus, theophylline, verapamil, warfarin, zidovudine, and zolpidem.*

2. *Other drugs that inhibit hepatic cytochromes P450 include chloramphenicol, cimetidine, clarithromycin, disulfiram, erythromycin, ethanol, ethinyl estradiol, fluconazole, furanocoumarins (in grapefruit juice), isoniazid, itraconazole, MAO inhibitors, phenylbutazone, and secobarbital.*

CHECKLIST

When you complete this chapter, you should be able to:

❑ Describe the mechanisms of action of the azole, polyene and echinocandin antifungal drugs.

❑ Identify the clinical uses of amphotericin B, flucytosine, individual azoles, caspofungin, griseofulvin, and terbinafine.

❑ Describe the pharmacokinetics and toxicities of amphotericin B.

❑ Describe the pharmacokinetics, toxicities, and drug interactions of the azoles.

❑ Identify the main topical antifungal agents.

DRUG SUMMARY TABLE: Antifungal Drugs

Drug/Drug Class	Mechanism of Action	Clinical Applications	Pharmacokinetics & Interactions	Toxicities
Amphotericin B	Binds to ergosterol in fungal cell membranes, forming "leaky pores"	Candidemia and infections caused by *Aspergillus, Blastomyces, Cryptococcus, Histoplasma, Mucor*, etc	Multiple forms, IV for systemic infections (liposomal forms less nephrotoxic) • topical for ocular/bladder infections	Nephrotoxicity is dose-limiting, additive with other nephrotoxic drugs; infusion reactions (chills, fever, muscle spasms, hypotension)
Azoles 　Ketoconazole 　Fluconazole 　Itraconazole 　Posaconazole 　Voriconazole	Inhibit fungal P450-dependent enzymes blocking ergosterol synthesis • resistance can occur with long-term use	Aspergillosis (voriconazole) • blastomycosis (itraconazole, fluconazole) • mucormycosis (posaconazole) • alternative drugs in candidemia and infections caused by *Aspergillus, Blastomyces, Cryptococcus*, and *Histoplasma*	Various topical and oral forms for dermatophytoses Oral, parenteral forms for mycoses (fluconazole, itraconazole, posaconazole, voriconazole) Most azoles undergo hepatic metabolism • fluconazole eliminated in urine unchanged	Ketoconazole rarely used in systemic fungal infections owing to its inhibition of hepatic and adrenal P450s • other azoles are less toxic, but may cause GI upsets and rash • voriconazole causes visual disturbances and is class D re pregnancy risk
Echinocandins 　Caspofungin 　Micafungin 　Anidulafungin	Inhibit β-glucan synthase decreasing fungal cell wall synthesis	Treatment of candidemia • caspofungin is also used as "salvage" therapy in apergillosis	IV forms • micafungin increases levels of nifedipine and cyclosporine	Gastrointestinal (GI) distress, flushing from histamine release
Flucytosine	Inhibits DNA and RNA polymerases	Synergistic with amphotericin B in candidemia and cryptococal infections	Oral; enters cerebrospinal fluid • renal elimination	Bone marrow suppression
Terbinafine	Inhibits epoxidation of squalene	Mucocutaneous fungal infections • accumulates in keratin	Oral • long duration of action (weeks)	GI upsets, headache

Antiviral Chemotherapy & Prophylaxis

As obligate intracellular parasites, the replication of viruses depends on synthetic processes of the host cell. Antiviral drugs can exert their actions at several stages of viral replication including viral entry, nucleic acid synthesis, late protein synthesis and processing, and in the final stages of viral packaging and virion release (Figure 49–1). Most of the drugs active against herpes viruses (HSV) and many agents active against human immunodeficiency virus (HIV) are antimetabolites, structurally similar to naturally occurring compounds. The selective toxicity of antiviral drugs usually depends on greater susceptibility of viral enzymes to their inhibitory actions than host cell enzymes.

One of the most important trends in viral chemotherapy, especially in the management of HIV infection, has been the introduction of combination drug therapy. This can result in greater clinical effectiveness in viral infections and can also prevent, or delay, the emergence of resistance.

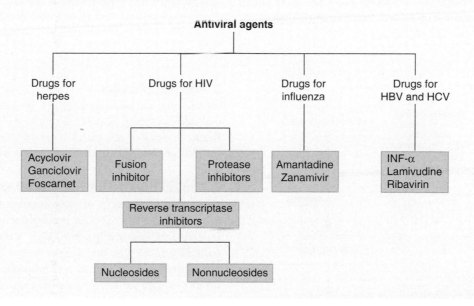

ANTIHERPES DRUGS

Most drugs active against herpes viruses are antimetabolites bioactivated via viral or host cell kinases to form compounds that inhibit viral DNA polymerases.

A. Acyclovir (Acycloguanosine)

1. Mechanisms—Acyclovir is a guanosine analog active against herpes simplex virus (HSV-1, HSV-2) and varicella-zoster virus (VZV).

The drug is activated to form acyclovir triphosphate, which interferes with viral synthesis in 2 ways. It acts as a competitive substrate for DNA polymerase, and it leads to chain termination after its incorporation into viral DNA (Figure 49–2). Resistance of HSV can involve changes in viral DNA polymerase. However, many resistant strains of HSV (TK⁻ strains) lack thymidine kinase, the enzyme involved in the initial *viral-specific* phosphorylation of acyclovir. Such strains are cross-resistant to famciclovir, ganciclovir, and valacyclovir.

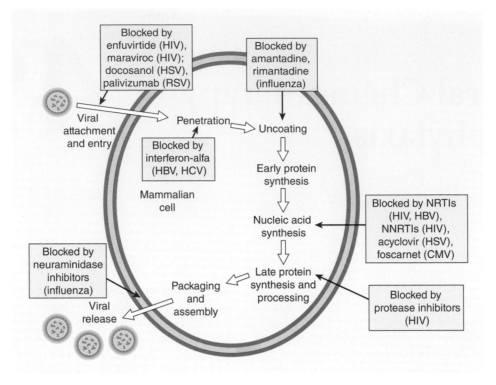

FIGURE 49–1   The major sites of antiviral drug action. Note: interferon-alfas are speculated to have multiple sites of action on viral replication. (Reproduced, with permission, from Katzung BG, editor: *Basic & Clinical Pharmacology*, 12th ed. McGraw-Hill, 2012: Fig. 49–1.)

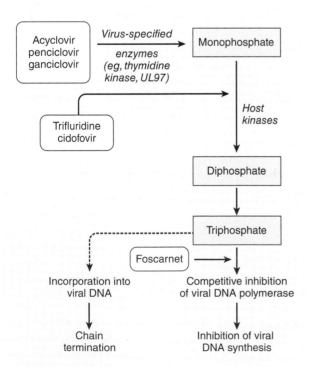

FIGURE 49–2   Mechanism of action of antiherpes agents. (Reproduced, with permission, from Katzung BG, editor: *Basic & Clinical Pharmacology*, 12th ed. McGraw-Hill, 2012: Fig. 49–3.)

2. Pharmacokinetics—Acyclovir can be administered by the topical, oral, and intravenous routes. Because of its short half-life, oral administration requires multiple daily doses of acyclovir. Renal excretion is the major route of elimination of acyclovir, and dosage should be reduced in patients with renal impairment.

3. Clinical uses and toxicity—Oral acyclovir is commonly used for the treatment of mucocutaneous and genital herpes lesions (Table 49–1) and for prophylaxis in AIDS and in other immunocompromised patients (eg, those undergoing organ transplantation). The oral drug is well tolerated but may cause gastrointestinal (GI) distress and headache. Intravenous administration is used for severe herpes disease, including encephalitis, and for neonatal HSV infection. Toxic effects with parenteral administration include delirium, tremor, seizures, hypotension, and nephrotoxicity. Acyclovir has no significant toxicity on the bone marrow.

4. Other drugs for HSV and VSV infections—Several newer agents have characteristics similar to acyclovir. **Valacyclovir** is a prodrug converted to acyclovir by hepatic metabolism after oral administration and reaches plasma levels 3–5 times greater than those achieved by acyclovir. Valacyclovir has a longer duration of action than acyclovir. **Penciclovir** undergoes activation by viral thymidine kinase, and the triphosphate form inhibits DNA polymerase but does not cause chain termination. **Famciclovir** is

TABLE 49–1 Important antiviral drugs.

Virus	Primary Drugs	Alternative or Adjunctive Drugs
CMV	Ganciclovir, valganciclovir	Cidofovir, foscarnet, fomiversin
HSV, VZV	Acyclovir[a]	Cidofovir, foscarnet, vidarabine
HBV	IFN-α, lamivudine	Adefovir dipivoxil, entacavir, lamivudine, telbivudine
HCV	IFN-α	Ribavirin
Influenza A	Oseltamivir	Amantadine, rimantadine, zanamivir
Influenza B	Oseltamivir	Zanamivir

[a]Anti-HSV drugs similar to acyclovir include famciclovir, penciclovir, and valacyclovir; IFN-α, interferon-α.

a prodrug converted to penciclovir by first-pass metabolism in the liver. Used orally in genital herpes and for herpes zoster, famciclovir is well tolerated and is similar to acyclovir in its pharmacokinetic properties. None of the acyclovir congeners has activity against TK⁻ strains of HSV. **Docosanol** is an aliphatic alcohol that inhibits fusion between the HSV envelope and plasma membranes. It prevents viral entry and subsequent replication. Used topically, docosanol shortens healing time.

B. Ganciclovir

1. Mechanisms—Ganciclovir, a guanine derivative, is triphosphorylated to form a nucleotide that inhibits DNA polymerases of cytomegalovirus (CMV), and HSV and causes chain termination. The first phosphorylation step is catalyzed by virus-specific enzymes in both CMV-infected and HSV-infected cells. CMV resistance mechanisms involve mutations in the genes that code for the activating viral phosphotransferase and the viral DNA polymerase. Thymidine kinase-deficient HSV strains are resistant to ganciclovir.

2. Pharmacokinetics—Ganciclovir is usually given intravenously and penetrates well into tissues, including the eye and the central nervous system (CNS). The drug undergoes renal elimination in direct proportion to creatinine clearance. Oral bioavailability is less than 10%. An intraocular implant form of ganciclovir can be used in CMV retinitis. **Valganciclovir**, a prodrug of ganciclovir, has high oral bioavailability and has decreased the use of intravenous forms of ganciclovir (and also of intravenous cidofovir and foscarnet) in end-organ CMV disease.

3. Clinical uses and toxicity—Ganciclovir is used for the prophylaxis and treatment of CMV retinitis and other CMV infections in immunocompromised patients. Systemic toxic effects include leukopenia, thrombocytopenia, mucositis, hepatic dysfunction, and seizures. The drug may cause severe neutropenia when used with zidovudine or other myelosuppressive agents.

C. Cidofovir

1. Mechanisms and pharmacokinetics—Cidofovir is activated exclusively by host cell kinases and the active diphosphate, which inhibits DNA polymerases of HSV, CMV, adenovirus, and papillomavirus (HPV). Because phosphorylation does not require viral kinase, cidofovir is active against many acyclovir and ganciclovir-resistant strains. Resistance is due to mutations in the DNA polymerase gene. The drug is given intravenously and undergoes renal elimination. Dosage should be adjusted in proportion to creatinine clearance and full hydration maintained.

2. Clinical uses and toxicity—Cidofovir is effective in CMV retinitis, in mucocutaneous HSV infections, including those resistant to acyclovir, and in genital warts. Nephrotoxicity is the major dose-limiting toxicity of cidofovir, additive with other nephrotoxic drugs including amphotericin B and aminoglycoside antibiotics.

D. Foscarnet

1. Mechanisms—Foscarnet is a phosphonoformate derivative that does not require phosphorylation for antiviral activity. Although it is not an antimetabolite, foscarnet inhibits viral RNA polymerase, DNA polymerase, and HIV reverse transcriptase. Resistance involves point mutations in the DNA polymerase gene.

2. Pharmacokinetics—Foscarnet is given intravenously and penetrates well into tissues, including the CNS. The drug undergoes renal elimination in direct proportion to creatinine clearance.

3. Clinical uses and toxicity—The drug is an alternative for prophylaxis and treatment of CMV infections, including CMV retinitis, and has activity against ganciclovir-resistant strains of this virus. Foscarnet inhibits herpes DNA polymerase in acyclovir-resistant strains that are thymidine kinase–deficient and may suppress such resistant herpetic infections in patients with AIDS. Adverse effects are severe and include nephrotoxicity (30% incidence) with disturbances in electrolyte balance (especially hypocalcemia), genitourinary ulceration, and CNS effects (headache, hallucinations, seizures).

E. Other Antiherpes Drugs

1. Vidarabine—Vidarabine is an adenine analog and has activity against HSV, VZV, and CMV. Its use for systemic infections is limited by rapid metabolic inactivation and marked toxic potential. Vidarabine is used topically for herpes keratitis but has no effect on genital lesions. Toxic effects with systemic use include GI irritation, paresthesias, tremor, convulsions, and hepatic dysfunction. Vidarabine is teratogenic in animals.

2. Idoxuridine and trifluridine—These pyrimidine analogs are used topically in herpes keratitis (HSV-1). They are too toxic for systemic use.

3. Fomivirsen—Fomivirsen is an antisense oligonucleotide that binds to mRNA of CMV, inhibiting early protein synthesis. The drug is injected intravitreally for treatment of CMV retinitis.

Cross-resistance between fomivirsen and other anti-CMV agents has not been observed. Concurrent systemic anti-CMV therapy is recommended to protect against extraocular and contralateral retinal CMV disease. Fomivirsen causes iritis, vitreitis, increased intraocular pressure and changes in vision.

ANTI-HIV DRUGS

The primary drugs effective against HIV are antimetabolite inhibitors of viral reverse transcriptase and inhibitors of viral aspartate protease (Table 49–2). The current approach to treatment of infection with HIV is the initiation of treatment with 3 or more antiretroviral drugs, if possible, before symptoms appear. Such combinations usually include nucleoside reverse transcriptase inhibitors (NRTIs) together with inhibitors of HIV protease (PI). Highly active antiretroviral therapy (HAART) involving drug combinations can slow or reverse the increases in viral RNA load that normally accompany progression of disease. In many AIDS patients, HAART slows or reverses the decline in CD4 cells and decreases the incidence of opportunistic infections.

Drug management of HIV infection is subject to change. Updated recommendations can be obtained at the following websites: ATIS, http://www.hivatis.org; and NPIN, http://www.cdcnpin.org.

A. Nucleoside Reverse Transcriptase Inhibitors (NRTIs)

To convert their RNA into dsDNA, retroviruses require virally encoded RNA-dependent DNA polymerase (reverse transcriptase). Mammalian RNA and DNA polymerases are sufficiently distinct to permit a selective inhibition of the viral reverse transcriptase.

NRTIs are prodrugs converted by host cell kinases to triphosphates, which not only competitively inhibit binding of natural nucleotides to the dNTP-binding site of reverse transcriptase but

TABLE 49–2 Major antiretroviral drugs.

Subclass	Prototype	Other Significant Agents
Nucleoside reverse transcriptase inhibitors	Zidovudine	Abacavir, didanosine, emtricitabine, lamivudine, stavudine, zalcitabine, zidovudine
Nonnucleoside reverse transcriptase inhibitors	Delavirdine	Efavirenz, etravirine, nevirapine, tenofovir
Protease inhibitors	Indinavir	Amprenavir, atazanavir, darunavir, indinavir, lopinavir, nelfinavir, ritonavir, saquinavir, tipranavir
CCR-5 antagonist	Maraviroc	
Fusion inhibitor	Enfuvirtide	

also act as chain terminators via their insertion into the growing DNA chain. Because NRTIs lack a 3'-hydroxyl group on the ribose ring, attachment of the next nucleotide is impossible. Resistance emerges rapidly when NRTIs are used as single agents via mutations in the *pol* gene; cross-resistance occurs but is not complete.

1. Abacavir—A guanosine analog, abacavir has good oral bioavailability and an intracellular half-life of 12–24 h. HIV resistance requires several concomitant mutations and tends to develop slowly. Hypersensitivity reactions, occasionally fatal, occur in 5% of HIV patients.

2. Didanosine (ddI)—Oral bioavailability of ddI is reduced by food and by chelating agents. The drug is eliminated by the kidney, and the dose must be reduced in patients with renal dysfunction. Pancreatitis is dose-limiting and occurs more frequently in alcoholic patients and those with hypertriglyceridemia. Other adverse effects include peripheral neuropathy, diarrhea, hepatic dysfunction, hyperuricemia, and CNS effects.

3. Emtricitabine—Good oral bioavailability and renal elimination with long half-life permits once-daily dosing of emtricitabine. Because of the propylene glycol in the oral solution, the drug is contraindicated in pregnancy and young children and in patients with hepatic or renal dysfunction. Common adverse effects of the drug include asthenia, GI distress, headache, and hyperpigmentation of the palms and/or the soles.

4. Lamivudine (3TC)—Lamivudine is 80% bioavailable by the oral route and is eliminated almost exclusively by the kidney. In addition to its use in HAART regimens for HIV, lamivudine is also effective in hepatitis B infections. Dosage adjustment is needed in patients with renal insufficiency. Adverse effects of lamivudine are usually mild and include GI distress, headache, insomnia, and fatigue.

5. Stavudine (d4T)—Stavudine has good oral bioavailability and penetrates most tissues, including the CNS. Dosage adjustment is needed in renal insufficiency. Peripheral neuropathy is dose-limiting and increased with coadministration of didanosine or zalcitabine. Lactic acidosis with hepatic steatosis occurs more frequently with stavudine than with other NRTIs.

6. Tenofovir—Although it is a nucleotide, tenofovir acts like NRTIs to competitively inhibit reverse transcript and cause chain termination after incorporation into DNA. Tenofovir also has activity against HBV (see below). Oral bioavailability of tenofovir is in the range 25–40%, the intracellular half-life is more than 60 h, and the drug undergoes renal elimination. Tenofovir may impede the renal elimination of acyclovir and ganciclovir. Adverse effects include GI distress, asthenia, and headache; rare cases of acute renal failure and Fanconi's syndrome have been reported.

7. Zalcitabine (ddC)—Zalcitabine has a high oral bioavailability. Dosage adjustment is needed in patients with renal insufficiency and nephrotoxic drugs (eg, amphotericin B, aminoglycosides) increase toxic potential. Dose-limiting peripheral neuropathy is the major adverse effect of ddC. Pancreatitis, esophageal ulceration, stomatitis, and arthralgias may also occur.

8. Zidovudine (ZDV)—Formerly called azidothymidine (AZT), zidovudine is active orally and is distributed to most tissues, including the CNS. Elimination of the drug involves both hepatic metabolism to glucuronides and renal excretion. Dosage reduction is necessary in uremic patients and those with cirrhosis. The primary toxicity of zidovudine is bone marrow suppression (additive with other immunosuppressive drugs) leading to anemia and neutropenia, which may require transfusions. GI distress, thrombocytopenia, headaches, myalgia, acute cholestatic hepatitis, agitation, and insomnia may also occur. Drugs that may increase plasma levels of zidovudine include azole antifungals and protease inhibitors. Rifampin increases the clearance of zidovudine.

9. NRTIs and lactic acidosis—NRTI agents, taken alone or in combination with other antiretroviral agents, may cause lactic acidemia and severe hepatomegaly with steatosis. Risk factors include obesity, prolonged treatment with NRTIs, and preexisting liver dysfunction. Consideration should be given to suspension of NRTI treatment in patients who develop elevated aminotransferase levels.

B. Nonnucleoside Reverse Transcriptase Inhibitors (NNRTIs)

NNRTIs bind to a site on reverse transcriptase different from the binding site of NRTIs. Nonnucleoside drugs do not require phosphorylation to be active and do not compete with nucleoside triphosphates. There is no cross-resistance with NRTIs. Resistance from mutations in the *pol* gene occur very rapidly if these agents are used as monotherapy.

1. Delavirdine—Drug interactions are a major problem with delavirdine, which is metabolized by both CYP3A4 and CYP2D6. Its blood levels are decreased by antacids, ddI, phenytoin, rifampin, and nelfinavir. Conversely, the blood levels of delavirdine are increased by azole antifungals and macrolide antibiotics. Delavirdine increases plasma levels of several benzodiazepines, nifedipine, protease inhibitors, quinidine, and warfarin. Delavirdine cause skin rash in up to 20% of patients, and the drug should be avoided in pregnancy because it is teratogenic in animals.

2. Efavirenz—Efavirenz can be given once daily because of its long half-life. Fatty foods may enhance its oral bioavailability. Efavirenz is metabolized by hepatic cytochromes P450 and is frequently involved in drug interactions. Toxicity of efavirenz includes CNS dysfunction, skin rash, and elevations of plasma cholesterol. The drug should be avoided in pregnancy, particularly in the first trimester because fetal abnormalities have been reported in animals at doses similar to those used in humans.

3. Etravirine—Etravirine, the newest NNRTI approved for treatment-experienced HIV patients, may be effective against HIV strains resistant to other drugs in the group. The drug causes rash, nausea, and diarrhea. Elevations in serum cholesterol, triglycerides, and transaminase levels may occur. Etravirine is a substrate as well as an inducer of CYP3A4 and also inhibits CYP2C9 and CYP2C19 and may be involved in significant drug–drug interactions.

4. Nevirapine—Nevirapine has good oral bioavailability, penetrates most tissues including the CNS, has a half-life of more than 24 h, and is metabolized by the hepatic CYP3A4 isoform. The drug is used in combination regimens and is effective in preventing HIV vertical transmission when given as single doses to mothers at the onset of labor and to the neonate. Hypersensitivity reactions with nevirapine include a rash, which occurs in 15–20% of patients, especially female. Stevens-Johnson syndrome and a life-threatening toxic epidermal necrolysis have also been reported. Nevirapine blood levels are increased by cimetidine and macrolide antibiotics and decreased by enzyme inducers such as rifampin.

C. Protease Inhibitors

The assembly of infectious HIV virions is dependent on an aspartate protease (HIV-1 protease) encoded by the *pol* gene. This viral enzyme cleaves precursor polyproteins to form the final structural proteins of the mature virion core. The HIV protease inhibitors are designer drugs based on molecular characterization of the active site of the viral enzyme. Resistance is mediated via multiple point mutations in the *pol* gene; the extent of cross-resistance is variable depending on the specific protease inhibitor. Protease inhibitors (PIs) have important clinical use in AIDS, most commonly in combinations with reverse transcriptase inhibitors as components of HAART. All of the PIs are substrates and inhibitors of CYP3A4 with ritonavir having the most pronounced inhibitory effect. The PIs are implicated in many drug–drug interactions with other antiretroviral agents and with commonly used medications.

1. Atazanavir—This is a PI with a pharmacokinetic profile that permits once-daily dosing. Oral absorption of atazanavir requires an acidic environment—antacid ingestion should be separated by 12 h. The drug penetrates cerebrospinal and seminal fluids and undergoes biliary elimination. Adverse effects include GI distress, peripheral neuropathy, skin rash, and hyperbilirubinemia. Prolongation of the QTc interval may occur at high doses. Unlike most PIs, atazanavir does not appear to be associated with dyslipidemias, fat deposition, or a metabolic syndrome. However, it is a potent inhibitor of CYP3A4 and CYP2C9.

2. Darunavir—This drug is used in combination with ritonavir in treatment-experienced patients with resistance to other PIs. The drug is a substrate of CYP3A4. GI adverse effects and rash occur, and liver toxicity has been reported. Darunavir contains a sulfonamide moiety and should be used with caution in sulfonamide allergy.

3. Fosamprenavir—Fosamprenavir is a prodrug forming amprenavir via its hydrolysis in the GI tract. The drug formulation includes propylene glycol and should not be used in children or in pregnant women. Fosamprenavir is often used in combination with low-dose ritonavir. The absorption of amprenavir is impeded by fatty foods. Amprenavir undergoes hepatic metabolism and is both an inhibitor and an inducer of CYP3A4. The drug causes GI distress, paresthesias, and rash, the latter sometimes severe enough to warrant drug discontinuation. Cross-allergenicity may occur with sulfonamides.

4. Indinavir—Oral bioavailability of indinavir is good except in the presence of food. Clearance is mainly via the liver, with about 10% renal excretion. Adverse effects include nausea, diarrhea, thrombocytopenia, hyperbilirubinemia, and nephrolithiasis. To reduce renal damage, it is important to maintain good hydration. Insulin resistance may be more common with indinavir than other PIs. Indinavir is a substrate for and an inhibitor of the cytochrome P450 isoform CYP3A4 and is implicated in drug interactions. Serum levels of indinavir are increased by azole antifungals and decreased by rifamycins. Indinavir increases the serum levels of antihistamines, benzodiazepines, and rifampin.

5. Lopinavir/ritonavir—In this combination, a subtherapeutic dose of ritonavir acts as a pharmacokinetic enhancer by inhibiting the CYP3A4-mediated metabolism of lopinavir. Patient compliance is improved owing to lower pill burden and the combination is usually well tolerated.

6. Nelfinavir—This PI is characterized by increased oral absorption in the presence of food, hepatic metabolism via CYP3A4 and a short half-life. As an inhibitor of drug metabolism, nelfinavir has been involved in many drug interactions. Adverse effects include diarrhea, which can be dose-limiting. The drug has the most favorable safety profile of the PIs in pregnancy.

7. Ritonavir—Oral bioavailability is good, and the drug should be taken with meals. Clearance is mainly via the liver, and dosage reduction is necessary in patients with hepatic impairment. The most common adverse effects of ritonavir are GI irritation and a bitter taste. Paresthesias and elevations of hepatic aminotransferases and triglycerides in the plasma also occur. Drugs that increase the activity of the cytochrome P450 isoform CYP3A4 (anticonvulsants, rifamycins) reduce serum levels of ritonavir, and drugs that inhibit this enzyme (azole antifungals, cimetidine, erythromycin) elevate serum levels of the antiviral drug. Ritonavir inhibits the metabolism of a wide range of drugs, including erythromycin, dronabinol, ketoconazole, prednisone, rifampin, and saquinavir.

Subtherapeutic doses of ritonavir inhibit the CYP3A-mediated metabolism of other protease inhibitors (eg, indinavir, lopinavir, saquinavir); this is the rationale for PI combinations that include ritonavir because it permits the use of lower doses of the other protease inhibitor.

8. Saquinavir—Original formulations of saquinavir had low and erratic oral bioavailability. Reformulation for once-daily dosing in combination with low-dose ritonavir has improved efficacy with decreased GI side effects. The drug undergoes extensive first-pass metabolism and functions as both a substrate and inhibitor of CYP3A4. Adverse effects of saquinavir include nausea, diarrhea, dyspepsia, and rhinitis. Saquinavir plasma levels are increased by azole antifungals, clarithromycin, grapefruit juice, indinavir, and ritonavir. Drugs that induce CYP3A4 decrease plasma levels of saquinavir.

9. Tipranavir—This is a newer drug used in combination with ritonavir in treatment-experienced patients with resistance to other PIs. The drug is a substrate and inducer of CYP3A4 and also induces P-glycoprotein transporters, possibly altering GI absorption of other drugs. For example, increased blood levels of the HMG-CoA reductase inhibitors (eg, lovastatin) may occur, thus increasing the risk for myopathy and rhabdomyolysis. GI adverse effects, rash, and liver toxicity have been reported.

10. Effects on carbohydrate and lipid metabolism—The use of PIs in HAART drug combinations has led to the development of disorders in carbohydrate and lipid metabolism. It has been suggested that this is due to the inhibition of lipid-regulating proteins, which have active sites with structural homology to that of HIV protease. The syndrome includes hyperglycemia and insulin resistance or hyperlipidemia, with altered body fat distribution. Buffalo hump, gynecomastia, and truncal obesity may occur with facial and peripheral lipodystrophy. The syndrome has been observed with PIs used in HAART regimens, with an incidence of 30–50% and a median onset time of approximately 1 yr duration of treatment.

D. Entry Inhibitors

1. Maraviroc—HIV-1 infection begins with attachment of an HIV envelope protein called gp120 to CD4 molecules on surfaces of helper T cells and other antigen-presenting cells such as macrophages and dendritic cells. The attachment of many HIV strains involves a transmembrane chemokine receptor CCR5. This receptor, a *human* protein, is the target for maraviroc, which blocks viral attachment. Although resistance has occurred, there is minimal cross-resistance with other antiretroviral drugs.

Maraviroc is used orally and has good tissue penetration. It is a substrate for CYP3A4, and dosage adjustments may be needed in the presence of drugs that induce or inhibit this enzyme. Adverse effects of maraviroc include cough, diarrhea, muscle and joint pain, and increases in hepatic transaminases.

2. Enfuvirtide—Enfuvirtide is a synthetic 36-amino-acid peptide. The drug binds to the gp41 subunit of the viral envelope glycoprotein, preventing the conformational changes required for the fusion of the viral and cellular membranes. There is no cross-resistance with other anti-HIV drugs, but resistance may occur via mutations in the *env* gene. Enfuvirtide is administered subcutaneously in combination with other anti-HIV agents in previously drug-treated patients with persistent HIV-1 replication despite ongoing therapy. Its metabolism via hydrolysis does not involve the cytochrome P450 system. Injection site reactions and hypersensitivity may occur. An increased incidence of bacterial pneumonia has been reported.

E. Integrase Strand Transfer Inhibitors

Raltegravir is a pyrimidine derivative that binds integrase, an enzyme essential to replication of both HIV-1 and HIV-2, inhibiting strand transfer. As a result, integration of reverse-transcribed HIV DNA into host cell chromosomes is inhibited. The drug has been used mainly in treatment-naïve HIV patients, usually in combination regimens. The drug is metabolized by glucuronidation and is not affected by agents that induce or inhibit hepatic cytochromes P450. However, if used with rifampin, which induces UDP-glucuronosyltransferase, the dose of raltegravir should be doubled. Adverse effects include nausea, diarrhea, dizziness, and fatigue. An increase in creatine kinase has been reported, with potential for myopathy or rhabdomyolysis.

ANTI-INFLUENZA AGENTS

A. Amantadine and Rimantadine

1. Mechanisms—Amantadine and rimantadine inhibit an early step in replication of the influenza A (but not influenza B) virus (Figure 49–1). They prevent "uncoating" by binding to a protein M2. This protein functions as a proton ion channel required at the onset of infection to permit acidification of the virus core, which in turn activates viral RNA transcriptase. Adamantine-resistant influenza A virus mutants are now common.

2. Clinical uses and toxicity—These drugs are prophylactic against influenza A virus infection and can reduce the duration of symptoms if given within 48 h after contact. However, adamantine-resistant influenza A virus mutants including H3N2 strains causing seasonal influenza in the United States have increased dramatically in the last 2–3 yr. The H1N1 strain responsible for the recent pandemic that contain genes derived from both avian and porcine influenza viruses is also resistant to the adamantines. Fortunately, there is minimal cross-resistance to the neuraminidase inhibitors. Toxic effects of these agents include GI irritation, dizziness, ataxia, and slurred speech. Rimantadine's activity is no greater than that of amantadine, but it has a longer half-life and requires no dosage adjustment in renal failure.

B. Oseltamivir and Zanamivir

1. Mechanisms—These drugs are inhibitors of neuraminidases produced by influenza A and B and are currently active against both H3N2 and H1N1 strains. These viral enzymes cleave sialic acid residues from viral proteins and surface proteins of infected cells. They function to promote virion release and to prevent clumping of newly released virions. By interfering with these actions, neuraminidase inhibitors impede viral spread. Decreased susceptibility to the drugs is associated with mutations in viral neuraminidase, but worldwide resistance remains rare.

2. Clinical use and toxicity—Oseltamivir is a prodrug used orally, activated in the gut and the liver. Zanamivir is administered intranasally. Both drugs decrease the time to alleviation of influenza symptoms and are more effective if used within 24 h after onset of symptoms. Taken prophylactically, oseltamivir significantly decreases the incidence of influenza. GI symptoms may occur with oseltamivir; zanamivir may cause cough and throat discomfort and has induced bronchospasm in asthmatic patients.

AGENTS USED IN VIRAL HEPATITIS

The agents available for use in the treatment of infections caused by hepatitis B virus (HBV) are suppressive rather than curative. The primary goal of drugs used for infections caused by hepatitis C virus (HCV) is viral eradication. The drugs available include interferon-α (IFN-α), lamivudine, adefovir dipivoxil, entacavir, telbivudine, tenofovir, and ribavirin.

A. IFN-α

1. Mechanisms—IFN-α is a cytokine that acts through host cell surface receptors increasing the activity of Janus kinases (JAKS). These enzymes phosphorylate signal transducers and activators of transcription (STATS) to increase the formation of antiviral proteins. The selective antiviral action of IFN-α is primarily due to activation of a host cell ribonuclease that preferentially degrades viral mRNA. IFN-α also promotes formation of natural killer cells that destroy infected liver cells.

2. Pharmacokinetics—There are several forms of IFN-α with minor differences in amino acid composition. Absorption from intramuscular or subcutaneous injection is slow; elimination of IFN-α is mainly via proteolytic hydrolysis in the kidney. Conventional forms of IFN-α are usually administered daily or 3 times a week. Pegylated forms of IFN-α conjugated to polyethylene glycol can be administered once a week.

3. Clinical uses—Interferon-α is used in chronic HBV as an individual agent or in combination with other drugs. When used in combinations with ribavirin, the progression of acute HCV infection to chronic HCV is reduced. Pegylated IFN-α together with ribavirin is superior to standard forms of IFN-α in chronic HCV. Other uses of IFN-α include treatment of Kaposi's sarcoma, papillomatosis, and topically for genital warts. Interferons also prevent dissemination of herpes zoster in cancer patients and reduce CMV shedding after renal transplantation.

4. Toxicity—Toxic effects of IFN-α include GI irritation, a flu-like syndrome, neutropenia, profound fatigue and myalgia, alopecia, reversible hearing loss, thyroid dysfunction, mental confusion, and severe depression. Contraindications include autoimmune disease, a history of cardiac arrhythmias, and pregnancy.

B. Adefovir Dipivoxil

1. Mechanisms—Adefovir dipivoxil is the prodrug of adefovir, which following its phosphorylation by cellular kinases, competitively inhibits HBV DNA polymerase and results in chain termination after incorporation into the viral DNA. HBV resistance to adefovir—though uncommon—has recently been reported.

2. Pharmacokinetics and clinical use—Adefovir has good oral bioavailability unaffected by foods. The drug is eliminated by the kidney, and dose reductions are required in renal dysfunction.

Adefovir suppresses HBV replication and improves liver histology and fibrosis. However, serum HBV DNA reappears after cessation of therapy. Adefovir has activity against lamivudine-resistant strains of HBV.

3. Toxicity—Nephrotoxicity is dose-limiting. Lactic acidosis and severe hepatomegaly with steatosis may also occur.

C. Entecavir

Entecavir is a guanosine nucleoside that inhibits HBV DNA polymerase. Effective orally, the drug has an intracellular half-life of more than 12 h and undergoes renal elimination in part via active tubular secretion. Clinical efficacy is similar to that of lamivudine and there is cross-resistance between the 2 drugs. The drug causes headache, dizziness, fatigue, and nausea.

D. Lamivudine

This nucleoside inhibitor of HIV reverse transcriptase (see prior discussion) is active in chronic HBV infection. Lamivudine has a longer intracellular half-life in HBV-infected cells than in HIV-infected cells (see prior discussion) and thus can be used in lower doses for hepatitis than for HIV infection. Used as monotherapy, lamivudine rapidly suppresses HBV replication and is remarkably nontoxic. However, coinfection with HIV may increase the risk of pancreatitis. Lamivudine–resistant HBV mutants emerge at a rate of about 20% per year if the drug is used alone. On reappearance of detectable levels of HBV DNA, patients should be switched to IFN-α or adefovir.

E. Ribavirin

1. Mechanisms—Ribavirin inhibits the replication of a wide range of DNA and RNA viruses, including influenza A and B, parainfluenza, respiratory syncytial virus (RSV), paramyxoviruses, HCV, and HIV. Although the precise antiviral mechanism of ribavirin is not known, the drug inhibits guanosine triphosphate formation, prevents capping of viral mRNA, and can block RNA-dependent RNA polymerases.

2. Pharmacokinetics and clinical uses—Ribavirin is effective orally (avoid antacids) and is also available in intravenous and aerosolic forms. It is eliminated by the kidney, necessitating dose reductions in renal dysfunction. Ribavirin is used adjunctively with IFN-α in chronic HCV infection in patients with compensated liver disease. Monotherapy with ribavirin alone is not effective. Early intravenous administration of ribavirin decreases mortality in viral hemorrhagic fevers. Despite its alleged activity against RSV, ribavirin has been shown to have no benefit in treatment of RSV infections, although it is still recommended by some authorities in immunocompromised children.

3. Toxicity—Systemic use results in dose-dependent hemolytic anemia. Aerosolic ribavirin may cause conjunctival and bronchial irritation. Ribavirin is a known human teratogen, absolutely contraindicated in pregnancy.

F. Newer Drugs for HBV

Telbivudine, a nucleoside analog, is phosphorylated by cellular kinases to the triphosphate form, which inhibits HBV DNA polymerase. The drug is at least as effective as lamivudine in chronic HBV infections and is similar in terms of its safety profile. However, like lamivudine, HBV mutants emerge at a rate of about 20% per year if the drug is used alone. **Tenofovir,** an antiretroviral drug, is also approved for chronic HBV infection and is active against lamivudine- and entecavir-resistant strains.

QUESTIONS

1. Which statement about the mechanisms of action of antiviral drugs is accurate?
   (A) Acyclovir has no requirement for activation by phosphorylation
   (B) An increase in activity of host cell ribonucleases that degrade viral mRNA is one of the antiviral actions of interferon-α
   (C) Ganciclovir inhibits viral DNA polymerase but does not cause chain termination
   (D) The initial step in activation of foscarnet in HSV-infected cells is its phosphorylation by thymidine kinase
   (E) The reverse transcriptase of HIV is 30–50 times more sensitive to inhibition by fosamprenavir than host cell DNA polymerases

Questions 2 and 3. A 30-year-old male patient who is HIV-positive and symptomatic has a CD4 count of 250/μL and a viral RNA load of 15,000 copies/mL. His treatment involves a 3-drug antiviral regimen consisting of zidovudine, didanosine, and ritonavir. In addition, the patient is taking oral valacyclovir for a herpes infection and ketoconazole for oral candidiasis. Because of weight loss, he is taking dronabinol. In addition, verapamil has been prescribed because he suffers from angina. He now complains of anorexia, nausea and vomiting, and abdominal pain. His abdomen is tender in the epigastric area. Laboratory results reveal an amylase activity of 220 units/L, and a preliminary diagnosis is made of acute pancreatitis.

2. If this patient has acute pancreatitis, the drug most likely to be responsible is
   (A) Didanosine
   (B) Ketoconazole
   (C) Ritonavir
   (D) Valacyclovir
   (E) Zidovudine

3. In the further treatment of this patient, the drug causing the pancreatitis should be withdrawn and replaced by
   (A) Atazanavir
   (B) Cidofovir
   (C) Foscarnet
   (D) Lamivudine
   (E) Ribavirin

4. In an accidental needlestick, an unknown quantity of blood from an AIDS patient is injected into a resident physician. The most recent laboratory report on the AIDS patient shows a CD4 count of 20/μL and a viral RNA load of greater than 10^7 copies/mL. The most appropriate course of action regarding treatment of the resident is to
   (A) Monitor the resident's blood to determine whether HIV transmission has occurred
   (B) Treat with single doses of ritonavir and zidovudine
   (C) Treat with full doses of zidovudine for 2 wk
   (D) Treat with full doses of zidovudine for 4 wk
   (E) Treat with zidovudine plus lamivudine plus a protease inhibitor for 4 wk

Questions 5 and 6. A patient with AIDS has a CD4 count of 45/μL. He is being maintained on a 3-drug regimen of indinavir, didanosine, and zidovudine. For prophylaxis against opportunistic infections, he is also receiving ganciclovir, fluconazole, rifabutin, and trimethoprim-sulfamethoxazole.

5. The drug most likely to suppress herpetic infections and provide prophylaxis against CMV retinitis in this patient is
   (A) Fluconazole
   (B) Ganciclovir
   (C) Indinavir
   (D) Rifabutin
   (E) Trimethoprim-sulfamethoxazole

6. The dose of indinavir in this patient may need to be increased above normal. This is because
   (A) Fluconazole slows gastric emptying
   (B) Ganciclovir increases the renal clearance of indinavir
   (C) Indinavir has to be taken with meals
   (D) Rifabutin increases liver drug-metabolizing enzymes
   (E) Sulfamethoxazole displaces indinavir from plasma proteins

7. A 27-year-old nursing mother is diagnosed as suffering from genital herpes. She has a history of this viral infection. Previously, she responded to a drug used topically. Apart from her current problem, she is in good health. Which drug to be used orally is most likely to be prescribed at this time?
   (A) Amantadine
   (B) Foscarnet
   (C) Ritonavir
   (D) Trifluridine
   (E) Valacyclovir

8. Oral formulations of this drug should not be used in a pregnant AIDS patient because they contain propylene glycol. One of the characteristic adverse effects of the drug is hyperpigmentation on the palms of the hands and soles of the feet especially in African-American patients.
   (A) Amprenavir
   (B) Efavirenz
   (C) Emtricitabine
   (D) Enfuvirtide
   (E) Zalcitabine

9. Regarding interferon-α, which of the following statements is false?
   (A) At the start of treatment, most patients experience flu-like symptoms
   (B) Indications include treatment of genital warts
   (C) It is used in the management of hepatitis B and C
   (D) Lamivudine interferes with its activity against hepatitis B
   (E) Toxicity includes bone marrow suppression

10. More than 90% of this drug is excreted in the urine in intact form. Because its urinary solubility is low, patients should be well hydrated to prevent nephrotoxicity. Which drug is described?
    (A) Acyclovir
    (B) Efavirenz
    (C) Indinavir
    (D) Trifluridine
    (E) Zidovudine

ANSWERS

1. Acyclovir is activated by host cell kinases. Like acyclovir, ganciclovir inhibits viral DNA polymerase and causes chain termination. However, foscarnet inhibits viral DNA polymerase without requiring bioactivation. Fosamprenavir is the prodrug of amprenavir, an inhibitor of HIV protease; it has no significant effect on reverse transcriptase. The answer is **B.**

2. Gastrointestinal problems occur with most antiviral drugs used in the HIV-positive patient, and acute pancreatitis has been reported for several reverse transcriptase inhibitors. However, didanosine is the drug most likely to be responsible because its most characteristic adverse effect is a dose-limiting acute pancreatitis. Other risk factors that are relative contraindications to didanosine are advanced AIDS, hypertriglyceridemia, and alcoholism. The answer is **A.**

3. Symptomatic AIDS patients should be treated with a HAART regimen regardless of a relatively high CD4 count or a relatively low HIV RNA load. Because didanosine must be discontinued, lamivudine would be the best choice for replacement in this case. Use of a second protease inhibitor (eg, atazanavir) with a single reverse transcriptase inhibitor could be as effective as regimens that include 2 reverse transcriptase inhibitors, although there may be an increased possibility of drug interactions. Atazanavir use is associated with electrocardiographic PR-interval prolongation, which may be exacerbated by other causative agents such as the calcium channel blocker verapamil, which the patient is taking for angina. The answer is **D.**

4. The viral RNA titer in the blood from the AIDS patient in this case is very high, and this needlestick must be considered as a high-risk situation. Although full doses of zidovudine for 4 wk has been shown to have prophylactic value, in high-risk situations combination regimens are favored. Optimal prophylaxis in this case might best be provided by the combination of zidovudine with lamivudine (basic regimen), plus the addition of protease inhibitors (expanded regimen). The answer is **E.**

5. Ganciclovir has been the most commonly used drug for prevention and treatment of CMV infections in the immunocompromised patient. Cidofovir (not listed) is also very effective in CMV retinitis and has good activity against many strains of HSV, including those resistant to acyclovir. The answer is **B.**

6. Drug interactions can be severe in the immunocompromised patient because many of the drugs administered can influence the pharmacokinetic properties of other drugs. Rifabutin, like rifampin, acts as an inducer of several isoforms of hepatic cytochrome P450. This action can result in an increased clearance of other drugs, including indinavir. The answer is **D.**

7. Three of the drugs listed (foscarnet, trifluridine, valacyclovir) are active against strains of herpes simplex virus. Foscarnet is not used in genital infections (HSV-2) because clinical efficacy has not been established, it has poor oral bioavailability and the drug causes many toxic effects. Trifluridine is used topically but only for herpes keratoconjunctivitis (HSV-1). Valacyclovir is converted to acyclovir by first-pass metabolism in the intestine and liver. The answer is **E.**

8. Three of the drugs listed should be avoided, or used with extreme caution, in the pregnant patient. Oral forms of amprenavir and emtricitabine both contain propylene glycol, a potentially toxic compound. Efavirenz has caused fetal abnormalities in pregnant monkeys. However, one of the distinctive adverse effects of emtricitabine is hyperpigmentation. The answer is **C.**

9. Lamivudine is used in monotherapy of HBV infections and does not oppose the beneficial effects of interferon-α when both agents are used together in the treatment of hepatitis B. The answer is **D.**

10. Acyclovir is eliminated in the urine by glomerular filtration and by active tubular secretion, which is inhibited by probenecid. Nephrotoxic effects, including hematuria and crystalluria, are enhanced in patients who are dehydrated or who have preexisting renal dysfunction. Adequate hydration is equally important in the case of indinavir because it causes nephrolithiasis. However, more than 80% of a dose of indinavir is eliminated via hepatic metabolism. Trifluridine is used topically to treat herpes keratoconjunctivitis. The answer is **A.**

CHECKLIST

When you complete this chapter, you should be able to:

❑ Identify the main steps in viral replication that are targets for antiviral drug action.

❑ Describe the mechanisms of action of antiherpes drugs and the mechanisms of HSV and CMV resistance.

❑ List the characteristic pharmacokinetic properties and toxic effects of acyclovir, ganciclovir, cidofovir, and foscarnet.

❑ Describe the mechanisms of anti-HIV action of zidovudine, indinavir, and enfuvirtide.

❑ Match a specific antiretroviral drug with each of the following, to be avoided in pregnancy: hyperpigmentation, neutropenia, pancreatitis, peripheral neuropathy, inhibition of P450, severe hypersensitivity reaction, injection site reactions.

❑ Identify the significant characteristics of 4 drugs active against HBV and HCV.

❑ Identify the significant characteristics of an anti-influenza drug acting at the stage of viral uncoating and another acting at the stage of viral release.

DRUG SUMMARY TABLE: Antivirals & Antiretrovirals

Drug Class	Mechanism of Action	Clinical Applications	Pharmacokinetics & Interactions	Toxicities
Antiviral Drugs				
Antiherpes drugs				
Acyclovir Valacyclovir (prodrug) Penciclovir Famciclovir (prodrug)	Activated by viral thymidine kinase (TK) to forms that inhibit viral DNA polymerase	Treatment and prophylaxis for HSV-I, HSV-2, and VZV None of these drugs is active against TK⁻ strains	Acyclovir: Topical, oral, and IV Penciclovir: Topical Famciclovir and valcyclovir: Oral	Oral forms cause nausea, diarrhea, and headache IV acyclovir may cause renal and CNS toxicity
Drugs for cytomegalovirus				
Ganciclovir Valganciclovir Cidofovir Foscarnet	Viral activation of ganciclovir to form inhibiting DNA polymerase; no viral bioactivation of cidofovir and foscarnet	Treatment of CMV infections in immuno-suppression (eg, AIDS) and organ transplantation	Ganciclovir: Oral, IV, intraocular forms Valganciclovir: Oral Cidofovir, foscarnet (IV)	Ganciclovir: Bone marrow suppression, hepatic and neurologic dysfunction Cidofovir and foscarnet: Nephrotoxicity Foscarnet: CNS effects and electrolyte imbalance
Antihepatitis drugs				
Interferon-α (IFN-α) Adefovir-dipivoxil Entecavir Lamivudine Ribavirin	Degrades viral RNA via activation of host cell RNAase (IFN-α) • inhibition of HBV polymerase (others) • multiple antiviral actions (ribavirin)	Suppressive treatment of HBV (all drugs except ribavirin) • treatment of HCV (ribavirin +/− IFN-α)	IFN-α: Parenteral Adefovir, entacavir, lamivudine, and ribavirin: Oral Ribavirin: Inhalational	IFN-α: Alopecia, myalgia, depression, flu-like syndrome Adefovir: lactic acidosis, renal and hepatic toxicity Ribavirin: Anemia, teratogen
Anti-influenza drugs				
Amantadine Rimantadine Oseltamivir Zanamivir	Amantadine and rimantidine: block of M2 proton channels Oseletamivir and zanamivir inhibit neuraminidase	M2 blockers virtually obsolete • others prophylaxis vs most current flu strains and shorten symptoms	Oral forms except zanamivir (inhalational)	Oseltamivir: Gastrointestinal effects Zanamivir: Bronchospasm in asthmatics
Antiretroviral Drugs				
Nucleoside/nucleotide reverse transcriptase inhibitor (NRTIs)ᵃ				
Abacavir Didanosine Emtricitabine Lamivudine Stavudine Tenofovir Zalcitabine Zidovudine	Inhibit HIV reverse transcriptase after phosphorylation by cellular enzymes • cross-resistance common, but incomplete	Duration of action usually longer than half-life • most undergo renal elimination especially, didanosine, emtricitabine, lamivudine, stavudine, tenofovir, and zidovudine	Zidovudine: Bone marrow suppression Abacavir: Hypersensitivity Didanosine: Pancreatitis Stavudine, zalcitabine: Peripheral neuropathy	Most NRTIs are not extensively metabolized by hepatic enzymes such as the CYP450 isoforms, so they have few interactions that concern their pharmacokinetic characteristics
Nonnucleoside reverse transcriptase inhibitors (NNRTIs)				
Delavirdine Efavirenz Etravirine Nevirapine	Inhibit HIV reverse transcriptase • no phosphorylation required • cross-resistance between NNRTIs but not with NRTIs	All current NNRTIs are metabolized via CYP450 isozymes • etravirine may induce formation of CYP3A4, but inhibits other CYP450s	Delavirdine, nevirapine: Rash, increased liver enzymes Efavirenz: Teratogenicity	Inducers of CYP450 isozymes (eg, phenytoin, rifampin) and inhibitors (eg, azoles, PIs) alter NNRTI duration of action • note etravirine

(Continued)

DRUG SUMMARY TABLE: Antivirals & Antiretrovirals (*Continued*)

Drug Class	Mechanism of Action	Clinical Applications	Pharmacokinetics & Interactions	Toxicities
Protease inhibitors (PIs)[b]				
Atazanavir Darunavir Fosamprenavir Indinavir Nelfinavir Ritonavir Saquinavir Tipranavir	Inhibit viral protein processing • cross-resistance between PIs common	Elimination mainly via metabolism by CYP450 isozymes • they act as substrates and inhibitors of P450 Fosamprenavir is a prodrug forming amprenavir, a substrate and inducer of CYP450	Atazanavir, fosamprenavir, lopinavir, nelfinavir, saquinavir: GI distress and diarrhea Atazanavir: Peripheral neuropathy Amprenavir: Rash Indinavir: Hyperbilirubinemia and nephrolithiasis	Ritonavir[c] and other PIs can inhibit CYP450 metabolism of many drugs including antihistamines, antiarrhythmics, HMG-CoA reductase inhibitors, oral contraceptives and sedative-hypnotics Drugs known to induce or inhibit CYP450 isoforms may alter the plasma levels of PIs
Entry inhibitors				
Enfuvirtide Maraviroc	Block fusion between viral and cellular membranes (enfuvirtide) • CCR5 receptor antagonist (maraviroc)	Extrahepatic hydrolysis of enfuvirtide (subcutaneous injection) • P450 metabolism (maraviroc)	Enfuvirtide: Hypersensitivity Maraviroc: Muscle/joint pain, diarrhea, and increased liver enzymes	Inducers and inhibitors of CYP450 alter elimination of maraviroc • no effects on enfuvirtide

[a]NRTIs, nucleoside/nucleotide reverse transcriptase inhibitors: Risk of lactic acidosis with hepatic steatosis is characteristic of the group.
[b]PIs, inhibitors: Risk of hyperlipidemia, fat maldistribution, hyperglycemia, and insulin resistance is characteristic of the group, with possible exception of fosamprenavir.
[c]Ritonavir is a potent inhibitor of the 3A4 isoform of CYP450, an action used to advantage in "boosting" effects of other PIs. Drug–drug interactions between PIs and many other medications occur commonly.

Miscellaneous Antimicrobial Agents & Urinary Antiseptics

This chapter includes miscellaneous agents that have antibacterial activity, urinary tract and other antiseptics, and disinfectants.

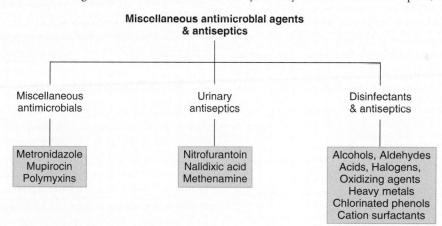

MISCELLANEOUS ANTIMICROBIAL AGENTS

This group includes imidazoles that have activity against several bacteria and protozoans, a drug that acts only on gram-positive cocci, and polypeptides that act on gram-negative bacilli.

A. Metronidazole and Tinidazole

1. Mechanisms—Metronidazole and tinidazole are imidazole derivatives with activity against protozoa and bacteria. The drugs undergo a reductive bioactivation of their nitro group by ferredoxin (present in anaerobic parasites) to form reactive cyto-toxic products that interfere with nucleic acid synthesis.

2. Pharmacokinetics—Metronidazole and tinidazole are effective orally and are distributed widely to tissues, achieving cerebrospinal fluid (CSF) levels similar to those in the blood. Metronidazole can also be given intravenously and is available in topical formulations. Elimination of the drugs require hepatic metabolism, and dosage reduction may be needed in patients with liver dysfunction. Tinidazole has a long elimination half-life permitting once-daily dosing.

3. Clinical use—As an antibacterial agent, metronidazole has greatest activity against *Bacteroides* and *Clostridium*. It is the drug of choice for treatment of pseudomembranous colitis resulting from *C difficile* and is effective in anaerobic or mixed intra-abdominal infections and in brain abscess. Tinidazole has similar activity versus anaerobic bacteria. Metronidazole is also used for infections involving *Gardnerella vaginalis* and in regimens for the eradication of *Helicobacter pylori* in gastric ulcers. As antiprotozoal drugs, metronidazole and tinidazole are effective drugs in trichomoniasis, giardiasis, and the treatment of intestinal amebiasis and amebic hepatic abscess.

4. Toxicity—Adverse effects include gastrointestinal irritation, headache, and dark coloration of urine. More serious toxicity includes leukopenia, dizziness, and ataxia. Opportunistic fungal infections may occur during treatment with metronidazole and tinidazole. Drug interactions with metronidazole include a disulfiram-like reaction with ethanol and potentiation of coumarin anticoagulant effects. Although metronidazole and tinidazole are not contraindicated in pregnancy, the drugs should be used with caution.

B. Mupirocin

1. Mechanisms—Mupirocin is a natural product from *Pseudomonas fluorescens*. It acts on gram-positive cocci and inhibits protein synthesis by specifically binding to isoleucyl-tRNA synthetase.

2. Pharmacokinetics and clinical use—Mupirocin is used topically and is not absorbed. This drug is indicated for impetigo caused by staphylococci (including methicillin-resistant strains), β-hemolytic streptococci, and *Streptococcus pyogenes*. It is also used intranasally to eliminate staphylococcal carriage by patients and medical personnel.

3. Toxicity—Local itching and burning sensations are common. Mupirocin may also cause rash, erythema, and contact dermatitis.

C. Polymyxins

1. Mechanisms—The polymyxins are polypeptides that are bactericidal against gram-negative bacteria. These drugs act like cationic detergents, disrupting bacterial cell membranes. They also bind and inactivate endotoxin.

2. Clinical use—Because of toxicity, clinical applications of the polymyxins are usually limited to topical therapy of resistant gram-negative infections, including those caused by *Enterobacter* and *Pseudomonas*. A parenteral form is also available.

3. Toxicity—If used parenterally or absorbed into the systemic circulation, adverse effects include neurotoxicity (paresthesias, dizziness, ataxia) and acute renal tubular necrosis (hematuria, proteinuria, nitrogen retention).

URINARY ANTISEPTICS

Urinary antiseptics are oral drugs that are rapidly excreted into the urine and act there to suppress bacteriuria. The drugs lack systemic antibacterial effects but may be toxic. Urinary antiseptics are often administered with acidifying agents because low pH is an independent inhibitor of bacterial growth in urine.

A. Nitrofurantoin

This drug is active against many urinary tract pathogens (but not *Proteus* or *Pseudomonas*), and resistance emerges slowly. Single daily doses of the drug can prevent recurrent urinary tract infections, and acidification of the urine enhances its activity. The drug is active orally and is excreted in the urine via filtration and secretion; toxic levels may occur in the blood of patients with renal dysfunction. Adverse effects of nitrofurantoin include gastrointestinal irritation, skin rashes, pulmonary infiltrates, phototoxicity, neuropathies, and hemolysis in patients with glucose-6-phosphate dehydrogenase (G6PD) deficiency.

B. Nalidixic Acid

This quinolone drug acts against many gram-negative organisms (but not *Proteus* or *Pseudomonas*) by mechanisms that may involve acidification or inhibition of DNA gyrase. Resistance emerges rapidly. The drug is active orally and is excreted in the urine partly unchanged and partly as the inactive glucuronide. Toxic effects include gastrointestinal irritation, glycosuria, skin rashes, phototoxicity, visual disturbances, and CNS stimulation. Nitrofurantoin may antagonize the action of nalidixic acid.

C. Methenamine

Methenamine mandelate and methenamine hippurate combine urine acidification with the release of the antibacterial compound formaldehyde at pH levels lower than 5.5. These drugs are not usually active against *Proteus* because these organisms alkalinize the urine. Insoluble complexes form between formaldehyde and sulfonamides, and the drugs should not be used together.

DISINFECTANTS, ANTISEPTICS, & STERILANTS

Although the terms are often used interchangeably, a **disinfectant** is a compound that is used to kill microorganisms in an inanimate environment, whereas an **antiseptic** is one that is used to inhibit bacterial growth both in vitro and in contact with the surfaces of living tissues. Disinfectants and antiseptics do not have selective toxicity. Most antiseptics delay wound healing. Sterilants kill both vegetative cells and spores when applied to materials for appropriate times and temperatures.

A. Alcohols, Aldehydes, and Acids

Ethanol (70%) and **isopropanol** (70–90%) are effective skin antiseptics because they denature microbial proteins. **Formaldehyde,** which also denatures proteins, is too irritating for topical use but is a disinfectant for instruments. **Acetic acid** (1%) is used in surgical dressings and has activity against gram-negative bacteria, including *Pseudomonas,* when used as a urinary irrigant and in the external ear. **Salicylic acid** and **undecylenic acid** are useful in the treatment of dermatophyte infections.

B. Halogens

Iodine tincture is an effective antiseptic for intact skin and, although it can cause dermatitis, is commonly used in preparing the skin before taking blood samples. Iodine complexed with povidone (**povidone-iodine**) is widely used, particularly as a preoperative skin antiseptic, but solutions can become contaminated with aerobic gram-negative bacteria.

Hypochlorous acid, formed when **chlorine** dissolves in water, is antimicrobial. This is the basis for the use of chlorine and **halazone** in water purification. Organic matter binds chlorine, thus preventing antimicrobial actions. In a given water sample, this process is referred to as the **chlorine demand** because the chlorine-binding capacity of the organic material must be exceeded before bacterial killing is accomplished. Many preparations of chlorine for water purification do not eradicate all bacteria or entamoeba cysts.

Sodium hypochlorite is the active component in household bleach, a 1:10 dilution of which is recommended by the Centers for Disease Control and Prevention (CDC) for the disinfection of blood spills that may contain HIV or hepatitis B virus (HBV).

C. Oxidizing Agents

Hydrogen peroxide exerts a short-lived antimicrobial action through the release of molecular oxygen. The agent is used as a mouthwash, for cleansing wounds, and for disinfection of contact lenses. **Potassium permanganate** is an effective bactericidal agent but has the disadvantage of causing persistent brown stains on skin and clothing.

D. Heavy Metals

Mercury and **silver** precipitate proteins and inactivate sulfhydryl groups of enzymes but are used rarely because of toxicity. Organic mercurials such as **nitromersol** and **thimerosal** frequently cause hypersensitivity reactions but continue to be used as preservatives for vaccines, antitoxins, and immune sera. **Merbromin** is a weak antiseptic and stains tissues a bright red color. In the past **silver nitrate** was commonly used for prevention of neonatal gonococcal ophthalmia, but it has been largely replaced by topical antibiotics. **Silver sulfadiazine** (a sulfonamide) is used to decrease bacterial colonization in burns.

E. Chlorinated Phenols

Owing to its toxicity, **phenol** itself is used only as a disinfectant of inanimate objects. Mixtures of phenolic derivatives are used in antiseptics but can cause skin irritation. **Hexachlorophene** has been widely used in surgical scrub routines and in deodorant soaps, where it forms antibacterial deposits on the skin, decreasing the population of resident bacteria. Repeated use on the skin in infants can lead to absorption of the drug, resulting in CNS white matter degeneration. Antiseptic soaps may also contain other chlorinated phenols such as **triclocarban** and **chlorhexidine.** Chlorhexidine is mainly active against gram-positive cocci and is commonly used in hospital scrub routines to cleanse skin sites. All antiseptic soaps may cause allergies or photosensitization.

F. Ectoparasiticides

Lindane (hexachlorocyclohexane) is used to treat infestations with mites or lice and is also an agricultural insecticide. The agent can be absorbed through the skin; if excessive amounts are applied, toxic effects, including blood dyscrasias and convulsions, may occur. **Crotamiton** is a scabicide with some antipruritic effects, which can be used as an alternative to lindane. Allergic contact hypersensitivity may occur. **Permethrin** is used topically in pediculosis and scabies; adverse effects include transient burning, stinging, and pruritus. The organophosphate cholinesterase inhibitor **malathion** is also used topically in pediculosis.

G. Cationic Surfactants

Benzalkonium chloride and **cetylpyridinium chloride** are used as disinfectants of surgical instruments and surfaces such as floors and bench tops. Because they are effective against most bacteria and fungi and are not irritating, they are also used as antiseptics. However, when used on the skin, the antimicrobial action of these agents is antagonized by soaps and multivalent cations. The CDC has recommended that benzalkonium chloride and similar quaternary compounds *not* be used as antiseptics because outbreaks of infection have resulted from growth of gram-negative bacteria (eg, *Pseudomonas*) in such antiseptic solutions.

QUESTIONS

1. Infections caused by gram-negative bacilli have occurred when this cationic surfactant has been used as a skin antiseptic.
   (A) Acetic acid
   (B) Cetylpyridinium chloride
   (C) Hexachlorophene
   (D) Merbromin
   (E) Thimerosal

Questions 2 and 3. A young woman is brought to a hospital emergency department with intense abdominal pain of 2 d duration. The pain has spread to the right lower quadrant and is accompanied by nausea, vomiting, and fever. She arrives at the emergency department with a blood pressure of 85/45, pulse 120/min, and temperature 40°C. Her abdomen has a board-like rigidity with diffuse pain to palpation. Laboratory values include the following: WBC 20,000/μL and creatinine 1.5 mg/dL. After abdominal x-ray films are taken, a preliminary diagnosis of abdominal sepsis is made, possibly resulting from bowel perforation. After appropriate samples are sent to the laboratory for culture, the patient is hospitalized, and antimicrobial therapy is started with intravenous ampicillin and gentamicin.

2. Regarding the treatment of this patient, which statement is accurate?
   (A) A Gram stain of the blood would provide positive identification of the specific organism involved in this infection
   (B) Cultures are pointless because this is probably a mixed infection
   (C) Empiric antimicrobial therapy of abdominal sepsis should always include a third-generation cephalosporin
   (D) The antibiotic regimen should include a drug active against anaerobes
   (E) The combination of ampicillin and gentamicin provides good coverage for all likely pathogens

3. If the antibiotic regimen in this patient is modified to include metronidazole
   (A) Ampicillin should be excluded from the regimen
   (B) Coverage will be extended to methicillin-resistant staphylococci
   (C) Gentamicin should be excluded from the regimen
   (D) Metronidazole should not be administered intravenously
   (E) The patient should be monitored for candidiasis

4. Which compound is used topically to treat scabies and pediculosis?
   (A) Benzoyl peroxide
   (B) Chlorhexidine
   (C) Mupirocin
   (D) Permethrin
   (E) Silver sulfadiazine

5. Methenamine salts are used as urinary antiseptics. The reason they lack systemic antibacterial action is that they are
   (A) Converted to formaldehyde only at low pH
   (B) Metabolized rapidly by hepatic drug-metabolizing enzymes
   (C) More than 98% bound to plasma proteins
   (D) Not absorbed into the systemic circulation after oral ingestion
   (E) Substrates for active tubular secretion

6. Which statement about the actions of antimicrobial agents is false?
   (A) Daptomycin has activity against strains of staphylococci resistant to vancomycin.
   (B) Neonatal gonococcal ophthalmia can be prevented by silver nitrate
   (C) Polymyxins act as cationic detergents to disrupt bacterial cell membranes
   (D) Resistance to nitrofurantoin emerges rapidly, and there is cross-resistance with sulfonamides
   (E) Salicylic acid has useful antidermatophyte activity when applied topically

7. Which antiseptic *promotes* wound healing?
   (A) Benzalkonium chloride
   (B) Chlorhexidine
   (C) Hexachlorophene
   (D) Iodine
   (E) None of the above

8. A 22-year-old man with gonorrhea is to be treated with cefixime and will need another drug to provide coverage for possible urethritis caused by *C trachomatis*. Which of the following drugs is *least* likely to be effective in nongonococcal urethritis?
   (A) Azithromycin
   (B) Clindamycin
   (C) Nitrofurantoin
   (D) Ofloxacin
   (E) Tetracycline

9. A patient with AIDS has an extremely high viral RNA titer. While blood is being drawn from this patient, the syringe is accidentally dropped, contaminating the floor, which is made of porous material. The best way to deal with this is to
   (A) Clean the floor with a 10% solution of household bleach
   (B) Clean the floor with soap and water
   (C) Completely replace the contaminated part of the floor
   (D) Neutralize the spill with a solution of potassium permanganate
   (E) Seal the room and decontaminate with ethylene oxide

10. Neuropathies are more likely to occur with this agent when it is used in patients with renal dysfunction. The drug may cause acute hemolysis in patients with glucose-6-phosphate dehydrogenase (G6PD) deficiency.
    (A) Chlorhexidine
    (B) Halazone
    (C) Methenamine
    (D) Metronidazole
    (E) Nitrofurantoin

ANSWERS

1. *Pseudomonas* and other gram-negative bacteria have caused infections after the use of cationic surfactants such as benzalkonium and cetylpyridinium chlorides, partly because they form a film on the skin under which microorganisms can survive. In addition, some gram-negative bacilli are able to grow in solutions containing benzalkonium salts. Bacterial growth may also occur in solutions of povidone-iodine. The answer is **B**.

2. Abdominal sepsis is commonly a mixed infection; the most likely pathogens are *Bacteroides fragilis, Enterobacteriaceae,* and *Enterococcus faecalis.* An antibiotic regimen that includes only ampicillin and gentamicin does not control *B fragilis.* Empiric treatment in this case should include a drug active against this pathogen (eg, metronidazole, cefoxitin, cefotetan, or clindamycin). The answer is **D**.

3. Fungal superinfections, especially from *Candida albicans,* occur frequently during treatment with metronidazole. In most cases of abdominal sepsis, metronidazole would be given by slow intravenous infusion. Both ampicillin and gentamicin should be maintained until the infection is controlled, at which time surgery is indicated. Metronidazole has no activity against aerobes. The combination of ampicillin, gentamicin, and

metronidazole does not provide coverage for methicillin-resistant staphylococci. The answer is **E.**

4. Of the agents listed, only permethrin is an effective scabicide and pediculicide. Lindane is also effective, but there is some concern about its systemic absorption if topically applied, which may cause neurotoxicity and hematotoxicity. Accidental ingestion of lindane in children has caused seizures. The answer is **D.**

5. Below pH 5.5, methenamine releases formaldehyde, which is antibacterial. This pH is achieved in the urine but nowhere else in the body. Ascorbic acid is sometimes given with methenamine salts to ensure a low urinary pH. The answer is **A.**

6. Resistance emerges very slowly when nitrofurantoin is used as a urinary antiseptic. There is no cross-resistance between the drug and other drugs used in the treatment of bacterial infections of the urinary tract. The answer is **D.**

7. No antiseptic in current use is able to promote wound healing, and most agents do the opposite. In general, cleansing of abrasions and superficial wounds with soap and water is just as effective as and less damaging than the application of topical antiseptics. The answer is **E.**

8. Urinary tract infections resulting from *C trachomatis* are likely to respond to all of the drugs listed except nitrofurantoin. However, nitrofurantoin is effective against many **bacterial** urinary tract pathogens with the exception of *Pseudomonas aeruginosa* and strains of *Proteus.* The answer is **C.**

9. Household bleach contains sodium hypochlorite. A 1:10 dilution of bleach is effective for disinfection of a direct blood spill on a porous surface. In addition to inactivating HIV, sodium hypochlorite solutions have disinfectant activity against other viruses, including hepatitis B virus. The answer is **A.**

10. Acute hemolytic reactions in G6PD deficiency occur with drugs that are oxidizing agents, including antimalarials, nalidixic acid, sulfonamides, and the nitrofurans. Severe polyneuropathies, with both motor and sensory nerve degeneration, may occur with nitrofurantoin. These reactions are more likely to occur in patients with renal dysfunction. The answer is **E.**

CHECKLIST

When you complete this chapter, you should be able to:

❑ Identify the clinical uses of metronidazole and its characteristic pharmacokinetics and toxicities.

❑ Describe the antimicrobial activity and clinical uses of daptomycin.

❑ List the clinical uses of mupirocin and polymyxins.

❑ Identify the major urinary antiseptics and their characteristic adverse effects.

❑ List the agents used as antiseptics and disinfectants and point out their limitations.

DRUG SUMMARY TABLE: Miscellaneous Antimicrobial Agents

Subclass	Mechanism of Action	Effects	Clinical Applications & Pharmacokinetics	Toxicities & Interactions
Nitroimidazoles				
Metronidazole Tinidazole	Disrupt electron transport	Bactericidal vs anaerobic bacteria and certain protozoa	Anaerobic bacterial infections and *Clostridium difficile* colitis • oral/IV, hepatic clearance Tinidazole: Longer half-life	Gastrointestinal (GI) upsets, metallic taste, neuropathy • disulfiram-like interaction with alcohol
Urinary antiseptics				
Nitrofurantoin Methenamine salts	Not identified (nitrofurantoin) • forms formaldehyde in urine (methenamine)	Bactericidal or bacteriostatic	Simple urinary tract (UT) infections and prophylaxis • methenamine is used for suppression in UT infections	Oral, low blood levels, high urine levels • GI upset; neuropathy (nitrofurantoin)
Macrolide				
Fidaxomicin	Inhibits bacterial RNA polymerase	Bactericidal	*C difficile* colitis	Oral, blood levels negligible

Clinical Use of Antimicrobials

C H A P T E R

51

A. Empiric Antimicrobial Therapy

Empiric antimicrobial therapy is begun before a specific pathogen has been identified and is based on the presumption of an infection that requires immediate drug treatment. Before initiation of such therapy, accepted practice involves making a clinical diagnosis of microbial infection, obtaining specimens for laboratory analyses, making a microbiologic diagnosis, deciding whether treatment should precede the results of laboratory tests, and, finally, selecting the optimal drug or drugs. A variety of publications provide annually updated lists of antimicrobial drugs of choice for specific pathogens. Such lists can provide a useful guide to empiric therapy based on presumptive microbiologic diagnosis. Tables 51–1 and 51–2 show examples of empiric antimicrobial therapy based on microbiologic etiology.

B. Principles of Antimicrobial Therapy

Antimicrobial therapy in established infections is guided by several principles.

1. Susceptibility testing—The results of susceptibility testing establish the drug sensitivity of the organism. These results usually predict the **minimum inhibitory concentrations (MICs)** of a drug for comparison with anticipated blood or tissue levels. The 2 most common methods of susceptibility testing are disk diffusion (Kirby-Bauer) and broth dilution. For severe infections caused by certain bacteria (eg, gram-positive cocci, *Haemophilus influenzae*), a direct test for beta-lactamase is used to aid in the selection of an appropriate antibiotic.

2. Drug concentration in blood—The measurement of drug concentration in the blood may be appropriate when using agents with a low therapeutic index (eg, aminoglycosides, vancomycin) and when investigating poor clinical response to a drug treatment regimen.

3. Serum bactericidal titers—In certain infections in which host defenses may contribute minimally to cure, the estimation of serum bactericidal titers can confirm the appropriateness of

choice of drug and dosage. Serial dilutions of serum are incubated with standardized quantities of the pathogen isolated from the patient; killing at a dilution of 1:8 is generally considered satisfactory.

4. Route of administration—Parenteral therapy is preferred in most cases of serious microbial infections. Chloramphenicol, the fluoroquinolones, and trimethoprim-sulfamethoxazole (TMP-SMZ) may be effective orally.

5. Monitoring of therapeutic response—Therapeutic responses to drug therapy should be monitored clinically and microbiologically to detect the development of resistance or superinfections. The duration of drug therapy required depends on the pathogen (eg, longer courses of therapy are required for infections caused by fungi or mycobacteria), the site of infection (eg, endocarditis and osteomyelitis require longer duration of treatment), and the immunocompetence of the patient.

6. Clinical failure of antimicrobial therapy—Inadequate clinical or microbiologic response to antimicrobial therapy can result from laboratory testing errors, problems with the drug (eg, incorrect choice, poor tissue penetration, inadequate dose), the patient (poor host defenses, undrained abscesses), or the pathogen (resistance, superinfection).

C. Factors Influencing Antimicrobial Drug Use

1. Bactericidal versus bacteriostatic actions—Antibiotics classified as bacteriostatic include clindamycin, macrolides, sulfonamides, and tetracyclines. For bacteriostatic drugs, the concentrations that inhibit growth are much lower than those that kill bacteria. Antibiotics classified as bactericidal include the aminoglycosides, beta-lactams, fluoroquinolones, metronidazole, most antimycobacterial agents, streptogramins, and vancomycin. For such drugs, there is little difference between the concentrations that inhibit growth and those that kill bacteria. Bactericidal drugs are preferred for the treatment of endocarditis and meningitis

High-Yield Terms to Learn

Antimicrobial prophylaxis	The use of antimicrobial drugs to decrease the risk of infection
Combination antimicrobial drug therapy	The use of 2 or more drugs together to increase efficacy more than can be accomplished with the use of a single agent
Empiric (presumptive) antimicrobial therapy	Initiation of drug treatment before identification of a specific pathogen
Minimum inhibitory concentration (MIC)	An estimate of the drug sensitivity of pathogens for comparison with anticipated levels in blood or tissues
Postantibiotic effect (PAE)	Antibacterial effect that persists after drug concentration falls below the minimum inhibitory concentration
Susceptibility testing	Laboratory methods to determine the sensitivity of the isolated pathogen to antimicrobial drugs

and for most infections in patients with impaired defense mechanisms, especially immunocompromised patients.

Some bactericidal agents (aminoglycosides, fluoroquinolones) cause **concentration-dependent** killing. Maximizing peak blood levels of such drugs increases the rate and the extent of their bactericidal effects. This is one of the factors responsible for the clinical effectiveness of high-dose, once-daily administration of aminoglycosides. Other bactericidal agents (beta-lactams, vancomycin) cause **time-dependent** killing. Their killing action is independent of drug concentration and continues only while blood levels are maintained above the minimal bactericidal concentration (MBC).

Inhibition of bacterial growth that continues after antibiotic blood concentrations have fallen to low levels is called the **postantibiotic effect (PAE).** The mechanisms of PAE are unclear but may reflect the lag time required by bacteria to synthesize new enzymes and cellular components, the possible persistence of antibiotic at the target site, or an enhanced susceptibility of bacteria to phagocytic and other defense mechanisms including postantibiotic

TABLE 51–1 Examples of empiric antimicrobial therapy based on microbiologic etiology.[a]

Pathogen	Drug(s) of First Choice	Alternative Drugs
Enterococcus spp	Ampicillin +/− gentamicin	Vancomycin +/− gentamicin
S aureus or *epidermidis*		
Methicillin-susceptible	Nafcillin	Cephalosporin, clindamycin, fluoroquinolone, imipenem
Methicillin-resistant	Vancomycin +/− gentamicin +/− rifampin	Daptomycin, doxycycline, fluoroquinolone, linezolid, streptogramins, tigecycline
S pneumoniae		
Penicillin-susceptible	Pen G, amoxicillin	Cephalosporin, clindamycin, fluoroquinolone, macrolide, TMP-SMZ
Penicillin-resistant	Vancomycin + ceftriaxone or cefotaxime +/− rifampin	Linezolid, streptogramins, third-generation fluoroquinolone
N gonorrhoeae	Ceftriaxone, cefixime	Spectinomycin, azithromycin
M meningitidis	Penicillin G	Third-generation cephalosporin, chloramphenicol
M catarrhalis	Cefuroxime, TMP-SMZ	Amoxicillin-clavulanate, third-generation fluoroquinolone, macrolide
C difficile	Metronidazole	Vancomycin, bacitracin
C trachomatis	Macrolide or tetracycline	Clindamycin, ofloxacin
C pneumoniae	Macrolide or tetracycline	Fluoroquinolone
M pneumoniae	Macrolide or tetracycline	Fluoroquinolone
T pallidum	Penicillin G	Doxycycline, ceftriaxone, azithromycin

[a]Based on various sources of treatment guidelines (USA) available in June 2011.

TABLE 51–2 Further examples of empiric antimicrobial therapy based on microbiologic etiology.[a]

Pathogen	Drug(s) of First Choice	Alternative Drugs
Bacteroides	Metronidazole	Carbapenems, penicillins + beta-lactamase inhibitor, chloramphenicol
Campylobacter jejuni	Macrolide	Fluoroquinolone, tetracycline
Enterobacter spp	Carbapenem, TMP-SMZ	Aminoglycoside, cefepime, fluoroquinolone, third-generation cephalosporin
E coli	Cephalosporin (first and second-generation), TMP-SMZ	Many penicillins +/− beta-lactamase inhibitor, fluoroquinolones, aminoglycosides
G vaginalis	Metronidazole	Clindamycin
K pneumoniae	Cephalosporin (first or second-generation), TMP-SMZ	Carbapenems, penicillins + beta-lactamase inhibitor, aminoglycosides, fluoroquinolones
P mirabilis	Ampicillin	Cephalosporins, penicillins + beta-lactamase inhibitor, aminoglycosides, TMP-SMZ, fluoroquinolones
Proteus-indole positive	Cephalosporin (first or second-generation), TMP-SMZ	Carbapenems, penicillins + beta-lactamase inhibitor, aminoglycosides, fluoroquinolones
S typhi	Ceftriaxone or fluoroquinolone	Chloramphenicol, TMP-SMZ, ampicillin
Serratia spp	Carbapenem	Aminoglycoside, third-generation cephalosporin, fluoroquinolone, TMP-SMZ
Shigella spp	Fluoroquinolone	Azithromycin, TMP-SMZ, ampicillin, ceftriaxone

[a]Based on various sources of treatment guidelines (USA) available in June 2011.

leucocyte enhancement. PAE is another factor contributory to the effectiveness of once-daily administration of aminoglycosides and may also contribute to the clinical efficacy of the fluoroquinolones.

2. Drug elimination mechanisms—Changes in hepatic and renal function—and the use of dialysis—can influence the pharmacokinetics of antimicrobials and may necessitate dosage modifications. The major mechanisms of elimination of commonly used antimicrobial drugs are shown in Table 51–3. In anuria (creatinine clearance <5 mL/min), the elimination half-life of drugs that are eliminated by the kidney is markedly increased, usually necessitating major reductions in drug dosage. Erythromycin, clindamycin, chloramphenicol, rifampin, and ketoconazole are notable exceptions, requiring no change in dosage in renal failure. Drugs contraindicated in renal impairment include cidofovir, nalidixic acid, long-acting sulfon-amides, and tetracyclines. Dosage adjustment may be needed in patients with hepatic impairment for drugs including amprenavir, chloramphenicol, clindamycin, erythromycin, indinavir, met-ronidazole, and tigecycline. Dialysis, especially hemodialysis, may markedly decrease the plasma levels of many antimicro-bials; supplementary doses of such drugs may be required to

TABLE 51–3 Elimination of commonly used antimicrobial agents.[a]

Mode of Elimination	Drugs or Drug Groups
Renal	Acyclovir, aminoglycosides, amphotericin B, most cephalosporins, fluconazole, fluoroquinolones, penicillins, sulfonamides, tetracyclines (except doxycycline), TMP-SMZ, vancomycin
Hepatic	Amphotericin B, ampicillin, cefoperazone, chloramphenicol, clindamycin, erythromycin, isoniazid, most azoles (not fluconazole), nafcillin, rifampin
Hemodialysis	Acyclovir (and most antiviral agents), aminoglycosides, cephalosporins (not cefonicid, cefoperazone, ceftriaxone), penicillins (not nafcillin), sulfonamides

[a]Dosage adjustments may be necessary, and in some cases drugs may be contraindicated, in patients with renal or hepatic impairment.

reestablish effective plasma levels after these procedures. Drugs that are *not* removed from the blood by hemodialysis include amphotericin B, cefonicid, cefoperazone, ceftriaxone, erythromycin, nafcillin, tetracyclines, and vancomycin.

3. Pregnancy and the neonate—Antimicrobial therapy during pregnancy and the neonatal period requires special consideration. Aminoglycosides (eg, gentamicin) may cause neurologic damage. Tetracyclines cause tooth enamel dysplasia and inhibition of bone growth. Sulfonamides, by displacing bilirubin from serum albumin, may cause kernicterus in the neonate. Chloramphenicol may cause gray baby syndrome. Other drugs that should be used with extreme caution during pregnancy include most antiviral and antifungal agents. The fluoroquinolones are not recommended for use in pregnancy or in small children because of possible effects on growing cartilage.

4. Drug interactions—Interactions sometimes occur between antimicrobials and other drugs (see also Chapter 61). Interactions include enhanced nephrotoxicity or ototoxicity when aminoglycosides are given with loop diuretics, vancomycin, or cisplatin. Several drug interactions with sulfonamides are based on competition for plasma protein binding; these include excessive hypoglycemia with sulfonylureas and increased hypoprothrombinemia with warfarin. Disulfiram-like reactions to ethanol occur with metronidazole, with TMP-SMZ, and with several cephalosporins (see Chapter 43). Erythromycin inhibits the hepatic metabolism of a number of drugs, including clozapine, lidocaine, loratadine, phenytoin, quinidine, sildenafil, theophylline, and warfarin. Ketoconazole inhibits the metabolism of caffeine, carbamazepine, cyclosporine, hepatic hydroxylmethylglutaryl coenzyme A (HMG-CoA) reductase inhibitors, methadone, oral contraceptives, phenytoin, sildenafil, verapamil, and zidovudine. Other azole antifungals are weaker inhibitors of drug metabolism.

Rifampin, an inducer of hepatic drug-metabolizing enzymes, decreases the effects of digoxin, ketoconazole, oral contraceptives, propranolol, quinidine, several antiretroviral drugs, and warfarin.

D. Antimicrobial Drug Combinations

Therapy with multiple antimicrobials may be indicated in several clinical situations.

1. Emergency situations—In severe infections (eg, sepsis, meningitis), combinations of antimicrobial drugs are used empirically to suppress all of the most likely pathogens.

2. To delay resistance—The combined use of drugs is valid when the rapid emergence of resistance impairs the chances for cure. For this reason, combined drug therapy is especially important in the treatment of tuberculosis.

3. Mixed infections—Multiple organisms may be involved in some infections. For example, peritoneal infections may be caused by several pathogens (eg, anaerobes and coliforms); a combination

of drugs may be required to achieve coverage. Skin infections are often due to mixed bacterial, fungal, or viral pathogens.

4. To achieve synergistic effects—The use of a drug combination against a specific pathogen may result in an effect greater than that achieved with a single drug. Examples include the use of penicillins with gentamicin in enterococcal endocarditis, the use of an extended-spectrum penicillin plus an aminoglycoside in *Pseudomonas aeruginosa* infections, and the combined use of amphotericin B and flucytosine in cryptococcal meningitis. Antibiotic combinations are also commonly used in the management of infections resulting from *S epidermidis* and penicillin-resistant pneumococci (eg, vancomycin plus rifampin). Several mechanisms, discussed next, may account for synergism.

a. Sequential blockade—The combined use of drugs may cause inhibition of 2 or more steps in a metabolic pathway. For example, trimethoprim and sulfamethoxazole (TMP-SMZ) block different steps in the formation of tetrahydrofolic acid.

b. Blockade of drug-inactivating enzymes—Clavulanic acid, sulbactam, and tazobactam inhibit penicillinases and are often used along with penicillinase-sensitive beta-lactam drugs.

c. Enhanced drug uptake—Increased permeability to aminoglycosides after exposure of certain bacteria to cell wall-inhibiting antimicrobials (eg, beta-lactams) is thought to underlie some synergistic effects.

E. Antimicrobial Chemoprophylaxis

The general principles of antimicrobial chemoprophylaxis can be summarized as follows: (1) Prophylaxis should always be directed toward a **specific pathogen**; (2) **no resistance** should develop during the period of drug use; (3) prophylactic drug use should be of **limited duration**; (4) conventional **therapeutic doses** should be used; and (5) prophylaxis should be used only in situations of documented **drug efficacy.**

Nonsurgical prophylaxis includes the prevention of cytomegalovirus (CMV), herpesvirus (HSV) infections, HIV infections in health care workers, influenza, malaria, meningococcal infections, and tuberculosis. In patients with AIDS, prophylactic measures are directed toward prevention of *Pneumocystis jiroveci* pneumonia (PCP) and toxoplasmosis. Though somewhat less effective, antimicrobial prophylaxis is also commonly used for animal or human bite wounds and chronic bronchitis. Severely leukopenic patients are often given prophylactic antibiotics.

Prophylaxis against postsurgical infections should be limited to procedures that are associated with infection in more than 5% of untreated cases under optimal conditions. Prophylaxis should embody the principles listed previously, with drug selection based on the most likely infecting organism and treatment initiated just before surgery and continued throughout the procedure. A first-generation cephalosporin (eg, cefazolin) is often the prophylactic drug of choice. Cefoxitin or cefotetan may be used for surgical patients at risk for infection caused by anaerobic bacteria. Situations in which surgical prophylaxis is of benefit (or commonly used) include gastrointestinal procedures, vaginal hysterectomy, cesarean section delivery, joint replacement, open fracture surgery, and dental procedures in patients with valvular disease or prostheses.

QUESTIONS

Questions 1–3. A hospitalized AIDS patient is receiving anti-retroviral drugs but no antimicrobial prophylaxis. He develops sepsis with fever, suspected to be caused by a gram-negative bacillus.

1. Antimicrobial treatment of this severely immune-depressed patient should *not* be initiated before
   (A) Antipyretic drugs have been given to reduce body temperature
   (B) Infecting organism(s) have been identified by the microbiology laboratory
   (C) Results of a Gram stain are available
   (D) Results of antibacterial drug susceptibility tests are available
   (E) Specimens have been taken for laboratory tests and examinations

2. If the aminoglycoside gentamicin is used in the treatment of this patient, monitoring of serum drug level may be advised because the drug
   (A) Does not penetrate into cerebrospinal fluid
   (B) Has a narrow therapeutic window
   (C) Is antagonized by beta-lactam antibiotics
   (D) Is metabolized by hepatic enzymes
   (E) Is hematotoxic

3. A combination of drugs might be given to this patient to provide coverage against multiple organisms or to obtain a synergistic action. Examples of antimicrobial drug synergism established at the clinical level include
   (A) Amphotericin B with flucytosine in cryptococcal meningitis
   (B) Carbenicillin with gentamicin in pseudomonal infections
   (C) Rifampin with vancomycin in enterococcal infections
   (D) Trimethoprim with sulfamethoxazole in coliform infections
   (E) All of the above

Questions 4 and 5. A 27-year-old pregnant patient with a history of pyelonephritis has developed a severe upper respiratory tract infection that appears to be due to a bacterial pathogen. The woman is hospitalized, and an antibacterial agent is to be selected for treatment.

4. Assuming that the physician is concerned about the effects of renal impairment on drug dosage in this patient, which drug would not require dosage modification in renal dysfunction?
   (A) Amikacin
   (B) Erythromycin
   (C) Ofloxacin
   (D) Trimethoprim-sulfamethoxazole
   (E) Vancomycin

5. Which antibacterial agent appears to be the safest to use in the pregnant patient?
   (A) Azithromycin
   (B) Clarithromycin
   (C) Kanamycin
   (D) Sulfadiazine
   (E) Tetracycline

Questions 6 and 7. A 48-year-old patient is scheduled for a vaginal hysterectomy. An antimicrobial drug will be used for prophylaxis against postoperative infection. It is proposed that cefazolin, a first-generation cephalosporin, be given intravenously at the normal therapeutic dose immediately before surgery and continued until the patient is released from the hospital.

6. Which statement about the proposed drug management of this patient is not accurate?
   (A) Enteric gram-negative rods, anaerobes, enterococci, and group B streptococci are likely pathogens
   (B) In this type of surgical procedure, antimicrobial prophylaxis has documented efficacy
   (C) Nosocomial (hospital-acquired) infection will be prevented by treatment throughout the period of hospitalization
   (D) This drug will not be effective against anaerobes
   (E) Without prophylaxis, the infection rate following this procedure exceeds 5% under optimal conditions

7. If the patient had been scheduled for elective colonic surgery, optimal prophylaxis against infection would be achieved by mechanical bowel preparation and the use of
   (A) Intravenous cefotetan
   (B) Intravenous third-generation cephalosporin
   (C) Oral ampicillin
   (D) Oral fluoroquinolone
   (E) Oral neomycin and erythromycin

8. Which drug increases the hepatic metabolism of other drugs?
   (A) Clarithromycin
   (B) Erythromycin
   (C) Ketoconazole
   (D) Rifampin
   (E) Ritonavir

9. If ampicillin and piperacillin are used in combination in the treatment of infections resulting from *Pseudomonas aeruginosa,* antagonism may occur. The most likely explanation is that
   (A) Ampicillin is bacteriostatic
   (B) Ampicillin induces beta-lactamase production
   (C) Autolytic enzymes are inhibited by piperacillin
   (D) Piperacillin blocks the attachment of ampicillin to penicillin-binding proteins
   (E) The 2 drugs form an insoluble complex

10. In a patient suffering from pseudomembranous colitis due to *C difficile* with established hypersensitivity to metronidazole the most likely drug to be of clinical value is
    (A) Chloramphenicol
    (B) Clindamycin
    (C) Doxycycline
    (D) Levofloxacin
    (E) Vancomycin

ANSWERS

1. To delay therapy until laboratory results are available is inappropriate in serious bacterial infections, but specimens for possible microbial identification must be obtained before drugs are administered. The answer is **E.**

2. Monitoring plasma aminoglycoside levels is important because aminoglycosides have a low therapeutic index; toxicity may occur when plasma levels are only 3–4 times higher than minimal inhibitory concentrations. Decreases in renal function may elevate the plasma levels of aminoglycosides to toxic levels within a few hours. Aminoglycosides undergo renal elimination, and they are not hematotoxic. The answer is **B.**

3. Combinations of antimicrobial drugs are not always synergistic and, in some cases, may even be antagonistic. However, all the choices listed are established examples of situations in which antimicrobial combinations have greater clinical efficacy than individual drugs. The answer is **E.**

4. Antimicrobial drugs that are eliminated via hepatic metabolism or biliary excretion include erythromycin, cefoperazone, clindamycin, doxycycline, isoniazid, ketoconazole, and nafcillin. The answer is **B.**

5. Several groups of antimicrobial drugs are best avoided in pregnancy if at all possible, including aminoglycosides, sulfonamides, and tetracyclines. The macrolide azithromycin appears to be safe, but studies in animals have shown that clarithromycin is potentially embryotoxic. The answer is **A.**

6. With few exceptions, the prophylactic use of antibiotics in surgery should not extend beyond the duration of the procedure. After routine surgical procedures, the risk of opportunistic infection (from disturbances in microbial flora) *increases* in a hospitalized patient if prophylaxis is prolonged; there is also more likelihood of drug toxicity. Cefazolin (or cefoxitin) constitutes the drug(s) of choice for prophylaxis in most hysterectomy procedures. The answer is **C.**

7. Second-generation cephalosporins, including cefoxitin and cefotetan, are more active than cefazolin against bowel anaerobes such as *Bacteroides fragilis* and are sometimes used for prophylaxis in "dirty" surgical procedures. However, for elective bowel surgery, most authorities favor the oral use of neomycin together with a poorly absorbed formulation of erythromycin, in conjunction with mechanical bowel preparation. In cases of bowel perforation, the use of a second- or third-generation cephalosporin is more appropriate. The answer is **E.**

8. Clarithromycin, erythromycin, ketoconazole, and ritonavir inhibit the hepatic metabolism of various drugs. Rifampin is an inducer of liver microsomal drug-metabolizing enzymes. The answer is **D.**

9. Gram-negative rods such as *Enterobacter* and *Pseudomonas aeruginosa* have inducible beta-lactamases. Several beta-lactam antibiotics, including ampicillin, cefoxitin, and imipenem, are potent inducers of beta-lactamase production. When such inducers are used in combination with a hydrolyzable penicillin (eg, piperacillin), antagonism may result. The answer is **B.**

10. Disturbances of gut flora occur commonly during treatment with antibiotics, and pseudomembranous colitis has been associated with the use of many agents including ampicillin and clindamycin. Vancomycin can be used in treatment of pseudomembranous colitis in patients with established hypersensitivity to metronidazole. The answer is **E.**

CHECKLIST

When you complete this chapter, you should be able to:

❏ List the steps that should be taken before the initiation of empiric antimicrobial therapy.

❏ Appreciate why susceptibility testing of isolates and the determination of antibiotic blood levels are important in the treatment of many infections.

❏ Identify the antibiotics of choice for treatment of infections resulting from *B fragilis,* atypical organisms (*Chlamydia, Mycoplasma*), enterococci, gonococci, pneumococci, staphylococci (including penicillin-resistant *Streptococcus pneumoniae* [PRSP] strains) and staphylococci (including methicillin-resistant *Streptococcus aureus* [MRSA] strains), and *Treponema pallidum.*

❏ Identify antibiotics that require major modifications of dosage in renal or hepatic dysfunction.

❏ List the reasons for use of antimicrobial drugs in combination and the probable mechanisms involved in drug synergy.

❏ Understand the principles underlying valid antimicrobial chemoprophylaxis and give examples of commonly used surgical and nonsurgical prophylaxis.

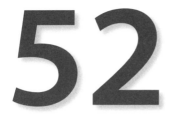
Antiprotozoal Drugs

Diseases caused by protozoans constitute a worldwide health problem. This chapter concerns the drugs used to combat malaria, amebiasis, toxoplasmosis, pneumocystosis, trypanosomiasis, and leishmaniasis.

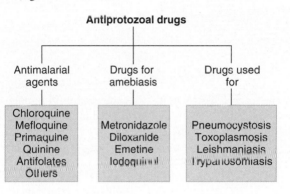

DRUGS FOR MALARIA

Malaria is one of the most common diseases worldwide and a leading cause of death. *Plasmodium* species that infect humans (*P falciparum, P malariae, P ovale, P vivax*) undergo a primary developmental stage in the liver and then parasitize erythrocytes. *P falciparum* and *P malariae* have only 1 cycle of liver cell invasion. The other species have a dormant hepatic stage responsible for recurrent infections and relapses. Primary **tissue schizonticides** (eg, primaquine) kill schizonts in the liver, whereas **blood schizonticides** (eg, chloroquine, quinine) kill these parasitic forms only in the erythrocyte. **Sporonticides** (proguanil, pyrimethamine) prevent sporogony and multiplication in the mosquito.

Drugs used for the treatment of malaria are shown in Table 52–1.

A. Chloroquine

1. Classification and pharmacokinetics— Chloroquine is a 4-aminoquinoline derivative. The drug is rapidly absorbed when given orally, is widely distributed to tissues, and has an extremely large volume of distribution. Antacids may decrease oral absorption of the drug. Chloroquine is excreted largely unchanged in the urine.

2. Mechanism of action— Chloroquine accumulates in the food vacuole of plasmodia and prevents polymerization of the hemoglobin breakdown product heme into hemozoin. Intracellular accumulation of heme is toxic to the parasite. Decreased intracellular accumulation via increased activity of membrane "pumps" is a mechanism of resistance to chloroquine and other antimalarial drugs. Resistance in *P falciparum* can also result from decreased intravacuolar accumulation of chloroquine via a transporter encoded by the *pfcrt* (*P falciparum* chloroquine-resistance transporter) gene.

3. Clinical use— Chloroquine is the drug of choice for acute attacks of nonfalciparum and sensitive falciparum malaria and for chemoprophylaxis, except in regions where *P falciparum* is resistant. The drug is solely a blood schizonticide. Chloroquine and hydroxychloroquine are also used in autoimmune disorders, including rheumatoid arthritis.

TABLE 52–1 Drugs used in the treatment of malaria.

Drug	Uses	Adverse Effects
Chloroquine	Prophylaxis and treatment in areas without resistant *P falciparum;* treatment of *P vivax* and *P ovale* malaria	GI distress, rash, headache; auditory dysfunction and retinal dysfunction (high dose)
Mefloquine	Prophylaxis and treatment in areas with resistant *P falciparum*	GI distress, rash, headache; cardiac conduction defects and neurologic symptoms (high dose)
Quinine[a]	Treatment of multidrug-resistant malaria	Cinchonism, hemolysis in G6PD deficiency, blackwater fever
Primaquine	Eradication of liver stages of *P vivax* and *P ovale*	GI distress, methemoglobinemia, hemolysis in G6PD deficiency
Antifolates	Prophylaxis and treatment of multidrug-resistant *P falciparum* malaria	GI distress, renal dysfunction, hemolysis, folate deficiency
Atovaquone-proguanil (Malarone)	Prophylaxis and treatment of multidrug-resistant *P falciparum* malaria	GI distress, headache, rash hemolysis, folate deficiency
Artesunate, Artemether	Treatment of multidrug-resistant malaria	GI distress

[a]In most cases quinine is used together with doxycycline or clindamycin, or an antifolate. Quinidine gluconate (IV) is used in severe infections or for patients unable to take oral quinine.

4. Toxicity—At low doses, chloroquine causes gastrointestinal irritation, skin rash, and headaches. High doses may cause severe skin lesions, peripheral neuropathies, myocardial depression, retinal damage, auditory impairment, and toxic psychosis. Chloroquine may also precipitate porphyria attacks.

B. Quinine

1. Classification and pharmacokinetics—Quinine is rapidly absorbed orally and is metabolized before renal excretion. Intravenous administration of quinine is possible in severe infections.

2. Mechanism of action—Quinine complexes with double-stranded DNA to prevent strand separation, resulting in block of DNA replication and transcription to RNA. Quinine is solely a blood schizonticide.

3. Clinical use—The main use of quinine is in *P falciparum* infections resistant to chloroquine in patients who can tolerate oral treatment. Quinine is commonly used with doxycycline or clindamycin to shorten the duration of therapy and limit toxicity. Quinidine, the dextrorotatory stereoisomer of quinine, is used intravenously in the treatment of severe or complicated falciparum malaria. To delay emergence of resistance, quinine should not be used routinely for prophylaxis.

4. Toxicity—Quinine commonly causes **cinchonism,** symptoms of which include gastrointestinal distress, headache, vertigo, blurred vision, and tinnitus. Severe overdose results in disturbances in cardiac conduction that resemble quinidine toxicity. Hematotoxic effects occur, including hemolysis in glucose-6-phosphate dehydrogenase (G6PD)-deficient patients. **Blackwater fever** (intravascular hemolysis) is a rare and sometimes fatal complication in quinine-sensitized persons. Quinine is contraindicated in pregnancy.

C. Mefloquine

1. Classification and pharmacokinetics—Mefloquine is a synthetic 4-quinoline derivative. Because of local irritation, mefloquine can only be given orally, although it is subject to variable absorption. Its mechanism of action is not known.

2. Clinical use—Mefloquine is a first-line drug (taken weekly) given for prophylaxis in all geographical areas with chloroquine resistance and an alternative drug to quinine in acute attacks and uncomplicated infections resulting from *P falciparum.* Resistance to mefloquine has emerged in regions of Southeast Asia.

3. Toxicity—Common adverse effects include gastrointestinal distress, skin rash, headache, and dizziness. At high doses, mefloquine has caused cardiac conduction defects, psychiatric disorders, neurologic symptoms, and seizures.

D. Primaquine

1. Classification and pharmacokinetics—Primaquine is a synthetic 8-aminoquinoline. Absorption is complete after oral administration and is followed by extensive metabolism.

2. Mechanism of action—Primaquine forms quinoline-quinone metabolites, which are electron-transferring redox compounds that act as cellular oxidants. The drug is a tissue schizonticide and also limits malaria transmission by acting as a gametocide.

3. Clinical use—Primaquine eradicates liver stages of *P vivax* and *P ovale* and should be used in conjunction with a blood schizonticide. Although not active alone in acute attacks of vivax and ovale malaria, a 14-d course of primaquine is standard after treatment with chloroquine, and the drug is also an alternative (daily) for primary prevention.

4. Toxicity—Primaquine is usually well tolerated but may cause gastrointestinal distress, pruritus, headaches, and methemoglobinemia. More serious toxicity involves hemolysis in G6PD-deficient patients. Primaquine is contraindicated in pregnancy.

E. Antifolate Drugs

1. Classification and pharmacokinetics—The antifolate group includes pyrimethamine, proguanil, sulfadoxine, and dapsone. All these drugs are absorbed orally and are excreted in the urine, partly in unchanged form. Proguanil has a shorter half-life (12–16 h) than other drugs in this subclass (half-life >100 h).

2. Mechanisms of action—Sulfonamides act as antimetabolites of PABA and block folic acid synthesis in certain protozoans by inhibiting dihydropteroate synthase. Proguanil (chloroguanide) is bioactivated to cycloguanil. Pyrimethamine and cycloguanil are selective inhibitors of protozoan dihydrofolate reductases. The combination of pyrimethamine with sulfadoxine has synergistic antimalarial effects through the **sequential blockade** of 2 steps in folic acid synthesis.

3. Clinical use—The antifols are blood schizonticides that act mainly against *P falciparum*. Pyrimethamine with sulfadoxine in fixed combination (Fansidar) is used in the treatment of chloroquine-resistant forms of this species, although the onset of activity is slow. Proguanil with atovaquone in fixed combination (Malarone) can be used (daily) for chemoprophylaxis of chloroquine-resistant malaria and is also protective against mefloquine-resistant falciparum strains.

4. Toxicity—The toxic effects of sulfonamides include skin rashes, gastrointestinal distress, hemolysis, kidney damage, and drug interactions caused by competition for plasma protein binding sites. Pyrimethamine may cause folic acid deficiency when used in high doses.

F. Other Antimalarial Drugs

1. Doxycycline—This tetracycline is chemoprophylactic (taken daily) for travelers to geographical areas with multidrug-resistant *P falciparum*.

2. Amodiaquine—This drug has been widely used to treat malaria in many countries because of its low cost and, in some geographical areas, effectiveness against chloroquine-resistant strains of *P falciparum*. It is also used in fixed combination with artusenate. Hematologic toxicity, including agranulocytosis and aplastic anemia, has been associated with the use of amodiaquine.

3. Atovaquone—This quinine derivative, a component of Malarone (proguanil), appears to disrupt mitochondrial electron transport in protozoa. Malarone is effective for both chemoprophylaxis (taken daily) and treatment of falciparum malaria. Abdominal pain and gastrointestinal effects occur at the higher doses needed for treatment. Atovaquone is an alternative treatment for *P jiroveci* infection.

4. Halofantrine—Although its mechanism of action is unknown, this drug is active against erythrocytic (but not other) stages of all 4 human malaria species, including chloroquine-resistant falciparum. Halofantrine is not used for chemoprophylaxis because of its potential for quinidine-like cardiotoxicity (QT prolongation) and embryotoxicity. **Lumefantrine**, a related drug with minimal cardiotoxicity, is now used in fixed combination with artemether (Coartem) for uncomplicated falciparum malaria in many countries.

5. Artesunate, artemether, dihydroartemisinin—These artemisinin derivatives are metabolized in the food vacuole of the parasite forming toxic free radicals. Artemisinins are blood schizonticides active against *P falciparum*, including multidrug-resistant strains. An intravenous form of artesunate is available for severe infections. These drugs are not used alone for chemoprophylaxis because of their short half-lives of 1–3 h. However, they are playing an increasingly important role in the treatment of malaria and are best used in combination with other agents. The artemisinins are the only drugs reliably effective against quinine-resistant strains. Adverse effects are mild, but include nausea, vomiting, and diarrhea. Rates of congenital abnormalities, stillbirths, and abortion do not appear to be elevated in women treated with artemisinins during pregnancy.

G. Drugs for the Prevention of Malaria in Travelers

Chloroquine (weekly) remains an appropriate agent for prophylaxis in regions without resistant *P falciparum* as does mefloquine (weekly) for regions with *P falciparum* resistance to chloroquine. In areas with multidrug-resistant malaria, the choice is either doxycycline or Malarone (atovaquone plus proguanil); both drugs must be taken daily. Primaquine (daily for 14 d) is recommended for terminal prophylaxis of *P vivax* and *P ovale* infections and is an alternative in primary prevention. (For updated information, check CDC guidelines at http://www.cdc.gov.)

DRUGS FOR AMEBIASIS

Tissue amebicides (**chloroquine, emetines, metronidazole, tindidazole**) act on organisms in the bowel wall and the liver; luminal amebicides (**diloxanide furoate, iodoquinol, paromomycin**) act only in the lumen of the bowel. The choice of a drug depends on the form of amebiasis. For asymptomatic disease, diloxanide furoate is the first choice. For mild to severe intestinal infection, metronidazole or tindidazole is used with a luminal agent, and this regimen is recommended in amebic

TABLE 52–2 Drugs used in the treatment of amebiasis.

Disease Form	Drug(s) of Choice	Alternative Drug(s)
Asymptomatic, Intestinal infection	Diloxanide furoate	Iodoquinol, paramomycin
Mild to moderate intestinal infection	Metronidazole *plus* luminal agent (see above)	Tinidazole, *or* tetracycline, *or* erythromycin *plus* luminal agent
Severe intestinal infection	Metronidazole *or* tinidazole *plus* luminal agent	Tetracycline *or* emetine *or* dihydroemetine *plus* luminal agent
Hepatic abscess and other extraintestinal disease	Metronidazole *or* tinidazole *plus* luminal agent	Emetine *or* dihydroemetine *plus* choroquine (for liver abscess) *plus* luminal agent

Adapted, with permission, from Katzung BG, editor: *Basic & Clinical Pharmacology*, 11th ed. McGraw-Hill, 2009.

hepatic abscess and other extraintestinal disease (Table 52–2). The mechanisms of amebicidal action of most drugs in this subclass are unknown.

A. Diloxanide Furoate

This drug is commonly used as the sole agent for the treatment of asymptomatic amebiasis and is also useful in mild intestinal disease when used with other drugs. Diloxanide furoate is converted in the gut to the diloxanide freebase form, which is the active amebicide. Toxic effects are mild and are usually restricted to gastrointestinal symptoms.

B. Emetines

Emetine and dehydroemetine inhibit protein synthesis by blocking ribosomal movement along messenger RNA. These drugs are used parenterally (subcutaneously or intramuscularly) as backup drugs for treatment of severe intestinal or hepatic amebiasis together with a luminal agent in hospitalized patients. The drugs may cause severe toxicity, including gastrointestinal distress, muscle weakness, and cardiovascular dysfunction (arrhythmias and congestive heart failure). The drugs are restricted to use in severe amebiasis when metronidazole cannot be used.

C. Iodoquinol

Iodoquinol, a halogenated hydroxyquinoline, is an orally active luminal amebicide used as an alternative to diloxanide for mild-to-severe intestinal infections. Adverse gastrointestinal effects are common but usually mild, especially when taken with meals. Systemic absorption after high doses may lead to thyroid enlargement, skin reactions due to iodine toxicity and possibly neurotoxic effects, including peripheral neuropathy and visual dysfunction.

D. Metronidazole and Tinidazole

1. Pharmacokinetics—Metronidazole and tinidazole are effective orally and distributed widely to tissues. The half-life of metronidazole is 6–8 h, and that of tinidazole 12–14 h. Elimination of the drugs requires hepatic metabolism.

2. Mechanism of action—Metronidazole undergoes a reductive bioactivation of its nitro group by ferredoxin (present in anaerobic parasites) to form reactive cytotoxic products. The mechanism of tinidazole is assumed to be similar.

3. Clinical use—Metronidazole or tinidazole is the drug of choice in severe intestinal wall disease and in hepatic abscess and other extraintestinal amebic disease. Both drugs are used with a luminal amebicide. The duration of treatment required with metronidazole is longer than with tinidazole. Metronidazole is the drug of choice for trichomoniasis: tinidazole may be effective against some metronidazole-resistant organisms. Other clinical uses of metronidazole include treatment of giardiasis (tinidazole is equally effective), and infections caused by *Gardnerella vaginalis* and anaerobic bacteria (*B fragilis, C difficile*). Metronidazole is also used in combination regimens for gastrointestinal ulcers associated with *H pylori*.

4. Toxicity—Adverse effects of metronidazole include gastrointestinal irritation (it is best taken with meals), headache, paresthesias, and dark coloration of urine. Tinidazole has a similar adverse effect profile but may be better tolerated than metronidazole. More serious toxicity includes neutropenia, dizziness, and ataxia. Drug interactions with metronidazole include a disulfiram-like reaction with ethanol and potentiation of coumarin anticoagulant effects. Safety of metronidazole and tinidazole in pregnancy and in nursing mothers has not been established.

E. Paromomycin

This drug is an aminoglycoside antibiotic used as a luminal amebicide and may be superior to diloxanide in asymptomatic infection. Paromomycin may also have some efficacy against cryptosporidiosis in the AIDS patient. Systemic absorption in renal insufficiency may lead to headaches, dizziness, rashes, and arthralgia. Tetracyclines (eg, doxycycline) are sometimes used with a luminal amebicide in mild intestinal disease.

F. Nitazoxanide

This agent has activity against various protozoans (including *Entamoeba*) and helminths. It is currently approved in the United

States for treatment of gastrointestinal infections caused by *G lamblia* and *Cryptosporidium parvum*. Nitazoxanide appears to have activity against metronidazole-resistant protozoal strains.

DRUGS FOR PNEUMOCYSTOSIS & TOXOPLASMOSIS

A. Pentamidine

1. Mechanism of action—Pentamidine's mechanism of action is unknown but may involve inhibition of glycolysis or interference with nucleic acid metabolism of protozoans and fungi. Preferential accumulation of the drug by susceptible parasites may account for its selective toxicity.

2. Clinical use—Aerosol pentamidine (once monthly) can be used in primary and secondary prophylaxis, although oral trimethoprim-sulfamethoxazole (TMP-SMZ) is usually preferred. Daily intravenous or intramuscular administration of the drug for 21 d is needed in the treatment of active pneumocystosis in the HIV-infected patient. Pentamidine is also used in trypanosomiasis (see later discussion).

3. Toxicity—Severe adverse effects follow parenteral use, including respiratory stimulation followed by depression, hypotension resulting from peripheral vasodilation, hypoglycemia, anemia, neutropenia, hepatitis, and pancreatitis. Systemic toxicity is minimal when pentamidine is used by inhalation.

B. TMP-SMZ

1. Clinical use—TMP-SMZ is the first choice in prophylaxis and treatment of pneumocystis pneumonia (PCP). Prophylaxis in AIDS patients is recommended when the CD4 count drops below 200 cells/μL. Oral treatment with the double-strength formulation 3 times weekly is usually effective. The same regimen of TMP-SMZ is prophylactic against toxoplasmosis and infections caused by *Isospora belli*. For treatment of active PCP, daily oral or intravenous administration of TMP-SMZ is required.

2. Toxicity—Adverse effects from TMP-SMZ occur in up to 50% of AIDS patients. Toxicity includes gastrointestinal distress, rash, fever, neutropenia, and thrombocytopenia. These effects may be serious enough to warrant discontinuance of TMP-SMZ and substitution of alternative drugs. (See Chapter 46 for additional information on TMP-SMZ.)

C. Antifols: Pyrimethamine and Sulfonamides

1. Clinical use—Combination of pyrimethamine with sulfadiazine has synergistic activity against *Toxoplasma gondii* through the **sequential blockade** of 2 steps in folic acid synthesis. Pyrimethamine plus clindamycin (or sulfadiazine) is a regimen of choice for prophylaxis against and treatment of toxoplasmosis. For treatment of active toxoplasmosis, the drug combination is given daily for 3–4 wk, with folinic acid to offset hematologic toxicity. For *Toxoplasma* encephalitis in AIDS, high-dose treatment with pyrimethamine plus sulfadiazine (or clindamycin) plus folinic acid must be maintained for at least 6 wk.

2. Toxicity—High doses of pyrimethamine plus sulfadiazine are associated with gastric irritation, glossitis, neurologic symptoms (headache, insomnia, tremors, seizures), and hematotoxicity (megaloblastic anemia, thrombocytopenia). Antibiotic-associated colitis may occur during treatment with clindamycin.

D. Atovaquone

1. Mechanism and pharmacokinetics—Atovaquone inhibits mitochondrial electron transport and probably folate metabolism. Used orally, it is poorly absorbed and should be given with food to maximize bioavailability. Most of the drug is eliminated in the feces in unchanged form.

2. Clinical use and toxicity—Atovaquone is approved for use in mild to moderate pneumocystis pneumonia. It is less effective than TMP-SMZ or pentamidine but is better tolerated. As noted, it is also used in combination with proguanil (as Malarone) for chemoprophylaxis and treatment of chloroquine-resistant malaria. Common adverse effects are rash, cough, nausea, vomiting, diarrhea, fever, and abnormal liver function tests. The drug should be avoided in patients with a history of cardiac conduction defects, psychiatric disorders, or seizures.

E. Miscellaneous Agents

Other alternative drug regimens for the treatment of pneumocystis pneumonia include trimethoprim plus dapsone, primaquine plus clindamycin, and trimetrexate plus leucovorin.

DRUGS FOR TRYPANOSOMIASIS

A. Pentamidine

Pentamidine is commonly used in the hemolymphatic stages of disease caused by *Trypanosoma gambiense* and *T rhodesiense*. Because it does not cross the blood-brain barrier, pentamidine is not used in later stages of trypanosomiasis. Other clinical uses include pneumocystosis and treatment of the kala azar form of leishmaniasis (Table 52–3).

B. Melarsoprol

This drug is an organic arsenical that inhibits enzyme sulfhydryl groups. Because it enters the CNS, melarsoprol is the drug of choice in African sleeping sickness. However, treatment failures do occur, possibly because of resistance. Melarsoprol is given parenterally because it causes gastrointestinal irritation; it may also cause a reactive encephalopathy that can be fatal.

TABLE 52–3 Drugs used in the treatment of other protozoal infections.

Drug	Indications
Melarsoprol	Mucocutaneous forms of trypanosomiasis and the CNS stage (African sleeping sickness)
Metronidazole	Drug of choice for infections caused by *Giardia lamblia* and *Trichomonas vaginalis*
Nifurtimox	Trypanosomiasis caused by *T cruzi*
Pentamidine	Hemolymphatic stage of trypanosomiasis and for *Pneumocystis jiroveci* infections
Pyrimethamine *plus* clindamycin *or* sulfadiazine *plus* folinic acid	Drug combinations used in treatment of toxoplasmosis
Sodium stibogluconate	Treatment of leishmaniasis (all stages)
Suramin	Drug of choice for hemolymphatic stage of trypanosomiasis (*T brucei gambiense, T rhodesiense*)
Trimethoprim-sulfamethoxazole	Drug combination of choice in *Pneumocystis jiroveci* infections

C. Nifurtimox

This drug is a nitrofurazone derivative that inhibits the parasite-unique enzyme trypanothione reductase. Nifurtimox is the drug of choice in American trypanosomiasis, an alternative agent in African forms of the disease, and has also been effective in mucocutaneous leishmaniasis. The drug causes severe toxicity, including allergies, gastrointestinal irritation, and CNS effects.

D. Suramin

This polyanionic compound is a drug of choice for the early hemolymphatic stages of African trypanosomiasis (before CNS involvement). It is also an alternative to ivermectin in the treatment of onchocerciasis (see Chapter 53). Suramin is used parenterally and causes skin rashes, gastrointestinal distress, and neurologic complications.

E. Eflornithine

This agent, a suicide substrate of ornithine decarboxylase, is effective in some forms of African trypanosomiasis. It is available for both oral and intravenous use and penetrates into the CNS. It causes gastrointestinal irritation and hematotoxicity; seizures have occurred in overdose.

DRUGS FOR LEISHMANIASIS

Leishmania, parasitic protozoa transmitted by flesh-eating flies, cause various diseases ranging from cutaneous or mucocutaneous lesions to splenic and hepatic enlargement with fever. **Sodium stibogluconate** (pentavalent antimony), the primary drug in all forms of the disease, appears to kill the parasite by inhibition of glycolysis or effects on nucleic acid metabolism. Stibogluconate must be administered parenterally and is potentially cardiotoxic (QT prolongation). Alternative agents include pentamidine or miltefosine (for visceral leishmaniasis), fluconazole or metronidazole (for cutaneous lesions), and amphotericin B (for mucocutaneous leishmaniasis).

QUESTIONS

1. Which statement about antiprotozoal drugs is accurate?
   (A) Chloroquine is an inhibitor of plasmodial dihydrofolate reductase
   (B) Mefloquine destroys secondary exoerythrocytic schizonts
   (C) Primaquine is a blood schizonticide and does not affect secondary tissue schizonts
   (D) Proguanil complexes with double-stranded DNA-blocking replication
   (E) Trimethoprim-sulfamethoxazole is the drug of choice for *Pneumocystis jiroveci* pneumonia

2. Plasmodial resistance to chloroquine is due to
   (A) Change in receptor structure
   (B) Increase in the activity of DNA repair mechanisms
   (C) Increased synthesis of dihydrofolate reductase
   (D) Induction of drug-inactivating enzymes
   (E) Reduced accumulation of the drug in the food vacuole

Questions 3–5. A traveler in a geographical region where chloroquine-resistant *P falciparum* is endemic used a drug for prophylaxis but nevertheless developed a severe attack of *P vivax* malaria.

3. The drug taken for chemoprophylaxis was probably
   (A) Atovaquone
   (B) Diloxanide furoate
   (C) Mefloquine
   (D) Proguanil
   (E) Quinine

4. Which drug should be used for oral treatment of the acute attack of *P vivax* malaria but does not eradicate exoerythrocytic forms of the parasite?
   (A) Chloroquine
   (B) Mefloquine
   (C) Primaquine
   (D) Pyrimethamine-sulfadoxine
   (E) Quinidine

5. Which drug should be given later to eradicate schizonts and latent hypnozoites in the patient's liver?
   (A) Amodiaquine
   (B) Halofantrine
   (C) Primaquine
   (D) Quinine
   (E) Sulfadoxine

Questions 6 and 7. A male patient presents with lower abdominal discomfort, flatulence, and occasional diarrhea. A diagnosis of intestinal amebiasis is made, and *E histolytica* is identified in his diarrheal stools. An oral drug is prescribed, which reduces his intestinal symptoms. Later he presents with severe dysentery, right upper quadrant pain, weight loss, fever, and an enlarged liver. Amebic liver abscess is diagnosed, and the patient is hospitalized. He has a recent history of drug treatment for a tachyarrhythmia.

6. The preferred treatment that he *should* have received for the initial symptoms (which were indicative of mild to moderate disease) is
   (A) Diloxanide furoate
   (B) Iodoquinol
   (C) Metronidazole
   (D) Metronidazole plus diloxanide furoate
   (E) Paromomycin

7. The drug regimen most likely to be effective in treating severe extraintestinal disease in this patient is
   (A) Chloroquine
   (B) Diloxanide furoate plus iodoquinol
   (C) Emetine plus diloxanide furoate plus chloroquine
   (D) Pentamidine followed by mefloquine
   (E) Tinidazole plus diloxanide furoate

8. After a backpacking trip in the mountains, a 24-year-old man develops diarrhea. He acknowledges drinking stream water without purification, and you suspect he is showing symptoms of giardiasis. Because you know that laboratory detection of cysts or trophozoites in the feces can be difficult, you decide to treat the patient empirically with
   (A) Chloroquine
   (B) Emetine
   (C) Metronidazole
   (D) Pentamidine
   (E) TMP-SMZ

9. This drug can clear trypanosomes from the blood and lymph nodes and is active in the late CNS stages of African sleeping sickness.
   (A) Emetine
   (B) Eflornithine
   (C) Melarsoprol
   (D) Nifurtimox
   (E) Suramin

10. Metronidazole is not effective in the treatment of
    (A) Amebiasis
    (B) Infections due to *Bacteroides fragilis*
    (C) Infections due to *Pneumocystis jiroveci*
    (D) Pseudomembranous colitis
    (E) Trichomoniasis

ANSWERS

1. Proguanil (not chloroquine) is an inhibitor of dihydrofolate reductase. Primaquine (not mefloquine) is the drug that destroys secondary exoerythrocytic schizonts. TMP-SMZ is the drug of choice for *Pneumocystis jiroveci* pneumonia. The answer is **E.**

2. Resistance to chloroquine in *P falciparum* can result from decreased accumulation of the drug in the food vacuole caused by the activity of a transporter system encoded by the *pfcrt* gene. The answer is **E.**

3. Mefloquine is a recommended drug for prophylaxis in regions of the world where chloroquine-resistant *P falciparum* is endemic. One dose of mefloquine weekly starting before travel and continuing until 4 wk after leaving the region is the preferred regimen. Doxycycline is an alternative drug for this indication, as is atovaquone plus proguanil (Malarone). The answer is **C.**

4. Chloroquine is the drug of choice for the oral treatment of an acute attack of malaria caused by *P vivax* but will not eradicate exoerythrocytic forms of the parasite. The answer is **A.**

5. Primaquine is the only antimalarial drug that reliably acts on tissue schizonts in liver cells. Quinine is a highly effective blood schizonticide against all 4 species of human malaria parasites, but it is not active against liver stages. Starting about day 4 after an acute attack, primaquine should be given daily for 2 wk. The answer is **C.**

6. Metronidazole plus a luminal amebicide is the treatment of choice in mild to moderate amebic colitis. Diloxanide furoate (or iodoquinol, or paramomycin) can be used as the sole agent in asymptomatic intestinal infection. The answer is **D.**

7. Metronidazole given for 10 d, or tinidazole for 5 d, plus a luminal agent is effective in most cases of hepatic abscess, and these regimens have the dual advantage of being both amebicidal and active against anaerobic bacteria. Though active in amebic hepatic abscess, treatment with emetine is contraindicated in patients with a history of cardiac disease. The answer is **E.**

8. Giardiasis is a common intestinal protozoan infection caused by *Giardia lamblia*. A large number of infections result from fecal contamination of food or water. Metronidazole has been considered the drug of choice. Tinidazole is equally effective. The answer is **C.**

9. In the advanced stages of African sleeping sickness, melarsoprol is the drug of choice because, unlike pentamidine or suramin, it effectively enters the CNS. Nifurtimox is the most commonly used drug for Chagas' disease. The answer is **C.**

10. Metronidazole is the drug of first choice for all of the conditions listed except pneumocystosis. The answer is **C.**

CHECKLIST

When you complete this chapter, you should be able to:

❑ Name the major antimalarial drugs. Know which are used for chemoprophylaxis, which are effective in chloroquine resistance, and which are exoerythrocytic schizonticides.

❑ Identify the characteristic adverse effects of the major antimalarial drugs.

❑ Describe the clinical uses and adverse effects of metronidazole.

❑ Be able to identify the intestinal amebicides.

❑ Identify the drugs used for prophylaxis and treatment of pneumocystosis and toxoplasmosis, and know their characteristic toxic effects.

❑ Identify the major drugs used for trypanosomiasis and leishmaniasis, and know their characteristic toxic effects.

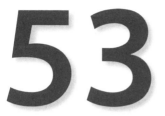

Antihelminthic Drugs

Antihelminthic drugs have diverse chemical structures, mechanisms of action, and properties. Most were discovered by empiric screening methods. Many act against specific parasites, and few are devoid of significant toxicity to host cells. In addition to the direct toxicity of the drugs, reactions to dead and dying parasites may cause serious toxicity in patients. In the text that follows, the drugs are divided into 3 groups on the basis of the type of helminth primarily affected (nematodes, trematodes, and cestodes). The drugs of choice and alternative agents for selected important helminthic infections are listed in Table 53–1.

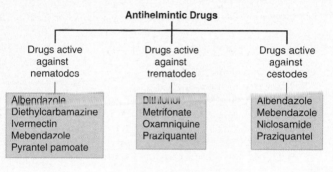

DRUGS THAT ACT AGAINST NEMATODES

The medically important intestinal nematodes responsive to drug therapy include *Enterobius vermicularis* (pinworm), *Trichuris trichiuria* (whipworm), *Ascaris lumbricoides* (roundworm), *Ancyclostoma* and *Necator* species (hookworms), and *Strongyloides stercoralis* (threadworm). More than 1 billion persons worldwide are estimated to be infected by intestinal nematodes. Pinworm infections are common throughout the United States, and hookworm and threadworm are endemic in the southern United States. Tissue nematodes responsive to drug therapy include *Ancyclostoma* species, which cause cutaneous larva migrans. Species of *Dracunculus, Onchocerca, Toxocara,* and *Wuchereria bancrofti* (the cause of filariasis) all are responsive to drug treatment. The number of persons worldwide estimated to be infected by tissue nematodes exceeds 0.5 billion.

A. Albendazole

1. Mechanisms—The action of albendazole is thought to involve inhibition of microtubule assembly. The drug is larvicidal in ascariasis, cystercercosis, hookworm, and hydatid disease and is ovicidal in ascariasis, ancyclostomiasis, and trichuriasis.

2. Clinical use—Albendazole has a wide antihelminthic spectrum. It is a primary drug for ascariasis, hookworm, pinworm, and whipworm infections and an alternative drug for treatment of threadworm infections, filariasis, and both visceral and cutaneous larva migrans. Albendazole is also used in hydatid disease and is active against the pork tapeworm in the larval stage (cysticercosis).

3. Toxicity—Albendazole has few toxic effects during short courses of therapy (1–3 d). However, a reversible leukopenia, alopecia, and elevation of liver function enzymes can occur with more prolonged use. Long-term animal toxicity studies have described bone marrow suppression and fetal toxicity. The safety of the drug in pregnancy and young children has not been established.

B. Diethylcarbamazine

1. Mechanisms—Diethylcarbamazine immobilizes microfilariae by an unknown mechanism, increasing their susceptibility to host defense mechanisms.

2. Clinical use—Diethylcarbamazine is the drug of choice for several filarial infections including those caused by *Wucheria bancrofti* and *Brugia malayi* and for eye worm disease (loa loa).

TABLE 53–1 Drugs for the treatment of helminthic infections.

Infecting Organism	Drugs of Choice	Alternative Drugs
Nematodes		
Ascaris lumbricoides (roundworm)	Albendazole *or* mebendazole *or* pyrantel pamoate	Ivermectin, piperazine
Necator americanus & *Ancylostoma duodenale* (hookworm)	Pyrantel pamoate *or* albendazole *or* mebendazole	
Trichuris trichiura (whipworm)	Albendazole *or* mebendazole	Ivermectin
Strongyloides stercoralis (threadworm)	Ivermectin	Albendazole, thiabendazole
Enterobius vermicularis (pinworm)	Mebendazole *or* pyrantel pamoate	Albendazole
Trichinella spiralis (trichinosis)	Mebendazole (+/– corticosteroids)	Albendazole
Cutaneous larva migrans	Albendazole *or* ivermectin	
Wuchereria bancrofti and *Brugia malayi* (filariasis)	Diethylcarbamazine	Ivermectin
Onchocerca volvulus (onchocerciasis)	Ivermectin	
Trematodes (flukes)		
Schistosoma haematobium	Praziquantel	Metrifonate
Schistosoma mansoni	Praziquantel	Oxamniquine
Schistosoma japonicum	Praziquantel	
Paragonimus westermani	Praziquantel	
Fasciola hepatica (sheep liver fluke)	Bithional *or* triclabendazole	
Fasciolopsis buski (large intestinal fluke)	Praziquantel *or* niclosamide	
Cestodes (tapeworms)		
Taenia saginata (beef tapeworm)	Praziquantel *or* niclosamide	Mebendazole
Taenia solium (pork tapeworm)	Praziquantel *or* niclosamide	
Cysticercosis (pork tapeworm larval stage)	Albendazole	Praziquantel
Diphylobothrium latum (fish tapeworm)	Praziquantel *or* niclosamide	
Echinococcus granulosus (hydatid disease)	Albendazole	

The drug undergoes renal elimination, and its half-life is increased significantly by urinary alkalinization.

3. Toxicity—Adverse effects include headache, malaise, weakness, and anorexia. Reactions to proteins released by dying filariae include fever, rashes, ocular damage, joint and muscle pain, and lymphangitis. In onchocerciasis, the reactions are more intense and include most of the symptoms described as well as hypotension, pyrexia, respiratory distress, and prostration.

C. Ivermectin

1. Mechanisms—Ivermectin intensifies γ-aminobutyric acid (GABA)-mediated neurotransmission in nematodes and causes

immobilization of parasites, facilitating their removal by the reticuloendothelial system. Selective toxicity results because in humans GABA is a neurotransmitter only in the CNS, and ivermectin does not cross the blood-brain barrier.

2. Clinical use—Ivermectin is the drug of choice for onchocerciasis, cutaneous larva migrans, strongyloidiasis, and some forms of filariasis.

3. Toxicity—Single-dose oral treatment in onchocerciasis results in reactions to the dying worms, including fever, headache, dizziness, rashes, pruritus, tachycardia, hypotension, and pain in joints, muscles, and lymph glands. These symptoms are usually of short duration, and most can be controlled with antihistamines and non-steroidal anti-inflammatory drugs. Avoid other drugs that enhance GABA activity. Ivermectin should not be used in pregnancy.

D. Mebendazole

1. Mechanism—Mebendazole acts by selectively inhibiting microtubule synthesis and glucose uptake in nematodes.

2. Clinical use—Mebendazole is a primary drug for treatment of ascariasis and for pinworm and whipworm infections. Mebendazole has also been used as a backup drug in visceral larval migrans. Less than 10% of the drug is absorbed systemically after oral use, and this portion is metabolized rapidly by hepatic enzymes. Plasma levels may be decreased by carbamazepine or phenytoin and increased by cimetidine.

3. Toxicity—Mebendazole toxicity is usually limited to gastrointestinal irritation, but at high doses agranulocytopenia and alopecia have occurred. The drug is teratogenic in animals and therefore contraindicated in pregnancy.

E. Piperazine

1. Mechanism—Piperazine paralyzes ascaris by acting as an agonist at GABA receptors. The paralyzed roundworms are expelled live by normal peristalsis.

2. Clinical use—Piperazine is an alternative drug for ascariasis.

3. Toxicity—Mild gastrointestinal irritation is the most common side effect. Piperazine should not be used in pregnant patients or those with hepatic or renal dysfunction or seizure disorders.

F. Pyrantel Pamoate

1. Mechanism—Pyrantel pamoate stimulates nicotinic receptors present at neuromuscular junctions of nematodes. Contraction of muscles occurs, followed by a depolarization-induced paralysis. The drug has no actions on flukes or tapeworms.

2. Clinical use—Pyrantel pamoate has wide activity against nematodes killing adult worms in the colon but not the eggs. It is a drug of choice for hookworm and roundworm infections and an alternative drug for pinworms. The drug is poorly absorbed when given orally.

3. Toxicity—Adverse effects are minor but include gastrointestinal distress, headache, and weakness. Use with caution in patients with hepatic dysfunction.

G. Thiabendazole

1. Mechanism—Thiabendazole is a structural congener of mebendazole and has a similar action on microtubules.

2. Clinical use—Because of its adverse effects, thiabendazole is an alternative drug in strongyloidiasis and trichinosis (adult worms).

Thiabendazole is rapidly absorbed from the gut and is metabolized by liver enzymes. The drug has anti-inflammatory and immunorestorative actions in the host.

3. Toxicity—Thiabendazole is much more toxic than other benzimidazoles or ivermectin, so these other drugs are preferred. Its toxic effects include gastrointestinal irritation, headache, dizziness, drowsiness, leukopenia, hematuria, and allergic reactions, including intrahepatic cholestasis. Reactions caused by dying parasites include fever, chills, lymphadenopathy, and skin rash. Irreversible liver failure and fatal Stevens-Johnson syndrome have also been reported. Avoid in pregnant patients or those with hepatic or renal disease.

SKILL KEEPER: ANTIMICROBIAL CHEMOTHERAPY IN PREGNANCY

Mebendazole is widely used for the treatment of nematode infections but is contraindicated in the pregnant patient because of possible embryotoxicity. Think back over the drugs used for the treatment of bacterial, fungal, protozoal, and viral infections.

1. *Which drugs are associated with a greater risk compared with benefit in pregnancy?*
2. *Which drugs are nominally contraindicated in pregnancy but might be used if the benefit were judged to outweigh the risk?*

The Skill Keeper Answers appear at the end of the chapter.

DRUGS THAT ACT AGAINST TREMATODES

The medically important trematodes include *Schistosoma* species (blood flukes, estimated to affect more than 150 million persons worldwide), *Clonorchis sinensis* (liver fluke, endemic in Southeast Asia), and *Paragonimus westermani* (lung fluke, endemic to both Asia and the Indian subcontinent). With few exceptions, fluke infections respond well to praziquantel.

A. Praziquantel

1. Mechanism—Praziquantel increases membrane permeability to calcium, causing marked contraction initially and then paralysis of trematode and cestode muscles; this is followed by vacuolization and parasite death.

2. Clinical use—Praziquantel has a wide antihelminthic spectrum that includes activity in both trematode and cestode infections. It is the drug of choice in schistosomiasis (all species), clonorchiasis, and paragonimiasis and for infections caused by small and large intestinal flukes. The drug is active against immature and adult schistosomal forms. Praziquantel is also 1 of 2 drugs of choice (with niclosamide) for infections caused by cestodes (all common tapeworms) and an alternative agent (to albendazole) in the treatment of cysticercosis.

3. Pharmacokinetics—Absorption from the gut is rapid, and the drug is metabolized by the liver to inactive products.

4. Toxicity—Common adverse effects include headache, dizziness and drowsiness, malaise, and less frequently, gastrointestinal irritation, skin rash, and fever. Neurologic effects can occur in the treatment of neurocyticercosis including intracranial hypertension and seizures. Corticosteroid therapy reduces the risk of the more serious reactions. Praziquantel is contraindicated in ocular cysticercosis. In animal studies, the drug increased abortion rate.

B. Bithionol

1. Clinical use—Bithionol is a codrug of choice (with triclabendazole) for treatment of fascioliasis (sheep liver fluke) and an alternative agent in paragonimiasis. The mechanism of action of the drug is unknown. Bithionol is orally effective and is eliminated in the urine.

2. Toxicity—Common adverse effects of bithionol include nausea and vomiting, diarrhea and abdominal cramps, dizziness, headache, skin rash (possibly a reaction to dying worms), and phototoxicity. Less frequently, pyrexia, tinnitus, proteinuria, and leukopenia may occur.

C. Metrifonate

Metrifonate is an organophosphate prodrug that is converted in the body to the cholinesterase inhibitor dichlorvos. The active metabolite acts solely against *Schistosoma haematobium* (the cause of bilharziasis). Toxic effects occur from excess cholinergic stimulation. The drug is contraindicated in pregnancy.

D. Oxamniquine

Oxamniquine is effective solely in *Schistosoma mansoni* infections (intestinal bilharziasis), acting on male immature forms and adult schistosomal forms. The drug causes paralysis of the worms, but its precise mechanism is unknown. Dizziness is a common adverse effect (no driving for 24 h); headache, gastrointestinal irritation, and pruritus may also occur. Reactions to dying parasites include eosinophilia, urticaria, and pulmonary infiltrates. It is not advisable to use the drug in pregnancy or in patients with a history of seizure disorders.

DRUGS THAT ACT AGAINST CESTODES (TAPEWORMS)

The 4 medically important cestodes are *Taenia saginata* (beef tapeworm), *Taenia solium* (pork tapeworm, which can cause cysticerci in the brain and the eyes), *Diphyllobothrium latum* (fish tapeworm),

and *Echinococcus granulosus* (dog tapeworm, which can cause hydatid cysts in the liver, lungs, and brain). The primary drugs for treatment of cestode infections are praziquantel (see prior discussion) and niclosamide.

A. Niclosamide

1. Mechanism—Niclosamide may act by uncoupling oxidative phosphorylation or by activating ATPases.

2. Clinical use—Niclosamide is an alternative drug to praziquantel for infections caused by beef, pork, and fish tapeworm. It is not effective in cysticercosis (for which albendazole or praziquantel is used) or hydatid disease caused by *Echinococcus granulosus* (for which albendazole is used). Scoleces and cestode segments are killed, but ova are not. Niclosamide is effective in the treatment of infections from small and large intestinal flukes.

3. Toxicity—Toxic effects are usually mild but include gastrointestinal distress, headache, rash, and fever. Some of these effects may result from systemic absorption of antigens from disintegrating parasites. Ethanol consumption should be avoided for 24–48 h.

QUESTIONS

1. A missionary from the United States is sent to work in a geographic region of a Central American country where *Onchocerca volvulus* is endemic. Infections resulting from this tissue nematode (onchocerciasis) are a cause of "river blindness," because microfilariae migrate through subcutaneous tissues and concentrate in the eyes. Which drug should be used prophylactically to prevent onchocerciasis?
   (A) Albendazole
   (B) Diethylcarbamazine
   (C) Ivermectin
   (D) Oxamniquine
   (E) Suramin

2. A nonindigenous person who develops onchocerciasis in an endemic region and receives drug treatment is likely to experience a severe reaction. Symptoms include headache, weakness, rash, muscle aches, hypotension, and peripheral edema. Which statement concerning this reaction is accurate?
   (A) Bithionol was prescribed
   (B) Extensive fluid replacement is essential
   (C) Symptoms are more intense in indigenous adults than expatriate adults
   (D) The reaction is due to drug toxicity
   (E) The reaction is due to killing of microfilariae

3. Which statement about pyrantel pamoate is accurate?
   (A) Acts as an antagonist at GABA receptors
   (B) Equivalent in efficacy to niclosamide in the treatment of tapeworm infections
   (C) Hepatotoxicity is dose-limiting
   (D) Kills adult worms in the colon but not the eggs
   (E) Synergistic with praziquantel in fluke infections

4. A student studying medicine at a Caribbean university develops fever, chills, and diarrhea resulting from *S mansoni,* and oxamniquine is prescribed. Which statement about the proposed drug therapy is accurate?
   (A) If the patient has a history of seizure disorders, hospitalization is recommended during treatment
   (B) It is not effective in the late stages of the disease
   (C) Oxamniquine is safe to use in pregnancy
   (D) The drug blocks GABA receptors in trematodes
   (E) The drug is also effective in tapeworm infections

5. A 22-year-old South Korean man has recently moved to Minnesota. He has symptoms of clonorchiasis (anorexia, upper abdominal pain, eosinophilia), presumably contracted in his homeland where the Oriental liver fluke is endemic. He also has symptoms of diphyllobothriasis (abdominal discomfort, diarrhea, megaloblastic anemia), probably caused by consumption of raw fish from lakes near the Canadian border. Which drug is most likely to be effective in the treatment of both clonorchiasis and diphyllobothriasis in this patient?
   (A) Ivermectin
   (B) Niclosamide
   (C) Praziquantel
   (D) Thiabendazole
   (E) Pyrantel pamoate

6. Which helminthic infection does not respond to treatment with praziquantel?
   (A) Hydatid disease
   (B) Opisthorchiasis
   (C) Paragonimiasis
   (D) Pork tapeworm infection
   (E) Schistosomiasis

7. Which drug causes muscle paralysis in nematodes by enhancing the actions of GABA?
   (A) Albendazole
   (B) Diethylcarbamazine
   (C) Ivermectin
   (D) Mebendazole
   (E) Pyrantel pamoate

8. Which parasite is susceptible to niclosamide?
   (A) *Ascaris lumbricoides*
   (B) *Echinococcus granulosus*
   (C) *Fasciola hepatica*
   (D) *Necator americanus*
   (E) *Taenia solium*

9. Which adverse effect occurs with the use of mebendazole during intestinal nematode therapy?
   (A) Cholestatic jaundice
   (B) Corneal opacities
   (C) Hirsutism
   (D) Peripheral neuropathy
   (E) None of the above

10. A malnourished 12-year-old child who lives in a rural area of the southern United States presents with weakness, fever, cough, abdominal pain, and eosinophilia. His mother tells you that she has seen long, thin worms in the child's stools, sometimes with blood. A presumptive diagnosis of ascariasis is confirmed by the presence of the ova of *A lumbricoides* in the stools. However, microscopy also reveals that the stools contain the eggs of *Necator americanus.* The drug most likely to be effective in the treatment of this child is
    (A) Albendazole
    (B) Diethylcarbamazine
    (C) Ivermectin
    (D) Niclosamide
    (E) Praziquantel

ANSWERS

1. Ivermectin prevents onchocerciasis and is the drug of choice in the individual and mass treatment of the disease. The only other drugs listed with any activity against *Onchocerca volvulus* are suramin and diethylcarbamazine. However, they are no longer recommended for onchocerciasis because they are less effective and more toxic than ivermectin. The answer is **C.**

2. The symptoms described are those of the so-called Mazzotti reaction. They are due to the killing action of ivermectin on microfilariae, and their intensity correlates with skin microfilaria load and is *not* a drug toxicity. The reaction occurs more frequently and with greater severity in nonindigenous persons than in the indigenous inhabitants of endemic areas. The answer is **E.**

3. Pyrantel pamoate, an activator of nicotinic receptors, is equivalent to albendazole and mebendazole in the treatment of common nematode infections. It acts on adult worms in the colon, but not on eggs. The drug causes only mild gastrointestinal side effects and is not hepatotoxic. It is not effective in the treatment of infections caused by cestodes or flukes. The answer is **D.**

4. Oxamniquine may cause seizures, especially in persons with a history of convulsive disorders. Such persons should be hospitalized or treated with praziquantel. Oxamniquine is effective in **all** stages of disease caused by *S mansoni,* including advanced hepatosplenomegaly, and it has been used extensively for mass treatment. The drug is not effective in other schistosomal diseases, and it is contraindicated in pregnancy. The answer is **A.**

5. Praziquantel is a primary drug for treatment of infections caused by the Oriental liver fluke and by the fish tapeworm. Both types of infection are transmitted mainly via the consumption of raw fish. Niclosamide is also a primary drug for fish tapeworm infections, but it is not active against *Clonorchis sinensis.* Albendazole is not effective in fish tapeworm infections, but it is useful in the pork tapeworm larval stage (cysticercosis). Pyrantel pamoate is not active against cestodes or trematodes. The answer is **C.**

6. In hydatid disease, praziquantel has marginal efficacy because it does not affect the inner germinal membrane of *Echinococcus granulosus* present in hydatid cysts. The answer is **A.**

7. Ivermectin and piperazine (not listed) both cause muscle paralysis in nematodes by acting through GABA receptors. Pyrantel pamoate relaxes muscles by blocking nicotinic receptors. Diethylcarbamazine also causes muscle relaxation, but the mechanism is unknown. The answer is **C**.

8. Niclosamide is not active against nematodes or flukes with the exception of the large intestinal fluke. It is considered a co-drug of choice (with praziquantel) to treat common tapeworm infections because it is usually effective in a single dose. The drug is minimally absorbed from the gastrointestinal tract and causes few side effects. The answer is **E**.

9. Doses of mebendazole required for intestinal nematode therapy are almost free of adverse effects even in the malnourished or debilitated patient. Gastrointestinal distress may occur in children with ascariasis who are heavily parasitized, together with a slight headache or dizziness. Avoid the drug in children under 2 yr of age because of rare reports of seizures. The answer is **E**.

10. Albendazole is effective against both nematodes causing infection in this child. Mebendazole and pyrantel pamoate (not listed in this question) are also primary drugs for the treatment of combined infections due to hookworm and roundworm. The answer is **A**.

SKILL KEEPER ANSWERS: ANTIMICROBIAL CHEMOTHERAPY IN PREGNANCY

1. *In the United States a drug is designated (by the FDA) as Pregnancy Risk Category **X** if the risk of its use in pregnancy is judged to be greater than any possible benefit. Such drugs have been established to cause fetal abnormalities or miscarriage in humans. This category includes the antiviral agent ribavirin and the antimalarial drug quinine. Clomiphene, ergots, ethionamide, HMG-CoA reductase inhibitors, isotretinoin, misoprostol, Premarin, and thalidomide are also category **X** drugs.*

2. *For drugs in FDA Pregnancy Risk Category **D**, there is evidence of human risk, but their potential benefit may outweigh such risk. In other words, they are not absolutely contraindicated in pregnancy. These include aminoglycosides (eg, gentamicin) and tetracyclines. Although they are not category **D** drugs, fluoroquinolones are not approved by the FDA for use in pregnancy, and many other drugs should be used with caution or avoided if alternatives are available.*

CHECKLIST

When you complete this chapter, you should be able to:

❑ List the clinical uses and the adverse effects of albendazole/mebendazole, diethylcarbamazepine, ivermectin, and pyrantel pamoate.

❑ Name the antihelminthic drug (or drugs) that (1) facilitate the actions of GABA, (2) increase calcium permeability in muscle, (3) activate nicotinic receptors, and (4) disruptmicrotubule function.

❑ Describe the clinical uses and adverse effects of both praziquantel and niclosamide.

Cancer Chemotherapy

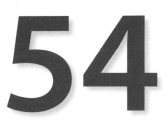

Cancer chemotherapy remains an intriguing area of pharmacology. On the one hand, use of anticancer drugs produces high rates of cure of diseases, which, without chemotherapy, result in extremely high mortality rates (eg, acute lymphocytic leukemia in children, testicular cancer, and Hodgkin's lymphoma). On the other hand, some types of cancer are barely affected by currently available drugs. Furthermore, as a group, the anticancer drugs are more toxic than any other pharmaceutic agents,

and thus their benefit must be carefully weighed against their risks. Many of the available drugs are cytotoxic agents that act on all dividing cells, cancerous or normal. The ultimate goal in cancer chemotherapy is to use advances in cell biology to develop drugs that selectively target specific cancer cells. A few such agents are in clinical use, and many more are in development.

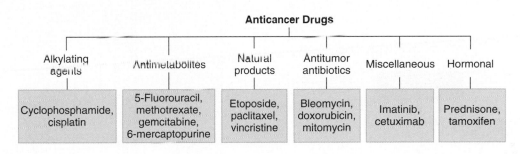

CANCER CELL CYCLE KINETICS

A. Cell Cycle Kinetics

Cancer cell population kinetics and the cancer cell cycle are important determinants of the actions and clinical uses of anticancer drugs. Some anticancer drugs exert their actions on cells undergoing cycling (cell cycle-specific [CCS] drugs), and others (cell cycle-nonspecific [CCNS] drugs) kill tumor cells in both cycling and resting phases of the cell cycle (although cycling cell are more sensitive). CCS drugs are usually most effective when cells are in a specific phase of the cell cycle (Figure 54–1). Both types of drugs are particularly effective when a large proportion of the tumor cells are proliferating (ie, when the growth fraction is high).

B. The Log-Kill Hypothesis

Cytotoxic drugs act with first-order kinetics in a murine model of leukemia. In this model system, in which all the cells are actively progressing through the cell cycle, a given dose kills a constant *proportion* of a cell population rather than a constant *number* of cells. The log-kill hypothesis proposes that the magnitude of tumor cell kill by anticancer drugs is a logarithmic function. For example, a 3-log-kill dose of an effective drug reduces a cancer cell population of 10^{12} cells to 10^9 (a total kill of 999×10^9 cells); the same dose would reduce a starting population of 10^6 cells to 10^3 cells (a kill of 999×10^3 cells). In both cases, the dose reduces the numbers of cells by 3 orders of magnitude, or "3 logs." A key principle that stems from this finding and that is applicable to hematologic

High-Yield Terms to Learn

Cell cycle-nonspecific (CCNS) drug	An anticancer agent that acts on tumor stem cells when they are traversing the cell cycle and when they are in the resting phase
Cell cycle-specific (CCS) drug	An anticancer agent that acts selectively on tumor stem cells when they are traversing the cell cycle and not when they are in the G_0 phase
Growth fraction	The proportion of cells in a tumor population that are actively dividing
Myelosuppressant	A drug that suppresses the formation of mature blood cells such as erythrocytes, leukocytes, and platelets. This effect is also known as "bone marrow suppression"
Oncogene	A mutant form of a normal gene that is found in naturally occurring tumors and which, when expressed in noncancerous cells, causes them to behave like cancer cells

malignancies is an inverse relationship between tumor cell number and curability (Figure 54–2). Mathematical modeling data suggest that most human solid tumors do not grow in such an exponential manner and rather that the growth fraction of the tumor decreases with time owing to blood supply limitations and other factors. In drug-sensitive solid tumors, the response to chemotherapy depends on where the tumor is in its growth curve.

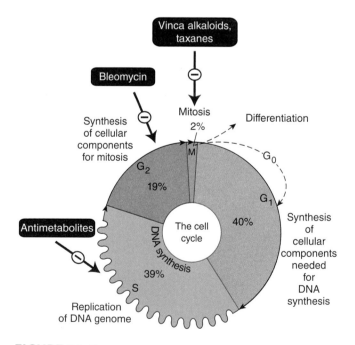

FIGURE 54–1 Phases of the cell cycle that are susceptible to the actions of cell cycle-specific (CCS) drugs. All dividing cells—normal and neoplastic—must traverse these cell cycle phases before and during cell division. Tumor cells are usually most responsive to specific drugs (or drug groups) in the phases indicated. Cell cycle-nonspecific (CCNS) drugs act on tumor cells while they are actively cycling and while they are in the resting phase (G_0). (Reproduced and modified, with permission, from Katzung BG, editor: *Basic & Clinical Pharmacology,* 12th ed. McGraw-Hill, 2012: Fig. 54–2.)

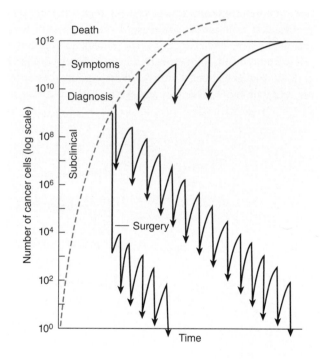

FIGURE 54–2 Relationship, based on the log-kill hypothesis, of tumor cell number to 3 approaches to drug treatment and to no treatment (*dashed line*). In the protocol diagrammed at the top, infrequent treatment (indicated by *arrows*) prolongs survival but with recurrence of symptoms between treatments and eventual death. With the regimen diagrammed in the middle section that is more intensive and begun earlier, cure results after many cycles of therapy. In the treatment diagrammed near the bottom of the graph, early surgery removes much of the tumor burden, and intensive adjuvant chemotherapy has been used long enough to produce a cure. (Reproduced with permission, from Katzung BG, editor: *Basic & Clinical Pharmacology,* 12th ed. McGraw-Hill, 2012: Fig. 54–1.)

C. Resistance to Anticancer Drugs

Drug resistance is a major problem in cancer chemotherapy. Mechanisms of resistance include the following:

1. Increased DNA repair—An increased rate of DNA repair in tumor cells can be responsible for resistance and is particularly important for alkylating agents and cisplatin.

2. Formation of trapping agents—Some tumor cells increase their production of thiol trapping agents (eg, glutathione), which interact with anticancer drugs that form reactive electrophilic species. This mechanism of resistance is seen with the alkylating agent bleomycin, cisplatin, and the anthracyclines.

3. Changes in target enzymes—Changes in the drug sensitivity of a target enzyme, dihydrofolate reductase, and increased synthesis of the enzyme are mechanisms of resistance of tumor cells to methotrexate.

4. Decreased activation of prodrugs—Resistance to the purine antimetabolites (mercaptopurine, thioguanine) and the pyrimidine antimetabolites (cytarabine, fluorouracil) can result from a decrease in the activity of the tumor cell enzymes needed to convert these prodrugs to their cytotoxic metabolites.

5. Inactivation of anticancer drugs—Increased activity of enzymes capable of inactivating anticancer drugs is a mechanism of tumor cell resistance to most of the purine and pyrimidine antimetabolites.

6. Decreased drug accumulation—This form of multidrug resistance involves the increased expression of a normal gene (*MDR1*) for a cell surface glycoprotein (P-glycoprotein). This transport molecule is involved in the accelerated efflux of many anticancer drugs in resistant cells.

STRATEGIES IN CANCER CHEMOTHERAPY

A. Cancer Treatment Modalities

Chemotherapy is used in three main clinical settings:

1. Primary induction chemotherapy—Drug therapy is administered as the primary treatment for many hematologic cancers and for advanced solid tumors for which no alternative treatment exists. Although primary induction can be curative in a small number of patients who present with advanced metastatic disease (eg, lymphoma, acute myelogenous leukemia, germ cell cancer, choriocarcinoma, and several childhood cancers), in many cases the goals of therapy are palliation of cancer symptoms, improved quality of life, and increased time to tumor progression.

2. Neoadjuvant chemotherapy—The use of chemotherapy in patients who present with localized cancer for which alternative local therapy, such as surgery, exist is known as neoadjuvant chemotherapy. The goal is to render the local therapy more effective.

3. Adjuvant chemotherapy—In the treatment of many solid tumors, chemotherapy serves as an important adjuvant to local treatment procedures such as surgery or radiation. The goal is to reduce the risk of local and systemic recurrence and to improve disease-free and overall survival.

B. Principles of Combination Therapy

Chemotherapy with combinations of anticancer drugs usually increases log-kill markedly, and in some cases synergistic effects are achieved. Combinations are often cytotoxic to a heterogeneous population of cancer cells and may prevent development of resistant clones. Drug combinations using CCS and CCNS drugs may be cytotoxic to both dividing and resting cancer cells. The following principles are important for selecting appropriate drugs to use in combination chemotherapy:

(1) Each drug should be active when used alone against the particular cancer.
(2) The drugs should have different mechanisms of action.
(3) Cross resistance between drugs should be minimal.
(4) The drugs should have different toxic effects (Table 54–1).

C. Rescue Therapy

Toxic effects of anticancer drugs can sometimes be alleviated by rescue strategy. For example, high doses of methotrexate may be given for 36–48 h to cells of the gastrointestinal tract and bone marrow and terminated before severe toxicity occurs. **Leucovorin,** a form of tetrahydrofolate that is accumulated more readily by normal than by neoplastic cells, is then administered. This results in rescue of the normal cells because leucovorin bypasses the dihydrofolate reductase step in folic acid synthesis.

Mercaptoethanesulfonate (**mesna**) "traps" acrolein released from cyclophosphamide and thus reduces the incidence of hemorrhagic cystitis. **Dexrazoxane** inhibits free radical formation and affords protection against the cardiac toxicity of anthracyclines (eg, doxorubicin).

ALKYLATING AGENTS

The alkylating agents include nitrogen mustards (**chlorambucil, cyclophosphamide, mechlorethamine**), nitrosoureas (**carmustine, lomustine**), and alkyl sulfonates (**busulfan**). Other drugs that act in part as alkylating agents include **cisplatin, dacarbazine,** and **procarbazine.**

The alkylating agents are CCNS drugs. They form reactive molecular species that alkylate nucleophilic groups on DNA bases, particularly the N-7 position of guanine. This leads to cross-linking of bases, abnormal base-pairing, and DNA strand breakage.

TABLE 54–1 Selected examples of cancer chemotherapy. (*Do not attempt to memorize type of treatment for each cancer. In this chapter focus on the drugs' mechanism of action, dose-limiting adverse effects and general mechanisms of resistance*).

Diagnosis	Examples of Commonly-Used Anticancer Drugs
Acute lymphocytic leukemia in children	Prednisone, vincristine, and asparaginase or an anthracycline, plus intrathecal methotrexate
Acute myelogenous leukemia in adults	Cytarabine and idarubicin or daunorubicin
Breast carcinoma	Cytotoxic agents, hormonal therapy with tamoxifen or an aromatase inhibitor (eg, anastrozole), trastuzumab
Chronic myelogenous leukemia	Imatinib, newer tyrosine kinase inhibitors, interferon
Colon carcinoma	Fluorouracil plus leucovorin plus oxaliplatin
Hodgkin's lymphoma	ABVD regimen: doxorubicin (Adriamycin), bleomycin, vincristine, dacarbazine, and prednisone
Non-Hodgkin's lymphoma	CHOP regimen (cyclophosphamide, doxorubicin, vincristine, and prednisone) plus rituximab
Ovarian carcinoma	Paclitaxel and carboplatin
Pancreatic carcinoma	Gemcitabine and erlotinib
Prostate carcinoma	GnRH agonist (eg, leuprolide) or antagonist (eg, abarelix) and androgen receptor antagonist
Lung carcinoma	Carboplatin, paclitaxel, and bevacizumab
Testicular carcinoma	PEB regimen: cisplatin (Platinol), etoposide, and bleomycin

GnRH, gonadotropin-releasing hormone.

Tumor cell resistance to the drugs occurs through increased DNA repair, decreased drug permeability, and the production of trapping agents such as thiols.

A. Cyclophosphamide

1. Pharmacokinetics—Hepatic cytochrome P450-mediated biotransformation of cyclophosphamide is needed for antitumor activity. One of the breakdown products is **acrolein**.

2. Clinical use—Uses of cyclophosphamide include leukemia, non-Hodgkin's lymphoma, breast and ovarian cancers, and neuroblastoma.

3. Toxicity—Gastrointestinal distress, myelosuppression, and alopecia are expected adverse effects of cyclophosphamide. Hemorrhagic cystitis resulting from the formation of acrolein may be decreased by vigorous hydration and by use of mercaptoethanesulfonate (mesna). Cyclophosphamide may also cause cardiac dysfunction, pulmonary toxicity, and a syndrome of inappropriate antidiuretic hormone (ADH) secretion.

B. Mechlorethamine

1. Mechanism and pharmacokinetics—Mechlorethamine spontaneously converts in the body to a reactive cytotoxic product.

2. Clinical use—Mechlorethamine is best known for use in regimens for Hodgkin's and non-Hodgkin's lymphoma.

3. Toxicity—Gastrointestinal distress, myelosuppression, alopecia, and sterility are common. Mechlorethamine has marked vesicant actions.

C. Platinum Analogs (Cisplatin, Carboplatin, Oxaliplatin)

1. Pharmacokinetics—Cisplatin is used intravenously; the drug distributes to most tissues and is cleared in unchanged form by the kidney.

2. Clinical use—Cisplatin is commonly used as a component of regimens for testicular carcinoma and for cancers of the bladder, lung, and ovary. Carboplatin has similar uses. Oxaliplatin is used in advanced colon cancer.

3. Toxicity—Cisplatin causes gastrointestinal distress and mild hematotoxicity and is neurotoxic (peripheral neuritis and acoustic nerve damage) and nephrotoxic. Renal damage may be reduced by the use of mannitol with forced hydration. Carboplatin is less nephrotoxic than cisplatin and is less likely to cause tinnitus and hearing loss, but it has greater myelosuppressant actions. Oxaliplatin causes dose-limiting neurotoxicity.

D. Procarbazine

1. Mechanisms—Procarbazine is a reactive agent that forms hydrogen peroxide, which generates free radicals that cause DNA strand scission.

2. Pharmacokinetics—Procarbazine is orally active and penetrates into most tissues, including the cerebrospinal fluid. It is eliminated via hepatic metabolism.

3. Clinical use—The primary use of the drug is as a component of regimens for Hodgkin's and non-Hodgkin's lymphoma, and brain tumors.

4. Toxicity—Procarbazine is a myelosuppressant and causes gastrointestinal irritation, CNS dysfunction, peripheral neuropathy, and skin reactions. Procarbazine inhibits many enzymes, including monoamine oxidase and those involved in hepatic drug metabolism. Disulfiram-like reactions have occurred with ethanol. The drug is leukemogenic.

E. Other Alkylating Agents

Busulfan is sometimes used in chronic myelogenous leukemia. It causes adrenal insufficiency, pulmonary fibrosis, and skin pigmentation. **Carmustine** and **lomustine** are highly lipid-soluble drugs used as adjuncts in the management of brain tumors. **Dacarbazine** is used in regimens for Hodgkin's lymphoma. It causes alopecia, skin rash, gastrointestinal distress, myelosuppression, phototoxicity, and a flu-like syndrome.

ANTIMETABOLITES

The antimetabolites are structurally similar to endogenous compounds and are antagonists of folic acid (**methotrexate**), purines (**mercaptopurine, thioguanine**), or pyrimidines (**fluorouracil, cytarabine, gemcitabine**). Antimetabolites are CCS drugs acting primarily in the S phase of the cell cycle. In addition to their cytotoxic effects on neoplastic cells, the antimetabolites also have immunosuppressant actions (see Chapters 36, 54, and 55).

A. Methotrexate

1. Mechanisms of action and resistance—Methotrexate is an inhibitor of dihydrofolate reductase. This action leads to a decrease in the synthesis of thymidylate, purine nucleotides, and amino acids and thus interferes with nucleic acid and protein metabolism (see Figure 33–2 for folate-dependent enzymatic reactions). The formation of polyglutamate derivatives of methotrexate appears to be important for cytotoxic actions. Tumor cell resistance mechanisms include decreased drug accumulation, changes in the drug sensitivity or activity of dihydrofolate reductase, and decreased formation of polyglutamates.

2. Pharmacokinetics—Oral and intravenous administration of methotrexate affords good tissue distribution except to the CNS. Methotrexate is not metabolized, and its clearance is dependent on renal function. Adequate hydration is needed to prevent crystallization in renal tubules.

3. Clinical use—Methotrexate is effective in choriocarcinoma, acute leukemias, non-Hodgkin's and primary central nervous

system lymphomas, and a number of solid tumors, including breast cancer, head and neck cancer, and bladder cancer. Methotrexate is used also in rheumatoid arthritis psoriasis (Chapter 36) and ectopic pregnancy.

4. Toxicity—Common adverse effects of methotrexate include bone marrow suppression and toxic effects on the skin and gastrointestinal mucosa (mucositis). The toxic effects of methotrexate on normal cells may be reduced by administration of folinic acid (leucovorin); this strategy is called **leucovorin rescue**. Long-term use of methotrexate has led to hepatotoxicity and to pulmonary infiltrates and fibrosis.

B. Mercaptopurine (6-MP) and Thioguanine (6-TG)

1. Mechanisms of action and resistance—Mercaptopurine and thioguanine are purine antimetabolites. Both drugs are activated by hypoxanthine-guanine phosphoribosyltransferases (HGPRTases) to toxic nucleotides that inhibit several enzymes involved in purine metabolism. Resistant tumor cells have a decreased activity of HGPRTase, or they may increase their production of alkaline phosphatases that inactivate the toxic nucleotides.

2. Pharmacokinetics—Mercaptopurine and thioguanine have low oral bioavailability because of first-pass metabolism by hepatic enzymes. The metabolism of 6-MP by xanthine oxidase is inhibited by the xanthine oxidase inhibitors allopurinol and febuxostat.

3. Clinical use—Purine antimetabolites are used mainly in the acute leukemias and chronic myelocytic leukemia.

4. Toxicity—Bone marrow suppression is dose limiting, but hepatic dysfunction (cholestasis, jaundice, necrosis) also occurs.

C. Fluorouracil (5-FU)

1. Mechanisms—Fluorouracil is converted in cells to 5-fluoro-2′-deoxyuridine-5′-monophosphate (5-FdUMP), which inhibits thymidylate synthase and leads to "thymineless death" of cells. Incorporation of FdUMP into DNA inhibits DNA synthesis and function while incorporation of 5-fluorouridine-5′-triphosphate (FUTP), another 5-FU metabolite, into RNA interferes with RNA processing and function. Tumor cell resistance mechanisms include decreased activation of 5-FU, increased thymidylate synthase activity, and reduced drug sensitivity of this enzyme.

2. Pharmacokinetics—When given intravenously, fluorouracil is widely distributed, including into the cerebrospinal fluid. Elimination is mainly by metabolism.

3. Clinical use—Fluorouracil is used in bladder, breast, colon, anal, head and neck, liver, and ovarian cancers. The drug can be used topically for keratoses and superficial basal cell carcinoma.

4. Toxicity—Gastrointestinal distress, myelosuppression, and alopecia are common.

D. Cytarabine (ARA-C)

1. Mechanisms of action and resistance—Cytarabine (cytosine arabinoside) is a pyrimidine antimetabolite. The drug is activated by kinases to AraCTP, an inhibitor of DNA polymerases. Of all the antimetabolites, cytarabine is the most specific for the S phase of the cell cycle. Resistance to cytarabine can occur as a result of its decreased uptake or its decreased conversion to AraCTP.

E. Gemcitabine

1. Mechanisms—Gemcitabine is a deoxycytidine analog that is converted into the active diphosphate and triphosphate nucleotide form. Gemcitabine diphosphate appears to inhibit ribonucleotide reductase and thereby diminish the pool of deoxyribonucleoside triphosphates required for DNA synthesis. Gemcitabine triphosphate can be incorporated into DNA, where it causes chain termination.

2. Pharmacokinetics—Elimination is mainly by metabolism.

3. Clinical use—Gemcitabine was initially approved for pancreatic cancer and now is used widely in the treatment of non-small cell lung cancer, bladder cancer, and non-Hodgkin's lymphoma.

4. Toxicity—Primarily myelosuppression occurs, mainly as neutropenia. Pulmonary toxicity has been observed.

NATURAL PRODUCT ANTICANCER DRUGS

The most important of these plant-derived, CCS drugs are the vinca alkaloids (**vinblastine, vincristine, vinorelbine**), the podophyllotoxins (**etoposide, teniposide**), the camptothecins (**topotecan, irinotecan**), the taxanes (**paclitaxel, docetaxel**).

A. Vinblastine, Vincristine, and Vinorelbine

1. Mechanisms—The **vinca alkaloids** block the formation of the mitotic spindle by preventing the assembly of tubulin dimers into microtubules. They act primarily in the M phase of the cancer cell cycle. Resistance can occur from increased efflux of the drugs from tumor cells via the membrane drug transporter.

2. Pharmacokinetics—These drugs must be given parenterally. They penetrate most tissues except the cerebrospinal fluid. They are cleared mainly via biliary excretion.

3. Clinical use—Vincristine is used in acute leukemias, lymphomas, Wilms' tumor, and neuroblastoma. **Vinblastine** is used for lymphomas, neuroblastoma, testicular carcinoma, and Kaposi's sarcoma. **Vinorelbine** is used in non-small cell lung cancer and breast cancer.

4. Toxicity—Vinblastine and vinorelbine cause gastrointestinal distress, alopecia, and bone marrow suppression. Vincristine does not cause serious myelosuppression but has neurotoxic actions and may cause areflexia, peripheral neuritis, and paralytic ileus.

B. Etoposide and Teniposide

1. Mechanisms—**Etoposide,** a semisynthetic derivative of podophyllotoxin, induces DNA breakage through its inhibition of topoisomerase II. The drug is most active in the late S and early G_2 phases of the cell cycle. **Teniposide** is an analog with very similar pharmacologic characteristics.

2. Pharmacokinetics—Etoposide is well absorbed after oral administration and distributes to most body tissues. Elimination of etoposide is mainly via the kidneys, and dose reductions should be made in patients with renal impairment.

3. Clinical use—These agents are used in combination drug regimens for therapy of lymphoma, and lung, germ cell, and gastric cancers.

4. Toxicity—Etoposide and teniposide are gastrointestinal irritants and cause alopecia and bone marrow suppression.

C. Topotecan and Irinotecan

1. Mechanisms—The 2 camptothecins, **topotecan** and **irinotecan**, produce DNA damage by inhibiting topoisomerase I. They damage DNA by inhibiting an enzyme that cuts and relegates single DNA strands during normal DNA repair processes.

2. Pharmacokinetics—Irinotecan is a prodrug that is converted in the liver into an active metabolite. Topotecan is eliminated renally, whereas irinotecan and its metabolite are eliminated in the bile and feces.

3. Clinical use—Topotecan is used as second-line therapy for advanced ovarian cancer and for small cell lung cancer. Irinotecan is used for metastatic colorectal cancer.

4. Toxicity—Myelosuppression and diarrhea are the 2 most common toxicities.

D. Paclitaxel and Docetaxel

1. Mechanisms—Paclitaxel and docetaxel interfere with the mitotic spindle. They act differently from vinca alkaloids, since they prevent microtubule *disassembly* into tubulin monomers.

2. Pharmacokinetics—Paclitaxel and docetaxel are given intravenously.

3. Clinical use—The taxanes have activity in a number of solid tumors, including breast, ovarian, lung, gastroesophageal, prostate, bladder, and head and neck cancers.

4. Toxicity—Paclitaxel causes neutropenia, thrombocytopenia, a high incidence of peripheral neuropathy, and possible hypersensitivity reactions during infusion. Docetaxel causes neurotoxicity and bone marrow depression.

ANTITUMOR ANTIBIOTICS

This category of antineoplastic drugs is made up of several structurally dissimilar microbial products and includes the **anthracyclines**, **bleomycin**, and **mitomycin**.

A. Anthracyclines

1. Mechanisms—The anthracyclines (**doxorubicin, daunorubicin, idarubicin, epirubicin, mitoxantrone**) intercalate between base pairs, inhibit topoisomerase II, and generate free radicals. They block the synthesis of RNA and DNA and cause DNA strand scission. Membrane disruption also occurs. Anthracyclines are CCNS drugs.

2. Pharmacokinetics—Doxorubicin and daunorubicin must be given intravenously. They are metabolized in the liver, and the products are excreted in the bile and the urine.

3. Clinical use—Doxorubicin is used in Hodgkin's and non-Hodgkin's lymphoma, myelomas, sarcomas, and breast, lung, ovarian, and thyroid cancers. The main use of daunorubicin is in the treatment of acute leukemias. Idarubicin, a newer anthracycline, is approved for use in acute myelogenous leukemia. Epirubicin is used in breast cancer and gastroesophageal cancer. Mitoxantrone is used in acute myeloid leukemias, non-Hodgkin's lymphoma, breast cancer, and gastroesophageal cancer.

4. Toxicity—These drugs cause bone marrow suppression, gastrointestinal distress, and severe alopecia. Their most distinctive adverse effect is cardiotoxicity, which includes initial electrocardiographic abnormalities (with the possibility of arrhythmias) and slowly developing, dose-dependent cardiomyopathy and congestive heart failure. **Dexrazoxane**, an inhibitor of iron-mediated free radical generation, may protect against the dose-dependent form of cardiotoxicity. Liposomal formulations of doxorubicin may be less cardiotoxic.

B. Bleomycin

1. Mechanisms—Bleomycin is a mixture of glycopeptides that generates free radicals, which bind to DNA, cause strand breaks, and inhibit DNA synthesis. Bleomycin is a CCS drug active in the G_2 phase of the tumor cell cycle.

2. Pharmacokinetics—Bleomycin must be given parenterally. It is inactivated by tissue aminopeptidases, but some renal clearance of intact drug also occurs.

3. Clinical use—Bleomycin is a component of drug regimens for Hodgkin's lymphoma and testicular cancer. It is also used for treatment of lymphomas and for squamous cell carcinomas.

4. Toxicity—The toxicity profile of bleomycin includes pulmonary dysfunction (pneumonitis, fibrosis), which develops slowly and is dose limiting. Hypersensitivity reactions (chills, fever, anaphylaxis) are common, as are mucocutaneous reactions (alopecia, blister formation, hyperkeratosis).

C. Mitomycin

1. Mechanisms and pharmacokinetics—Mitomycin is a CCNS drug that is metabolized by liver enzymes to form an alkylating agent that cross-links DNA. Mitomycin is given intravenously and is rapidly cleared via hepatic metabolism.

2. Clinical use—Mitomycin acts against hypoxic tumor cells and is used in combination regimens for adenocarcinomas of the cervix, stomach, pancreas, and lung.

3. Toxicity—Mitomycin causes severe myelosuppression and is toxic to the heart, liver, lung, and kidney.

MISCELLANEOUS ANTICANCER AGENTS

A. Tyrosine Kinase Inhibitors

Imatinib is an example of a selective anticancer drug whose development was guided by knowledge of a specific oncogene. It inhibits the tyrosine kinase activity of the protein product of the *bcr-abl* oncogene that is commonly expressed in chronic myelogenous leukemia (CML). In addition to its activity in CML, imatinib is effective for treatment of gastrointestinal stromal tumors that express the *c-kit* tyrosine kinase, which is also inhibited. Resistance may occur from mutation of the *bcr-abl* gene. Toxicity of imatinib includes diarrhea, myalgia, fluid retention, and congestive heart failure. **Dasatinib** and **nilotinib** are newer anticancer kinase inhibitors.

B. Growth Factor Receptor Inhibitors

Trastuzumab, a monoclonal antibody, recognizes a surface protein in breast cancer cells that overexpress the HER-2/*neu* receptor for epidermal growth factor. Acute toxicity of this antibody includes nausea and vomiting, chills, fevers, and headache. Trastuzumab may cause cardiac dysfunction, including congestive heart failure.

Several drugs inhibit the epidermal growth factor receptor (EGFR), which is distinct from the HER-2/*neu* receptor for epidermal growth factor that is targeted by trastuzumab. The EGFR regulates signaling pathways involved in cellular proliferation, invasion and metastasis, and angiogenesis. It is also implicated in inhibiting the cytotoxic activity of some anticancer drugs and radiation therapy. **Cetuximab** is a chimeric monoclonal antibody directed to the extracellular domain of the EGFR. It is used in combination with irinotecan and oxaliplatin for metastatic colon cancer and is used in combination with radiation for head and neck cancer. Its primary toxicity is skin rash and a hypersensitivity infusion reaction. **Panitumumab** is a fully human antibody directed against the EGFR; it is approved for refractory metastatic colorectal cancer. **Gefitinib** and **erlotinib** are small molecule inhibitors of the EGFR's tyrosine kinase domain. Both are used as second-line agents for non-small cell lung cancer, and erlotinib is also used in combination therapy of advanced pancreatic cancer. Rash and diarrhea are the main toxicities.

Bevacizumab is a monoclonal antibody that binds to **vascular endothelial growth factor** (**VEGF**) and prevents it from interacting with VEGF receptors. VEGF plays a critical role in the angiogenesis required for tumor metastasis. Bevacizumab has activity in colorectal, breast, non-small cell lung, and renal cancer. Adverse effects include hypertension, infusion reactions, arterial thrombosis, impaired wound healing, gastrointestinal perforation, and proteinuria.

Sorafenib, sunitinib, and **pazopanib** are small molecules that inhibit multiple receptor tyrosine kinases (RTKs), including those associated with the VEGF receptor family. They are metabolized by CYP3A4, and elimination is primarily hepatic. Hypertension, bleeding complications, and fatigue are the most common adverse effects.

C. Rituximab

Rituximab is a monoclonal antibody that binds to a surface protein in non-Hodgkin's lymphoma cells and induces complement-mediated lysis, direct cytotoxicity, and induction of apoptosis. It is currently used with conventional anticancer drugs (eg, cyclophosphamide plus vincristine plus prednisone) in low-grade lymphomas. Rituximab is associated with hypersensitivity reactions and myelosuppression.

D. Interferons

The interferons are endogenous glycoproteins with antineoplastic, immunosuppressive, and antiviral actions. Alpha-interferons (see Chapter 55) are effective against a number of neoplasms, including hairy cell leukemia, the early stage of chronic myelogenous leukemia, and T-cell lymphomas. Toxic effects of the interferons include myelosuppression and neurologic dysfunction.

E. Asparaginase

Asparaginase is an enzyme that depletes serum asparagine; it is used in the treatment of T-cell auxotrophic cancers (leukemia and lymphomas) that require exogenous asparagine for growth.

Asparaginase is given intravenously and may cause severe hypersensitivity reactions, acute pancreatitis, and bleeding.

F. Proteasome Inhibitors

Bortezomib is a reversible inhibitor of the chymotrypsin-like activity of the 26S proteasome in mammalian cells. The 26S proteasome is a large protein complex that degrades ubiquitinated proteins, such as cyclin-dependent kinases. Adverse effects include peripheral neuropathy, thrombocytopenia, and hypotension. It is currently used for the treatment of multiple myeloma.

> ### SKILL KEEPER: MANAGEMENT OF ANTICANCER DRUG HEMATOTOXICITY (SEE CHAPTER 33)
>
> *Bone marrow suppression is a characteristic toxicity of most cytotoxic anticancer drugs. What agents are available for the treatment of anemia and neutropenia, and for platelet restoration in patients undergoing cancer chemotherapy?*
>
> The Skill Keeper Answer appears at the end of the chapter.

HORMONAL ANTICANCER AGENTS

A. Glucocorticoids

Prednisone is the most commonly used glucocorticoid in cancer chemotherapy and is widely used in combination therapy for leukemias and lymphomas. Toxicity is described in Chapter 39.

B. Gonadal Hormone Antagonists

Tamoxifen, a selective estrogen receptor modulator (see Chapter 40), blocks the binding of estrogen to receptors of estrogen-sensitive cancer cells in breast tissue. The drug is used in receptor-positive breast carcinoma and has been shown to have a preventive effect in women at high risk for breast cancer. Because it has agonist activity in the endometrium, tamoxifen increases the risk of endometrial hyperplasia and neoplasia. Other adverse effects include nausea and vomiting, hot flushes, vaginal bleeding, and venous thrombosis. **Toremifene** is a newer estrogen receptor antagonist used in advanced breast cancer. **Flutamide** is an androgen receptor antagonist used in prostatic carcinoma (see Chapter 40). Adverse effects include gynecomastia, hot flushes, and hepatic dysfunction.

C. Gonadotropin-Releasing Hormone (GnRH) Analogs

Leuprolide, goserelin, and **nafarelin** are GnRH agonists, effective in prostatic carcinoma. When administered in constant doses so as to maintain stable blood levels, they *inhibit* release of pituitary luteinizing hormone (LH) and follicle-stimulating hormone (FSH). Leuprolide may cause bone pain, gynecomastia, hematuria, impotence, and testicular atrophy (see Chapters 37 and 40).

D. Aromatase Inhibitors

Anastrozole and letrozole inhibit aromatase, the enzyme that catalyzes the conversion of androstenedione (an androgenic precursor) to estrone (an estrogenic hormone). Both drugs are used in advanced breast cancer. Toxicity includes nausea, diarrhea, hot flushes, bone and back pain, dyspnea, and peripheral edema.

QUESTIONS

Questions 1–3. A 32-year-old woman underwent segmental mastectomy for a breast tumor of 3 cm diameter. Lymph node sampling revealed 2 involved nodes. Because chemotherapy is of established value in her situation, she underwent postoperative treatment with antineoplastic drugs. The regimen consisted of doxorubicin followed by cyclophosphamide/methotrexate/fluorouracil. Adjunctive drugs included tamoxifen because the tumor cells were hormone receptor-positive.

1. Which of the following best describes the mechanism of anti-cancer action of cellular metabolites of fluorouracil?
   (A) Cross-linking of double-stranded DNA
   (B) Inhibition of DNA-dependent RNA synthesis
   (C) Interference with the activity of topoisomerases I
   (D) Irreversible inhibition of thymidylate synthase
   (E) Selective inhibition of DNA polymerases

2. The chemotherapy undertaken by this patient caused acute hemorrhagic cystitis. Which drug was most likely to be responsible for this toxicity?
   (A) Cyclophosphamide
   (B) Doxorubicin
   (C) Fluorouracil
   (D) Methotrexate
   (E) Tamoxifen

3. After several cycles of chemotherapy, the patient was found to have a high resting pulse rate. A noninvasive radionuclide scan revealed evidence of cardiomyopathy. The drug that is most likely responsible for the cardiac toxicity is
   (A) Cyclophosphamide
   (B) Doxorubicin
   (C) Fluorouracil
   (D) Methotrexate
   (E) Tamoxifen

4. Which of the following is a cell cycle-specific anticancer drug that acts mainly in the M phase of the cell cycle?
   (A) Bleomycin
   (B) Cisplatin
   (C) Etoposide
   (D) Methotrexate
   (E) Paclitaxel

5. An adult patient is being treated for acute leukemia with a combination of anticancer drugs that includes cyclophosphamide, mercaptopurine, methotrexate, vincristine, and prednisone. He is also using ondansetron for emesis, a chlorhexidine mouthwash to reduce mucositis, and laxatives. The patient complains of "pins and needle" sensations in the extremities and muscle weakness. He is not able to execute a deep knee bend or get up out of a chair without using his arm muscles. He is also very constipated. If these problems are related to the chemotherapy, which of the following is the most likely causative agent?
   (A) Cyclophosphamide
   (B) Mercaptopurine
   (C) Methotrexate
   (D) Prednisone
   (E) Vincristine

6. Which of the following is a drug that is used in combination therapy for testicular carcinoma and is also associated with nephrotoxicity?
   (A) Bleomycin
   (B) Cisplatin
   (C) Etoposide
   (D) Leuprolide
   (E) Vinblastine

7. A cancer cell that is resistant to the effects of both vincristine and methotrexate probably has developed the resistance as a result of which of the following mechanisms?
   (A) Changes in the properties of a target enzyme
   (B) Decreased activity of an activating enzyme
   (C) Increased expression of a P-glycoprotein transporter
   (D) Increased production of drug-trapping molecules
   (E) Increase in proteins that are involved in DNA repair

Questions 8 and 9. A 23-year-old man with Hodgkin's lymphoma was treated unsuccessfully with the MOPP regimen (mechlorethamine, vincristine, prednisone, procarbazine). He subsequently underwent a successful course of therapy with the ABVD regimen (doxorubicin, bleomycin, vinblastine, dacarbazine).

8. Which of the following classes of anticancer drugs used in the treatment of this patient is cell cycle specific (CCS) and used in both the MOPP and ABVD regimens?
   (A) Alkylating agents
   (B) Antibiotics
   (C) Antimetabolites
   (D) Glucocorticoids
   (E) Plant alkaloids

9. During the second course of drug treatment (ABVD regimen), this patient developed dyspnea, a nonproductive cough, and intermittent fever. Chest x-ray film revealed pulmonary infiltration. If these problems are due to the anticancer drugs to which he has been exposed, which of the following is the most likely causative agent?
   (A) Bleomycin
   (B) Dacarbazine
   (C) Doxorubicin
   (D) Prednisone
   (E) Vinblastine

10. All the following agents have been used in drug regimens for the treatment of breast carcinoma. Which one has specific activity in a subset of female breast cancers?
(A) Cyclophosphamide
(B) Doxorubicin
(C) Fluoxymesterone
(D) Methotrexate
(E) Trastuzumab

DIRECTIONS: 11–13. For each numbered item, select the ONE lettered option from the following list that is most closely associated with it. Each lettered option may be selected once, more than once, or not at all.
(A) Bleomycin
(B) Cytarabine
(C) Dacarbazine
(D) Doxorubicin
(E) Etoposide
(F) Flutamide
(G) Fluorouracil
(H) Leuprolide
(I) Mechlorethamine
(J) Mercaptopurine
(K) Methotrexate
(L) Paclitaxel
(M) Procarbazine
(N) Tamoxifen
(O) Vincristine

11. If allopurinol is used adjunctively in cancer chemotherapy to offset hyperuricemia, the dosage of this anticancer drug should be reduced to 25% of normal.

12. This drug is used in combination therapy for testicular carcinoma. It is a CCS drug that acts in the late S and early G_0 phases of the tumor cell cycle via interactions with topoisomerase II.

13. This antimetabolite inhibits DNA polymerase and is one of the most active drugs in leukemias. Although myelosuppression is dose limiting, the drug may also cause cerebellar dysfunction, including ataxia and dysarthria.

ANSWERS

1. Fluorouracil (5-FU) undergoes metabolism to form 5-fluoro-2′-deoxyuridine 5′-phosphate (5-dUMP). This metabolite forms a covalently bound ternary complex with thymidylate synthase and its coenzyme *N*-methylenetetrahydrofolate. The synthesis of thymine nucleotides is blocked, DNA synthesis is inhibited, and a "thymineless death" of cells results. The answer is **D.**

2. Acrolein, a toxic metabolite of cyclophosphamide that is concentrated in the urine, is associated with hemorrhagic cystitis. Mesna, a sulfur-containing substance that also concentrates in urine, can be administered in an attempt to prevent this complication. The answer is **A.**

3. A high resting pulse rate is one of the first signs of cardiotoxicity resulting from anthracyclines, which can include arrhythmias, cardiomyopathies, and congestive heart failure. The risk of cardiotoxicity depends on cumulative dosage, so doxorubicin should be discontinued. The answer is **B.**

4. The taxanes, paclitaxel and docetaxel, interfere with the separation of chromosomes during mitosis because of their effects on microtubules. The answer is **E.**

5. Neuropathy is a toxic side effect of vincristine. In its mildest form, paresthesias occur, but it progresses to significant muscle weakness, initially in the quadriceps muscle group. Constipation is the most common symptom of autonomic neuropathy. The answer is **E.**

6. Nephrotoxicity is a characteristic toxicity of cisplatin. Renal toxicity can be reduced by slow intravenous infusion, maintenance of good hydration, and administration of mannitol to maximize urine flow. For testicular cancer, cisplatin is used in combination with etoposide and bleomycin. The answer is **B.**

7. The P-glycoprotein family of transporters moves foreign molecules out of cells. Cancer cells acquire resistance to multiple drugs that act through different mechanisms by increasing the expressions of genes encoding these transporters. The answer is **C.**

8. The cell cycle-specific drugs used in standard treatment protocols for Hodgkin's lymphoma are bleomycin and the vinca alkaloids. Vinblastine is used in the ABVD regimen, and vincristine (Oncovin) is used in the MOPP regimen. The answer is **E.**

9. The anticancer drug most commonly associated with pulmonary toxicity is bleomycin. The answer is **A.**

10. Each of the drugs listed has been used in drug regimens for breast cancer, but only trastuzumab has specificity in its actions. The drug is a monoclonal antibody to a surface protein in breast cancer cells that overexpress the HER-2 protein. Consequently, trastuzumab has value in a specific subset of breast cancers. The answer is **E.**

11. Allopurinol, a xanthine oxidase inhibitor, is given to control the hyperuricemia that occurs as a result of large cell kills in the successful drug therapy of malignant diseases. The antimetabolite mercaptopurine is metabolized by xanthine oxidase and, in the presence of an inhibitor of this enzyme (eg, allopurinol), toxic levels of the drug may be reached rapidly. The answer is **J.**

12. Bleomycin, etoposide, and vinblastine are all CCS drugs used for the treatment of testicular carcinoma. Bleomycin is an antibiotic, not a plant alkaloid. Vinblastine is a mitotic spindle poison that acts in the M phase of the cell cycle. The answer is **E.**

13. The pyrimidine antimetabolite cytarabine (Ara-C) is commonly used in drug regimens for the acute leukemias. Cytarabine is dose-limited by hematotoxicity. Cerebellar dysfunction may also occur with Ara-C, especially if the drug is used at high doses. The answer is **B.**

SKILL KEEPER ANSWER: MANAGEMENT OF ANTICANCER DRUG HEMATOTOXICITY (SEE CHAPTER 33)

Recombinant DNA technology has provided several agents that have value in the management of hematotoxicity caused by anticancer drugs. Erythropoietin stimulates red cell formation by interaction with receptors on erythroid progenitors in bone marrow. Myeloid growth factors filgrastim (G-CSF) and sargramostim (GM-CSF) stimulate the production and function of neutrophils. Megakaryocyte growth factor oprelvekin (IL-11) stimulates the growth of platelet progenitors.

CHECKLIST

When you complete this chapter, you should be able to:

❑ Name 3 anticancer drugs that are cell cycle-specific and act at different phases of the cell cycle.

❑ Describe the relevance of cell cycle kinetics to the modes of action and clinical uses of anticancer drugs.

❑ List the mechanisms by which tumor cells develop drug resistance.

❑ Describe the rationale underlying strategies of combination drug chemotherapy and rescue therapies.

❑ Identify the major subclasses of anticancer drugs and describe the mechanisms of action of the main drugs in each subclass.

❑ Identify a distinctive "characteristic" dose-limiting toxicity for each of the following anticancer drugs: bleomycin, cisplatin, cyclophosphamide, doxorubicin, and vincristine.

DRUG SUMMARY TABLE: Cancer Chemotherapy Drugs

Subclass	Mechanism of Action	Clinical Applications	Acute Toxicities	Chronic Toxicities
Alkylating agents				
Cyclophosphamide	Forms DNA cross-links, resulting in inhibition of DNA synthesis and function	Breast cancer, ovarian cancer, non-Hodgkin's lymphoma, chronic lymphocytic leukemia, neuroblastoma	Nausea and vomiting	Myelosuppression, alopecia, hemorrhagic cystitis
Other major alkylating agents: Mechlorethamine, procarbazine, busulfan carmustine, lomustine, dacarbazine				
Platinum analogs: Cisplatin, carboplatin, oxaliplatin				
Antimetabolites				
Methotrexate	Inhibits DHFR, resulting in inhibition of synthesis of thymidylate, purine nucleotides, serine, and methionine	Breast cancer, head and neck cancer, primary CNS lymphoma, non-Hodgkin's lymphoma, bladder cancer, chorio-carcinoma	Mucositis, diarrhea	Myelosuppression
6-Mercaptopurine	Inhibits de novo purine synthesis	Acute myelogenous leukemia	Nausea and vomiting	Myelosuppression, immunosuppression, hepatotoxicity
5-Fluorouracil	Inhibits thymidylate synthase, and its metabolites are incorporated into RNA and DNA, all resulting in inhibition of DNA synthesis and function and in RNA processing	GI cancers, breast cancer, head and neck cancer, hepatocellular cancer	Nausea, mucositis, diarrhea	Myelosuppression, neurotoxicity
Other antimetabolites: Cytarabine, gemcitabine				
Vinca alkaloids				
Vincristine	Interferes with microtubule function, resulting in impaired mitosis	Acute lymphocytic leukemia, Hodgkin's and non-Hodgkin's lymphoma, Wilms' tumor, neuroblastoma	None	Neurotoxicity with peripheral neuropathy, paralytic ileus, myelosuppression, alopecia, inappropriate ADH secretion
Other vinca alkaloids: Vinblastine, vinorelbine				
Podophyllotoxins				
Etoposide	Inhibits topoisomerase II, resulting in DNA damage	Lung cancer, non-Hodgkin's lymphoma, gastric cancer	Nausea, vomiting	Alopecia, myelosuppression
Other podophyllotoxins: Teniposide				
Camptothecins				
Topotecan	Inhibits topoisomerase I, resulting in DNA damage	Small cell lung cancer, ovarian cancer	Nausea, vomiting, diarrhea	Myelosuppression
Other camptothecins: Irinotecan				
Taxanes				
Paclitaxel	Interferes with microtubule function, resulting in impaired mitosis	Breast, lung, ovarian, gastroesophageal, prostate, bladder, and head and neck cancers	Nausea, vomiting, hypotension, arrhythmias, hypersensitivity	Myelosuppression, peripheral sensory neuropathy
Other taxanes: Docetaxel				

(Continued)

DRUG SUMMARY TABLE: Cancer Chemotherapy Drugs (*Continued*)

Subclass	Mechanism of Action	Clinical Applications	Acute Toxicities	Chronic Toxicities
Anthracyclines				
Doxorubicin	Oxygen free radicals bind to DNA causing strand breakage; inhibits topoisomerase II; intercalates into DNA	Lymphomas, myelomas, sarcomas, and breast, lung, ovarian and thyroid cancers	Nausea, arrhythmias	Alopecia, myelosuppression, cardiomyopathy, myelosuppression
Other anthracyclines: Daunorubicin, idarubicin, epirubicin, mitoxantrone Other antitumor antibiotics: Bleomycin, mitomycin				
Tyrosine kinase inhibitors				
Imatinib	Inhibits bcr-*abl* tyrosine kinase and other receptor tyrosine kinases	Chronic myelogenous leukemia, gastrointestinal stromal tumor	Nausea, vomiting	Fluid retention with ankle and periorbital edema, diarrhea, myalgias, congestive heart failure
Other tyrosine kinase inhibitors: Dasatinib, nilotinib, sorafenib*, sunitinib*, and pazopanib*				
Growth factor receptor inhibitors				
Trastuzumab	Inhibits the binding of EGF to the HER-2/*neu* growth receptor	HER-2/*neu* receptor + breast cancer	Nausea, vomiting, chills, fever, headache	Cardiac dysfunction
Other growth factor receptor inhibitors: Cetuximab, panitumumab, gefitinib, erlotinib				
Vascular endothelial growth factor (VEGF) inhibitors				
Bevacizumab	Inhibits binding of VEGF to its receptor, resulting in inhibition of tumor vascularization	Colorectal, breast, non-small cell lung, and renal cancer	Hypertensin, infusion reaction	Arterial thromboembolic events, gastrointestinal perforations, wound healing complications, proteinuria
Proteasome Inhibitors				
Bortezomib	Reversibly inhibits chymotrypsin-like activity of the 26S proteasome	Multiple myeloma	Hypotension, edema, GI upset	Peripheral neuropathy, cardiac dysfunction,
Hormone agonists				
Prednisone	See Chapter 39			
Hormone antagonists				
Tamoxifen	See Chapter 40			
Other hormonal antagonists: Aromatase inhibitors, GnRH agonist and antagonists, androgen receptor antagonists (see Chapter 40)				

DHFR, dihydrofolate reductase; EGF, epidermal growth factor; GnRH, gonadotropin-releasing hormone; VEGF, vascular endothelial growth factor.
These small molecules all inhibit VEGF-R2 VEGF-R3 receptor tyrosine kinases (RTKs). In addition they each inhibit a different spectrum of multiple other RTKs.

Immunopharmacology

Although the immune system is essential for protection against pathogens, in certain instances its powerful destructive mechanisms do more harm than good. Examples include hypersensitivity reactions, autoimmune disorders, and rejection reactions to transplanted tissues. Drugs that suppress immune mechanisms play an important role in treating these conditions. Increasingly, monoclonal antibodies targeting proteins with key roles in immune responses are being developed as immunosuppressive agents. In some situations, drugs that potentiate the immune response provide benefit.

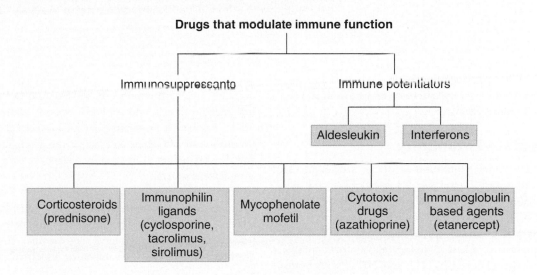

IMMUNE MECHANISMS

A. Overview

Using the concerted actions of complement components, phagocytic cells, and natural killer (NK) cells, the *innate* immune system initiates the defense against pathogens and antigenic insult. If the innate response is inadequate, the *adaptive* immune response is mobilized. This culminates in activation of T lymphocytes, the effectors of **cell-mediated immunity,** and production of antibodies by activated B lymphocytes, the effectors of **humoral immunity.** The subsets of lymphocytes that mediate different parts of the immune response can be identified by specific cell surface components or **clusters of differentiation (CDs).** For example, helper T (TH) cells bear the CD4 protein complex, whereas cytotoxic T lymphocytes express the CD8 protein complex.

B. Antigen Recognition and Processing

This critical inaugural step in the adaptive immune response involves **antigen-presenting cells (APCs),** which process antigens into small peptides recognized by T-cell receptors (TCRs) on the surface of CD4 TH cells (Figure 55–1). The most important antigen-presenting cell surface molecules are the **major histocompatibility complex (MHC) class I** and **II** proteins. The activation of TH cells by the class II MHC-peptide complex requires

479

participation of costimulatory and adhesion molecules in addition to activation of T-cell receptors.

C. Cell-Mediated Immunity

Activated TH cells secrete interleukin-2 (IL-2), a cytokine that initiates proliferation and activation of 2 subsets of helper T cells, TH1 and TH2 (Figure 55–1). TH1 cells orchestrate cell-mediated immunity and delayed hypersensitivity reactions. They produce interferon (IFN)-γ, IL-2, and tumor necrosis factor (TNF)-β (also known as lymphotoxin). These cytokines activate macrophages, CD8 cytotoxic T lymphocytes (CTLs), and NK cells. Activated CTLs recognize processed peptides that are bound to class I MHC molecules on the surface of virus-infected or tumor cells. The CTLs induce target cell death via lytic enzyme and nitric oxide production and by stimulation of apoptosis pathways in the target cells. CTLs also play a role in autoimmune diseases by reacting against normal tissues, such as the synovium in rheumatoid arthritis and myelin in multiple sclerosis. NK cells kill both virus-infected and neoplastic cells.

D. Humoral Immunity

The **B lymphoid cells,** which are capable of differentiating into antibody-forming cells, mediate humoral immunity. The humoral response is triggered when B lymphocytes bind antigen via their surface immunoglobulins. The antigens are internalized, processed into peptides, bound to MHC class II molecules, and presented on the B-cell surface. When T-cell receptors on TH2 cells are activated by the MHC II–peptide complex, they release interleukins (IL-4, IL-5, IL-6, IL-10, IL-13). These cytokines induce B-lymphocyte proliferation and differentiation into memory B cells and antibody-secreting plasma cells (Figure 55–1). Antibodies produced by plasma cells bind to antigens on the surface of pathogens and trigger the precipitation of viruses and the destruction of bacteria by phagocytic cells or lysis by the complement system.

The proliferation and differentiation of both B and T lymphocytes are under the control of a complex interplay between the cytokines (Table 55–1) and other endogenous molecules, including leukotrienes, and prostaglandins. For example, IL-10 and IFN-γ downregulate TH1 and TH2 responses, respectively (Figure 55–1).

E. Abnormal Immune Responses

Abnormal immune responses include hypersensitivity, autoimmunity, and immunodeficiency states. Immediate hypersensitivity is usually antibody-mediated and includes anaphylaxis and hemolytic disease of the newborn. Delayed hypersensitivity, associated with extensive tissue damage, is cell-mediated. Autoimmunity arises from lymphocytes that react to one's own molecules, or self antigens. Examples of autoimmune diseases that are amenable to drug treatment include rheumatoid arthritis and systemic lupus erythematosus. Immunodeficiency states can be genetically acquired (eg, DiGeorge syndrome) or can result from extrinsic factors (eg, HIV infection).

IMMUNOSUPPRESSIVE AGENTS

The primary immunosuppressive agents are a diverse group of drugs that range from the corticosteroid hormonal drugs

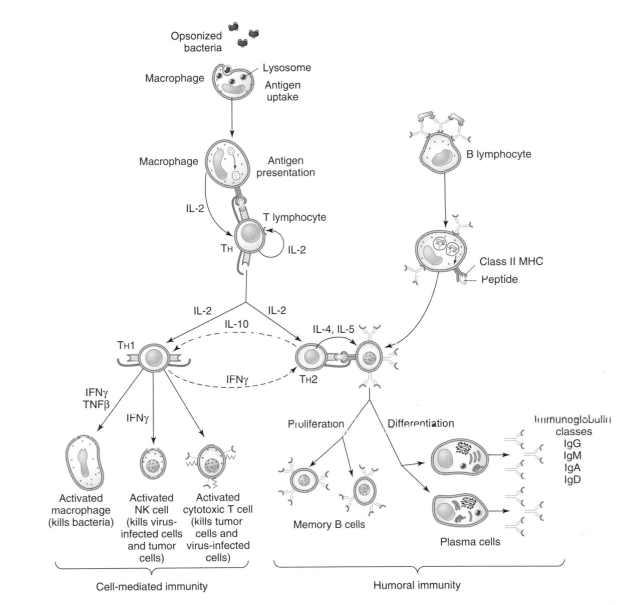

FIGURE 55–1 Scheme of cell-mediated and humoral immune responses. An immune response is initiated by internalization and processing of antigen by an antigen-presenting cell such as a macrophage. The class II MHC-peptide complex is recognized by the T cell receptor (TCR) on T-helper (TH) lymphocytes, resulting in T-cell activation. Activated (TH) cells secrete cytokines such as IL-2, which cause proliferation and activation of TH1 and TH2 cells. TH1 cells produce IFN-γ and TNF-β, which activate macrophages and NK cells. A humoral response is triggered when B lymphocytes bind antigen via their surface immunoglobulins. They are then induced by TH2-derived cytokines (eg, IL-4, IL-5) to proliferate and differentiate into memory cells and antibody-secreting plasma cells. (Modified and reproduced, with permission, from Katzung BG, editor: *Basic & Clinical Pharmacology,* 12th ed. McGraw-Hill, 2012: Fig. 55–3.)

(discussed also in Chapter 39) to antimetabolite anticancer drugs (discussed also in Chapter 54) to drugs that more selectively target cells of the immune system.

A. Corticosteroids

1. Mechanism of action—Glucocorticoids act at multiple cellular sites to produce broad effects on inflammatory and immune processes (see Chapter 39). At the biochemical level, their actions on gene expression decrease the synthesis of prostaglandins, leukotrienes, cytokines, and other signaling molecules that participate in immune responses (eg, platelet activating factor). At the cellular level, the glucocorticoids inhibit the proliferation of T lymphocytes and are cytotoxic to certain subsets of T cells. Although glucocorticoids impair cell-mediated immunity to the greatest extent, humoral immunity is also dampened and continuous therapy lowers IgG levels by increasing the catabolic rate of this class of immunoglobulins.

2. Clinical use—Glucocorticoids are used alone or in combination with other agents in a wide variety of medical conditions

TABLE 55–1 Cytokines that modulate immune responses.

Cytokine	Characteristic Properties
Interferon-α (IFN-α)	Activates NK cells, antiviral, oncostatic
Interferon-β (IFN-β)	Activates NK cells, antiviral, oncostatic
Interferon-γ (IFN-γ)	Activates TH1, NK, cytotoxic T cells, and macrophages; antiviral, oncostatic
Interleukin-1 (IL-1)	T-cell activation, B-cell proliferation and differentiation
Interleukin-2 (IL-2)	T-cell proliferation, activation of TH1, NK, and LAK cells
Interleukin-4 (IL-4)	TH2 and CTL activation, B-cell proliferation
Interleukin-5 (IL-5)	Eosinophil proliferation, B-cell proliferation and differentiation
Interleukin-10 (IL-10)	TH1 suppression, CTL activation, B-cell proliferation
Interleukin-11 (IL-11)	B-cell differentiation, megakaryocyte proliferation (see Chapter 33)
Tumor necrosis factor-α (TNF-α)	Proinflammatory, macrophage activation, oncostatic
Tumor necrosis factor-β (TNF-β)	Proinflammatory, chemotactic, oncostatic
Granulocyte colony-stimulating factor (G-CSF)	Granulocyte production (see Chapter 33)
Granulocyte-macrophage colony-stimulating factor (GM-CSF)	Granulocyte, monocyte, eosinophil production (see Chapter 33)

Modified and reproduced, with permission, from Katzung BG, editor: *Basic & Clinical Pharmacology*, 12th ed. McGraw-Hill, 2012: Table 55–2.

that have an underlying undesirable immunologic reaction (see Chapter 39). They are also used to suppress immunologic reactions in patients who undergo organ transplantation and to treat hematologic cancers (see Chapter 54).

3. Toxicity—Predictable adverse effects include adrenal suppression, growth inhibition, muscle wasting, osteoporosis, salt retention, glucose intolerance, and behavioral changes (see Chapter 39).

B. Immunophilin Inhibitors

1. Mechanism of action—These immunosuppressants interfere with T-cell function by binding to **immunophilins,** small cytoplasmic proteins that play critical roles in T-cell responses to T-cell receptor activation and to cytokines. **Cyclosporine** binds to cyclophilin and **tacrolimus** binds to FK-binding protein (FKBP). Both complexes inhibit **calcineurin,** a cytoplasmic phosphatase. Calcineurin regulates the ability of the nuclear factor of activated T cells (NF-AT) to translocate to the nucleus and increase the production of key cytokines such as IL-2, IL-3, and IFN-γ. Cyclophilin and tacrolimus prevent the increased production of cytokines that normally occurs in response to T-cell receptor activation. **Sirolimus** and its analogs (everolimus, temsirolimus) also bind to FKBP-binding protein 12. Instead of inhibiting calcineurin, these drug–protein complexes inhibit the kinase activity of mammalian target of rapamycin (mTOR), a key regulator of a complex intracellular signaling pathway involved in cell growth and proliferation, angiogenesis, and metabolism. By inhibiting the mTOR pathway, sirolimus inhibits the T-cell proliferation response to IL-2.

2. Clinical uses and pharmacokinetics—Use of these immunosuppressants is a major factor in the success of solid organ transplantation. They are used in solid organ transplantation and to prevent and treat graft-versus-host (GVH) disease in recipients of allogeneic stem cell transplantation. These agents, particularly cyclosporine and tacrolimus, are also used in some autoimmune diseases, including rheumatoid arthritis, uveitis, psoriasis, asthma, and type 1 diabetes. Sirolimus-eluting stents are used to prevent restenosis after coronary angioplasty. Like sirolimus, everolimus is used as an immunosuppressant. Everolimus and temsirolimus are used for various cancers.

Cyclosporine and tacrolimus are available as oral or intravenous agents, whereas sirolimus and everolimus are available only as oral drugs. Temsirolimus is available as an intravenous agent. Because cyclosporine exhibits erratic bioavailability, serum levels are routinely monitored. The drug undergoes slow hepatic metabolism by the cytochrome P450 system and has a long half-life. Its metabolism is affected by a host of other drugs.

3. Toxicity—Cyclosporine and tacrolimus have similar toxicity profiles. The most common adverse effects are renal dysfunction, hypertension, and neurotoxicity. These drugs can also cause hyperglycemia, hyperlipidemia, and cholelithiasis. Sirolimus and its analogs are more likely than the other agents to cause hypertriglyceridemia, hepatotoxicity, diarrhea, and myelosuppression.

C. Mycophenolate Mofetil

1. Mechanism of action—This drug is rapidly converted into mycophenolic acid, which inhibits inosine monophosphate dehydrogenase, an enzyme in the de novo pathway of guanosine triphosphate (GTP) synthesis. This action suppresses both B- and T-lymphocyte activation. Lymphocytes are particularly susceptible to inhibitors of the de novo pathway because they lack the enzymes necessary for the alternative salvage pathway for GTP synthesis.

2. Clinical use—Mycophenolate mofetil has been used successfully as a sole agent in kidney, liver, and heart transplantations. In renal transplantations, its use with low-dose cyclosporine has reduced cyclosporine-induced nephrotoxicity.

3. Toxicity—This drug can cause gastrointestinal disturbances and myelosuppression, especially neutropenia.

D. Thalidomide

This sedative drug, notorious for its teratogenic effects, has complex immune effects that include suppression of TNF-α production, increased IL-10, reduced neutrophil phagocytosis, altered adhesion molecule expression, and enhanced cell-mediated immunity. Thalidomide is used for some forms of leprosy reactions, for immunologic diseases (eg, systemic lupus), and as an anticancer drug. It is also effective in treating aphthous ulcers and the wasting syndrome in AIDS patients. Lenalidomide, one of many immunomodulatory derivatives of thalidomide (IMiDs) under investigation, is an oral drug approved for multiple myeloma.

E. Other Immunosuppressive Agents

A variety of other anticancer drugs (Chapter 54) and antirheumatic drugs (Chapter 36) have clinically useful immunosuppressive actions. Several of the most important of these are listed in Table 55–2.

ANTIBODY-BASED IMMUNOSUPPRESSIVE AGENTS

A. Antilymphocyte Globulin and Antithymocyte Globulin

1. Mechanism of action—Two types of antisera directed against lymphocytes are available. Antilymphocyte globulin (ALG) and antithymocyte globulin (ATG) are produced in horses or sheep by immunization against human thymus cells. Antibodies in these preparations bind to T cells involved in antigen recognition and initiate their destruction by serum complement. These antibodies selectively block cellular immunity rather than antibody formation, which accounts for their ability to suppress organ graft rejection, a cell-mediated process.

2. Clinical use—ALG and ATG are used before allogeneic stem cell transplantation to prevent graft-versus-host reaction. They are also used in combination with other immunosuppressants for solid organs transplantation.

3. Toxicity—Because humoral immunity may remain intact, injection of ALG or ATG can cause hypersensitivity reactions, including serum sickness and anaphylaxis. Pain and erythema occur at injection sites, and lymphoma has been noted as a late complication.

B. Immune Globulin Intravenous (IGIV)

1. Mechanism of action—Intravenous use of this immunoglobulin preparation (usually IgG) prepared from pools of thousands of healthy donors is believed to have a normalizing effect on an individual's immune networks. Its precise mechanism of action is not known.

TABLE 55–2 Other drugs used as immunosuppressive agents.

Drug	Characteristics
Azathioprine	Prodrug of the anticancer drug mercaptopurine, which interferes with purine nucleic acid metabolism used for rheumatic diseases and organ transplantation (see Chapter 36)
Cyclophosphamide	Anticancer alkylating agent used in organ transplantation and rheumatic diseases (see Chapters 36 and 54)
Leflunomide	Inhibitor of dihydroorotate dehydrogenase, an enzyme involved in de novo pyrimidine synthesis. Used in rheumatoid arthritis (see Chapter 36)
Hydroxychloroquine	Antimalarial drug with immunosuppressive activity used for rheumatoid arthritis and systemic lupus erythematosus (see Chapters 36 and 52)
Methotrexate	Anticancer drug that inhibits dihydrofolate reductase used for rheumatoid arthritis and hematopoietic stem cell transplantation (see Chapters 36 and 54)
Sulfasalazine	Prodrug metabolized to sulfapyridine and 5-aminosalisylic acid (5-ASA). Used for rheumatoid arthritis and inflammatory bowel disease (see Chapters 36 and 59)

2. Clinical use—IGIV has proved useful in a wide range of conditions including immunoglobulin deficiencies, autoimmune disorders, HIV disease, and stem cell transplantation.

3. Toxicity—Renal toxicity, including acute renal failure, is a particular concern with IGIV.

C. Rh$_o$(D) Immune Globulin

1. Mechanism of action—Rh$_o$GAM is a human IgG preparation that contains antibodies against red cell Rh$_o$(D) antigens. Administration of this antibody to Rh$_o$(D)-negative mothers at time of antigen exposure (ie, birth of an Rh$_o$(D)-positive child) blocks the primary immune response to the foreign cells.

2. Clinical use—Rh$_o$(D) immune globulin is used for prevention of Rh hemolytic disease of the newborn. In women treated with Rh$_o$(D) immune globulin, maternal antibodies to Rh-positive cells are not produced in subsequent pregnancies, and hemolytic disease of the neonate is averted.

D. Monoclonal Antibodies

Monoclonal antibodies (MAbs) have the advantage of high specificity because they can be developed for interaction with a single molecule. "Humanization" of murine monoclonal antibodies and wholly human monoclonal antibodies (based on genetic engineering of transgenic mice that make human antibodies, Figure 55–2) have reduced the likelihood of formation of neutralizing antibodies and of immune reactions. Three types of MAbs used as immunosuppressive agents are described in the text that follows, and characteristics of some other therapeutic MAbs, including some used for nonimmunologic purposes, are listed in Table 55–3.

1. Muromonab-CD3—This MAb binds to the CD3 antigen on the surface of human thymocytes and mature T cells. It blocks the killing action of cytotoxic T cells and probably interferes with other T-cell functions. Muromonab-CD3 is used to manage renal, cardiac, and liver transplant rejection crises. Serious anaphylactic reactions can occur, especially with the first few doses. Neuropsychiatric and hypersensitivity reactions may also occur.

2. Infliximab—This humanized MAb (Figure 55–2) is targeted against TNF-α, a proinflammatory cytokine, and thereby decreases formation of interleukins and adhesion molecules involved in leukocyte activation. Infliximab induces remissions in treatment-resistant Crohn's disease. In combination with methotrexate, infliximab improves symptoms in patients with rheumatoid arthritis. It also is effective in the treatment of ulcerative colitis, ankylosing spondylitis, and psoriatic arthritis. Infusion reactions and an increased rate of infection may occur. **Adalimumab** (Figure 55–2) is a completely human IgG monoclonal antibody that binds to TNF-α and is approved for treatment of rheumatoid arthritis. Though not a true MAb, **etanercept** (Figure 55–2) is an immunoglobulin-based agent that also binds with high affinity and thereby sequesters TNF-α. It is a dimer of identical chains of a human TNF receptor fused to a human IgG constant region. Etanercept is used in arthritis, psoriasis, and ankylosing spondylitis, and it is being investigated in other inflammatory diseases. Injection site reactions and hypersensitivity may occur.

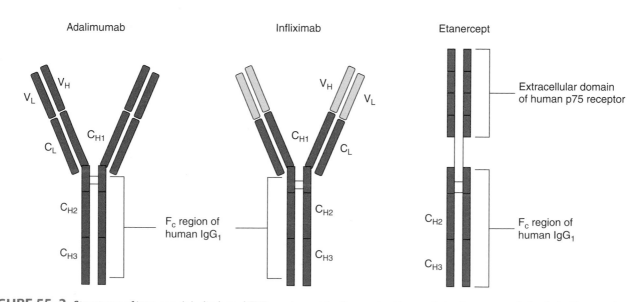

FIGURE 55–2 Structures of immunoglobulin-based TNF-α antagonists. C$_H$, constant heavy chain; C$_L$, constant light chain; Fc, complex immunoglobulin region; V$_H$, variable heavy chain; V$_L$, variable light chain. Red regions, human derived; blue regions, mouse derived. (Reproduced, with permission, from Katzung BG, editor: *Basic & Clinical Pharmacology*, 12th ed. McGraw-Hill, 2012: Fig. 36–4.)

TABLE 55–3 **Characteristics of selected monoclonal antibodies (MAbs) and immunoglobulin-based agents.**

MAb	Characteristics and Clinical Uses
Abatacept	Extracellular domain of cytotoxic T-lymphocyte-associated antigen 4 (CTLA-4) fused to human IgG Fc. Blocks T-cell activation by interfering with the interaction of T-cell CD28 to APC CD 80/86 (Figure 55–3). Used for severe rheumatoid arthritis
Abciximab	Antagonist of glycoprotein IIb1/IIIa receptor, preventing cross-linking reaction in platelet aggregation. Used post-angioplasty and in acute coronary syndromes
Alefacept	Fusion of a fragment of leukocyte-function-associated antigen-3 (LFA-3) to human IgG Fc region that prevents T-cell CD2 from binding to APC LFA-3. Approved for psoriasis
Efalizumab	MAb to CD-11a, the alpha subunit of T-cell leukocyte-function-associated antigen-1 (LFA-1). Inhibits binding of LFA-1 to APC intercellular adhesion molecule-1 (ICAM-1; Figure 55–3). Approved for psoriasis
Ipilimumab	Anti-CTLA-4 antibody that prolongs T-cell activation. Approved for melanoma (Figure 55–3)
Omalizumab	Anti-IgE MAb used to treat severe asthma (see Chapter 20)
Palivizumab	Antibody to surface protein of respiratory syncytial virus (RSV). Used for prophylaxis and treatment of RSV infection
Rituximab	Binds to the CD20 antigen on B lymphocytes and recruits immune effector functions to mediate lysis. Used in B-cell non-Hodgkin's lymphoma and with methotrexate for rheumatoid arthritis
Trastuzumab	Binds to the HER-2 protein on the surface of tumor cells. Cytotoxic for breast tumors that overexpress HER-2 protein

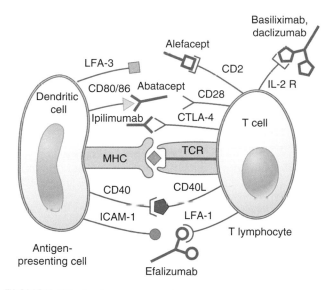

FIGURE 55–3 The activation of a T cell by an antigen-presenting cell (APC) involves engagement of the T-cell receptor (TCR) by the MHC-peptide complex plus secondary costimulatory signals based on interactions between APC and T-cell surface proteins. Alefacept inhibits the interaction between T-cell CD2 and APC LF-3. Abatacept prevents T-cell CD28 from binding APC CD80/86, efalizumab interferes with the binding of T-cell FLA-1 to APC ICAM-1, and basiliximab and daclizumab inhibit the IL-2 receptor. Ipilimumab helps maintain T-cell activation by inhibiting CTLA-4 interaction with CD80/86. (Modified and reproduced, with permission, from Katzung BG, editor: *Basic & Clinical Pharmacology*, 11th ed. McGraw-Hill, 2009: Fig. 55–7.)

All of the anti-TNF-α agents increase the risk of serious infection and lymphoma.

3. Daclizumab—Daclizumab is a highly specific MAb that binds to the alpha subunit of the IL-2 receptor displayed on the surface of T cells and prevents activation by IL-2 (Figure 55–3). It is used in combination with other immunosuppressants to prevent renal transplant rejection. In contrast to cyclosporine, tacrolimus, or cytotoxic immunosuppressants, the adverse effects of daclizumab are equivalent to those of placebo. **Basiliximab** is a chimeric human-mouse IgG with an action that is equivalent to that of daclizumab.

IMMUNOMODULATING AGENTS

Agents that stimulate immune responses represent a newer area in immunopharmacology with the potential for important therapeutic uses, including the treatment of immune deficiency diseases, chronic infectious diseases, and cancer.

A. Aldesleukin

Aldesleukin is recombinant **interleukin-2 (IL-2),** an endogenous lymphokine that promotes the production of cytotoxic T lymphocytes and activates NK cells (Table 55–1). Aldesleukin is indicated for the adjunctive treatment of renal cell carcinoma and malignant melanoma. It is investigational for possible efficacy in restoring immune function in AIDS and other immune deficiency disorders.

B. Interferons

Interferon-α-2a inhibits cell proliferation and is used in hairy cell leukemia, chronic myelogenous leukemia, malignant melanoma, Kaposi's sarcoma, and hepatitis B and C. **Interferon-β-1b** has some beneficial effects in relapsing multiple sclerosis. **Interferon-γ-1b** has greater immune-enhancing actions than the other interferons and appears to act by increasing the synthesis of TNF. The recombinant form is used to decrease the incidence and severity of infections in patients with chronic granulomatous disease.

MECHANISMS OF DRUG ALLERGY

Immunologic reactions to drugs can fall into any of the 4 categories of hypersensitivity reactions.

A. Type I (Immediate) Drug Allergy

This form of drug allergy involves **IgE**-mediated reactions to animal and plant stings and pollens as well as to drugs. Such reactions include anaphylaxis, urticaria, and angioedema. When linked to carrier proteins, small drug molecules can act as haptens and initiate B-cell proliferation and formation of IgE antibodies. These antibodies bind to Fc receptors on tissue mast cells and blood basophils. On subsequent exposure, the antigenic drug cross-links the IgE antibodies on the surface of mast cells and basophils and triggers release of mediators of vascular responses and tissue injury, including histamine, kinins, prostaglandins, and leukotrienes. Drugs that commonly cause type I reactions include penicillins and sulfonamides.

SKILL KEEPER: ANAPHYLAXIS AND SYMPATHOMIMETIC DRUGS (SEE CHAPTERS 6 AND 9)

In severe anaphylactic reactions, the life-threatening events commonly involve airway obstruction, laryngeal edema, and vascular collapse resulting from peripheral vasodilation and reduction in blood volume. Hypoxemia can contribute to cardiac events, including arrhythmias and myocardial infarction. Drugs used to treat anaphylaxis mainly target the receptors used by neurotransmitters of the sympathetic nervous system.

1. *Why is epinephrine rather than norepinephrine used in anaphylaxis?*
2. *What other sympathomimetic drugs might be useful in the treatment of anaphylaxis?*

The Skill Keeper Answers appear at the end of the chapter.

B. Type II Drug Allergy

Type II allergy involves IgG or IgM antibodies that are bound to circulating blood cells. On reexposure to the antigen, complement-dependent cell lysis occurs. Type II reactions include autoimmune syndromes such as hemolytic anemia from methyldopa, systemic lupus erythematosus from hydralazine or procainamide, thrombocytopenic purpura from quinidine, and agranulocytosis from exposure to many drugs.

C. Type III Drug Allergy

Type III hypersensitivity is a complex type of drug allergy reaction that involves complement-fixing IgM or IgG antibodies and, possibly, IgE antibodies. Drug-induced serum sickness and vasculitis are examples of type III reactions; Stevens-Johnson syndrome (associated with sulfonamide therapy) may also result from type III mechanisms.

D. Type IV Drug Allergy

Type IV allergy is a cell-mediated reaction that can occur from topical application of drugs. It results in contact dermatitis.

E. Modification of Drug Allergies

Drugs that modify allergic responses to other drugs or toxins act at several steps of the immune mechanism. For example, corticosteroids inhibit lymphoid cell proliferation and reduce tissue injury and edema. However, most drugs that are useful in type I reactions (eg, epinephrine, H_1 antagonists, corticosteroids) block mediator release or act as physiologic antagonists of the mediators.

QUESTIONS

1. Cyclosporine is effective in organ transplantation. Which of the following most accurately describes the immunosuppressant action of cyclosporine?
   (A) Activation of NK cells
   (B) Blockade of tissue responses to inflammatory mediators
   (C) Increased catabolism of IgG antibodies
   (D) Inhibition of the gene transcription of interleukins
   (E) Interference with MHC II-peptide activation of T cells

2. Which of the following is a widely used drug that suppresses cellular immunity, inhibits prostaglandin and leukotriene synthesis, and increases the catabolism of IgG antibodies?
   (A) Cyclophosphamide
   (B) Cyclosporine
   (C) Infliximab
   (D) Mycophenolate mofetil
   (E) Prednisone

3. Which of the following drugs is used to prevent the primary immune response of an Rh-negative mother to an Rh-positive newborn?
   (A) Cyclosporine
   (B) Cyclophosphamide
   (C) Methotrexate
   (D) $Rh_o(D)$ immune globulin
   (E) Tacrolimus

4. Tumor necrosis factor (TNF)-α appears to play an important role in autoimmunity and inflammatory diseases. Which of the following is a humanized monoclonal antibody that binds to TNF-α and inhibits its action?
   (A) Etanercept
   (B) Infliximab
   (C) Muromonab-CD3
   (D) Sirolimus
   (E) Thalidomide

Questions 5 and 6. A patient was treated for a bacterial infection with a penicillin. Within a few minutes of the antibiotic injection, he developed severe bronchoconstriction, laryngeal edema, and hypotension. Because of the rapid administration of epinephrine, the patient survived. Unfortunately, a year later he was treated with an antipsychotic drug and developed agranulocytosis.

5. Which type of immunologic process was triggered by the penicillin injection?
   (A) An autoimmune syndrome
   (B) A cell-mediated reaction
   (C) A type II drug allergy
   (D) Mediated by IgE
   (E) Serum sickness

6. Which type of immunologic process was triggered by the antipsychotic drug?
   (A) A type III drug reaction
   (B) A type IV drug reaction
   (C) Delayed-type hypersensitivity
   (D) Mediated by IgG or IgM antibodies
   (E) Stevens-Johnson syndrome

7. Which of the following is an immunosuppressant that suppresses both B and T lymphocytes via inhibition of de novo synthesis of purines?
   (A) Cyclophosphamide
   (B) Methotrexate
   (C) Mycophenolate mofetil
   (D) Prednisone
   (E) Tacrolimus

8. Recombinant interleukin-2 has proved useful in the treatment of which of the following diseases?
   (A) Graft-versus-host disease in patients with hematopoietic stem cell transplantation
   (B) Psoriasis
   (C) Renal cell carcinoma
   (D) Rheumatoid arthritis
   (E) Superficial bladder carcinoma

9. Although sirolimus and cyclosporine have similar immunosuppressant effects, their toxicity profiles differ. Which of the following toxicities is more likely to be associated with sirolimus than with cyclosporine?
   (A) An anaphylactic reaction
   (B) Hypertension
   (C) Osteoporosis
   (D) Renal insufficiency
   (E) Thrombocytopenia

10. Which of the following is an immune modulator that increases phagocytosis by macrophages in patients with chronic granulomatous disease?
    (A) Aldesleukin
    (B) Interferon-γ
    (C) Lymphocyte immune globulin
    (D) Prednisone
    (E) Trastuzumab

ANSWERS

1. Cyclosporine inhibits calcineurin, a serine phosphatase that is needed for activation of T-cell-specific transcription factors. Gene transcription of IL-2, IL-3, and interferon-γ is inhibited. The answer is **D**.

2. The corticosteroid prednisone is used extensively as an immunosuppressant in autoimmune diseases and organ transplantation. Glucocorticoids have multiple actions, including those described. The answer is **E**.

3. Rh_o(D) immune globulin contains antibodies against Rh_o(D) antigens. Administration to an Rh-negative mother within 72 h after the birth of an Rh-positive infant prevents Rh hemolytic disease of the newborn in subsequent pregnancies. The answer is **D**.

4. Infliximab is a humanized monoclonal antibody that binds to TNF-α. Etanercept also binds to TNF-α, but it is a chimeric protein containing a portion of the human TNF-α receptor linked to the Fc region of a human IgG. Thalidomide is a small molecule that appears to inhibit production of TNF-α. The answer is **B**.

5. The patient experienced an anaphylactic response to the penicillin. This is a type I (immediate) drug reaction, mediated by IgE antibodies. The answer is **D**.

6. Agranulocytosis (and systemic lupus erythematosus) are autoimmune syndromes that can be drug-induced. They are type II reactions involving IgM and IgG antibodies that bind to circulating blood cells. The patient was probably treated with clozapine for his psychosis (see clozapine toxicity, Chapter 29). The answer is **D**.

7. Mycophenolic acid, formed from mycophenolate mofetil, inhibits inosine monophosphate dehydrogenase, the rate-limiting enzyme in the de novo pathway of purine synthesis. This action suppresses both B- and T-lymphocyte activation. Mycophenolate mofetil is used in organ transplantation. The answer is **C**.

8. Interleukin-2 is a cytokine that stimulates T-cell proliferation and activates TH1, NK, and LAK cells. It has shown efficacy in renal cell carcinoma and malignant melanoma, 2 cancers that respond poorly to conventional cytotoxic anticancer drugs. The answer is **C**.

9. Cyclosporine and tacrolimus both are associated with renal toxicity and hypertension. In contrast, sirolimus appears to spare the kidney and instead is more likely to cause gastrointestinal disturbance, hypertriglyceridemia, and myelosuppression, especially in the form of thrombocytopenia. The answer is **E**.

10. Interferon-γ is approved for use in chronic granulomatous disease, a condition that results from phagocyte deficiency. The agent markedly reduces the frequency of recurrent infections. The answer is **B**.

SKILL KEEPER ANSWERS: ANAPHYLAXIS AND SYMPATHOMIMETIC DRUGS (SEE CHAPTERS 6 AND 9)

1. *Epinephrine activates all adrenoceptors, whereas norepinephrine has minimal agonist activity at β_2 adrenoceptors. This difference is important in anaphylaxis because β_2 adrenoceptor activation is needed to provide a bronchodilatory effect that will oppose the anaphylaxis-induced airway obstruction. The α_1 adrenoceptor agonist effect of epinephrine opposes the anaphylaxis-induced vasodilation and, to some extent, the vascular leak (administration of fluid is also a cornerstone of the treatment of anaphylaxis), whereas the β_1 adrenoceptor agonist effect helps maintain cardiac output.*

2. *If bronchospasm is predominant, then administration by inhalation of a β_2-selective agonist such as albuterol may be useful. If cardiovascular collapse is predominant and does not respond adequately to fluid resuscitation, then vasopressor drugs may be helpful; these include α adrenoceptor agonists such as phenylephrine and β_1-adrenoceptor agonists such as dobutamine or dopamine.*

CHECKLIST

When you complete this chapter, you should be able to:

❏ Describe the primary features of cell-mediated and humoral immunity.

❏ Name 7 immunosuppressants and, for each, describe the mechanism of action, clinical uses, and toxicities.

❏ Describe the mechanisms of action, clinical uses, and toxicities of antibodies used as immunosuppressants.

❏ Identify the major cytokines and other immunomodulating agents and know their clinical applications.

❏ Describe the different types of allergic reactions to drugs.

DRUG SUMMARY TABLE: Drugs That Modulate Immune Function

Subclass	Mechanism of Action	Clinical Applications	Pharmacokinetics	Toxicities, Interactions
Glucocorticoids				
Prednisone	Activation of glucocorticoid receptor leads to altered gene transcription	Many inflammatory conditions, organ transplantation, hematologic cancers	Duration of activity is longer than pharmacokinetic half-life of drug owing to gene transcription effects	Adrenal suppression, growth inhibition, muscle wasting, osteoporosis, salt retention, glucose intolerance, behavioral changes

Many other glucocorticoids available for oral and parenteral use. See Chapter 39

Subclass	Mechanism of Action	Clinical Applications	Pharmacokinetics	Toxicities, Interactions
Immunophilin ligands				
Cyclosporine	The complex of cyclosporine-cyclophilin inhibits calcineurin	Organ transplantation, graft-versus-host disease, some autoimmune diseases	Metabolized by CYP450 system • many drug-drug interactions	Renal dysfunction, hypertension, neurotoxicity

Tacrolimus: like cyclosporine but inhibits calcineurin by binding to FK506 immunophilin
Sirolimus: its binding to cyclophilin inhibits the IL-2 signaling pathway; toxicity effects include hypertriglyceridemia, hepatotoxicity, diarrhea, and myelosuppression. Everolimus and temsirolimus are similar

Subclass	Mechanism of Action	Clinical Applications	Pharmacokinetics	Toxicities, Interactions
Purine antagonist				
Mycophenolate mofetil	Blocks de novo GTP synthesis by inhibiting inosine monophosphate dehydrogenase	Organ transplantation, graft-versus-host disease, some autoimmune diseases	Oral, parenteral	Gastrointestinal disturbances, myelosuppression

Subclass	Mechanism of Action	Clinical Applications	Pharmacokinetics	Toxicities, Interactions
Miscellaneous				
Thalidomide	Complex immune effects including reduction in TNF-α production	Erythema nodosum leprosum, multiple myeloma	Oral	Teratogen, somnolence, peripheral neuropathy, neutropenia

Lenalidomide: thalidomide analog approved for multiple myeloma

Subclass	Mechanism of Action	Clinical Applications	Pharmacokinetics	Toxicities, Interactions
CD-2 receptor antagonist				
Alefacept	Binds to T-cell CD2 receptor and blocks its association with LFA-3	Psoriasis	Recombinant protein • parenteral	Reduced T-cell count, hepatotoxicity, hypersensitivity reaction, infection, malignancy

Subclass	Mechanism of Action	Clinical Applications	Pharmacokinetics	Toxicities, Interactions
Immunosuppressive antisera				
Antithymocyte globulin	Binds to T cells and triggers complement-based cytotoxicity	Transplantation	Parenteral	Hypersensitivity reaction, injection site reaction, malignancy

Antilymphocyte globulin: like antithymocyte globulin
Immune globulin intravenous (IGIV): immunoglobulin preparation of pooled IgG from healthy donors. Wide range of clinical applications including immunoglobulin deficiencies and autoimmune disorders

Subclass	Mechanism of Action	Clinical Applications	Pharmacokinetics	Toxicities, Interactions
Anti-Rh$_0$(D) antibody				
Rh$_0$GAM	Prevents Rh sensitization by binding to Rh$_0$(D) antigens	Administered to Rh$_0$(D)-negative mothers who carry a Rh$_0$(D)-positive fetus	Parenteral	Injection-site reactions, hemolysis if given to Rh-positive person

(Continued)

DRUG SUMMARY TABLE: Drugs That Modulate Immune Function (*Continued*)

Subclass	Mechanism of Action	Clinical Applications	Pharmacokinetics	Toxicities, Interactions
CD3 antagonist				
Muromonab-CD3	MAb that inhibits cytotoxic T cells by binding to CD3	Allograft rejection	Parenteral	Anaphylactic reactions, neuropsychiatric effects, hypersensitivity reactions
IL-2 antagonists				
Daclizumab	MAb that blocks the T-cell IL-2 receptor	Renal transplantation	Parenteral	Hypersensitivity reactions, infection, malignancy
Basiliximab: chimeric MAb similar to daclizumab				
Anti-TNF-α agents				
Infliximab	MAb binds to TNF-α and prevents it from activating TNF-α receptor	Inflammatory bowel disease, rheumatoid arthritis, ankylosing spondylitis, psoriatic arthritis	Parenteral	Hypersensitivity reactions, infection, malignancy
Adalimumab: human MAb similar to daclizumab *Etanercept*: dimer of human TNF receptor fused to IgG constant region				
Recombinant IL-2				
Aldesleukin	Activates IL-2 receptors on T, B, and NK cells	Renal cell carcinoma, melanoma	Parenteral	Capillary leak syndrome, exacerbation of preexisting inflammatory/autoimmune diseases, hypersensitivity reactions
Interferons (IFNs)				
Interferon-α-2a	Enhances immune responses by activating IFN-α receptors	Leukemia, melanoma, hepatitis B and C	Parenteral	
Interferon-α-1b: used for multiple sclerosis *Interferon-γ-1b*: used for chronic granulomatous disease				

GTP, guanosine triphosphate; LFA, lymphocyte-associated antigen; MAb, monoclonal antibody; TNF, tumor necrosis factor.

Environmental and Occupational Toxicology

56

Toxicology is the branch of pharmacology that encompasses the deleterious effects of chemicals on biologic systems. A number of chemicals in the environment (eg, atmosphere, home, workplace) pose important health hazards.

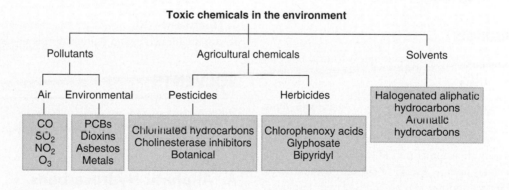

Toxic chemicals in the environment

- Pollutants
  - Air
    - CO
    - SO_2
    - NO_2
    - O_3
  - Environmental
    - PCBs
    - Dioxins
    - Asbestos
    - Metals
- Agricultural chemicals
  - Pesticides
    - Chlorinated hydrocarbons
    - Cholinesterase inhibitors
    - Botanical
  - Herbicides
    - Chlorophenoxy acids
    - Glyphosate
    - Bipyridyl
- Solvents
  - Halogenated aliphatic hydrocarbons
  - Aromatic hydrocarbons

AIR POLLUTANTS

A. Classification and Prototypes

The major air pollutants in industrialized countries include carbon monoxide (which accounts for about 50% of the total amount of air pollutants), sulfur oxides (18%), hydrocarbons (12%), particulate matter (eg, smoke particles, 10%), and nitrogen oxides (6%).

Air pollution appears to be a contributing factor in bronchitis, obstructive pulmonary disease, and lung cancer.

B. Carbon Monoxide

Carbon monoxide (CO) is an odorless, colorless gas that competes avidly with oxygen for hemoglobin. The affinity of CO for hemoglobin is more than 200-fold greater than that of oxygen.

491

High-Yield Terms to Learn

Bioaccumulation	The increasing concentration of a substance in the environment as the result of environmental persistence and physical properties (eg, lipid solubility) that leads to accumulation in biologic tissues
Endocrine disruptors	Chemicals in the environment that have estrogen-like or antiandrogen activity or disrupt thyroid function. There is concern that exposure to endocrine disruptors may increase reproductive cancers, impair fertility, and have teratogenic effects
Environmental toxicology	The area of toxicology that deals with the effects of agents found in the environment; regulated by the Environmental Protection Agency (EPA) in the United States
Occupational toxicology	The area of toxicology that deals with the toxic effects of chemicals found in the workplace; regulated by the Occupational Safety and Health Administration (OSHA) in the United States
Threshold limit value	The amount of exposure to a given agent that is deemed safe for a stated time period. It is higher for shorter periods than for longer periods

The threshold limit value of CO for an 8-h workday is 25 parts per million (ppm); in heavy traffic, the concentration of CO may exceed 100 ppm.

1. Effects—CO causes tissue hypoxia. Headache occurs first, followed by confusion, decreased visual acuity, tachycardia, syncope, coma, seizures, and death. Collapse and syncope occur when approximately 40% of hemoglobin has been converted to carboxyhemoglobin. Prolonged hypoxia can result in irreversible damage to the brain and the myocardium.

2. Treatment—Removal of the source of CO and 100% oxygen are the main features of treatment. Hyperbaric oxygen accelerates the clearance of carbon monoxide.

C. Sulfur Dioxide

Sulfur dioxide (SO_2) is a colorless, irritating gas formed from the combustion of fossil fuels.

1. Effects—SO_2 forms sulfurous acid on contact with moist mucous membranes; this acid is responsible for most of the pathologic effects. Conjunctival and bronchial irritation (especially in individuals with asthma) are the primary signs of exposure. Presence of 5–10 ppm in the air is enough to cause severe bronchospasm. Heavy exposure may lead to delayed pulmonary edema. Chronic low-level exposure may aggravate cardiopulmonary disease.

2. Treatment—Removal from exposure to SO_2 and relief of irritation and inflammation constitute the major treatment.

D. Nitrogen Oxides

Nitrogen dioxide (NO_2), a brownish irritant gas, is the principal member of this group. It is formed in fires and in silage on farms.

1. Effects—NO_2 causes deep lung irritation and pulmonary edema. Farm workers exposed to high concentrations of the gas

within enclosed silos may die rapidly of acute pulmonary edema. Irritation of the eyes, nose, and throat is common.

2. Treatment—No specific treatment is available. Measures to reduce inflammation and pulmonary edema are important.

E. Ozone

Ozone (O_3) is a bluish irritant gas produced in air and water purification devices and in electrical fields.

1. Effects—Exposure to 0.01–0.1 ppm may cause irritation and dryness of the mucous membranes. Pulmonary function may be impaired at higher concentrations. Chronic exposure leads to bronchitis, bronchiolitis, pulmonary fibrosis, and emphysema.

2. Treatment—No specific treatment is available. Measures that reduce inflammation and pulmonary edema are emphasized.

SOLVENTS

Solvents used in industry and solvents to clean clothing are a major source of direct exposure to hydrocarbons and also contribute to air pollution.

A. Aliphatic Hydrocarbons

This group includes halogenated solvents such as carbon tetrachloride, chloroform, and trichloroethylene.

1. Effects—Solvents are potent CNS depressants. The acute effects of excessive exposure are nausea, vertigo, locomotor disturbances, headache, and coma. Chronic exposure leads to hepatic dysfunction and nephrotoxicity. Long-term exposure to tetrachloroethylene or to trichloroethane has caused peripheral neuropathy.

2. Treatment—Removal from exposure is the only specific treatment available. Serious CNS depression must be treated with support of vital signs (see Chapter 58).

B. Aromatic Hydrocarbons

Benzene, toluene, and xylene are important aromatic hydrocarbons.

1. Effects—Acute exposure to any of these hydrocarbons leads to CNS depression with ataxia and coma. Long-term exposure to benzene is associated with hematotoxicity (thrombocytopenia, aplastic anemia, pancytopenia) and various types of hematologic cancers, especially leukemia.

2. Treatment—Removal from exposure is the only specific way to reduce toxicity. CNS depression is managed by support of vital signs.

SKILL KEEPER: SAFETY OF NEW DRUGS (SEE CHAPTER 5)

The FDA requires evidence of the relative safety of a new drug before its clinical evaluation. If a new drug is destined for chronic systemic administration, what animal toxicity testing is required? The Skill Keeper Answer appears at the end of the chapter.

PESTICIDES

A. Classification and Prototypes

The 3 major classes of pesticides are chlorinated hydrocarbons (DDT and its analogs), acetylcholinesterase inhibitors (carbamates, organophosphates), and botanical agents (nicotine, rotenone, pyrethrum alkaloids).

B. Chlorinated Hydrocarbons

These agents are persistent, poorly metabolized, lipophilic chemicals that exhibit significant bioaccumulation.

1. Effects—Chlorinated hydrocarbons block physiologic inactivation in the sodium channels of nerve membranes and cause uncontrolled firing of action potentials. Tremor is usually the first sign of acute toxicity and may progress to seizures. Chronic exposure of animals to these pesticides is tumorigenic. The toxicologic impact of long-term exposure in humans is unclear. Although no relationship has been shown in humans between the risk of breast cancer and serum levels of DDT metabolites, recent evidence suggests an association with brain and testicular cancer.

2. Treatment—No specific treatment is available for the acute toxicity caused by chlorinated hydrocarbons. Because of their extremely long half-lives in organisms and in the environment (years), their use in North America and Europe has been curtailed.

C. Cholinestersase Inhibitors

The carbamates (eg, aldicarb, carbaryl) and organophosphates (eg, dichlorvos, malathion, parathion) are effective pesticides with short environmental half-lives. These inexpensive drugs are heavily used in agriculture.

1. Effects—As described in Chapter 7, cholinesterase inhibitors increase muscarinic and nicotinic cholinergic activity. The signs and symptoms include pinpoint pupils, sweating, salivation, bronchoconstriction, vomiting and diarrhea, CNS stimulation followed by depression, and muscle fasciculations, weakness, and paralysis. The most common cause of death is respiratory failure.

2. Treatment—Atropine is used in large doses to control muscarinic excess; pralidoxime is used to regenerate cholinesterase. Mechanical ventilation may be necessary.

D. Botanical Insecticides

1. Nicotine—Nicotine has the same effects on nicotinic cholinoceptors in insects as in mammals and probably kills by the same mechanism (ie, excitation followed by paralysis of ganglionic, CNS, and neuromuscular transmission). Treatment is supportive.

2. Rotenone—This plant alkaloid pesticide causes gastrointestinal distress when ingested and conjunctivitis and dermatitis after direct contact with exposed body surfaces. Treatment is symptomatic.

3. Pyrethrum—The most common toxic effect of this mixture of plant alkaloids is contact dermatitis. Ingestion or inhalation of large quantities may cause CNS excitation (including seizures) and peripheral neurotoxicity. Treatment is symptomatic, with anticonvulsants if necessary.

HERBICIDES

A. Chlorophenoxy Acids

The 2 most important members of this group are 2,4-dichlorophenoxyacetic acid and 2,4,5-trichlorophenoxyacetic acid, the compound in Agent Orange. 2,4,5-Trichlorophenoxyacetic acid is longer used because it is often contaminated during manufacturing with dioxin and other polychlorinates (see following text). Large doses of these drugs cause muscle hypotonia and coma. Long-term exposure has been associated with an increased risk of non-Hodgkin's lymphoma.

B. Glyphosate

Glyphosate is the most widely used herbicide in the world. It is a key enzyme involved in aromatic amino acid biosynthesis in plants.

1. Effects—Glyphosate exposure causes significant eye and skin irritation.

2. Treatment—No specific treatment is available.

C. Paraquat

Paraquat, a bipyridyl herbicide, is used extensively to kill weeds on farms and for highway maintenance.

1. Effects—The compound is relatively nontoxic unless ingested. After ingestion, the initial effect is gastrointestinal irritation with hematemesis and bloody stools. Within a few days, signs of pulmonary impairment occur and are usually progressive, resulting in severe pulmonary fibrosis and often death.

2. Treatment—No antidote is available; the best supportive treatment, including gastric lavage and dialysis, still results in less than 50% survival after ingestion of as little as 50–500 mg/kg.

ENVIRONMENTAL POLLUTANTS

Chemical compounds that contribute to environmental pollution include the polychlorinated biphenyls, dioxins, asbestos, and the heavy metals discussed in Chapter 57.

A. Polychlorinated Biphenyls

1. Source—The polychlorinated biphenyls (PCBs) were used extensively in manufacturing electrical equipment until their potential for environmental damage was recognized. PCBs are among the most stable organic compounds known. They are poorly metabolized and lipophilic. They are therefore highly persistent in the environment, and they accumulate in the food chain.

2. Effects—In workers exposed to PCBs, the most common effect is dermatotoxicity (acne, erythema, folliculitis, hyperkeratosis). Less frequently, mild increases in plasma triglycerides and elevated liver enzymes have been observed.

B. Dioxins

1. Source—The polychlorinated dibenzo-*p*-dioxins (dioxins) are a large group of related compounds of which the most important is 2,3,7,8-tetrachlorodibenzo-*p*-dioxin (TCDD). The dioxins have appeared in the environment as unwanted by-products of the chemical industry. They are chemically stable and highly resistant to environmental degradation.

2. Effects—In laboratory animals, exposure to TCDD causes a wasting syndrome, hepatotoxicity, immune dysfunction, teratogenicity, and cancer. In humans, the most common signs of toxicity are dermatitis and chloracne, which are cystic acneiform lesions that typically form on the face and upper body. Epidemiologic evidence suggests that the dioxins also have carcinogenic and teratogenic effects in humans.

C. Asbestos

1. Source—Asbestos is a group of naturally occurring long, flexible mineral fibers, most commonly containing silicon.

Asbestos has been used widely in manufacturing and building. Because it is poorly metabolized and lipophilic, it is highly persistent in the environment and accumulates in the food chain. Many countries have banned all use of asbestos because of its toxicity and strictly regulate handling of preexisting asbestos building products.

2. Effects—Inhalation of asbestos fibers can cause a fibrotic lung disorder called asbestosis, which is characterized by shortness of breath. Asbestos is also associated with several cancers including lung cancer, mesothelioma, and cancers of the gastrointestinal tract.

QUESTIONS

1. The light brownish color of smog often apparent in a major metropolitan area on a hot summer day is mainly due to
   (A) Carbon monoxide
   (B) Hydrocarbons
   (C) Ozone
   (D) Nitrogen dioxide
   (E) Sulfur dioxide

2. You are stuck in traffic in New York City in summer for 3 or 4 h and you begin to get a headache, a feeling of tightness in the temporal region, and an increased pulse rate. The most likely cause of these effects is inhalation of
   (A) Carbon monoxide
   (B) Nicotine
   (C) Nitrogen dioxide
   (D) Ozone
   (E) Sulfur dioxide

3. Toxicity that stems from exposure to parathion is treated with
   (A) Antiseizure drugs
   (B) Atropine and pralidoxime
   (C) Hemodialysis
   (D) Hyperbaric oxygen
   (E) Measures to reduce pulmonary edema

4. A compound that is toxic to bone marrow cells in the early stages of development and that may also be leukemogenic is
   (A) Benzene
   (B) Carbon monoxide
   (C) Glyphosate
   (D) DDT
   (E) Pyrethrum

5. A compound or group of compounds that damages the skin and whose use in manufacturing has largely been eliminated because of extensive persistence in the environment and bioaccumulation is
   (A) Aromatic hydrocarbons such as benzene
   (B) Dichlorvos
   (C) Phenoxyacetic acids such as 2,4-dichlorophenoxyacetic acid
   (D) Polychlorinated biphenyls (PCBs)
   (E) 2,3,7,8-tetrachlorodibenzo-*p*-dioxin (TCDD)

6. An employee of a company engaged in clearing vegetation from county roadsides accidentally ingested a small quantity of an herbicidal solution that contained paraquat. Within 2 h, he was admitted to the emergency department of a nearby hospital. Which of the following best describes his probable signs and symptoms in the emergency department?
(A) Diarrhea, vomiting, sweating, and profound skeletal muscle weakness
(B) Dizziness, nausea, agitation, and hyperreflexia
(C) Dyspnea, pulmonary dysfunction, and elevated body temperature
(D) Gastrointestinal irritation with hematemesis and bloody stools
(E) Hypotension, tachycardia, and respiratory impairment

7. Chemical warfare agents that had been manufactured in the 1950s were being stored at a military installation. Several civilian workers at the facility began to feel unwell, with symptoms that included dyspnea, abdominal cramps, and diarrhea. They also had copious nasal and tracheobronchial secretions. Which type of toxic compound is most likely to be the cause of these effects?
(A) Aliphatic hydrocarbons
(B) Botulinum toxins
(C) Nitrogen mustards
(D) Organophosphates
(E) Rotenones

DIRECTIONS: 8–10. The matching questions in this section consist of a list of lettered options followed by several numbered items. For each numbered item, select the ONE lettered option that is most closely associated with it. Each lettered option may be selected once, more than once, or not at all.
(A) Aldicarb
(B) Benzene
(C) Carbon monoxide
(D) Carbon dioxide
(E) DDT
(F) Dioxin
(G) Malathion
(H) Nitrogen dioxide
(I) Paraquat
(J) Pyrethrum
(K) Rotenone
(L) Sulfur dioxide
(M) Tetrachloroethylene
(N) Toluene

8. Asthma is often exacerbated in patients exposed to this reducing agent when concentrations in the air are as low as 1–2 ppm. It is formed mainly from combustion of fossil fuels.

9. Acute exposure to this *aliphatic* hydrocarbon solvent causes CNS depression; chronic exposure has led to impairment of memory and peripheral neuropathy.

10. This compound is a potential environmental hazard that is formed as a contaminating by-product in the manufacture of herbicides.

ANSWERS

1. Smog color is derived in part from suspended particulate matter. When smog is light brown, the color derives from nitrogen oxides. All of the other air pollutants listed are colorless. The answer is **D.**

2. The symptoms described are those of carbon monoxide inhalation. The answer is **A.**

3. Organophosphate poisoning is treated with the muscarinic receptor antagonist atropine and pralidoxime, which regenerates cholinesterase. The answer is **B.**

4. The aromatic hydrocarbon benzene is used as a solvent in industry. Long-term exposure is associated with increased risk of leukemia. The answer is **A.**

5. The polychlorinated biphenyls (PCBs) are dermatotoxic drugs that persist in the environment and accumulate in living organisms. PCBs have been banned from manufacture in the United States since 1979. However, many electrical transformers still retain traces of them. The answer is **D.**

6. Paraquat is highly corrosive to the gastrointestinal tract. Oral ingestion of the herbicide leads to marked gastrointestinal irritation, hematemesis, and usually blood in the stools. Signs of pulmonary impairment do not appear for several days and are usually progressive, resulting in severe pulmonary fibrosis and, often, death. The answer is **D.**

7. Highly potent organophosphate inhibitors of acetylcholinesterase (eg, sarin, tabun) have been developed for chemical warfare purposes. Their storage represents a potential toxicologic hazard. It is important to recognize the signs and symptoms of excess acetylcholine (DUMBBELSS; see Chapter 7), which include those described. The answer is **D.**

8. Sulfur dioxide is a reducing agent that forms sulfurous acid on contact with moist surfaces. This is responsible for irritant effects on mucous membranes of the eye, the oropharyngeal cavity, and the respiratory tract. Nitrogen dioxide causes similar problems, but it is an oxidizing agent formed from fires and in silage on farms. The answer is **L.**

9. Three hydrocarbon solvents are listed: benzene, tetrachloroethylene, and toluene. Each can cause CNS effects such as headache, fatigue, and loss of appetite. However, benzene and toluene are *aromatic* hydrocarbons. The answer is **M.**

10. Dioxin is a contaminant formed in the manufacture of chlorophenoxy acid herbicides, including 2,4-dichlorophenoxyacetic acid and 2,4,5-trichlorophenoxyacetic acid. The answer is **F.**

SKILL KEEPER ANSWER: SAFETY OF NEW DRUGS (SEE CHAPTER 5)

Acute toxicity studies in 2 animal species are required by the FDA for all new drugs before their use in humans. Subacute and chronic toxicity studies are required for drugs that are intended for chronic systemic use. Toxicity testing in animals usually involves the determination of lethal dose, monitoring of blood, hepatic, renal, and respiratory functions, gross and histopathologic examination of tissues, and tests of reproductive effects and potential carcinogenicity.

CHECKLIST

When you complete this chapter, you should be able to:

❏ List the major air pollutants and their clinical effects.

❏ Describe the signs and symptoms of carbon monoxide poisoning.

❏ Identify the major organ system toxicities of common solvents.

❏ Describe the signs, symptoms, and treatment of toxicity resulting from cholinesterase inhibitor insecticides.

❏ Identify the toxic effects of chlorinated hydrocarbons and botanical insecticides.

❏ List 2 important herbicides and their major toxicities.

❏ Appreciate the toxicologic significance of environmental pollution resulting from dioxins and polychlorinated biphenyls (PCBs).

Heavy Metals

The heavy metals discussed in this chapter—lead, arsenic, mercury, and iron—frequently cause toxicity in humans. The toxicity profiles of metals differ, but most of their effects appear to result from interaction with sulfhydryl groups of enzymes and regulatory proteins. Chelators are organic compounds with 2 or more electronegative groups that form stable bonds with cationic metal atoms. These stable complexes lack the toxicity of the free metals and often are excreted readily. Chelators, which function as chemical antagonists, are used as antidotes in the treatment of heavy metal poisoning.

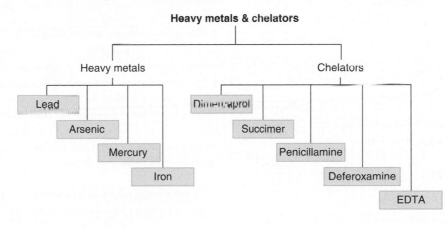

TOXICOLOGY OF HEAVY METALS

A. Lead

Lead serves no useful purpose in the body and can damage the hematopoietic tissues, liver, nervous system, kidneys, gastrointestinal tract, and reproductive system (Table 57–1). Lead is a major environmental hazard because it is present in the air and water throughout the world.

1. Acute lead poisoning—Because of the ban on lead over 20 years ago in gasoline, and because of bans on other industrial products that previously contained lead, acute inorganic lead poisoning is no longer common in the United States. It can occur rarely from industrial exposures (usually via the inhalation of dust) and in children who have ingested large quantities of chips or flakes from surfaces in older houses covered with lead-containing paint. The primary signs of this syndrome are acute abdominal colic and central nervous system (CNS) changes, including,

particularly in children, acute encephalopathy. The mortality rate is high in those with lead encephalopathy, and prompt chelation therapy is mandatory.

2. Chronic lead poisoning—Chronic inorganic lead poisoning (plumbism) is much more common than the acute form. Signs include peripheral neuropathy (wrist-drop is characteristic), anorexia, anemia, tremor, weight loss, and gastrointestinal symptoms. Treatment involves removal from the source of exposure, and chelation therapy, usually with oral succimer in outpatients and with parenteral agents (eg, EDTA with or without dimercaprol) in more severe cases. Chronic lead poisoning in children presents as growth retardation, neurocognitive deficits, and developmental delay. Succimer is generally used in such children. In workers exposed to lead, prophylaxis with oral chelating agents is contraindicated because some evidence suggests that lead absorption may be enhanced by the presence of chelators. In contrast, high dietary calcium is indicated because it impedes lead absorption.

3. Organic lead poisoning—Now rare, poisoning by organic lead was usually due to tetraethyl lead or tetramethyl lead contained in "antiknock" gasoline additives, which are no longer used. This form of lead is readily absorbed through the skin and lungs. The primary signs of intoxication include hallucinations, headache, irritability, convulsions, and coma. Treatment consists of decontamination and seizure control.

B. Arsenic

Arsenic is widely used in industrial processes and is also an environmental pollutant released during the burning of coal.

1. Acute arsenic poisoning—Acute arsenic poisoning results in severe gastrointestinal discomfort, vomiting, "rice-water" stools, and capillary damage with dehydration and shock. A sweet, garlicky odor may be detected in the breath and the stools. Treatment consists of supportive therapy to replace water and electrolytes, and chelation therapy with dimercaprol.

2. Chronic arsenic poisoning—Chronic arsenic intoxication causes skin changes, hair loss, bone marrow depression and anemia, and chronic nausea and gastrointestinal disturbances. Dimercaprol therapy appears to be of value. Arsenic is a known human carcinogen.

3. Arsine gas—Arsine gas (AsH_3), an occupational hazard, is formed during the refinement and processing of certain metals and is used in the semiconductor industry. Arsine causes a unique form of toxicity characterized by massive hemolysis. Pigment overload from erythrocyte breakdown can cause renal failure. Treatment is supportive.

C. Mercury

The main source of inorganic mercury as a toxic hazard is through the use of mercury-containing materials in dental laboratories and in the manufacture of wood preservatives, insecticides, and batteries. Organic mercury compounds are used as seed dressings (treatments to prevent fungal and bacterial infection of seed and to improve the seed's dispersion and adhesiveness) and fungicides.

1. Acute mercury poisoning—Acute mercury poisoning usually occurs through inhalation of inorganic elemental mercury. It causes chest pain, shortness of breath, nausea and vomiting, kidney damage, gastroenteritis, and CNS damage. In addition to intensive supportive care, prompt chelation with oral succimer or with intramuscular dimercaprol is essential. Acute ingestion of mercuric chloride causes a severe, life-threatening hemorrhagic gastroenteritis followed by renal failure.

2. Chronic mercury poisoning—Chronic mercury poisoning may occur with inorganic or organic mercury. Poisoning from inhalation of mercury vapor presents as a diffuse set of symptoms involving the gums and teeth, gastrointestinal disturbances, and neurologic and behavioral changes (erethism). Chronic mercury intoxication has been treated with succimer and unithiol, but their efficacy has not been established. Dimercaprol may redistribute mercury to the CNS and should not be used in chronic exposure to elemental mercury.

3. Organic mercury poisoning—Intoxication with organic mercury compounds was first recognized in connection with an epidemic of neurologic and psychiatric disease in the village of Minamata, Japan, which was first noticed in the 1950s. The outbreak was a result of consumption of fish containing a high content of methylmercury, which was produced by bacteria in seawater from mercury in the effluent of a nearby vinyl plastics-manufacturing plant. Similar epidemics have resulted from the consumption of grain that was intended for use as seed and treated with fungicidal organic mercury compounds. Treatment with chelators has been tried, but the benefits are uncertain.

D. Iron

Acute poisoning from the ingestion of ferrous sulfate tablets occurs frequently in small children, although the incidence of poisonings dropped dramatically in the United States after iron supplements were required to be packed in unit-dose packing. The initial symptoms of iron poisoning include vomiting, gastrointestinal bleeding, lethargy, and gray cyanosis. These can be followed by signs of severe gastrointestinal necrosis, pneumonitis, jaundice, seizures, and coma. Deferoxamine is the chelating agent of choice. Chronic excessive intake of iron can lead to hemosiderosis or hemochromatosis (see Chapter 33).

CHELATORS

Chelators used clinically include dimercaprol (BAL), succimer, unithiol, penicillamine, edetate (EDTA), deferoxamine, and deferasirox. Variations among these agents in their affinities for specific metals govern their clinical applications (Table 57–1).

A. Dimercaprol

Dimercaprol (2,3-dimercaptopropanol; BAL [British antilewisite]) is a bidentate chelator; that is, a chelator that forms 2 bonds with the metal ion, preventing the metal's binding to tissue proteins and permitting its rapid excretion.

1. Clinical use—Dimercaprol is used in acute arsenic and mercury poisoning and, in combination with EDTA, for lead poisoning. It is an oily liquid that must be given parenterally.

2. Toxicity—Dimercaprol causes a high incidence of adverse effects, possibly because it is highly lipophilic and readily enters cells. Its toxicity includes transient hypertension, tachycardia, headache, nausea and vomiting, paresthesias, and fever (especially in children). It may cause pain and hematomas at the injection site. Long-term use is associated with thrombocytopenia and increased prothrombin time.

B. Succimer

Succimer (2,3-dimercaptosuccinic acid; DMSA) is a water-soluble bidentate congener of dimercaprol.

1. Clinical use—Succimer is used for the oral treatment of lead toxicity in children and adults. It is as effective as parenteral EDTA in reducing blood lead concentration. Succimer is also effective in arsenic and mercury poisoning, if given within a few hours of exposure.

2. Toxicity—Although succimer appears to be less toxic than dimercaprol, gastrointestinal distress, CNS effects, skin rash, and elevation of liver enzymes may occur.

C. Unithiol

A water-soluble derivative of dimercaprol, unithiol can be administered orally or intravenously.

1. Clinical use—Intravenous unithiol is used in the initial treatment of severe acute poisoning by inorganic mercury or arsenic. Oral unithiol is an alternative to succimer in the treatment of lead intoxication.

2. Toxicity—Unithiol causes a low incidence of dermatological reactions, usually mild. Vasodilation and hypotension may occur with rapid intravenous infusion.

D. Penicillamine

Penicillamine, a derivative of penicillin, is another bidentate chelator.

1. Clinical use—The major uses of penicillamine are in the treatment of copper poisoning and Wilson's disease. It is sometimes used as adjunctive therapy in gold, arsenic, and lead intoxication and in rheumatoid arthritis. The agent is water-soluble, well absorbed from the gastrointestinal tract, and excreted unchanged.

TABLE 57–1 Important characteristics of the toxicology of arsenic, iron, lead, and mercury.

Metal	Form Entering Body	Route of Absorption	Target Organs for Toxicity	Treatment[a]
Lead	Inorganic lead oxides and salts	Gastrointestinal, respiratory, skin (minor)	Hematopoietic system, CNS, kidneys	Dimercaprol, EDTA, succimer, unithiol
	Tetraethyl lead	Skin (major), gastrointestinal	CNS	Seizure control
Arsenic	Inorganic arsenic salts	All mucous surfaces	Capillaries, gastrointestinal tract, hematopoietic system	Dimercaprol, unithiol, succimer, penicillamine
	Arsine gas	Inhalation	Erythrocytes	Supportive
Mercury	Elemental	Inhalation	CNS, kidneys	Succimer, unithiol
	Inorganic salts	Gastrointestinal	Kidneys, gastrointestinal tract	Succimer, unithiol, penicillamine, dimercaprol
	Organic mercurials	Gastrointestinal	CNS	Supportive
Iron	Ferrous sulfate	Gastrointestinal	Gastrointestinal, CNS, blood	Deferoxamine

[a]In all cases, removal of the person from the source of toxicity is the first requirement of management.

2. Toxicity—Adverse effects are common and may be severe. They include nephrotoxicity with proteinuria, pancytopenia, and autoimmune dysfunction, including lupus erythematosus and hemolytic anemia.

E. Ethylenedinitrilotetraacetic Acid

Ethylenedinitrilotetraacetic acid (EDTA; edetate) is an efficient polydentate chelator of many divalent cations, including calcium, and trivalent cations.

1. Clinical use—The primary use of EDTA is in the treatment of lead poisoning. Because the agent is highly polar, it is given parenterally. To prevent dangerous hypocalcemia, EDTA is given as the calcium disodium salt.

2. Toxicity—The most important adverse effect of the agent is nephrotoxicity, including renal tubular necrosis. This risk can be reduced by adequate hydration and restricting treatment with EDTA to 5 d or less. Electrocardiographic changes can occur at high doses.

F. Deferoxamine and Deferasirox

Deferoxamine is a polydentate bacterial product with an extremely high and selective affinity for iron and a much lower affinity for aluminum. Fortunately, the drug competes poorly for heme iron in hemoglobin and cytochromes. Deferasirox is a newer tridentate chelator with selectively high affinity for iron.

1. Clinical use—Deferoxamine is used parenterally in the treatment of acute iron intoxication and in the treatment of iron overload caused by blood transfusions in patients with diseases such as thalassemia or myelodysplastic syndrome (see Chapter 33). Deferasirox is an oral drug approved for treatment of iron overload.

2. Toxicity—Skin reactions (blushing, erythema, urticaria) may occur. With long-term use, neurotoxicity (eg, retinal degeneration), hepatic and renal dysfunction, and severe coagulopathies have been reported. Rapid intravenous administration of deferoxamine can cause histamine release and hypotensive shock.

QUESTIONS

1. A small child is brought to a hospital emergency department suffering from severe gastrointestinal distress and abdominal colic. If this patient has severe acute lead poisoning with signs and symptoms of encephalopathy, treatment should be instituted immediately with
   (A) Acetylcysteine
   (B) Deferoxamine
   (C) EDTA
   (D) Penicillamine
   (E) Succimer

2. A young woman employed as a dental laboratory technician complains of conjunctivitis, skin irritation, and hair loss. On examination, she has perforation of the nasal septum and a "milk and roses" complexion. These signs and symptoms are most likely due to
   (A) Acute mercury poisoning
   (B) Chronic inorganic arsenic poisoning
   (C) Chronic mercury poisoning
   (D) Excessive use of supplementary iron tablets
   (E) Lead poisoning

3. A patient complains of chronic headache, fatigue, loss of appetite, and constipation. He has slight weakness of the extensor muscles in the upper limbs. Based on the laboratory data in the table below, the most reasonable diagnosis is chronic poisoning caused by
   (A) Arsenic
   (B) Hexane
   (C) Inorganic lead
   (D) Iron
   (E) Mercuric chloride

Test	Result in Patient	Normal
Hemoglobin	<13 g/dL	>14 g/dL
Urinary coproporphyrin	>80 mcg/100 mg creatinine	<10 mcg/100 mg creatinine
Urinary aminolevulinic acid	>2 mg/100 mg creatinine	<0.5 mg/100 mg creatinine

4. In the treatment of acute inorganic arsenic poisoning, the most likely drug to be used is
   (A) Deferoxamine
   (B) Dimercaprol
   (C) EDTA
   (D) Penicillamine
   (E) Succimer

5. A 24-year-old man was employed in the supply department of a company that manufactures semiconductors. After an accident at the plant, he presented with nausea and vomiting, headache, hypotension, and shivering. Laboratory analyses showed hemoglobinuria and a plasma free hemoglobin level greater than 1.4 g/dL. This young man was probably exposed to
   (A) Arsine
   (B) Inorganic arsenic
   (C) Mercury vapor
   (D) Methylmercury
   (E) Tetraethyl lead

6. A 2-year-old child was brought to the emergency department 1 h after ingestion of tablets he had managed to obtain from a bottle on top of the refrigerator. His symptoms included marked gastrointestinal distress, vomiting (with hematemesis), and epigastric pain. Metabolic acidosis and leukocytosis were also present. This patient is most likely to have ingested tablets containing
   (A) Acetaminophen
   (B) Aspirin
   (C) Diphenhydramine
   (D) Iron
   (E) Vitamin C

DIRECTIONS: 7–10. The matching questions in this section consist of a list of lettered options followed by several numbered items. For each numbered item, select the ONE lettered option that is most closely associated with it. Each lettered option may be selected once, more than once, or not at all.

(A) Arsine
(B) Deferoxamine
(C) Dimercaprol
(D) Edetate calcium disodium
(E) Inorganic mercury
(F) Iron
(G) Methylmercury
(H) Mercury vapor
(I) Penicillamine
(J) Succimer
(K) Tetraethyl lead
(L) Trivalent arsenic

7. This toxic compound can be produced in seawater by the action of bacteria and algae. It is also synthesized chemically for commercial use as a fungicide.

8. This agent has been reported to cause lupus erythematosus and hemolytic anemia.

9. High doses of this agent can cause histamine release and extreme vasodilation.

10. Gingivitis, discolored gums, and loose teeth are common symptoms of chronic exposure to this agent.

ANSWERS

1. Encephalopathy in severe lead poisoning is a medical emergency. Of the drugs listed, intravenous EDTA is the most effective chelating agent. Oral succimer is used in children with mild to moderate lead poisoning and may be initiated 4–5 d after the parenteral use of EDTA or dimercaprol in severe poisoning. The answer is **C**.

2. The "milk and roses" complexion, which results from vasodilation and anemia, is a characteristic of chronic inorganic arsenic poisoning, whereas patients with lead poisoning often have a gray pallor. Other signs and symptoms of arsenic poisoning include gastrointestinal distress, hyperpigmentation, and white lines on the nails. We hope you were not led astray by her employment. The answer is **B**.

3. Of the agents listed, lead is most likely to cause a decrease in heme biosynthesis. The urinary concentrations of lead before and after EDTA treatment can confirm the diagnosis. The answer is **C**.

4. The treatment of choice in acute arsenic poisoning is intramuscular dimercaprol. Although succimer is less toxic, it is only available in an oral formulation, and its absorption may be impaired by the severe gastroenteritis that occurs in acute arsenic poisoning. The answer is **B**.

5. From the signs and symptoms alone, a diagnosis of arsine gas poisoning cannot be made. However, clues to the cause of poisoning are often provided by a patient's occupation. The laboratory reports suggest marked hemolysis. Arsine gas binds to hemoglobin and decreases erythrocyte glutathione levels, causing membrane fragility and resulting hemolysis. The answer is **A**.

6. This question emphasizes that the ingestion of iron tablets is a relatively common cause of accidental poisoning in young children. The signs and symptoms described usually occur in the first 6 h after ingestion. In a child whose body weight is 22 lb, the ingestion of 600 mg can cause severe, perhaps lethal, toxicity. The answer is **D**.

7. Methylmercury is used as a fungicide to prevent mold growth in seed grain. The answer is **G**.

8. Autoimmune diseases such as lupus erythematosus and hemolytic anemia have occurred during the treatment of Wilson's disease with penicillamine. The answer is **I**.

9. Deferoxamine can cause shock if given by rapid intravenous infusion. The answer is **B**.

10. Oral and gastrointestinal complaints are common in chronic mercury poisoning, and tremor involving the fingers and arms is often present. The answer is **E**.

SKILL KEEPER ANSWERS: IRON DEFICIENCY (SEE CHAPTER 33)

1. *Regulation of total body iron occurs through a tightly regulated system of intestinal absorption. Iron is absorbed and either stored in mucosal cells as ferritin or transported into blood and distributed throughout the body bound to transferrin. Most of the iron in the body is present in hemoglobin. Small quantities of iron are eliminated in sweat, saliva, and the exfoliation of skin and mucosal cells*

2. *Iron deficiency can be diagnosed from red blood cell changes, including microcytic size and decreased hemoglobin content, and from measurement of serum and bone marrow iron stores. Iron deficiency anemia is treated by dietary oral ferrous iron supplements or, in severe cases, parenteral administration of a colloid containing a core of iron oxyhydroxide surrounded by a core of carbohydrate.*

CHECKLIST

When you complete this chapter, you should be able to:

❑ Describe the general mechanism of metal chelation.

❑ Identify the clinically useful chelators and know their indications and their adverse effects.

❑ Describe the major clinical features and treatment of acute and chronic lead poisoning.

❑ Describe the major clinical features and treatment of arsenic poisoning.

❑ Describe the major clinical features and treatment of inorganic and organic mercury poisoning.

❑ Describe the major clinical features and treatment of iron poisoning.

DRUG SUMMARY TABLE: Heavy Metal Chelators

Drugs	Mechanism of Action	Clinical Applications	Pharmacokinetics	Toxicities, Interactions
EDTA (ethylenediamine-tetraacetic acid; edetate)	Chelator of many divalent and trivalent metals	Lead poisoning • poisoning by zinc, manganese, and certain heavy radionuclides	Parenteral	Administered as calcium disodium salt to avoid calcium depletion • nephrotoxicity, ECG changes
Deferoxamine	Chelates excess iron	Acute iron poisoning • inherited or acquired hemochromatosis	Preferred route of administration: Intramuscular or subcutaneous	Rapid IV administration may cause hypotension • neurotoxicity and increased susceptibility to certain infections have occurred with long-term use
Deferasirox: oral iron chelator for treatment of hemochromatosis				
Dimercaprol	Bidentate chelator forms 2 bonds with metal ions	Arsenic and inorganic mercury poisoning • combined with EDTA for lead poisoning	Parenteral	Transient hypertension, tachycardia, headache, nausea, vomiting, paresthesias, fever • thrombocytopenia and increased prothrombin time with long-term use
Succimer: water-soluble congener of dimercaprol used for oral treatment of lead poisoning *Unithiol*: water-soluble congener of dimercaprol used intravenously for initial treatment of severe mercury or arsenic poisoning and used orally for lead poisoning				
Penicillamine	Bidentate chelator	Copper poisoning and Wilson's disease	Oral	Nephrotoxicity, pancytopenia, autoimmune dysfunction, including lupus erythematosus and hemolytic anemia

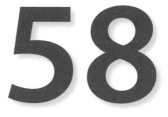

Management of the Poisoned Patient

Toxic substances include therapeutic agents as well as agricultural and industrial chemicals that have no medical applications. Most chemicals are capable of causing toxic effects when given in excessive dosage; even for therapeutic drugs, the difference between a therapeutic action and a toxic one is most often a matter of dose. Many toxic effects of therapeutic agents have been discussed in previous chapters. Common toxic syndromes associated with major drug groups are summarized in this chapter. This chapter also reviews the principles of management of the poisoned patient.

TOXICOKINETICS, TOXICODYNAMICS, & CAUSE OF DEATH

A. Toxicokinetics

This term denotes the disposition of poisons in the body (ie, their pharmacokinetics). Knowledge of a toxin's absorption, distribution, and elimination permits assessment of the value of procedures designed to remove it from the skin or gastrointestinal tract. For example, drugs with large apparent volumes of distribution, such as antidepressants and antimalarials, are not amenable to dialysis procedures for drug removal. Drugs with low volumes of distribution, including lithium, phenytoin, and salicylates, are more readily removed by dialysis and diuresis procedures. In some cases, renal elimination of weak acids can be accelerated by urinary alkalinization, whereas renal elimination of some weak bases can be accelerated by urinary acidification. The clearance of drugs may be different at toxic concentrations than at therapeutic concentrations. For example, in overdoses of phenytoin or salicylates, the capacity of the liver to metabolize the drugs is usually exceeded, and elimination changes from first-order (constant half-life) to zero-order (variable half-life) kinetics.

B. Toxicodynamics

Toxicodynamics denotes the injurious effects of toxins (pharmacodynamic effects). A knowledge of toxicodynamics can be useful in the diagnosis and management of poisoning. For example, hypertension and tachycardia are typically seen in overdoses with amphetamines, cocaine, and antimuscarinic drugs. Hypotension with bradycardia occurs with overdoses of calcium channel blockers, β blockers, and sedative-hypnotics. Hypotension with tachycardia occurs with tricyclic antidepressants, phenothiazines, and theophylline. Hyperthermia is most frequently a result of overdose of drugs with antimuscarinic actions, the salicylates, or sympathomimetics. Hypothermia is more likely to occur with toxic doses of ethanol and other central nervous system (CNS) depressants. Increased respiratory rate is often a feature of overdose with carbon monoxide, salicylates, and other drugs that cause metabolic acidosis or cellular asphyxia. Overdoses of agents that depress the heart are likely to affect the functions of all organ systems that are critically dependent on blood flow, including the brain, liver, and kidney.

C. Cause of Death in Intoxicated Patients

The most common causes of death from drug overdose reflect the drug groups most often selected for abuse or for suicide. Sedative-hypnotics and opioids cause respiratory depression, coma, aspiration of gastric contents, and other respiratory malfunctions. Drugs such as cocaine, phencyclidine (PCP), tricyclic antidepressants, and theophylline cause seizures, which may lead to vomiting and aspiration of gastric contents and to postictal respiratory depression. Tricyclic antidepressants and cardiac glycosides cause dangerous and frequently lethal arrhythmias. Severe hypotension can occur with any of these drugs. A few intoxicants directly damage the liver and kidney. These include acetaminophen, mushroom poisons of the *Amanita phalloides* type, certain inhalants, and some heavy metals. (see Chapter 57).

MANAGEMENT OF THE POISONED PATIENT

Management of the poisoned patient consists of maintenance of vital functions, identification of the toxic substance, decontamination procedures, enhancement of elimination, and, in a few instances, administration of a specific antidote.

High-Yield Terms to Learn

ABCDs	Mnemonic for the supportive initial treatment of all poisoned patients that stands for **A**irway, **B**reathing, **C**irculation, and **D**extrose or **D**econtamination
Anion gap	The difference between the serum concentrations of the major cations (Na^+/K^+) and (HCO_3^-/Cl^-); an increased anion gap indicates the presence of extra anions and is most commonly caused by metabolic acidosis
Antidote	A substance that counteracts the effect of a poison
Osmolar gap	The difference between the measured serum osmolality and the osmolality that is calculated from serum concentrations of sodium, glucose, and BUN; an increased osmolar gap is associated with poisoning due to ethanol and other alcohols

A. Vital Functions

The most important aspect of treatment of a poisoned patient is maintenance of vital functions, as indicated by the mnemonic, ABCDs. The most commonly endangered or impaired vital function is respiration. Therefore, an open and protected airway (**A**) must be established first and effective ventilation (**B** for breathing) must be ensured. The circulation (**C**) should be evaluated and supported as needed. The cardiac rhythm should be determined, and if ventricular fibrillation is present, it must be corrected at once. The blood pressure should be measured but rarely needs immediate treatment except in cases of traumatic hemorrhage. Because of the danger of brain damage from hypoglycemia, intravenous 50% dextrose (**D**) should be given to comatose patients immediately after blood has been drawn for laboratory tests and before laboratory results have been obtained. Thiamine should be administered to prevent Wernicke's syndrome in patients with suspected alcoholism or malnourishment. In patients with signs of respiratory or CNS depression, intravenous naloxone offsets possible toxic effects of opioid analgesic overdose.

B. Identification of Poisons

Many intoxicants cause a characteristic syndrome of clinical and laboratory changes. Table 58–1 summarizes toxic syndromes associated with major drug groups and the key interventions called for. The toxic features of selected individual agents are listed in Table 58–2. When the toxic agent cannot be directly examined and identified, the clinician must rely on indirect means to identify the type of intoxication and the progress of therapy. In addition to the history and physical examination, certain laboratory examinations may be useful. A few intoxicants can be directly identified in the blood or urine, especially when information in the history narrows the search. In the more common situation of a comatose patient unable to provide a history, general tests for replacement of anions or osmotic equivalents in the blood (anion gap, osmolar gap) may be useful. A few intoxicants can be identified or strongly suspected on the basis of electrocardiographic or radiologic findings.

1. Osmolar gap—The osmolar gap is the difference between the measured serum osmolarity (measured by the freezing point depression method) and the osmolarity predicted by measured serum concentrations of sodium glucose and BUN:

$$Gap = Osm \text{ (measured)} - [(2 \times Na^+ \text{ [mEQ/L]})$$
$$+ (Glucose \text{ [mg/dL]} \div 18) + (BUN \text{[mg/dL]} \div 3)]$$

This gap is normally zero. A significant gap is produced by high serum concentrations of intoxicants of low molecular weight such as ethanol, methanol, and ethylene glycol.

2. Anion gap—The anion gap is the difference between the sum of the measured serum concentrations of the 2 primary cations, sodium and potassium, and the sum of the measured serum concentrations of the 2 primary anions, chloride and bicarbonate:

$$Anion \text{ } gap = (Na^+ + K^+) - (HCO_3^- + Cl^-)$$

This gap is normally 12–16 mEq/L. A significant increase can be produced by diabetic ketoacidosis, renal failure, or drug-induced metabolic acidosis. Drugs that cause an anion gap include cyanide, ethanol, ethylene glycol, ibuprofen, isoniazid, iron, methanol, phenelzine, salicylates, tranylcypromine, valproic acid, and verapamil.

3. Serum potassium—Myocardial function is critically dependent on serum potassium level. Drugs that cause hyperkalemia include β-adrenoceptor blockers, digitalis (in overdose), fluoride, lithium, and potassium-sparing diuretics. Drugs associated with hypokalemia include barium, β-adrenoceptor agonists, methylxanthines, most diuretics, and toluene.

C. Decontamination

Decontamination is the removal of any unabsorbed poison from the skin or gastrointestinal tract (Figure 58–1). In the case of topical exposure (insecticides, solvents), the clothing should be removed and the patient washed to remove any chemical still

TABLE 58–1 Toxic syndromes caused by major drug groups.

Drug Group	Clinical Features	Key Interventions
Antimuscarinic drugs (anticholinergics)	Delirium, hallucinations, seizures, coma, tachycardia, hypertension, hyperthermia, mydriasis, decreased bowel sounds, urinary retention	Control hyperthermia; physostigmine may be helpful, but not for tricyclic overdose
Cholinomimetic drugs (carbamate or organophosphate cholinesterase inhibitors)	Anxiety, agitation, seizures, coma, bradycardia or tachycardia, pinpoint pupils, salivation, sweating, hyperactive bowel, muscle fasciculations, then paralysis	Support respiration. Treat with atropine and pralidoxime. Decontaminate
Opioids (eg, heroin, morphine, methadone)	Lethargy, sedation, coma, bradycardia, hypotension, hypoventilation, pinpoint pupils, cool skin, decreased bowel sounds, flaccid muscles	Provide airway and respiratory support. Give naloxone as required
Salicylates (eg, aspirin)	Confusion, lethargy, coma, seizures, hyperventilation, hyperthermia, dehydration, hypokalemia, anion gap metabolic acidosis	Correct acidosis and fluid and electrolyte imbalance. Alkaline diuresis or hemodialysis to aid elimination
Sedative-hypnotics (barbiturates, benzodiazepines, ethanol)	Disinhibition initially, later lethargy, stupor, coma. Nystagmus is common, decreased muscle tone, hypothermia. Small pupils, hypotension, and decreased bowel sounds in severe overdose	Provide airway and respiratory support. Avoid fluid overload. Consider flumazenil for benzodiazepine overdose
Stimulants (amphetamines, cocaine, phencyclidine [PCP])	Agitation, anxiety, seizures. Hypertension, tachycardia, arrhythmias. Mydriasis, vertical and horizontal nystagmus with PCP. Skin warm and sweaty, hyperthermia, increased muscle tone, possible rhabdomyolysis	Control seizures, hypertension, and hyperthermia
Tricyclic antidepressants	Antimuscarinic effects (see above). The "3 C's" of coma, convulsions, cardiac toxicity (widened QRS, arrhythmias, hypotension)	Control seizures. Correct acidosis and cardiotoxicity with ventilation, sodium bicarbonate, and norepinephrine (for hypotension). Control hyperthermia

TABLE 58–2 Toxic features of selected agents.

Agent	Toxic Features
Acetaminophen	Mild anorexia, nausea, vomiting, delayed jaundice, hepatic and renal failure
Botulism	Dysphagia, dysarthria, ptosis, ophthalmoplegia, muscle weakness; incubation period 12–36 h
Carbon monoxide	Coma, metabolic acidosis, retinal hemorrhages
Cyanide	Bitter almond odor, seizures, coma, abnormal ECG
Ethylene glycol	Renal failure, crystals in urine, increased anion and osmolar gap, initial CNS excitation; eye examination normal
Iron	Bloody diarrhea, coma, radiopaque material in gut (seen on x-ray), high leukocyte count, hyperglycemia
Lead	Abdominal pain, hypertension, seizures, muscle weakness, metallic taste, anorexia, encephalopathy, delayed motor neuropathy, changes in renal and reproductive function
Lysergic acid (LSD)	Hallucinations, dilated pupils, hypertension
Mercury	Acute renal failure, tremor, salivation, gingivitis, colitis, erethism (fits of crying, irrational behavior), nephrotic syndrome
Methanol	Rapid respiration, visual symptoms, osmolar gap, severe metabolic acidosis
Mushrooms (*Amanita phalloides* type)	Severe nausea and vomiting 8 h after ingestion; delayed hepatic and renal failure
Phencyclidine (PCP)	Coma with eyes open, horizontal and vertical nystagmus

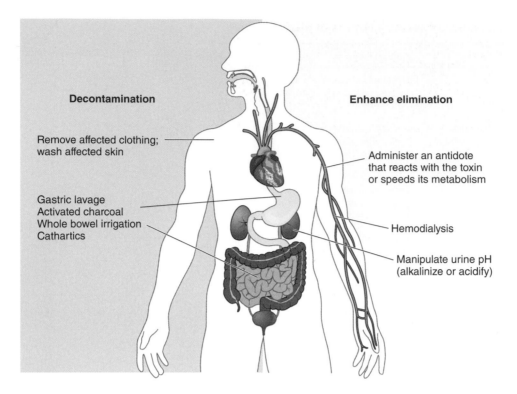

FIGURE 58-1 Important measures for the decontamination and enhanced elimination in poisonings.

present on the skin. Medical personnel must be careful not to contaminate themselves during this procedure. For most cases of ingested toxins, **activated charcoal,** given orally or by stomach tube, is very effective in adsorbing any toxin remaining in the gut. Poisons that can be removed by multiple treatments with activated charcoal include amitriptyline, barbiturates, carbamazepine, digitalis glycosides, phencyclidine, propoxyphene, theophylline, tricyclic antidepressants, and valproic acid. Charcoal does *not* bind iron, lithium, or potassium, and it binds alcohols and cyanide poorly. Less commonly, **gastric lavage** with a large-bore tube is used to remove noncorrosive drugs from the stomach of an awake patient or from a comatose patient whose airway has been protected with a cuffed endotracheal tube. In the past, decontamination was attempted by inducing vomiting (emesis), mostly by administering **syrup of ipecac** in a conscious patient. (*Fluid extract* of ipecac should not be used because it contains cardiotoxic alkaloids.) However, this approach has fallen out of favor because the risks involved, particularly of aspiration, have been shown to outweigh the benefits. **Whole bowel irrigation** with a balanced polyethylene-glycol electrolyte solution can enhance gut decontamination of iron tablets, enteric-coated pills, and illicit drug-filled packets. **Cathartics** such as sorbitol can decrease absorption and hasten removal of toxins from the gastrointestinal tract.

D. Enhancement of Elimination

Enhancement of elimination is possible for some toxins (Figure 58–1), including manipulation of urine pH to accelerate renal excretion of weak acids and bases. For example, alkaline diuresis is effective in

toxicity caused by fluoride, isoniazid, fluoroquinolones, phenobarbital, and salicylates. Urinary acidification may be useful in toxicity caused by weak bases, including amphetamines, nicotine, and phencyclidine, but care must be taken to prevent acidosis and renal failure in rhabdomyolysis. **Hemodialysis,** an extracorporeal circulation procedure in which a patient's blood is pumped through a column containing a semipermeable membrane that allows the removal of many toxic compounds, is used commonly to remove toxins such as ethylene glycol, lithium, metformin, procainamide, salicylates, and valproic acid, and to correct fluid and electrolyte imbalances.

SKILL KEEPER: CYANIDE POISONING (SEE CHAPTERS 11, 12, AND 33)

Cyanide forms a stable complex with the ferric ion of cytochrome oxidase enzymes and inhibits cellular respiration. What is the connection between the management of cyanide poisoning and the drugs amyl nitrite and nitroprusside? The Skill Keeper Answer appears at the end of the chapter.

E. Antidotes

Antidotes exist for several important poisons (Table 58–3). Since the duration of action of some antidotes is shorter than that of the intoxicant, the antidotes may need to be given repeatedly. The use of chelating agents for metal poisoning is discussed in Chapter 57.

TABLE 58–3 Important antidotes.

Antidote	Poison(s)
Acetylcysteine	Acetaminophen; best given within 8–10 h of overdose
Atropine	Cholinesterase inhibitors
Bicarbonate, sodium	Membrane-depressant cardiotoxic drugs (eg, quinidine, tricyclic antidepressants)
Calcium	Fluoride; calcium channel blockers
Deferoxamine	Iron salts
Digoxin antibodies	Digoxin and related cardiac glycoside
Esmolol	Caffeine, theophylline, sympathomimetics
Ethanol	Methanol, ethylene glycol
Flumazenil	Benzodiazepines, zolpidem
Fomepizole	Methanol, ethylene glycol
Glucagon	Beta adrenoceptor blockers
Glucose	Hypoglycemics
Hydroxocobalamin	Cyanide
Naloxone	Opioid analgesics
Oxygen	Carbon monoxide
Physostigmine	"Suggested" for muscarinic receptor blockers, NOT tricyclics
Pralidoxime	Organophosphate cholinesterase inhibitors

(Modified and reproduced, with permission, from Katzung BG, editor: *Basic & Clinical Pharmacology*, 12th ed. McGraw-Hill, 2012: Table 58–4.)

QUESTIONS

1–3. A 2-yr-old girl presented with lethargy, increased respiratory rate, and an elevated temperature that appeared to result from a drug poisoning. Laboratory testing revealed the following serum concentrations: glucose, 36 mg/dL; Na$^+$, 148 mEq/L; K$^+$, 5 mEq/L; Cl$^-$, 111 mEq/L; HCO$_3^-$, 12 mEq/L; BUN, 21 mg/dL; osmolality, 300 mOsm/L.

1. The anion gap in this patient is
   (A) −60 mEq/L
   (B) −20 mEq/L
   (C) +5 mEq/L
   (D) +30 mEq/L
   (E) +304 mEq/L

2. The osmolar gap in this patient is
   (A) −40 mOsm/L
   (B) −5 mOsm/L
   (C) +15 mOsm/L
   (D) +60 mOsm/L
   (E) +305 mOsm/L

3. The patient's signs, symptoms, and laboratory values are *most* consistent with an overdose of
   (A) Acetaminophen
   (B) Aspirin
   (C) Ethylene glycol
   (D) Lead
   (E) Phencyclidine

4. An 18-month-old boy presented in a semiconscious state with profound hypotension and bradycardia after ingesting a number of his grandmother's metoprolol tablets. In this case, the *most* appropriate antidote is
   (A) Atropine
   (B) Esmolol
   (C) Glucagon
   (D) Naloxone
   (E) Neostigmine

5. An 81-year-old woman with type 2 diabetes presents to the emergency department in a coma and with tachypnea, tachycardia, hypotension, and severe lactic acidosis approximately 9 hr after ingesting a number of her metformin tablets. Her serum glucose concentration was 148 mg/dL. Metformin is a base with a pK_a of 12.4. The procedure that is *most* likely to improve her condition is
   (A) Administration of activated charcoal
   (B) Administration of glucagon
   (C) Administration of syrup of ipecac
   (D) Gastric lavage
   (E) Hemodialysis

6. Which drug is *most* likely to cause hypotension, seizures, and cardiac arrhythmia when taken in overdose?
   (A) Acetaminophen
   (B) Diazepam
   (C) Ethylene glycol
   (D) Morphine
   (E) Tricyclic antidepressant

7. A patient with heart failure has accidentally taken an overdose of digoxin. The blood concentration of the drug is 8 times the threshold for toxicity. Pharmacokinetic parameters for digoxin include a clearance of 7 L/h and an elimination half-life of 56 h. If no procedures are instituted to decontaminate this patient, the time taken to reach a safe level of digoxin will be approximately
   (A) 3.5 d
   (B) 7 d
   (C) 14 d
   (D) 28 d
   (E) 56 d

Questions 8 and 9. A patient is brought to the emergency department having taken an overdose (unknown quantity) of a sustained-release preparation of theophylline by oral administration 2 h previously. He has marked gastrointestinal distress with vomiting and is agitated and exhibits hyperreflexia, and hypotension.

8. The plasma level of theophylline measured immediately upon hospitalization was 80 mg/L. If the oral bioavailability of theophylline is 98%, the clearance is 50 mL/min, volume of distribution is 35 L, and the elimination half-life is 7.5 h, the amount ingested must have been at least
   (A) 0.3 g
   (B) 0.6 g
   (C) 1.6 g
   (D) 2.8 g
   (E) 8.0 g

9. A short-acting antidote that can reduce this patient's tachycardia is
   (A) Acetylcysteine
   (B) Deferoxamine
   (C) Esmolol
   (D) Fomepizole
   (E) Pralidoxime

10. A contraindication to the use of gastric lavage for the removal of drugs from the stomach of victim of poisoning is
   (A) An overdose of iron pills
   (B) An unconscious patient
   (C) Ingestion of a corrosive
   (D) Overdose with a sustained-release formulation

ANSWERS

1. Anion gap is calculated by subtracting measured serum anions (bicarbonate plus chloride) from cations (potassium plus sodium). Increases in anion gap above normal are due to the presence of unmeasured anions that accompany acidosis. The gap in this case is 30 mEq/L, a value that is well in excess of the normal gap (12–16 mEq/L). The answer is **D**.

2. The osmolar gap is the difference between the measured serum osmolality and the osmolarity calculated from the serum sodium, glucose, and BUN concentrations according to the equation above for calculating the osmolar gap. In this case, the measured osmolality is 300 mOsm/L, whereas the calculated osmolality is 305 mOsm/L; the difference is −5 mOsm/L. The answer is **B**.

3. Of the drugs listed, the 2 that are likely to cause an anion gap are aspirin and ethylene glycol. However, if the child had ingested ethylene glycol, she would be expected to exhibit a significant osmolar gap. The anion gap, lethargy, tachypnea, and hyperthermia all are consistent with aspirin poisoning. The answer is **B**.

4. Glucagon (Chapter 41) stimulates heart rate and contractility through cardiac glucagon receptors that are coupled to adenylyl cyclase and the cAMP signaling pathway. This ability to increase cardiac cAMP without requiring access to β receptors makes it valuable for β-blocker overdose. The answer is **C**.

5. In this woman with severe signs of poisoning due to the ingestion of metformin, hemodialysis can be used to accelerate the elimination of both metformin and lactic acid. Since most of the metformin has been absorbed by the time she presented (9 hrs after drug ingestion), efforts to decontaminate her gastrointestinal tract with activated charcoal, gastric lavage, or syrup of ipecac are unlikely to be beneficial. Furthermore, syrup of ipecac has fallen out of favor and should not be used in unconscious patient. Unlike other drugs used to treat type 2 diabetes, metformin in overdose is unlikely to cause hypoglycemia (see Chapter 41), and this patient's serum glucose is in the normal range so that glucagon administration is not required. The answer is **E**.

6. Tricyclic antidepressants are extremely toxic in overdose because of their effects in the CNS and cardiovascular systems. In addition to hypotension, seizures, and cardiac arrhythmias, the tricyclics have strong antimuscarinic effects. The answer is **E**.

7. Estimations of the time period required for drug or toxin elimination may be of value in the management of the poisoned patient. If no procedures were used to hasten the elimination of digoxin in this patient, the time taken to reach a safe plasma level of the drug (12.5% of the measured level) is 3 half-lives, or approximately 7 d. The answer is **B**.

8. Estimations of the quantity of a drug or toxin ingested may be of value in the management of the poisoned patient. Applying toxicokinetic principles, a rough estimate of ingested dose of theophylline could be made by multiplying the peak plasma level of the drug (80 mg/L) by its volume of distribution (35 L) to give a value of 2800 mg, or 2.8 g. Because only about one-fourth of a half-life has passed since ingestion, the amount eliminated since that time will be rather small. The answer is **D**.

9. The short-acting β blocker esmolol helps reverse the tachycardia and possibly the vasodilation associated with an overdose of theophylline. The answer is **C.**

10. Neither gastric lavage nor syrup of ipecac should be used in patients who have ingested a corrosive because of the risk of esophageal damage. Gastric lavage can be used in a comatose patient if the airway has been protected with a cuffed endotracheal tube. The answer is **C.**

> ## SKILL KEEPER ANSWER: CYANIDE POISONING (SEE CHAPTERS 11, 12, AND 33)
>
> *The conventional cyanide antidote kit contains amyl nitrite, sodium nitrite, and sodium thiosulfate. The nitrites convert hemoglobin to methemoglobin, which has a higher affinity for the cyanide ion (forming cyanomethemoglobin) than cytochrome oxidase. It is the inhibition by cyanide of cytochrome oxidase that blocks oxidative metabolism and causes much of the toxicity. The sodium thiosulfate reacts with cyanide to form nontoxic thiocyanate ions. A newer cyanide antidote kit contains hydroxocobalamin, a form of vitamin B12 that rapidly reacts with cyanide to form the nontoxic cyanocobalamin. Nitroprusside, a compound with 5 cyanide molecules complexed to a central iron atom, is often considered the drug of choice in severe hypertension. Prolonged use of nitroprusside may result in toxicity caused by the release of cyanide.*

CHECKLIST

When you complete this chapter, you should be able to:

❏ Describe the steps involved in the supportive care of the poisoned patient.

❏ Identify toxic syndromes associated with overdose of the major drugs or drug groups frequently involved in poisoning.

❏ Outline methods for identifying toxic compounds, including descriptive signs and symptoms and laboratory methods.

❏ Describe the methods available for decontamination of poisoned patients and for increasing the elimination of toxic compounds.

❏ List the antidotes available for management of the poisoned patient.

Drugs Used in Gastrointestinal Disorders

C H A P T E R

59

The gastrointestinal tract serves many important functions: digestive, excretory, endocrine, exocrine, and so on. These functions are the targets of several important classes of drugs.

Some of these drugs have been discussed previously. This chapter mentions them and discusses in more detail others that do not fall into the classes of agents described previously.

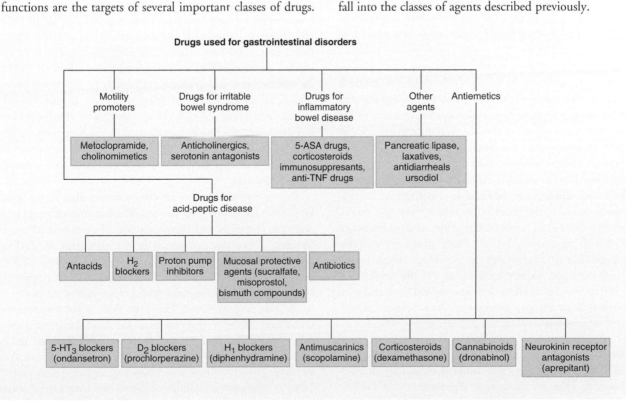

Acid-peptic disease	A group of disorders involving erosion or ulceration of the mucosal lining of the gastrointestinal tract; includes GERD, gastric and duodenal ulcers, nonulcer dyspepsia, and stress-related gastritis
Antiemetic	A drug that reduces nausea and vomiting
Gastroesophageal reflux disease (GERD)	Esophageal irritation or inflammation due to reflux of stomach acid; also known as heartburn
Gastroparesis	Paralysis of the muscles of the stomach and possibly other parts of the gastrointestinal tract due to damage to gastrointestinal nerves or muscle; common in advanced diabetes and advanced Parkinson disease
Inflammatory bowel disease (IBD)	Inflammatory disorder involving irritation and ulceration of the colon and rectum (ulcerative colitis) or the colon plus more proximal parts of the gastrointestinal tract (Crohn's disease)
Irritable bowel syndrome (IBS)	Disease of unknown origin characterized by episodes of abdominal discomfort and abnormal bowel function (diarrhea, constipation, or both)
Prokinetic	A drug that promotes gastrointestinal motility
Proton pump	The parietal cell H^+/K^+ ATPase that uses the energy of ATP to secrete protons into the stomach (Figure 59–1); final common target of drugs that suppress acid secretion

A. Drugs Used in Acid-Peptic Disease

Ulceration and erosion of the lining of the upper portion of the gastrointestinal tract are common problems that manifest as gastroesophageal reflux disease (GERD), gastric and duodenal peptic ulcers, and stress-related mucosal injury. Drugs used in acid-peptic disease reduce intragastric acidity by manipulating systems controlling hydrogen acid secretion (Figure 59–1), promote mucosal defense or, in the case of peptic ulcers, eradicate the bacterium *Helicobacter pylori,* which is detectable in over 80% of patients with duodenal ulcers.

1. Antacids—Antacids are weak bases that neutralize stomach acid by reacting with protons in the lumen of the gut and may also stimulate the protective functions of the gastric mucosa. When used regularly in the large doses needed to significantly raise the stomach pH, antacids reduce the recurrence rate of peptic ulcers.

The antacids differ mainly in their absorption and effects on stool consistency. Popular antacids include **magnesium hydroxide** ($Mg[OH]_2$) and **aluminum hydroxide** ($Al[OH]_3$). Neither of these weak bases is significantly absorbed from the bowel. Magnesium hydroxide has a strong laxative effect, whereas aluminum hydroxide has a constipating action. These drugs are available as single-ingredient products and as combined preparations. Calcium carbonate and sodium bicarbonate are also weak bases, but they differ from aluminum and magnesium hydroxides in being absorbed from the gut. Because of their systemic effects, calcium and bicarbonate salts are less popular as antacids.

2. H_2-receptor antagonists—**Cimetidine** and other H_2 antagonists (ranitidine, famotidine, and nizatidine) inhibit stomach acid production. They are effective in the treatment of GERD, peptic ulcer disease, and nonulcer dyspepsia and in the prevention of stress-related gastritis in seriously ill patients. Although they are still used widely, their clinical use is being supplanted by the more effective and equally safe proton pump inhibitors. The H_2 antagonists are described in detail in Chapter 16.

3. Proton pump inhibitors—**Omeprazole** and other proton pump inhibitors (esomeprazole, lansoprazole, pantoprazole, and rabeprazole) are lipophilic weak bases that diffuse into the parietal cell canaliculi, where they become protonated and concentrated more than 1000-fold. There they undergo conversion to compounds that irreversibly inactivate the parietal cell H^+/K^+ ATPase, the transporter that is primarily responsible for producing stomach acid. Oral formulations of these drugs are enteric coated to prevent acid inactivation in the stomach. After absorption in the intestine, they are rapidly metabolized in the liver, with half-lives of 1–2 h. However, their durations of action are approximately 24 h, and they may require 3–4 d of treatment to achieve their full effectiveness.

Proton pump inhibitors are more effective than H_2 antagonists for GERD and peptic ulcer and equally effective in the treatment of nonulcer dyspepsia and the prevention of stress-related mucosal bleeding. They are also useful in the treatment of Zollinger-Ellison syndrome. Adverse effects of proton pump inhibitors occur infrequently and include diarrhea, abdominal pain, and headache. Chronic treatment with proton pump inhibitors may result in hypergastrinemia. However, there is no documentation that the use of these drugs increases the incidence of carcinoid or colon cancer. Proton pump inhibitors may decrease the oral bioavailability of vitamin B_{12} and certain drugs that require acidity for their gastrointestinal absorption (eg, digoxin, ketoconazole). Patients taking proton pump inhibitors may have a small increase in the risk of respiratory and enteric infections.

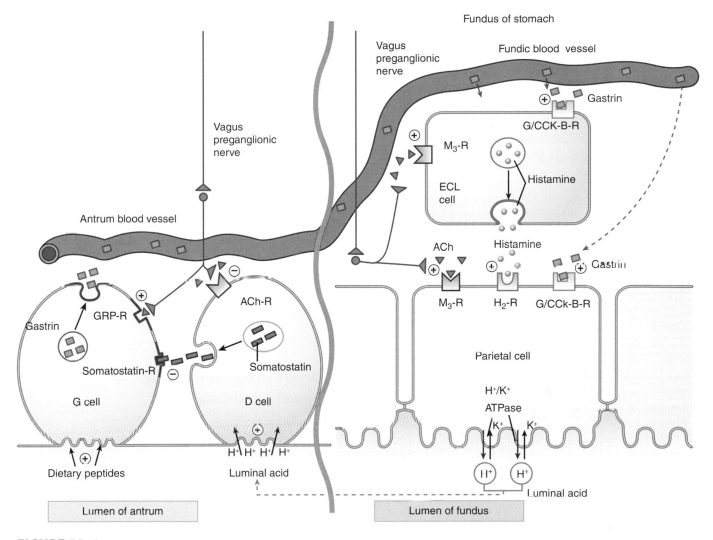

FIGURE 59-1 Schematic model of physiologic control of hydrogen ion (acid) secretion by the gastric parietal cells, which are stimulated by gastrin (acting on gastrin/CCK-B receptors), acetylcholine (ACh; M_3 receptor), and histamine (H_2 receptor). Acid is secreted across the parietal cell canalicular membrane by the H^+/K^+ ATPase proton pump into the gastric lumen. The gastrin that is secreted by antral G cells in response to intraluminal dietary peptides acts directly on parietal cells and also stimulates release of histamine from enterochromaffin-like (ECL) cells. The vagus nerve stimulates postganglionic neurons of the enteric nervous system to release acetylcholine ACh, which acts on parietal and ECL cells. In the antrum, release of gastrin-releasing peptide (GRP) from postganglionic neurons directly increases gastrin release, whereas release of ACh indirectly increases gastrin secretion by inhibiting release of somatostatin from antral D cells. The increase in intraluminal H^+ concentration causes D cells to release somatostatin and thereby inhibit gastrin release from G cells. CCK, cholecystokinin; R, receptor. (Reproduced, with permission, from Katzung BG, editor: *Basic & Clinical Pharmacology*, 12th ed. McGraw-Hill, 2012: Fig. 62–1.)

4. Sucralfate—An aluminum sucrose sulfate, sucralfate is a small, poorly soluble molecule that polymerizes in the acid environment of the stomach. The polymer binds to injured tissue and forms a protective coating over ulcer beds. Sucralfate accelerates the healing of peptic ulcers and reduces the recurrence rate. Unfortunately, sucralfate must be taken 4 times daily. Sucralfate is too insoluble to have significant systemic effects when taken by the oral route; toxicity is very low.

5. Misoprostol—An analog of PGE_1, misoprostol increases mucosal protection and inhibits acid secretion. It is effective in reducing the risk of ulcers in users of nonsteroidal anti-inflammatory

drugs (NSAIDs) but is not widely used because of the need for multiple daily dosing and poorly tolerated adverse effects (gastrointestinal upset and diarrhea). Misoprostol is discussed in detail in Chapter 18.

6. Colloidal bismuth—Bismuth has multiple actions, including formation of a protective coating on ulcerated tissue, stimulation of mucosal protective mechanisms, direct antimicrobial effects, and sequestration of enterotoxins. Bismuth subsalicylate, a nonprescription formulation of bismuth and salicylate, reduces stool frequency and liquidity in infectious diarrhea. Bismuth causes black stools.

7. Antibiotics—Chronic infection with *H pylori* is present in most patients with recurrent non-NSAID-induced peptic ulcers. Eradication of this organism greatly reduces the rate of recurrence of ulcer in these patients. One regimen of choice consists of a proton pump inhibitor plus a course of clarithromycin and amoxicillin (or metronidazole in patients with penicillin allergy).

B. Drugs That Promote Upper Gastrointestinal Motility

Prokinetic drugs that stimulate upper gastrointestinal motility are helpful for gastroparesis and for postsurgical gastric emptying delay. Their ability to increase lower esophageal sphincter pressures also makes them useful for some patients with GERD. In the past, cholinomimetic agonists such as bethanechol were used for GERD and gastroparesis, but the availability of less toxic agents has supplanted their use. The acetylcholinesterase inhibitor neostigmine is still used for the treatment of hospitalized patients with acute large bowel distention. The cholinomimetics are discussed in Chapter 7.

In the enteric nervous system, dopamine serves as an inhibitory function by inhibiting cholinergic stimulation of smooth muscle contraction. **Metoclopramide** and **domperidone** are D_2 dopamine receptor antagonists that promote gastrointestinal motility. The D_2 receptor-blocking action of these drugs in the area postrema is also of value in preventing emesis after surgical anesthesia and emesis induced by cancer chemotherapeutic drugs. When used chronically, metoclopramide can cause symptoms of parkinsonism, other extrapyramidal effects, and hyperprolactinemia. Because it does not cross the blood-brain barrier, domperidone is less likely to cause CNS toxicity.

The macrolide antibiotic **erythromycin** (Chapter 44) promotes motility by stimulating motilin receptors. It may have benefit in some patients with gastroparesis.

C. Laxatives

Laxatives increase the probability of a bowel movement by several mechanisms: an irritant or stimulant action on the bowel wall; a bulk-forming action on the stool that evokes reflex contraction of the bowel; a softening action on hard or impacted stool; and a lubricating action that eases passage of stool through the rectum. Examples of drugs that act by these mechanisms are listed in Table 59–1.

D. Antidiarrheal Agents

The most effective antidiarrheal drugs are the opioids and derivatives of opioids that have been selected for maximal antidiarrheal and minimal CNS effect. Of the latter group, the most important are **diphenoxylate** and **loperamide,** meperidine analogs with very weak analgesic effects. Diphenoxylate is formulated with antimuscarinic alkaloids (eg, atropine) to reduce the likelihood of abuse; loperamide is formulated alone. **Kaolin**, a naturally occurring hydrated magnesium aluminum silicate, is combined with **pectin**, an indigestible carbohydrate derived from apples in a popular nonprescription preparation that absorbs bacterial toxins

TABLE 59–1 The major laxative mechanisms and some representative laxative drugs.

Mechanism	Examples
Bulk-forming	Psyllium, methylcellulose, polycarbophil
Stool-softening	Docusate, glycerin, mineral oil
Osmotic	Magnesium oxide, sorbitol, lactulose, magnesium citrate, sodium phosphate, polyethylene glycol
Stimulant	Aloe, senna, cascara, castor oil, bisacodyl
Chloride channel activator	Lubiprostone
Opioid receptor antagonists	Methylnaltrexone, alvimopan

and fluid, resulting in decreased stool liquidity. They can cause constipation and interfere with absorption of other drugs.

E. Drugs Used for Irritable Bowel Syndrome

Irritable bowel syndrome (IBS) is associated with relapsing episodes of abdominal discomfort (pain, bloating, distention, or cramps) plus diarrhea or constipation (or both). The pharmacologic strategy is tailored to patients' symptoms and includes antidiarrheal agents and laxatives, and for the treatment of abdominal pain, low doses of tricyclic antidepressants (Chapter 30). The anticholinergic drugs **dicyclomine** and **hyoscyamine** are used as antispasmodics to relieve abdominal pain; however, their efficacy has not been convincingly demonstrated. **Alosetron**, a potent $5\text{-}HT_3$ antagonist, is approved for treatment of women with severe IBS with diarrhea. Alosetron can cause constipation, including rare complications of severe constipation that have required hospitalization or surgery, and rare cases of ischemic colitis. For this reason, its use is restricted. **Lubiprostone,** a laxative that activates the type 2 chloride channels in the small intestine, is approved for treatment of women with IBS with predominant constipation.

F. Drugs With Antiemetic Actions

A variety of drugs are valuable in the prevention and treatment of vomiting, especially cancer chemotherapy-induced vomiting. In addition to **metoclopramide** and other D_2 dopamine receptor antagonists, useful antiemetics are drugs with H_1 histamine-blocking activity (Chapter 16), including **diphenhydramine** and several **phenothiazines** (Chapter 29); **antimuscarinic drugs** such as **scopolamine** (Chapter 8); the corticosteroid **dexamethasone** (Chapter 39); and the cannabinoid receptor agonists **dronabinol** and nabilone (Chapter 32). The $5\text{-}HT_3$ antagonists (Chapter 16) **ondansetron, granisetron, dolasetron,** and **palonosetron** are particularly useful in preventing nausea and vomiting after general anesthesia and in patients receiving cancer chemotherapy. **Aprepitant** a newer antiemetic is an antagonist of the neurokinin 1 (NK_1) receptor, a receptor in the area postrema of the CNS that is activated by substance P and other tachykinins (see Chapter 17). Aprepitant is approved for use in combination with other antiemetics for prevention of the nausea and vomiting associated with highly emetogenic chemotherapeutic regimens. Aprepitant can cause fatigue, dizziness, and diarrhea. As a substrate and an inhibitor of CYP3A4, aprepitant participates in many drug interactions.

SKILL KEEPER: 5-HT AGONISTS AND ANTAGONISTS (SEE CHAPTERS 16 AND 30)

List the various 5-HT receptor agonists and antagonists in current use. Describe their clinical applications. The Skill Keeper Answer appears at the end of the chapter.

G. Drugs Used in Inflammatory Bowel Disease (IBD)

1. Aminosalicylates—Drugs containing **5-aminosalicylic acid (5-ASA)** are used as topical therapy for IBD. The precise mechanism of 5-ASA action is uncertain but may involve inhibiting the synthesis of prostaglandins and inflammatory leukotrienes, and interfering with the production of inflammatory cytokines. 5-ASA, known generically as mesalamine, is readily absorbed from the small intestine whereas absorption from the colon is extremely low. Proprietary formulations of 5-ASA (Pentasa, Asacol, Lialda) deliver 5-ASA to different segments of the small and large intestine (Figure 59–2). **Balsalazide, olsalazine,** and **sulfasalazine** contain 5-ASA bound by an azo (N=N) bond to an inert compound, another 5-ASA molecule, or sulfapyridine. The azo structure is poorly absorbed in the small intestine. **Sulfasalazine** (a combination of 5-ASA and sulfapyridine) has a higher incidence of adverse effects that the other 5-ASA drugs, due to the systemic absorption of the sulfapyridine moiety.

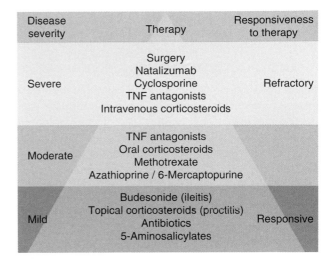

FIGURE 59–3 Therapeutic pyramid approach to inflammatory bowel disease. Treatment choice is predicted on both the severity of the illness and responsiveness to therapy. Agents at the bottom of the pyramid are less efficacious but carry a lower risk of serious adverse effects. TNF, tumor necrosis factor. (Reproduced, with permission, from Katzung BG, editor: *Basic & Clinical Pharmacology*, 12th ed. McGraw-Hill, 2012: Fig. 62–9.)

These effects are dose related and include nausea, gastrointestinal upset, headaches, arthralgias, myalgias, bone marrow suppression, malaise, and severe hypersensitivity reactions. Other aminosalicylates, which do not contain sulfapyridine, are well tolerated.

2. Other agents—Other drugs used in the treatment of ulcerative colitis and Crohn's disease (Figure 59–3) include antibiotics, **glucocorticoids** (Chapters 39 and 55), **immunosuppressive antimetabolites** (eg, azathioprine, 6-mercaptopurine, methotrexate; Chapters 54 and 55), anti-tumor necrosis factor [TNF] drugs (eg, infliximab, Chapters 36 and 55). **Natalizumab** is a humanized monoclonal antibody that blocks integrins on circulating leukocytes. Because of a possible association of natalizumab

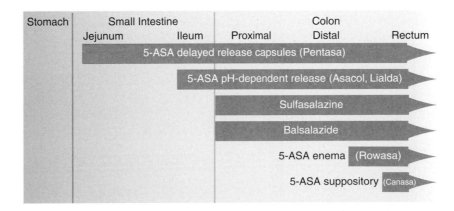

FIGURE 59–2 Sites of 5-aminosalicyclic acid (5-ASA) release from different formulations in the small and large intestines. (Reproduced, with permission, from Katzung BG, editor: *Basic & Clinical Pharmacology*, 12th ed. McGraw-Hill, 2012: Fig. 62–7.)

with multifocal leukoencephalopathy, it is carefully restricted to patients with severe refractory Crohn's disease.

H. Pancreatic Enzyme Replacements

Steatorrhea, a condition of decreased fat absorption together with an increase in stool fat excretion, results from inadequate pancreatic secretion of lipase. The abnormality of fat absorption can be significantly relieved by oral administration of pancreatic lipase (**pancrelipase** or **pancreatin**) obtained from pigs. Pancreatic lipase is inactivated at a pH lower than 4.0; the enzyme should be taken as enteric-coated capsules unless the pH is raised with antacids or drugs that reduce acid secretion.

I. Drugs That Inhibit the Formation of Gallstones

The formation of cholesterol gallstones can be inhibited by the bile acid derivative ursodiol, which decreases the cholesterol content of bile by decreasing hepatic cholesterol secretion and other effects on hepatocyte canalicular membranes. Toxicity due to the drug is uncommon.

QUESTIONS

1. A 55-year-old woman with type 1 diabetes of 40 yrs' duration complains of severe bloating and abdominal distress, especially after meals. Evaluation is consistent with diabetic gastroparesis. Which of the following is a prokinetic drug that could be used in this situation?
   (A) Alosetron
   (B) Cimetidine
   (C) Loperamide
   (D) Metoclopramide
   (E) Sucralfate

2. A patient who is taking verapamil for hypertension and angina has become constipated. Which of the following drugs is an osmotic laxative that could be used to treat the patient's constipation?
   (A) Aluminum hydroxide
   (B) Diphenoxylate
   (C) Magnesium hydroxide
   (D) Metoclopramide
   (E) Ranitidine

3. Which drug accumulates in parietal cell canaliculi and undergoes conversion to a derivative that irreversibly inhibits H^+/K^+ ATPase?
   (A) Cimetidine
   (B) Diphenoxylate
   (C) Esomeprazole
   (D) Metoclopramide
   (E) Sulfasalazine

4. Which drug is most likely to be useful in the treatment of inflammatory bowel disease?
   (A) Diphenhydramine
   (B) Diphenoxylate
   (C) Mesalamine
   (D) Ondansetron
   (E) Ursodiol

5. A 34-year-old woman has irritable bowel syndrome with diarrhea that is not responsive to conventional therapies. Despite the small risk of severe constipation and ischemic colitis, the patient decides to begin therapy with alosetron. Alosetron has which of the following receptor actions?
   (A) $5\text{-}HT_3$ receptor antagonist
   (B) $5\text{-}HT_4$ receptor agonist
   (C) D_2 receptor antagonist
   (D) NK_1 receptor antagonist
   (E) Muscarinic receptor antagonist

6. On your way to an examination, you experience the vulnerable feeling that an attack of diarrhea is imminent. If you stopped at a drugstore, which one of the following antidiarrheal drugs could you buy without a prescription even though it is related chemically to the strong opioid analgesic meperidine?
   (A) Aluminum hydroxide
   (B) Diphenoxylate
   (C) Loperamide
   (D) Magnesium hydroxide
   (E) Metoclopramide

7. A 45-year-old man with a duodenal ulcer was treated with a combination of drugs intended to heal the mucosal damage and to eradicate *Helicobacter pylori*. Which of the following antibacterial drugs is used commonly to eradicate intestinal *Helicobacter pylori*?
   (A) Cefazolin
   (B) Ciprofloxacin
   (C) Clarithromycin
   (D) Clindamycin
   (E) Vancomycin

8. A patient is receiving highly emetogenic chemotherapy for metastatic carcinoma. To prevent chemotherapy-induced nausea and vomiting, she is likely to be treated with which of the following?
   (A) Levodopa
   (B) Methotrexate
   (C) Misoprostol
   (D) Ondansetron
   (E) Sucralfate

DIRECTIONS: 9 and 10. The following matching questions consist of a list of lettered options followed by several numbered items. For each numbered item, select the ONE option that is most closely associated with it.

(A) Aluminum hydroxide
(B) Balsalazide
(C) Castor oil
(D) Cimetidine
(E) Dexamethasone
(F) Methotrexate
(G) Metoclopramide
(H) Mineral oil
(I) Omeprazole
(J) Ondansetron
(K) Pancrelipase
(L) Sucralfate

9. Management of steatorrhea is best accomplished by the use of this agent.

10. This is a small molecule that polymerizes in stomach acid and coats the ulcer bed, resulting in accelerated healing and reduction of symptoms.

ANSWERS

1. Of the drugs listed, only metoclopramide is considered a prokinetic agent (ie, one that increases propulsive motility in the gut). The answer is **D**.

2. A laxative that mildly stimulates the gut would be most suitable in a patient taking a smooth muscle relaxant drug such as verapamil. By holding water in the intestine, magnesium hydroxide provides additional bulk and stimulates increased contractions. The answer is **C**.

3. Esomeprazole, the (S) isomer of omeprazole, is a prodrug converting spontaneously in the parietal cell canaliculus to a sulfonamide that irreversibly inactivates the proton pump. The answer is **C**.

4. Mesalamine is a form of aminosalicylate that releases 5-aminosalicyclic acid in the large intestine and thereby provides a local anti-inflammatory effect that is useful in inflammatory bowel disease. The answer is **C**.

5. Serotonin plays a major regulatory role in the enteric nervous system, and the potent 5-HT$_3$ receptor antagonist alosetron has shown efficacy in treating women with IBS that is accompanied by diarrhea. The answer is **A**.

6. Aluminum hydroxide is constipating but is not related chemically to meperidine; magnesium hydroxide is a strong laxative. The 2 antidiarrheal drugs that are structurally related to opioids are diphenoxylate and loperamide. Loperamide is available over-the-counter; diphenoxylate is mixed with atropine alkaloids, and the product (Lomotil, others) requires a prescription. The answer is **C**.

7. The macrolide antibiotic clarithromycin is commonly used in antibiotic regimens designed to treat duodenal ulcers caused by *H pylori*. The other antibiotics that are used include amoxicillin, tetracycline, and metronidazole. Bismuth also has an antibacterial action. The answer is **C**.

8. The 5-HT$_3$ receptor antagonists are highly effective at preventing chemotherapy-induced nausea and vomiting, which can be a dose-limiting toxicity of anticancer drugs. The answer is **D**.

9. Steatorrhea is due to decreased fat absorption as a result of inadequate pancreatic secretion of lipase. The answer is **K**.

10. Sucralfate is a small molecule that polymerizes in stomach acid and forms a protective coat over the ulcer bed. The answer is **L**.

SKILL KEEPER ANSWER: 5-HT AGONISTS & ANTAGONISTS (SEE CHAPTERS 16 AND 30)

The only serotonin agonists in common use are the 5-HT$_{1D}$-selective agonists such as sumatriptan and its congeners (see Chapter 16) that are used in migraine. Ergot alkaloids are partial agonists at several 5-HT receptors and are also used in migraine and other conditions. Several valuable antidepressants are inhibitors of the serotonin reuptake pump in neurons (see Chapter 30). Serotonin antagonists include cyproheptadine (also an H$_1$ blocker), phenoxybenzamine (also an α blocker), and several of the atypical antipsychotic drugs (eg, olanzapine, aripiprazole; see Chapter 29), which have high affinity for HT$_{2A}$ receptors. Cyproheptadine is used for pruritus and sometimes for carcinoid tumor. Phenoxybenzamine is used for carcinoid tumor as well as for pheochromocytoma. 5-HT$_3$ receptors are blocked by ondansetron and its congeners. These drugs are extremely useful in preventing postoperative and cancer chemotherapy-induced nausea and vomiting.

CHECKLIST

When you complete this chapter, you should be able to:

❑ Identify 5 different groups of drugs used in peptic ulcer disease.

❑ Describe the mechanism of action of omeprazole and related drugs.

❑ List 7 different drugs used in the prevention of chemotherapy- or radiation-induced emesis and identify the receptors with which they interact.

❑ Describe the mechanism of action, clinical uses, and adverse effects of metoclopramide.

❑ Identify 2 drugs commonly used as antidiarrheal agents and 4 drugs with different mechanisms that are used as laxatives.

❑ Identify drugs used in the management of inflammatory bowel disease and irritable bowel syndrome.

DRUG SUMMARY TABLE: Gastrointestinal Drugs

Subclass	Mechanism of Action	Clinical Applications	Pharmacokinetics	Toxicities, Interactions
Drugs used in acid-peptic diseases				
Proton pump inhibitors (PPIs; eg, omeprazole)	Irreversible blockade of H^+/K^+ ATPase in active gastric parietal cells	Peptic ulcer, GERD, erosive gastritis	Half-lives much shorter than duration of action	Low toxicity • reduction of stomach acid may reduce absorption of some drugs and increase that of others

Other PPIs: esomeprazole, dexlansoprazole, lansoprazole, pantoprazole, rabeprazole
H_2-*receptor blockers*: cimetidine, famotidine, nizatidine, ranitidine reduce nocturnal acid but less effective than PPIs against stimulated secretion; very safe, available over the counter (OTC). Cimetidine, but not other H_2 blockers, is a weak antiandrogenic agent and a potent CYP enzyme inhibitor
Sucralfate: polymerizes at site of tissue damage and protects against further damage; very insoluble with no systemic effects; must be given 4 times daily
Antacids: popular OTC medication for symptomatic relief of heartburn; not as useful as PPIs and H_2 blockers in peptic diseases

Prokinetic agents				
Metoclopramide	D_2 receptor blocker • increases gastric emptying and intestinal motility	Gastric paresis (eg, in diabetes) • antiemetic	Oral and parenteral formulations	Parkinsonian symptoms due to block of CNS D_2 receptors

Domperidone: like metoclopramide but less CNS effect; not available in United States
Cholinomimetics: neostigmine used for colonic pseudo-obstruction in hospitalized patients
Macrolides: erythromycin useful in diabetic gastroparesis but tolerance develops

Laxatives				
Magnesium hydroxide, other nonabsorbable salts and sugars	Osmotic agents increase water content of stool	Simple constipations • bowel prep for endoscopy (especially PEG solutions)	Oral	Magnesium may be absorbed and cause toxicity in renal impairment

Bulk-forming: methylcellulose, psyllium, etc; increase volume, stimulate evacuation
Stool surfactants: docusate, mineral oil; lubricate stool, ease passage
Stimulants: senna, cascara; stimulate activity; may cause cramping
Chloride channel activator: lubiprostone, prostanoic acid derivative, stimulates chloride secretion into intestine, increasing fluid content
Opioid receptor antagonists: alvimopan, methylnaltrexone, block intestinal μ opioid receptors but do not enter CNS, so analgesia is maintained

(Continued)

DRUG SUMMARY TABLE: Gastrointestinal Drugs (*Continued*)

Subclass	Mechanism of Action	Clinical Applications	Pharmacokinetics	Toxicities, Interactions
Antidiarrheal drugs				
Loperamide	Activates μ opioid receptors in enteric nervous system and slows motility with negligible CNS effects	Nonspecific, noninfectious diarrhea	Oral	Mild cramping but little or no CNS toxicity

Diphenoxylate: similar to loperamide, but high doses can cause CNS opioid effects and toxicity
Colloidal bismuth compounds: subsalicylate and citrate salts available as OTC products; have some value in travelers' diarrhea due to absorption of toxins
Kaolin + pectin: adsorbent compounds available OTC

Drugs for irritable bowel syndrome (IBS)				
Alosetron	5-HT$_3$ receptor antagonist of high potency and duration of binding • reduces smooth muscle activity in GI tract	Severe diarrhea-predominant IBS in women	Oral	Rare but serious constipation; ischemic colitis • bowel infarction

Anticholinergics: nonselective action on GI activity; associated with typical antimuscarinic toxicity
Chloride channel activator: lubiprostone is useful in constipation-predominant IBS in women

Antiemetics				
5-HT$_3$ antagonists (eg, ondansetron)	5-HT$_3$ receptor block in GI and CNS	Prevention of chemotherapy-induced and postoperative nausea and vomiting	Oral and parenteral formulations	May slow colonic transit

Other 5-HT$_3$ antagonist antiemetics: dolasetron, granisetron, palonosetron; see Chapter 16
Corticosteroids: mechanism not known but useful in antiemetic IV cocktails; see Chapter 39
Antimuscarinics (eg, scopolamine): effective in emesis due to motion sickness; not other types; see Chapter 8
Phenothiazines: act primary through block of D$_2$ and muscarinic receptors; see Chapter 16
Cannabinoids: dronabinol is available for use in chemotherapy-induced nausea and vomiting, but is associated with CNS marijuana effects (see Chapter 32)
Aprepitant: A neurokinin 1 (NK$_1$) antagonist available for use in chemotherapy-induced nausea and vomiting; associated with fatigue, dizziness, diarrhea, and CYP interactions

Drugs for inflammatory bowel disease (IBD)				
Mesalamine (5-aminosalicylate)	Mechanism uncertain • may be inhibition of eicosanoid inflammatory mediators	Mild to moderately severe Crohn's disease and ulcerative colitis	Various formulations designed to deliver drug to distal ileum and colon	Little or no toxicity

Azo compounds: dalsalazide, olsalazine, sulfasalazine; colonic bacterial azoreductase enzymes release 5-aminosalicylate in the colon; sulfasalazine can cause sulfonamide toxicity due to absorption of the sulfapyridine moiety
Glucocorticoids: see Chapters 30 and 55
Immunosuppressant antimetabolites: see Chapters 54 and 55
Anti-TNF drugs: see Chapters 36 and 55
Natalizumab: antibody that blocks leukocyte integrins; may cause multifocal leukoencephalopathy

Pancreatic supplements				
Pancrelipase	Replacement enzymes from animal pancreatic extracts that improve digestion of fat, protein, and carbohydrate	Pancreatic insufficiency due to cystic fibrosis, pancreatitis, pancreatectomy	Taken with every meal	May increase incidence of gout

Pancreatin: similar pancreatic extracts but much lower potency; rarely used

Bile acid therapy for gallstones				
Ursodiol	Reduces cholesterol secretion into bile	Gallstones in patients refusing or not eligible for surgery	Oral	Little or no toxicity

GERD, gastrointestinal reflux disease; PEG, pegylated.

Dietary Supplements & Herbal Medications

Dietary supplements, which include substances known as botanical and herbal medications, are available without prescription and, unlike over-the-counter medications, are considered to be nutritional supplements rather than drugs. These substances are marketed in the United States without FDA or other governmental premarketing review of efficacy or safety, and with little government oversight of purity, variations in potency, or adverse effects. Purified nonherbal nutritional supplements such as dehydroepiandrosterone (DHEA) and melatonin are also used widely by the general public in pursuit of "alternative medicine." In the case of many herbal products and nutritional supplements, evidence from controlled clinical studies for their medical effectiveness is incomplete or nonexistent. A summary of the intended uses of some herbal products and nutritional supplements is presented in Table 60–1.

BOTANICAL SUBSTANCES

A. Echinacea

1. Nature—Leaves and roots of echinacea species (eg, *Echinacea purpurea*) contain flavonoids, polyacetylenes, and caffeoyl conjugates.

2. Pharmacology—In vitro studies have shown that echinacea has cytokine activation and anti-inflammatory properties. There is some evidence for the efficacy of aerial (above-ground) parts of *E purpurea* plants in the early treatment of colds.

3. Toxicity and drug interactions—Unpleasant taste and gastrointestinal effects may occur, sometimes with dizziness or headache. Some preparations have a high alcohol content, but no drug interactions have been reported.

B. Ephedra (Ma Huang)

1. Nature—Ma huang is one of many names given to various plants of the genus *Ephedra,* the major chemical constituents of which are ephedrine and pseudoephedrine (see Chapter 9). Ephedrine is a prescription drug in the United States; pseudoephedrine is available in over-the-counter decongestants. In the

United States, the FDA has banned the marketing of dietary supplements containing ephedrine alkaloids, which are considered to pose an unreasonable cardiovascular risk. The ban is not applicable to Chinese herbal remedies.

2. Pharmacology—The actions of ephedra products are those of ephedrine and pseudoephedrine, which are indirect-acting sympathomimetics that release norepinephrine from sympathetic nerve endings (see Chapter 9). In addition to nasal decongestion, the established clinical use of ephedrine is as a pressor agent. Ephedra herbal products are commonly used for treatment of respiratory dysfunction, including bronchitis and asthma, and as mild CNS stimulants. In Chinese medicine, ephedra products are also used for relief of cold and flu symptoms, for diuresis, and for bone or joint pain. Dietary supplements containing ephedrine alkaloids have been widely promoted for weight loss and for enhancement of athletic performance.

3. Toxicity and drug interactions—Toxic effects are those of ephedrine and include dizziness, insomnia, anorexia, flushing, palpitations, tachycardia, and urinary retention. In high doses, ephedra can cause a marked increase in blood pressure, cardiac arrhythmias, and a toxic psychosis. Contraindications are those for ephedrine and include anxiety states, bulimia, cardiac arrhythmias, diabetes, heart failure, hypertension, glaucoma, hyperthyroidism, and pregnancy. As a weak base, renal elimination of ephedrine in overdose can be facilitated by urinary acidification.

C. Garlic

1. Nature—Garlic (*Allium sativum*) contains organic thiosulfinates that can form allicin (responsible for the characteristic odor) via enzymes activated by disruption of the garlic bulb.

2. Pharmacology—In vitro studies show that allicin inhibits hepatic hydroxymethylglutaryl coenzyme A (HMG-CoA) reductase and angiotensin-converting enzyme (ACE), blocks platelet aggregation, increases nitric oxide (NO), is fibrinolytic, has antimicrobial activity, and reduces carcinogen activation. There is some evidence from clinical trials that garlic is more effective than

Alternative medicine	Treatments that are not generally recognized by the medical community as standard or conventional medical approaches
Controlled clinical trial	A clinical trial that compares a group of subjects who are receiving a treatment with a closely matched group of individuals who are not receiving a treatment. Chapter 5 describes clinical trials in more detail
Herbal medication	Plants or plant extracts that people use to improve their health
Nutritional supplement	A substance that is added to the diet to improve health and which usually contains dietary ingredients such as vitamins, minerals, amino acids, and enzymes
Placebo	An inactive medication made to resemble the investigational formulation as much as possible

placebo at lowering total cholesterol, although a trial in adults with moderately elevated low-density lipoprotein (LDL) cholesterol failed to find an LDL cholesterol-lowering effect. A randomized study of garlic in patients with advanced coronary artery disease showed a reduction in plaque accumulation but primary end points (death, stroke, myocardial infarction) were not studied.

3. Toxicity and drug interactions—Nausea, hypotension, and allergic reactions may occur. Possible antiplatelet action warrants

TABLE 60–1 Common intended uses of some botanical or nutritional supplements.

Botanical or Nutritional Supplement	Common Intended Use
Echinacea	Decrease duration and intensity of cold symptoms
Ephedra (ma huang)	Treatment of respiratory ailments such as bronchitis and asthma, and as a CNS stimulant
Garlic	For cholesterol lowering and atherosclerosis
Ginkgo	Treatment of intermittent claudication, and cerebral insufficiency and dementia
Ginseng	Improvement of physical and mental performance
Milk thistle	Limitation of hepatic injury and as an antidote to *Amanita* mushroom poisoning
Saw palmetto	Improvement in symptoms of benign prostatic hyperplasia
St. John's wort	Treatment of mild to moderate depression
Coenzyme Q10	Improvement of ischemic heart disease and for Parkinson's disease
Glucosamine	Reduction of pain associated with osteoarthritis
Melatonin	Decrease jet lag symptoms and as a sleep aid

caution in patients receiving anticoagulants or conventional antiplatelet drugs.

D. Ginkgo

1. Nature—Prepared from the leaves of *Ginkgo biloba,* ginkgo contains flavone glycosides and terpenoids.

2. Pharmacology—In in vitro studies, ginkgo exhibits anti-oxidant and radical-scavenging effects and increases nitric oxide formation. Animal studies have revealed reduced blood viscosity and changes in CNS neurotransmitters. At the clinical level, ginkgo may have value in intermittent claudication, and its use as a pretreatment may reduce markers of oxidative stress associated with coronary artery bypass surgery. Although several studies have shown a mild benefit of ginkgo in patients with cognitive impairment and dementia, the effects are unpredictable and unlikely to be clinically significant. A large trial investigating ginkgo as a prophylactic agent for dementia failed to show a benefit after 6 yr of treatment.

3. Toxicity and drug interactions—Gastrointestinal effects, anxiety, insomnia, and headache occur. Possible antiplatelet action suggests caution in patients receiving anticoagulants or antiplatelet drugs. Ginkgo may be epileptogenic and should be avoided in persons with a history of seizure disorders.

E. Ginseng

1. Nature—Most ginseng products are derived from plants of the genus *Panax,* which contain multiple triterpenoid saponin glycosides (ginsenosides). Siberian or Brazilian ginseng does not contain these chemicals.

2. Pharmacology—Ginseng is purported to improve mental and physical performance, but the clinical evidence for such effects is limited. There is some evidence that ginseng may have some effect in cold prevention and in lowering postprandial glucose.

3. Toxicity and drug interactions—Estrogenic effects include mastalgia and vaginal bleeding. Insomnia, nervousness, and hypertension have been reported. Ginseng should be used cautiously in patients receiving anticoagulant, antihypertensive, hypoglycemic, or psychiatric medications.

F. Milk Thistle

1. Nature—Milk thistle is derived from the fruit and seeds of *Silybum marianum,* which contain flavonolignans such as silymarin.

2. Pharmacology—In vitro studies show that milk thistle reduces lipid peroxidation, scavenges free radicals, enhances superoxide dismutase, inhibits formation of leukotrienes, and increases hepatocyte RNA polymerase activity. In animal models, milk thistle protects against liver injury caused by alcohol, acetaminophen, and *Amanita* mushrooms. A systematic review of randomized trials of milk thistle in patients with alcoholic liver disease or viral hepatitis found no significant reduction in all-cause mortality, liver histopathology, or complications of liver disease. A commercial preparation of silybin (an isomer of silymarin) is available in some countries as an antidote to *Amanita phalloides* mushroom poisoning.

3. Toxicity and drug interactions—Other than loose stools, milk thistle does not cause significant toxicity, and there are no reports of drug interactions.

G. St. John's Wort

1. Nature—St. John's wort is made from dried flowers of *Hypericum perforatum,* which contains the active constituents hypericin and hyperforin.

2. Pharmacology—In vitro studies with hyperforin have shown decreased activity of serotonergic reuptake systems. In animals, chronic treatment with commercial extracts led to downregulation of adrenoceptors and upregulation of 5-HT receptors. Some (but not all) clinical trials of the extract in patients with mild to moderate depression have shown efficacy that is greater than placebo and, in some trials, similar to those of prescription antidepressants for mild or moderate depression. Hypericin, when photoactivated, may have antiviral and anticancer effects.

3. Toxicity and drug interactions—Mild gastrointestinal side effects occur, and photosensitization has been reported with St. John's wort. It should be avoided in patients using selective serotonin reuptake inhibitors (SSRIs) or monoamine oxidase (MAO) inhibitors and in those with a history of bipolar or psychotic disorder. Constituents in St. John's wort induce the formation of cytochrome P450 isoforms and P-glycoprotein drug transporters. Decreases in effectiveness of birth control pills, cyclosporine, digoxin, HIV protease inhibitors, and warfarin have been reported in patients who regularly use St. John's wort.

H. Saw Palmetto

1. Nature—Saw palmetto is derived from the berries of *Serenoa repens* or *Sabal serrulata* and contains phytosterols, aliphatic alcohols, polyprenes, and flavonoids.

2. Pharmacology—In vitro studies have shown inhibition of 5α-reductase and antagonistic effects at androgen receptors. Clinical trials of saw palmetto in benign prostatic hyperplasia (BPH) have been mixed. Some have shown improvement in urologic function and in urinary flow. Others, including a recent well-controlled, double-blind 1-yr study in moderate to severe BPH, have shown no significant effects on symptoms or objective measures.

3. Toxicity and drug interactions—Abdominal pain with gastrointestinal distress, decreased libido, headache, and hypertension occur; overall incidence was less than 3%. Saw palmetto has no effect on the prostate specific antigen (PSA) marker.

SKILL KEEPER: DRUGS FROM PLANT SOURCES

Many conventional drugs, strictly regulated by governmental agencies such as the FDA, originated from plant sources. How many of these compounds can you identify? The Skill Keeper Answer appears at the end of the chapter.

PURIFIED NUTRITIONAL SUBSTANCES

A. Coenzyme Q10

1. Nature—Coenzyme Q10, also known as ubiquinone, is a benzoquinone that serves as a cofactor in the mitochondrial electron transport chain and, in its reduced form of ubiquinol, serves as an important antioxidant. After ingestion, the reduced form predominates in the circulation.

2. Pharmacology—Coenzyme Q10 may have a small degree of efficacy in reducing systolic and diastolic blood pressure and in treating coronary artery disease and chronic stable angina, but it does not appear to be useful as adjunctive therapy of heart failure. Coenzyme Q10 may have some efficacy in reducing muscle pain in patients with statin-related myopathy.

3. Toxicity—Coenzyme Q10 is well tolerated. The most common adverse effect is gastrointestinal disturbances. Rare effects include rash, thrombocytopenia, irritability, dizziness, and headache. Coenzyme Q10 has structural similarity to vitamin K and can decrease the effects of warfarin.

B. Glucosamine

1. Nature—Glucosamine is an amino sugar that serves as the precursor of nitrogen-containing sugars, including the glycosaminoglycans that are a major constituent of connective tissue, including the cartilage in joints.

2. Pharmacology—Glucosamine is primarily used for pain associated with osteoarthritis. The many clinical trials examining the use of oral or intra-articular glucosamine have produced mixed results. Although some early trials and a meta-analysis found a beneficial effect in osteoarthritis, a recent large placebo-controlled, double-blind trial failed to find a benefit for glucosamine in treating osteoarthritis.

3. Toxicity—Glucosamine can occasionally cause diarrhea and nausea but otherwise is well tolerated. Because glucosamine is commercially prepared from crustaceans, there is some concern about cross-allergenicity in people with shellfish allergy.

C. Melatonin

1. Nature—Melatonin is a serotonin derivative produced mainly in the pineal gland. It appears to regulate sleep–wake cycles, and its release coincides with darkness (9 PM to 4 AM). Other purported activities include contraception, prevention of aging, protection against oxidative stress, and the treatment of cancer, major depression, and HIV infection.

2. Pharmacology—Melatonin has been used extensively for jet lag and insomnia. In jet lag, clinical studies have shown subjective improvements in mood, more rapid recovery times, and reductions in daytime fatigue. Melatonin improves sleep onset, duration, and quality when given to patients with sleep disorders. **Ramelteon**, an agonist of melatonin receptors, has been FDA approved for insomnia (see Chapter 22).

3. Toxicity—Sedation and next-day drowsiness and headache have been reported. Melatonin can suppress the midcycle surge of luteinizing hormone (LH) and should not be used in pregnancy or in women attempting to conceive. Because it can decrease prolactin levels, melatonin should not be used by nursing mothers. In healthy men, chronic melatonin use decreases sperm quality.

QUESTIONS

1. A patient has accidentally ingested mushrooms identified as *Amanita phalloides*. Which herbal substance is most likely to protect against hepatic dysfunction?
   (A) Echinacea
   (B) Ginkgo
   (C) Melatonin
   (D) Milk thistle
   (E) Saw palmetto

2. There may be a link between this important endogenous antioxidant and statin-induced myopathy because statins reduce the synthesis of this compound and some clinical trials suggest that patients with statin-associated myopathy had reduced muscle pain after receiving this supplement. The supplement is which of the following?
   (A) Coenzyme Q10
   (B) Glucosamine
   (C) Melatonin
   (D) Tyrosine
   (E) Vitamin E

3. Which drug has a biochemical effect that most closely resembles the proposed mechanism of action of the psychoactive constituent(s) of St. John's wort?
   (A) Alprazolam
   (B) Fluoxetine
   (C) Levodopa
   (D) Methylphenidate
   (E) Morphine

4. An alternative medicine that is commonly used to treat the urinary symptoms associated with benign prostatic hyperplasia (BPH) is
   (A) Echinacea
   (B) Ephedra
   (C) Ginseng
   (D) Milk thistle
   (E) Saw palmetto

5. Which of the following is a derivative of serotonin that may have value in managing symptoms of jet lag?
   (A) Ephedra
   (B) Garlic
   (C) Ginseng
   (D) Glucosamine
   (E) Melatonin

6. Which compound enhances immune function in vitro and is used to decrease the symptoms of the common cold?
   (A) Echinacea
   (B) Ginkgo
   (C) Garlic
   (D) Melatonin
   (E) Milk thistle

7. Rejection of heart transplants has occurred in patients being treated with standard doses of cyclosporine when they also used which of the following dietary supplements?
   (A) Echinacea
   (B) Ginkgo
   (C) Milk thistle
   (D) St. John's wort
   (E) Saw palmetto

8. In 2003, a study published in the *Annals of Internal Medicine* found that this botanical substance accounted for more than 60% of adverse events associated with dietary supplements used in the United States. The "herbal" in question, which is used to aid weight loss and promote sports performance, is which of the following?
   (A) Echinacea
   (B) Ephedra
   (C) Ginkgo
   (D) Ginseng
   (E) Saw palmetto

9. Which of the following is a popular supplement whose purported efficacy in osteoarthritis is believed to be due to its role as a precursor to the glycosaminoglycans that form joint cartilage?
   (A) Coenzyme Q10
   (B) Dehydroepiandrosterone (DHEA)
   (C) Glycosamine
   (D) Nicotinic acid
   (E) Melatonin

10. Couples who are attempting to conceive a child should avoid chronic use of which of the following?
(A) Echinacea
(B) Ephedra
(C) Ginkgo
(D) Ginseng
(E) Melatonin

ANSWERS

1. Milk thistle contains compounds that may have cytoprotective actions against liver toxins, including those present in *Amanita* mushrooms. The answer is **D.**

2. HMG-CoA reductase, the enzyme required for coenzyme Q10 synthesis, is inhibited by statins (see Chapter 35). This inhibition may contribute to statin-associated myopathy. A small double-blind clinical trial found a significant reduction in muscle pain in patients with statin-associated myopathy who were treated with coenzyme Q10. The answer is **A.**

3. Extracts of the flowers of St. John's wort contain chemicals with possible antidepressant activity. In vitro studies have shown that these chemicals interfere with the neuronal reuptake of amine neurotransmitters in a fashion similar to the proposed mechanism of antidepressant actions of tricyclic antidepressants and SSRIs such as fluoxetine. The answer is **B.**

4. Saw palmetto, a complex extract from the berries of *Serenoa repens* or *Sabal serrulata*, is widely believed to improve the symptoms of BPH. The answer is **E.**

5. Garlic might get you a row of seats to yourself, but the compound that will help in jet lag is melatonin. The answer is **E.**

6. The freshly pressed juice of the aerial parts of *Echinacea purpurea* is purported to reduce the symptoms of the common cold and the time of recovery if ingested within 24 h of onset. The answer is **A.**

7. St. John's wort induces the formation of hepatic enzymes that metabolize cyclosporine, and its use can decrease the effectiveness of the immunosuppressant drug in organ and tissue transplantation. The answer is **D.**

8. Concern about the risks of using products containing ephedra during heavy workouts or in diet programs that stress the cardiovascular system has led to a ban on such nutritional supplements in the United States. The answer is **B.**

9. The amino sugar glucosamine, a building block for glycosaminoglycans, has become popular among people with osteoarthritis of the knee. The answer is **C.**

10. Chronic use of melatonin appears to suppress LH secretion in women and to decrease sperm quality in men. The answer is **E.**

SKILL KEEPER ANSWER: DRUGS FROM PLANT SOURCES

The clinical application of drugs that originated from plant sources has contributed greatly to conventional medicine. Such compounds include aspirin, atropine, cocaine, codeine, colchicine, digoxin, ephedrine, etoposide, methysergide, morphine, nicotine, physostigmine, pilocarpine, quinidine, quinine, reserpine, scopolamine, taxanes (eg, paclitaxel), tubocurarine, vinblastine, and vincristine.

CHECKLIST

When you complete this chapter, you should be able to:

❏ Contrast the regulations in the United States of botanicals and nutritional supplements with those of therapeutic drugs with regard to efficacy and safety.

❏ List several of the most widely used botanical products, and describe their purported medical uses, adverse effects, and potential for drug interactions.

❏ Describe the proposed medical uses and adverse effects of several purified nutritional supplements.

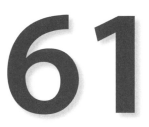

Drug Interactions

Drug interactions occur when one drug modifies the actions of another drug in the body. Drug interactions can result from pharmacokinetic alterations, pharmacodynamic changes, or a combination of both. Interactions between drugs in vitro (eg, precipitation when mixed in solutions for intravenous administration) are usually classified as *drug incompatibilities,* not drug interactions.

Although hundreds of drug interactions have been documented, relatively few are of enough clinical significance to constitute a contraindication to simultaneous use or to require a change in dosage. Some of these are listed in Table 61–1. In patients taking many drugs, however, the likelihood of significant drug interactions is increased. Elderly patients have a high incidence of drug interactions because they often have age-related changes in drug clearance and commonly take multiple medications.

PHARMACOKINETIC INTERACTIONS

A. Interactions Based on Absorption

Absorption from the gastrointestinal tract may be influenced by agents that bind drugs (eg, resins, antacids, calcium-containing foods), by agents that increase or decrease gastrointestinal motility (eg, metoclopramide or antimuscarinics, respectively), and by drugs that alter the P-glycoprotein and organic anion transporters in the intestine. Concomitant use of antacids, which increase gastric pH, can decrease gastrointestinal absorption of digoxin, ketoconazole, quinolone antibiotics, and tetracyclines. Compounds in grapefruit juice and some drugs inhibit the P-glycoprotein drug transporter in the intestinal epithelium and may increase the net absorption of drugs that are normally expelled by the transporter. Absorption from subcutaneous sites can be slowed predictably by vasoconstrictors given simultaneously (eg, local anesthetics and epinephrine) and by cardiac depressants that decrease tissue perfusion (eg, β blockers).

B. Interactions Based on Distribution and Binding

Distribution of a drug can be altered by other drugs that compete for binding sites on plasma proteins. For example, antibacterial sulfonamides can displace methotrexate, phenytoin, sulfonylureas, and warfarin from binding sites on albumin. However, it is difficult to document many clinically significant interactions of this type, and they seem to be the exception rather than the rule. Changes in drug distribution can occur if one agent alters the size of the physical compartment in which another drug distributes. For example, diuretics, by reducing total body water, can increase plasma levels of aminoglycosides and lithium, possibly enhancing drug toxicities.

C. Interactions Based on Metabolic Clearance

Drug interactions of this type are well documented and have considerable clinical significance. The metabolism of many drugs can be increased by other agents that induce hepatic drug-metabolizing enzymes, especially cytochrome P450 isozymes. Induction of drug-metabolizing enzymes occurs predictably with chronic administration of **barbiturates, carbamazepine, ethanol, phenytoin,** or **rifampin.** Conversely, the metabolism of some drugs may be decreased by other drugs that inhibit drug-metabolizing enzymes. Such inhibitors of drug-metabolizing enzymes include **cimetidine, disulfiram, erythromycin, furanocoumarins** (in grapefruit juice), **ketoconazole, quinidine, ritonavir, sulfonamides,** and many others. The CYP3A4 isozyme of cytochrome P450, the dominant form in the human liver, is particularly sensitive to such inhibitory actions.

Drugs that reduce hepatic blood flow (eg, **propranolol**) may reduce the clearance of other drugs metabolized in the liver, especially those subject to flow-limited hepatic clearance such as morphine and verapamil.

A modified form of an interaction based on metabolic clearance results from the ability of some drugs to increase the stores of endogenous substances by blocking their metabolism. These endogenous compounds may subsequently be released by other exogenous drugs, resulting in an unexpected action. The best-documented reaction of this type is the sensitization of patients taking **MAO inhibitors** to indirectly acting sympathomimetics (eg, amphetamine, phenylpropanolamine). Such patients may suffer a severe hypertensive reaction in response to ordinary doses of cold remedies, decongestants, and appetite suppressants.

High-Yield Terms to Learn

Additive effects	The effect of 2 drugs given together is equal to the sum of the responses to the same doses given separately
Antagonism	The effect of 2 drugs given together is less than the sum of the responses to the same doses given separately
Pharmacodynamic interaction	A change in the pharmacodynamics of 1 drug caused by the interacting drug (eg, additive action of 2 drugs having similar effects)
Pharmacokinetic interaction	A change in the pharmacokinetics of 1 drug caused by the interacting drug (eg, an inducer of hepatic enzymes)
Synergism	The effect of 2 drugs given together is greater than the sum of the 2 responses when they are given separately

TABLE 61–1 Some important drug interactions.

Drug Causing the Interaction	Examples of Drugs Affected	Comments
Alcohol	CNS depressants	Additive CNS depression, sedation, ataxia, increased risk of accidents
	Acetaminophen	Increased formation of hepatotoxic metabolites of acetaminophen
Antacids	Digoxin, iron supplements, fluoroquinolones, ketoconazole, tetracyclines, thyroxine	Decreased gut absorption due either to reaction with the affected drug or due to reduced acidity
Antihistamines (H₁ blockers)	Antimuscarinics, sedatives	Additive effects with the drugs affected
Antimuscarinic drugs	Drugs absorbed from the small intestine	Slowed onset of effect because stomach emptying is delayed
Barbiturates, especially phenobarbital	Azoles, calcium channel blockers, cyclosporine, propranolol, protease inhibitors, quinidine, steroids, warfarin, and many other drugs metabolized in the liver	Increased clearance of the affected drugs due to enzyme induction, possibly leading to decreases in drug effectiveness
Beta blockers	Insulin Prazosin	Masking of symptoms of hypoglycemia Increased first-dose syncope
Bile acid-binding resins	Acetaminophen, digitalis, thiazides, thyroxine	Reduced absorption of the affected drug
Carbamazepine	Cyclosporine, doxycycline, estrogen, haloperidol, theophylline, warfarin	Reduced effect of other drugs because of induction of metabolism
Cimetidine	Benzodiazepines, lidocaine, phenytoin, propranolol, quinidine, theophylline, warfarin	Risk of toxicity due to inhibition of metabolism
Disulfiram, metronidazole, certain cephalosporins	Ethanol	Increased hangover effect due to inhibition of aldehyde dehydrogenase
Erythromycin	Carbamazepine, cisapride, quinidine, sildenafil, SSRIs	Risk of toxicity due to inhibition of metabolism
Furanocoumarins (grapefruit juice)	Alprazolam, atorvastatin, cyclosporine, midazolam	Risk of toxicity due to inhibition of metabolism
Ketoconazole and other azoles	Benzodiazepines, cisapride cyclosporine, fluoxetine, lovastatin, omeprazole, quinidine, tolbutamide, warfarin	Risk of toxicity due to inhibition of metabolism
MAO inhibitors	Catecholamine releasers (amphetamine, ephedrine) Tyramine-containing foods and beverages	Increased norepinephrine in sympathetic nerve endings released by the interacting drugs Hypertensive crisis
NSAIDs	Anticoagulants Angiotensin-converting enzyme (ACE) inhibitors Loop diuretics, thiazides	Increased bleeding tendency because of reduced platelet aggregation Decreased antihypertensive efficacy of ACE inhibitor Reduced diuretic efficacy

(Continued)

TABLE 61–1 Some important drug interactions. (*Continued*)

Drug Causing the Interaction	Examples of Drugs Affected	Comments
Phenytoin	Doxycycline, methadone, quinidine, steroids, verapamil	Reduced effect of other drugs because of induction of metabolism
Rifampin	Azole antifungal drugs, corticosteroids, methadone, sulfonylureas	Reduced effect of other drugs because of induction of metabolism
Ritonavir	Benzodiazepines, cyclosporine, diltiazem, HMG-CoA reductase inhibitors, lidocaine, metoprolol, other HIV protease inhibitors, SSRIs	Risk of toxicity due to inhibition of metabolism
Salicylates	Corticosteroids Heparin, warfarin Methotrexate Sulfinpyrazone, probenecid	Additive toxicity to gastric mucosa Increased bleeding tendency Decreased clearance, causing greater methotrexate toxicity Decreased uricosuric effect
Selective serotonin reuptake inhibitors (SSRIs)	Monoamine oxidase (MAO) inhibitors, meperidine, tricyclic antidepressants, St. John's wort	Serotonin syndrome (hypertension, tachycardia, muscle rigidity, hyperthermia, seizures)
Thiazides	Digitalis Lithium	Increased risk of digitalis toxicity because thiazides diminish potassium stores Increased plasma levels of lithium due to decreased total body water
Warfarin	Amiodarone, cimetidine, erythromycin, fluconazole, lovastatin, metronidazole Aspirin, NSAIDs, quinidine, thyroxine Barbiturates, carbamazepine, phenytoin, rifabutin, rifampin, St. John's wort	Increased anticoagulant effect via inhibition of warfarin metabolism Increased anticoagulant effects via pharmacodynamic mechanisms Decreased anticoagulant effect due to increased metabolism

SKILL KEEPER: WARFARIN (SEE CHAPTER 34)

When describing pharmacokinetic drug interactions, the anticoagulant warfarin inevitably springs to mind. This is because warfarin has such a narrow therapeutic window and because its metabolism depends on CYP450 activity. How does this important anticoagulant work, how is its action monitored, and if a drug interaction leads to an excessive effect, how is its action reversed? The Skill Keeper Answer appears at the end of the chapter.

D. Interactions Based on Renal Function

Excretion of drugs by the kidney can be changed by drugs that reduce renal blood flow (eg, β blockers) or inhibit specific renal transport mechanisms (eg, the action of aspirin on uric acid secretion in the proximal tubule). Drugs that alter urinary pH can alter the ionization state of drugs that are weak acids or weak bases, leading to changes in renal tubular reabsorption.

PHARMACODYNAMIC INTERACTIONS

A. Interactions Based on Opposing Actions or Effects

Antagonism, the simplest type of drug interaction, is often predictable. For example, antagonism of the bronchodilating effects of β$_2$-adrenoceptor activators used in asthma is to be anticipated if a β blocker is given for another condition. Likewise, the action of a catecholamine on heart rate (via β-adrenoceptor activation) is antagonized by an inhibitor of acetylcholinesterase that acts through acetylcholine (via muscarinic receptors). Antagonism by mixed agonist-antagonist drugs (eg, pentazocine) or by partial agonists (eg, pindolol) is not as easily predicted but should be expected when such drugs are used with pure agonists. Some drug antagonisms do not appear to be based on receptor interactions. For example, nonsteroidal anti-inflammatory drugs (NSAIDs) may decrease the antihypertensive action of angiotensin-converting enzyme (ACE) inhibitors by reducing renal elimination of sodium.

B. Interactions Based on Additive Effects

Additive interaction describes the algebraic summing of the effects of 2 drugs. The 2 drugs may or may not act on the same receptor

TABLE 61-2 Selected interactions of herbals with other drugs.

Herbal Medication	Other Drugs	Interaction
Dong quai	Warfarin	Increased anticoagulant effect of warfarin; bleeding
Garlic, ginkgo	Anticoagulants, antiplatelet agents	Increased risk of bleeding
Ginseng	Antidepressants	Increased antidepressant effect, mania
Kava	Sedative-hypnotics	Additive sedation
Liquorice root	Aldosterone, antihypertensive drugs	Liquorice root extract (not candy) increases salt retention; hypertension
Ma huang, other ephedra preparations	Sympathomimetics	Ephedrine in ma huang is additive with other sympathomimetics; hypertension, stroke
St. John's wort	Oral contraceptives, cyclosporine digoxin, HIV protease inhibitors, warfarin	Increased metabolism of drug, decreased efficacy
	Antidepressants	Increased antidepressant effect; serotonin syndrome with selective serotonin reuptake inhibitors

to produce such effects. The combination of tricyclic antidepressants with diphenhydramine or promethazine predictably causes excessive atropine-like effects because all these drugs have significant muscarinic receptor-blocking actions. Tricyclic antidepressants may increase the pressor responses to sympathomimetics by interference with amine transporter systems.

One of the most common and important drug interactions is the additive depression of CNS function caused by concomitant administration of sedatives, hypnotics, and opioids with each other or associated with the consumption of ethanol. Similarly, the patient with moderate to severe hypertension maintained on one drug is at risk of excessive lowering of blood pressure if another drug with a different site of action is added at high dosage. Additive effects of anticoagulant drugs can lead to bleeding complications. In the case of warfarin, the potential for such adverse effects is enhanced by aspirin (via an antiplatelet action), thrombolytics (via plasminogen activation), and the thyroid hormones (via enhanced clotting factor catabolism).

Supra-additive interactions and potentiation appear to be much less common than antagonism and the simple additive interactions described previously. Supra-additive (synergistic) interaction is said to occur when the result of interaction is greater than the sum of the drugs used alone; the best example is the therapeutic synergism of certain antibiotic combinations such as sulfonamides and dihydrofolic acid reductase inhibitors such as trimethoprim. Potentiation is said to occur when a drug's effect is increased by another agent that has no such effect. The best example of this type of interaction is the therapeutic interaction of β-lactamase inhibitors such as clavulanic acid with β-lactamase-susceptible penicillins.

INTERACTIONS OF HERBAL MEDICATIONS WITH OTHER DRUGS

Because of the marked increase in use of herbal medications, more interactions of these agents with purified drugs are being

reported. Some of the reported or suspected interactions are listed in Table 61–2. Several herbals listed are known to enhance the actions of anticoagulants. Many other herbs, or edible plants, also contain compounds with anticoagulant or antiplatelet potential, including anise, arnica, capsicum, celery, chamomile, clove, feverfew, garlic, ginger, horseradish, meadowsweet, onion, passion flower, turmeric, and wild lettuce.

QUESTIONS

1. A 55-year-old patient currently receiving a drug for a psychiatric condition is to be started on diuretic therapy for mild heart failure. Consideration should be given to the fact that thiazides are known to reduce the excretion of which of the following?
    (A) Diazepam
    (B) Fluoxetine
    (C) Imipramine
    (D) Lithium
    (E) Trifluoperazine

2. A hypertensive patient has been using nifedipine for some time without untoward effects. If he experiences a rapidly developing enhancement of the antihypertensive effect of the drug, it is most likely due to which of the following?
    (A) Concomitant use of antacids
    (B) Foods containing tyramine
    (C) Furanocoumarins in grapefruit juice
    (D) Induction of drug metabolism
    (E) Over-the-counter decongestants

3. A patient suffering from a depressive disorder is being treated with imipramine. If he uses diphenhydramine for allergic rhinitis, a drug interaction is likely to occur because
    (A) Both drugs block muscarinic receptors
    (B) Both drugs block reuptake of norepinephrine released from sympathetic nerve endings
    (C) Diphenhydramine inhibits imipramine metabolism
    (D) Imipramine inhibits the metabolism of diphenhydramine
    (E) The drugs compete with each other for renal elimination

4. If phenelzine is administered to a patient taking fluoxetine, which of the following is most likely to occur?
   (A) A decrease in the plasma levels of fluoxetine
   (B) Antagonism of the antidepressant action of fluoxetine
   (C) Agitation, muscle rigidity, hyperthermia, seizures
   (D) Decreased metabolism of fluoxetine
   (E) Priapism

5. Which antibiotic is a potent inducer of hepatic drug-metabolizing enzymes?
   (A) Ciprofloxacin
   (B) Cyclosporine
   (C) Erythromycin
   (D) Rifampin
   (E) Tetracycline

6. The antihypertensive effects of captopril can be antagonized (reduced) by which of the following?
   (A) Angiotensin II receptor blockers
   (B) Loop diuretics
   (C) NSAIDs
   (D) Sulfonylurea hypoglycemics
   (E) Thiazides

7. Which drug has resulted in severe hematotoxicity when administered to a patient being treated with azathioprine?
   (A) Allopurinol
   (B) Cholestyramine
   (C) Digoxin
   (D) Lithium
   (E) Theophylline

DIRECTIONS: 8–10. The following section consists of a list of lettered options followed by several numbered items. For each numbered item, select the ONE option that is most closely associated with it.
   (A) Allopurinol
   (B) Carbamazepine
   (C) Cholestyramine
   (D) Cimetidine
   (E) Clarithromycin
   (F) Cyclosporine
   (G) Digoxin
   (H) Erythromycin
   (I) Fluoxetine
   (J) Ibuprofen
   (K) Lovastatin
   (L) Phenelzine
   (M) Rifampin
   (N) Ritonavir
   (O) Theophylline

8. In patients with HIV infection, the inhibitory action of this agent on drug metabolism has clinical value.

9. This drug enhances the toxicity of methotrexate by decreasing its renal clearance.

10. Concomitant use of St. John's wort is reported to increase the effectiveness of this drug.

ANSWERS

1. Thiazides reduce the clearance of lithium by about 25%. They do not alter the clearance of the other agents listed. The answer is **D**.

2. Compounds in grapefruit juice can increase the rate and extent of bioavailability of several dihydropyridine calcium channel blockers, including felodipine and nifedipine. This interaction may be due to inhibition of the metabolism of the dihydropyridines by intestinal wall CYP3A4 or inhibition of the P-glycoprotein transporter in the same location. The answer is **C**.

3. This is a good example of an additive drug interaction resulting from 2 drugs acting on the same type of receptor. Most tricyclic antidepressants, phenothiazines, and older antihistaminic drugs (those available without prescription) are blockers of muscarinic receptors. Used concomitantly, any pair of these agents will demonstrate a predictable increase in atropine-like adverse effects. The answer is **A**.

4. The drug interaction between the inhibitors of monoamine oxidase used for depression and the drugs that selectively block serotonin reuptake (SSRIs) is called the serotonin syndrome. In the case of phenelzine and fluoxetine, the interaction has resulted in a fatal outcome. Key interventions include control of hyperthermia and seizures. The answer is **C**.

5. Rifampin is an effective inducer of hepatic P450 isozymes. Cyclosporine and tetracycline have no significant effects on drug metabolism. Ciprofloxacin and erythromycin are inhibitors of drug metabolism. The answer is **D**.

6. NSAIDs interfere with the antihypertensive action of angiotensin-converting enzyme inhibitors; the other drugs listed enhance the blood pressure-lowering effects of captopril and other members of the "pril" drug family. The answer is **C**.

7. Azathioprine is converted to mercaptopurine, which is responsible for both its immunosuppressant action and its hematotoxicity. Allopurinol inhibits xanthine oxidase, the enzyme that metabolizes mercaptopurine. The answer is **A**.

8. Ritonavir inhibits the metabolism of other HIV protease inhibitors and is used in low-dose combinations with indinavir or lopinavir. The answer is **N**.

9. Several NSAIDs, including aspirin, ibuprofen, and piroxicam, increase serum levels of methotrexate by interfering with its renal clearance. The adverse effects of methotrexate, including its hematotoxicity, are predictably increased. The answer is **J**.

10. Concomitant use of St. John's wort enhances the effects of selective serotonin reuptake inhibitors. In contrast, the herb decreases the effectiveness of other drugs (including cyclosporine, estrogens, and protease inhibitors) via its induction of drug-metabolizing enzymes. The answer is **I**.

SKILL KEEPER ANSWER: WARFARIN (SEE CHAPTER 34)

Warfarin inhibits coagulation by interfering with the vitamin K-dependent post-translational modification of several clotting factors (prothrombin and factors VII, IX and X) and the anticoagulant proteins C and S. Without this post-translational modification, these proteins are inactive. Because warfarin inhibits the synthesis of coagulation factors and not the function of preformed factors, it has a relatively slow onset and offset of activity. The anticoagulant effect of warfarin is monitored by the prothrombin time (PT) test. Excessive anticoagulation can be reversed by administration of vitamin K or by transfusion with fresh or frozen plasma, which contains functional clotting factors.

CHECKLIST

When you complete this chapter, you should be able to:

❑ Describe the primary pharmacokinetic mechanisms that underlie drug interactions.

❑ Describe how the pharmacodynamic characteristics of different drugs administered concomitantly may lead to additive, synergistic, or antagonistic effects.

❑ Identify specific drug interactions that involve (1) alcohol, (2) antacids, (3) cimetidine, (4) ketoconazole, (5) NSAIDs, (6) phenytoin, (7) rifampin, and (8) warfarin.

❑ List specific drug interactions that can occur in the management of HIV patients.

❑ Identify specific drug interactions that involve commonly used herbals.

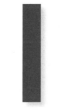

Key Words for Key Drugs

The following list is a compilation of the drugs that are most likely to appear on examinations. The brief descriptions should serve as a rapid review. The list can be used in 2 ways. First, cover the column of properties and test your ability to recall descriptive information about drugs picked at random from the left column; second, cover the left column and try to name a drug that fits the properties described. The numbers in parentheses at the end of each drug description denote relevant chapter.

Common abbreviations and acronyms: ACE, angiotensin converting enzyme; ADHD, attention deficit hyperactivity disorder; ANS, autonomic nervous system; AV, atrioventricular; BP, blood pressure; CNS, central nervous system; COMT, catechol-O-methyl transferase; DMARD, disease-modifying antirheumatic drug; ENS, enteric nervous system; EPS, extrapyramidal system; GABA, γ-aminobutyric acid; GI, gastrointestinal; HF, heart failure; HR, heart rate; HTN, hypertension; LMW, low molecular weight; MAO, monoamine oxidase; MI, myocardial infarct; NSAID, nonsteroidal anti-inflammatory drug; PANS, parasympathetic autonomic nervous system; RA, rheumatoid arthritis; SANS, sympathetic autonomic nervous system; TCA, tricyclic antidepressant; TNF, tumor necrosis factor; Tox, toxicity; WBCs, white blood cells.

Drug	Properties
Abciximab	Monoclonal antibody that inhibits the binding of platelet glycoprotein IIb/IIIa (GPIIb/IIIa) to fibrinogen. Used to prevent clotting after coronary angioplasty and in acute coronary syndrome. **Eptifibatide** and **tirofiban** are also GPIIb/IIIa inhibitors. (34)
Acetaminophen	Antipyretic analgesic: very weak cyclooxygenase inhibitor; not anti-inflammatory. Less GI distress than aspirin but dangerous in overdose. Tox: hepatic necrosis. Antidote: **acetylcysteine**. (36)
Acetazolamide	Carbonic anhydrase-inhibiting diuretic acting in the proximal convoluted tubule: produces a $NaHCO_3$ diuresis, results in bicarbonate depletion and metabolic acidosis. Has self-limited diuretic but persistent bicarbonate-depleting action. Used in glaucoma and mountain sickness. Tox: paresthesias, hepatic encephalopathy. **Dorzolamide** and **brinzolamide** are topical analogs for glaucoma. (15)
Acetylcholine	Cholinomimetic prototype: transmitter in CNS, ENS, all ANS ganglia, parasympathetic postganglionic synapses, sympathetic postganglionic fibers to sweat glands, and skeletal muscle end plate synapses. (6, 7)
Acyclovir	Antiviral: inhibits DNA synthesis in herpes simplex virus (HSV) and varicella-zoster virus (VZV). Requires activation by viral thymidine kinase (TK⁻ strains are resistant). Tox: behavioral effects and nephrotoxicity (crystalluria) but minimal myelosuppression. **Famciclovir, penciclovir**, and **valacyclovir** are similar but with longer half-lives. (49)
Adenosine	Antiarrhythmic: miscellaneous group; parenteral only. Hyperpolarizes AV nodal tissue, blocks conduction for 10–15 s. Used for nodal reentry arrhythmias. Tox: hypotension, flushing, chest pain. (14)
Albuterol	Prototypic rapid-acting β_2 agonist; important use in acute asthma. Tox: tachycardia, arrhythmias, tremor. Other drugs with similar action: **metaproterenol, terbutaline**. Slow-acting analogs: formoterol, salmeterol; used for prophylaxis. (9, 20)
Alendronate	Bisphosphonate: chronic treatment with low doses increases bone mineral density and reduces fractures. Higher doses lower serum calcium. Used in osteoporosis and for the hypercalcemia in Paget's disease and malignancies. Tox: esophageal irritation at low oral doses. Renal dysfunction and osteonecrosis of the jaw in high doses. Other bisphosphonates include **etidronate, pamidronate, risedronate,** etc. (42)

Allopurinol	Irreversible inhibitor of xanthine oxidase; reduces production of uric acid. Used in gout and adjunctively in cancer chemotherapy. Inhibits metabolism of purine analogs (eg, mercaptopurine, azathioprine). **Febuxostat** is similar. (36)
Alteplase (t-PA)	Thrombolytic: human recombinant tissue plasminogen activator. Used to recanalize occluded blood vessels in acute MI, severe pulmonary embolism, stroke. **Reteplase** and **tenecteplase** are similar. **Streptokinase** is a bacterial protein with thrombolytic properties. *Tox:* bleeding. (34)
Amiloride	K^+-sparing diuretic: blocks epithelial Na^+ channels in cortical collecting tubules. *Tox:* hyperkalemia. (15)
Amiodarone	Group 3 (and other groups) antiarrhythmic: broad spectrum; blocks sodium, potassium, calcium channels, β receptors. High efficacy and very long half-life (weeks to months). *Tox:* deposits in tissues; skin coloration; hypo- or hyperthyroidism; pulmonary fibrosis; optic neuritis. (14)
Amphetamine	Indirect-acting sympathomimetic: displaces stored catecholamines in nerve endings. Marked CNS stimulant actions; high abuse liability. Used in ADHD, for short-term weight loss, and for narcolepsy. *Tox:* psychosis, HTN, MI, seizures. Other indirect-acting sympathomimetics that displace catecholamines: **ephedrine, pseudoephedrine, methylphenidate, tyramine.** (9, 32)
Amphotericin B	Antifungal: polyene commonly a drug of choice for systemic mycoses; binds to ergosterol to disrupt fungal cell membrane permeability. *Tox:* chills and fever, hypotension, nephrotoxicity (dose limiting; less with liposomal forms). (48)
Ampicillin	Penicillin: wider spectrum than penicillin G, susceptible to penicillinases unless used with sulbactam. Activity similar to that of penicillin G, plus *E coli, H influenzae, P mirabilis, Shigella.* Synergy with aminoglycosides versus *Enterococcus* and *Listeria.* *Tox:* penicillin allergy; more adverse effects on GI tract than other penicillins; maculopapular skin rash. **Amoxicillin** has greater oral bioavailability and less GI effects; also used with clavulanate, a penicillinase inhibitor. (43)
Anastrozole	Aromatase inhibitor: prototype inhibitor of the enzyme that converts testosterone to estradiol. Used in estrogen-dependent breast cancer. **Letrozole** is similar; **exemestane** is an irreversible aromatase inhibitor. (40, 54)
Aspirin	NSAID prototype: inhibits cyclooxygenase (COX)-1 and -2 irreversibly. Antiplatelet agent as well as antipyretic, analgesic and anti-inflammatory drug. *Tox:* GI ulcers, nephrotoxicity, rash, hypersensitivity leading to bronchoconstriction, salicylism. Other NSAIDs: **ibuprofen, indomethacin, ketorolac,** and **naproxen.** (34, 36)
Atenolol	Beta$_1$-selective blocker: low lipid solubility, less CNS effect; used for HTN, angina. (**Mnemonic:** Generic names of β$_1$-selective blockers start with A through M except for carteolol, carvedilol, and labetalol.) *Tox:* asthma, bradycardia, AV block, heart failure. (10)
Atropine	Muscarinic cholinoceptor blocker prototype: lipid-soluble, CNS effects; antidote for cholinesterase poisoning. *Tox:* "red as a beet, dry as a bone, blind as a bat, mad as a hatter," urinary retention, mydriasis. **Cyclopentolate, tropicamide:** antimuscarinics for ophthalmology; cause cycloplegia and mydriasis. **Glycopyrrolate:** antimuscarinic with decreased CNS effects. (8, 58)
Azithromycin	Macrolide antibiotic: similar to erythromycin but greater activity against *H influenzae,* chlamydiae, and streptococci; long half-life with renal elimination. *Tox:* GI distress but no inhibition of drug metabolism. **Clarithromycin** is similar but has a shorter half-life, and inhibits drug metabolism. (44)
Baclofen	GABA analog, orally active: spasmolytic; activates GABA$_B$ receptors in the spinal cord. (27)
Benztropine	Muscarinic cholinoceptor blocker: centrally acting antimuscarinic prototype for parkinsonism. *Tox:* excess antimuscarinic effects. (8, 28)
Botulinum	Toxins produced by *Clostridium botulinum:* enzymes that cleave proteins (synaptobrevin, others) and block transmitter release from acetylcholine vesicles. Injected to treat muscle spasm, smooth wrinkles, and reduce excessive sweating. *Tox:* paralysis. (6, 27)
Bromocriptine	Ergot derivative: prototype dopamine agonist in CNS; inhibits prolactin release. Used in hyperprolactinemia and a rarely used alternative drug in parkinsonism. *Tox:* CNS, dyskinesias, hypotension. (16, 28, 37)
Bupivacaine	Long-acting amide local anesthetic prototype. *Tox:* greater cardiovascular toxicity than most local anesthetics. (26)
Buprenorphine	Opioid: long-acting partial agonist of μ receptors. Analgesic (not equivalent to morphine) and effective for detoxification and maintenance in opioid dependence. Other mixed agonist-antagonists: **nalbuphine** activates κ and weakly blocks μ receptors; **pentazocine,** κ agonist and weak μ antagonist or partial agonist. (31)
Bupropion	Antidepressant & used in smoking cessation: mechanism uncertain, but no direct actions on CNS amines. *Tox:* agitation, anxiety, aggravation of psychosis and, at high doses, seizures. (30)

Captopril	ACE inhibitor prototype: used in HTN, diabetic nephropathy, and HF. *Tox:* hyperkalemia, fetal renal damage, cough ("sore throat"). Other "prils" include **benazepril, enalapril, lisinopril, quinapril**. (11, 13, 17)
Carbamazepine	Antiseizure drug: used for tonic-clonic and partial seizures; blocks Na^+ channels in neuronal membranes. Drug of choice for trigeminal neuralgia; backup drug in bipolar disorder. *Tox:* CNS depression, myelotoxic, induces liver drug-metabolizing enzymes, teratogenicity. (24, 29)
Carvedilol	Adrenoceptor blocker: racemic mixture, one isomer a nonselective β blocker and the other an α_1 blocker. Used in HTN, prolongs survival in HF. *Tox:* cardiovascular depression, asthma. **Labetalol** is similar. (10, 11, 13)
Caspofungin	Antifungal: echinocandin prototype, inhibitor of β (1-3)-glucan synthesis, a cell wall component. Used IV for disseminated *Candida* and *Aspergillus* infections. *Tox:* GI effects, flushing. Increases cyclosporine levels (avoid combination). (48)
Cefazolin	First-generation cephalosporin prototype: bactericidal beta-lactam inhibitor of cell wall synthesis. Active against gram-positive cocci, *E coli, K pneumoniae*, but does not enter the CNS. *Tox:* potential allergy; partial cross-reactivity with penicillins. (43)
Ceftriaxone	Third-generation cephalosporin: active against many bacteria, including pneumococci, gonococci (a drug of choice), and gram-negative rods. Enters the CNS and is used in bacterial meningitis. **Cefotaxime** and **ceftazidime** are other third-generation cephalosporins. (43)
Celecoxib	Selective COX-2 inhibitor. Less GI toxicity than nonselective NSAIDs. *Tox:* nephrotoxicity, increased risk of myocardial thrombosis and stroke. (36)
Chloramphenicol	Antibiotic: broad-spectrum agent; inhibits protein synthesis (50S); uses restricted to backup drug for bacterial meningitis, infections due to anaerobes, *Salmonella*. *Tox:* reversible myelosuppression, aplastic anemia, gray baby syndrome. (44)
Chloroquine	Antimalarial: blood schizonticide used for treatment and prophylaxis in areas in which *P falciparum* is susceptible. Binds to hemin, causing dysfunctional cell membranes; resistance resulting from efflux via P-glycoprotein pump. *Tox:* GI distress and skin rash at low doses; peripheral neuropathy, skin lesions, auditory and visual impairment, quinidine-like cardiotoxicity at high doses. (52)
Chlorpheniramine	Antihistamine first-generation H_1 blocker prototype. *Tox:* less sedation and ANS-blocking action than **diphenhydramine**. (16)
Chlorpromazine	Phenothiazine antipsychotic drug prototype: blocks most dopamine receptors in CNS. *Tox:* atropine-like, EPS dysfunction, hyperprolactinemia, postural hypotension, sedation, seizures (in overdose), additive effects with other CNS depressants. Other phenothiazines: **fluphenazine**, **trifluoperazine** (antipsychotics), **prochlorperazine** (antiemetic), **promethazine** (preoperative sedation). (29)
Cholestyramine	Antihyperlipidemic: bile acid-binding resin prototype that sequesters bile acids in gut and diverts more cholesterol from the liver to bile acids instead of circulating lipoproteins. Used for hypercholesterolemia *Tox:* constipation, bloating; interferes with absorption of some drugs. **Colestipol** and **colesevelam** are similar. (35)
Cimetidine	H_2 blocker prototype: used in acid-peptic disease. *Tox:* inhibits hepatic drug metabolism; antiandrogen effects. Less toxic analogs: **ranitidine, famotidine, nizatidine**. (16, 59)
Ciprofloxacin	Second-generation fluoroquinolone antibiotic: bactericidal inhibitor of topoisomerases; active against *E coli, H influenzae, Campylobacter, Enterobacter, Pseudomonas, Shigella*. *Tox:* CNS dysfunction, GI distress, superinfection, collagen dysfunction (caution in children and pregnant women). *Interactions:* inhibits metabolism of caffeine, theophylline, warfarin. See also **levofloxacin**. (46)
Cisplatin	Antineoplastic: platinum-containing alkylating anticancer drug. Used for solid tumors (eg, testes, lung). *Tox:* Neurotoxic and nephrotoxic. **Carboplatin, oxaliplatin** are similar. (54)
Clindamycin	Lincosamide antibiotic: bacteriostatic inhibitor of protein synthesis (50S); active against gram-positive cocci, *B fragilis*. *Tox:* GI distress, pseudomembranous colitis. (44)
Clomiphene	Selective estrogen receptor modulator (SERM): synthetic, used in infertility to induce ovulation by blocking pituitary estrogen receptors. May result in multiple births. (40)
Clonidine	Alpha$_2$ agonist: acts centrally to reduce SANS outflow, lowers BP. Used in HTN and in drug dependency states. *Tox:* mild sedation in normal doses, rebound HTN if stopped suddenly. See also **methyldopa**. (9, 11, 32)
Clopidogrel	Antiplatelet agent: irreversibly inhibits platelet ADP receptors and platelet aggregation. Used in transient ischemic attacks and to prevent strokes and restenosis after placement of coronary stents. *Tox:* bleeding, neutropenia. **Ticlopidine** is similar, but higher risk of neutropenia and thrombotic thrombocytopenic purpura (TTP). (34)

Cocaine	Indirect-acting sympathomimetic that blocks amine reuptake into nerve endings: local anesthetic (ester type). Marked CNS stimulation, euphoria; high abuse and dependence liability. *Tox:* psychosis, HTN, cardiac arrhythmias, seizures. (9, 26, 32)
Colchicine	Microtubule assembly inhibitor: reduces macrophage mobility and phagocytosis; used in chronic gout. *Tox:* GI (often severe), hepatic, renal damage. (36)
Cyclophosphamide	Antineoplastic, immunosuppressive: cell cycle-nonspecific alkylating agent. *Tox:* alopecia, GI distress, hemorrhagic cystitis (use **mesna**), myelosuppression. (54, 55)
Cyclosporine	Immunosuppressant: immunophilin ligand; inhibits T-cell synthesis of cytokines. *Tox:* nephrotoxicity, hypertension, peripheral neuropathy, seizures. **Tacrolimus** is similar. **Sirolimus** binds to same immunophilin as tacrolimus (FKBP12), but this complex inhibits mammalian target of rapamycin (mTOR) kinase and T-cell response to IL-2. (36, 55)
Cytokines, recombinant	DNA technology products: aldesleukin (IL-2, used in renal cancer); **erythropoietin** (epoetin alfa, used in anemias); **filgrastim** (G-CSF, used in neutropenia); **interferon-α** (used in hepatitis B and C and in cancer); **interferon-β** (used in multiple sclerosis); **interferon-γ** (used in chronic granulomatous disease); **oprelvekin** (IL-11, used in thrombocytopenia); and **sargramostim** (GM-CSF, used in neutropenia). (33, 36, 49, 54, 55)
Dantrolene	Muscle relaxant: blocks Ca^{2+} release from sarcoplasmic reticulum of skeletal muscle. Used in muscle spasm (cerebral palsy, multiple sclerosis, cord injury) and in emergency treatment of malignant hyperthermia. (25, 27, 29)
Desmopressin	Vasopressin (ADH) analog, more selective for V_2 receptors: used for pituitary diabetes insipidus and mild hemophilia A or von Willebrand disease. **Vasopressin** (ADH), an agonist for V_1 and V_2 receptors, is used in pituitary diabetes insipidus and bleeding esophageal varices. **Conivaptan**, an *antagonist* at V_{1a} and V_2 receptors and **tolvaptan**, an antagonist at V_2 receptors, are used for hyponatremia. (15, 34, 37)
Diazepam	Benzodiazepine (BZ) prototype: binds to BZ receptors of the $GABA_A$ receptor-chloride ion channel complex; facilitates the inhibitory actions of GABA by increasing the *frequency* of channel opening (compare phenobarbital). Uses: anxiety states, ethanol detoxification, muscle spasticity, status epilepticus. Other benzodiazepines include **alprazolam**, **lorazepam**, **midazolam** & **triazolam**. *Tox:* dependence, additive effects with other CNS depressants. (22, 24, 27, 32)
Digoxin	Cardiac glycoside prototype: positive inotropic drug for HF, half-life 40 h; inhibits Na^+/K^+-ATPase. *Tox:* calcium overload arrhythmias, GI upset. (13, 14)
Diphenhydramine	Antihistamine (first-generation) H_1 blocker: used in hay fever, motion sickness, dystonias. *Tox:* antimuscarinic, α adrenoceptor blocker, strong sedative. **Doxylamine** is similar. (16, 59)
Dopamine	Neurotransmitter and agonist drug at dopamine receptors: used in shock to increase renal blood flow (low dose) and cardiac output (moderate dose). (6, 9, 13, 21, 28, 29, 37)
Doxorubicin	Antineoplastic: anthracycline drug (cell cycle-nonspecific); intercalates between base pairs to disrupt DNA functions, inhibits topoisomerases, and forms cytotoxic free radicals. *Tox:* cardiomyopathy (**dexrazoxane** is antidote), myelosuppression. **Daunorubicin** is similar. (54)
Doxycycline	Tetracycline antibiotic: protein synthesis inhibitor (30S), more effective than other tetracyclines against chlamydia and in Lyme disease; malaria prophylaxis. Unlike other tetracyclines, it is eliminated mainly in the feces and has longer half-life. *Tox:* see **tetracycline**. (44, 53)
Edrophonium	Cholinesterase inhibitor: very short duration of action (15 min). Used in diagnosis of myasthenia gravis and to distinguish myasthenic crisis from cholinergic crisis. (7)
Efavirenz	Nonnucleoside reverse transcriptase inhibitor (NNRTI): used in combination regimens for HIV. *Tox:* skin rash, CNS effects, avoid in pregnancy. Other NNRTIs: **delavirdine, nevirapine**. (49)
Enfuvirtide	Antiviral: HIV fusion inhibitor used in combination regimens. *Tox:* injection site reactions and rare hypersensitivity. (49)
Enoxaparin	LMW heparin: used parenterally for anticoagulation. Primary effect is on factor Xa, less on thrombin. The aPTT test is unreliable. Other LMW heparins include **dalteparin, tinzaparin**. *Tox:* bleeding. (34)
Entacapone	COMT inhibitor: enhances levodopa access to CNS neurons; adjunctive use in Parkinson's disease. *Tox:* exacerbates levodopa effects. **Tolcapone** is similar in action and use but can be hepatotoxic. (28)
Ephedrine	Indirectly acting sympathomimetic: like **amphetamine** but less CNS stimulation, more smooth muscle effects. In botanicals (eg, ma huang) and products for weight loss that are banned in the United States. *Tox:* hypertension, stroke, MI. (9, 61)
Epinephrine	Adrenoceptor agonist prototype: product of adrenal medulla, some CNS neurons. Affinity for all α and all β receptors. Drug of choice in anaphylaxis; used as hemostatic and as adjunct with local anesthetics; cardiac stimulant; traditional use in asthma. *Tox:* tachycardia, hypertension, MI, pulmonary edema, and hemorrhage. (6, 9)

Ergot alkaloids   **Ergonovine, ergotamine**: cause prolonged vasoconstriction and uterine contraction. Used in migraine and obstetrics. *Tox*: vasospasm (including coronaries). (16, 28)

Erythromycin   Macrolide antibiotic: bacteriostatic inhibitor of protein synthesis (50S); activity includes gram-positive cocci and bacilli, *M pneumoniae, Legionella pneumophila, C trachomatis. Tox*: cholestatic jaundice (avoid estolate in pregnancy), inhibits liver drug-metabolizing enzymes, interactions with cisapride, theophylline, warfarin. Other macrolide antibiotics include **azithromycin** and **clarithromycin**. (44)

Erythropoietin   Hematopoietic growth factor: stimulates RBC production and release from bone marrow. Used in anemia associated with renal failure and anemias secondary to cancer chemotherapy. **Darbepoetin alfa** has a longer half-life. (33)

Etanercept   DMARD: recombinant protein that binds TNF-α. **Infliximab** and **adalimumab** have a similar mechanism of action. Effective in rheumatoid arthritis and other chronic inflammatory diseases. *Tox*: injection site reactions include erythema, itching, and swelling; possible increased rates of infection and malignancy. (36, 55)

Ethambutol   Antimycobacterial: inhibitor of arabinogalactan synthesis, a cell wall component; commonly used in standard antitubercular drug regimens. *Tox*: dose-dependent ocular dysfunction, dizziness, headache, hyperuricemia. (47)

Ethanol   Sedative-hypnotic: acute actions include impaired judgment, ataxia, loss of consciousness, vasodilation, and cardiovascular and respiratory depression. Chronic use leads to dependence and dysfunction of multiple organ systems; fetal alcohol syndrome. *Note*: zero-order elimination kinetics. (23, 32)

Ethinyl estradiol   Synthetic estrogen: used in many hormonal contraceptives. **Mestranol** is similar. (40)

Ethosuximide   Anticonvulsant: used in absence seizures; may block T-type Ca^{2+} channels in thalamic neurons. *Tox*: GI distress; safe in pregnancy. (24)

Ezetimibe   Antihyperlipidemic: cholesterol-lowering drug that inhibits GI transporter of dietary cholesterol and the cholesterol secreted in bile. Used for hypercholesterolemia, usually in combination with a statin. *Tox*: possible increased risk of hepatic damage when combined with statin. (35)

Fentanyl   Short-acting potent opioid agonist (see morphine) used commonly in anesthesia and for chronic pain (transdermal form). **Remifentanil** and **sufentanil** are similar. (25, 31, 32)

Finasteride   Antiandrogen: steroid inhibitor of 5α-reductase that inhibits synthesis of dihydrotestosterone. Used in benign prostatic hyperplasia and male-pattern baldness. **Dutasteride** is similar. (40)

Flecainide   Group 1C antiarrhythmic prototype: used in ventricular tachycardia and rapid atrial arrhythmias with Wolff-Parkinson-White syndrome. *Tox*: arrhythmogenic, CNS excitation. (14)

Fluconazole   Imidazole antifungal: inhibits ergosterol synthesis. CNS entry and renal elimination. Used in esophageal and vaginal candidiasis, in coccidioidomycosis, and in the prophylaxis and treatment of fungal meningitis. Adverse effects similar to those of **ketoconazole** but less severe. (48)

Fludrocortisone   Synthetic corticosteroid: high mineralocorticoid and moderate glucocorticoid activity; long duration of action. Used in Addison's disease. (39)

Flumazenil   Benzodiazepine receptor antagonist: used to reverse CNS depressant effects of benzodiazepines, zolpidem, eszopiclone and zaleplon. (22, 58)

Fluorouracil   Antineoplastic: pyrimidine antimetabolite (cell cycle-specific), irreversibly inhibits thymidylate synthase, resulting in dTMP deficiency and "thymine-less" cell death; used mainly for solid tumors. *Tox*: GI distress, myelosuppression, neurotoxicity. (54)

Fluoxetine   Antidepressant: selective serotonin reuptake inhibitor (SSRI) prototype. Less ANS adverse effects and cardiotoxic potential than tricyclics. *Tox*: CNS stimulation, sexual dysfunction, seizures in overdose, serotonin syndrome. Other SSRIs: **citalopram, escitalopram, fluvoxamine, paroxetine, sertraline**. (30)

Flutamide   Antiandrogen: prototype androgen receptor antagonist used in prostatic carcinoma. Others: **bicalutamide, nilutamide**. (40)

Furosemide   Loop diuretic prototype: blocks $Na^+/K^+/2Cl^-$ transporter in thick ascending limb; high efficacy; used in acute pulmonary edema, refractory edematous states, hypercalcemia, and HTN. *Tox*: ototoxicity, K^+ wasting, hypovolemia, increased serum uric acid. **Bumetanide** and **torsemide** differ only in half-life. **Ethacrynic acid** is similar but causes less hyperuricemia and may even reduce uric acid levels. (13, 15)

Gabapentin   Anticonvulsant: structural analog of GABA that facilitates its inhibitory actions in the CNS; used for partial seizures, for neuropathic pain, and in bipolar disorder. *Tox*: sedation, movement disorders. (24, 27, 29)

Ganciclovir   Antiviral: effective against herpesviruses (cytomegalovirus [CMV] and herpes simplex virus [HSV]); for CMV requires bioactivation via viral phosphotransferase. *Tox*: myelosuppression, nephrotoxicity, neurotoxicity. (49)

Gemfibrozil	Antihyperlipidemic: fibrate prototype used for hypertriglyceridemia. Lowers serum VLDL and triglycerides and increases HDL by activating peroxisome proliferator-activated receptor-α nuclear receptors. *Tox:* GI distress, cholelithiasis, increased risk of myopathy when combined with statins or niacin. (35)
Gentamicin	Aminoglycoside prototype: bactericidal inhibitor of protein synthesis (30S); active against many aerobic gram-negative bacteria. Narrow therapeutic window; dose reduction required in renal impairment. *Tox:* renal dysfunction, ototoxicity; once-daily dosing is effective (postantibiotic effect) and less toxic. **Amikacin** and **tobramycin** are similar. (45, 51)
Glipizide	Oral antidiabetic: second-generation, potent sulfonylurea secretagogue. Blocks K^+ channels in pancreatic B cells, causing depolarization and release of insulin. *Tox:* hypoglycemia, weight gain. Related drugs: **glyburide** and older sulfonylureas such as chlorpropamide and tolbutamide; short-acting secretagogues include **repaglinide** and nateglinide. (41)
Glucagon	Hormone from pancreatic A cells. Increases blood glucose via increased cyclic adenosine monophosphate. Used in severe hypoglycemia and as an antidote in β-blocker overdose. (41, 58)
Haloperidol	Antipsychotic butyrophenone: blocks brain dopamine D_2 receptors. *Tox:* marked EPS dysfunction, hyperprolactinemia; fewer ANS adverse effects than phenothiazines. (29)
Halothane	General anesthetic prototype: inhaled halogenated hydrocarbon. *Tox:* cardiovascular and respiratory depression and relaxation of skeletal and smooth muscle. Use is declining because of sensitization of heart to catecholamines and occurrence (rare) of hepatitis. Other inhaled anesthetics: **isoflurane** and **sevoflurane.** (25)
Heparin	Anticoagulant: large polymeric molecule with activity against thrombin and factor X. Rapid onset, parenteral administration. LMW heparins (eg, enoxaparin) and fondaparinux have a similar mechanism of action, although they are more selective for factor X. *Tox:* bleeding. *Antidote:* **protamine.** (34)
Hexamethonium	Prototypic ganglion blocker, now obsolete except for research use. Causes marked block of both PANS and SANS, hypotension. Newer analogs **trimethaphan, mecamylamine** are rarely used. (6)
Hydralazine	Antihypertensive: arteriolar vasodilator, orally active; used in severe HTN, HF. **Minoxidil**, a similar but more powerful antihypertensive, is also used topically in baldness. *Tox:* tachycardia, salt and water retention, lupus-like syndrome (hydralazine). (11, 13)
Hydrochlorothiazide	**Thiazide** diuretic prototype: acts in distal convoluted tubule to block Na^+/Cl^- transporter; used in HTN, HF, nephrolithiasis. *Tox:* hypersensitivity reactions; increased serum lipids, uric acid, glucose; K^+ wasting. (11, 13, 15)
Hydroxychloroquine	DMARD: immunosuppressant used for rheumatoid arthritis. *Tox:* rash, GI distress, ocular toxicity, myopathy, neuropathy. Other DMARDs: **methotrexate, sulfasalazine, gold salts, penicillamine.** (36)
Ibuprofen	NSAID: nonselective COX inhibitor with analgesic, antipyretic, and anti-inflammatory actions similar to aspirin, but no low-dose antiplatelet effect. *Tox:* GI, renal. (36)
Imipenem	Prototype carbapenem antibiotic: active against many aerobic and anaerobic bacteria, including penicillinase-producing organisms; a bactericidal inhibitor of cell wall synthesis. Used with cilastatin (which inhibits metabolism by renal dehydropeptidases). *Tox:* allergy (partial cross-reactivity with penicillins), seizures. **Meropenem** and **ertapenem** are similar but do not require cilastatin and are less likely to cause seizures. (43)
Imipramine	Tricyclic antidepressant (TCA): blocks reuptake of norepinephrine and serotonin. *Tox:* atropine-like, postural hypotension, sedation, cardiac arrhythmias in overdose, additive effects with other CNS depressants. Other TCAs: **amitriptyline, clomipramine, doxepin**. (30)
Indinavir	Antiviral: HIV protease inhibitor (PI) used as a component of combination regimens in AIDS. *Tox:* anemia, nephrolithiasis, metabolic disorders, inhibits P450 drug metabolism. Other PIs: **amprenavir, nelfinavir, ritonavir** (major P450 inhibitor, see below), and **saquinavir**. (49)
Indomethacin	NSAID: highly potent. Usually reserved for acute inflammation (eg, acute gout); neonatal patent ductus arteriosus. *Tox:* GI toxicity, renal damage. (36)
Interferon α	Cytokine: treatment of hepatitis B and C viral infections and some malignancies. *Tox:* "flu-like" syndrome, myelosuppression, neurotoxicity. (49, 55)
Ipratropium	Antimuscarinic agent: aerosol for asthma, chronic obstructive pulmonary disease (COPD). Good bronchodilator in 30–60% of patients. **Tiotropium** is similar with longer action. Not as efficacious as β_2 agonists but less toxic in COPD. *Tox:* dry mouth. (8, 20)
Isoniazid	Antimycobacterial: primary drug in combination regimens for tuberculosis; used as sole agent in treatment of latent infection. Metabolic clearance via *N*-acetyltransferases (genetic variability). *Tox:* hepatotoxicity (age-dependent), peripheral neuropathy (reversed by pyridoxine), hemolysis (in glucose-6-phosphate dehydrogenase deficiency [G6PD] deficiency). (47)

Isoproterenol	Beta$_1$ and β$_2$ agonist catecholamine prototype: bronchodilator, cardiac stimulant. Always causes tachycardia because both direct and reflex actions increase HR. *Tox:* arrhythmias, tremor, angina. (9)
Ivermectin	Antihelminthic: drug of choice for onchocerciasis and threadworm infections. Intensifies GABA-mediated neurotransmission in nematodes, but no access to CNS in humans. *Tox:* in onchocerciasis causes headache, fever, hypotension, joint pain. (53)
Ketoconazole	Antifungal azole prototype: active systemically; inhibits the synthesis of ergosterol. Used for *C albicans,* dermatophytosis, and non-life-threatening systemic mycoses. Is sometimes used to suppress adrenocorticoid or gonadal hormone synthesis. *Tox:* hepatic dysfunction, inhibits steroid synthesis and CYP450-dependent drug metabolism. Others: **fluconazole, itraconazole, and voriconazole** have a wider spectrum and less inhibitory effects on hepatic cytochromes P450. (39, 40, 48)
Ketorolac	NSAID: mainly used as a systemic analgesic; only NSAID available in parenteral form; see also aspirin. (36)
Lamivudine	Nucleoside reverse transcriptase inhibitor (NRTI) also known as 3TC. Least toxic NRTI. Notable for use in chronic hepatitis B in addition to HIV infection. (49)
Lamotrigine	Antiepileptic drug for absence and partial seizures; also used in bipolar affective disorder. *Tox:* rash, possibly life threatening, especially in pediatric patients. (24, 29)
Latanoprost	Prostaglandin F$_{2\alpha}$ analog used topically in closed angle glaucoma. **Bimatoprost, travoprost** are similar. (18)
Lepirudin	Antithrombotic: recombinant form of a medicinal leech protein that directly inhibits thrombin; rapid onset; parenteral administration. Used in heparin-induced thrombocytopenia (HIT). *Tox:* bleeding; monitor with aPTT. **Bivalirudin** is similar, used for PCI. **Argatroban** is a small molecule used parenterally for PCI. **Dabigatran** is oral thrombin inhibitor. (34)
Leuprolide	GnRH analog: continuous therapy used to suppress gonadotropin and gonadal hormone synthesis, especially in concert with gonadotropins for ovulation induction and in advanced prostate cancer. **Goserelin** and **nafarelin** are similar. **Ganirelix** is a GnRH receptor *antagonist* with similar effects. *Tox:* hot flushes, decreased bone density with prolonged use, gynecomastia (men). (37, 40, 54)
Levodopa	Dopamine precursor: used in parkinsonism, usually in combination with carbidopa (a peripheral inhibitor of dopamine metabolism). *Tox:* dyskinesias, hypotension, on-off phenomena, behavioral changes. (28)
Levofloxacin	Fluoroquinolone: Bactericidal inhibitor of topoisomerases; one of several "respiratory" fluoroquinolones (**gemifloxacin, moxifloxacin**) with greater activity than ciprofloxacin against pneumococci. *Tox:* see **ciprofloxacin**. (46)
Levonorgestrel	Progestin: used in many contraceptives including combined oral contraceptives, progestin-only oral contraceptives, the levonorgestrel IUD, subcutaneous implants, and the Plan B emergency contraceptive. (40)
Lidocaine	Amide local anesthetic, medium-duration amide prototype: highly selective use-dependent group 1B antiarrhythmic; used for nerve block and acute post-MI ischemic ventricular arrhythmias. Parenteral only. *Tox:* CNS excitation. **Mexiletine:** like lidocaine, but orally active, longer duration. (14, 26)
Lithium	Antimanic prototype: a primary drug in mania and bipolar affective disorders; blocks recycling of the phosphatidylinositol second messenger system. *Tox:* tremor, diabetes insipidus, goiter, seizures (in overdose). (29)
Loratadine	Second-generation H$_1$ antihistamine: used in hay fever. *Tox:* much less sedation than first-generation antihistamines; no ANS effects. Others: **desloratadine, cetirizine, fexofenadine**. (16)
Losartan	Angiotensin AT$_1$ receptor blocker (ARB) prototype: used in HTN. Effects and toxicity similar to those of ACE inhibitors but causes less cough. Other AT$_1$ blockers: **candesartan, eprosartan, irbesartan, olmesartan, telmisartan, valsartan**. (11, 13, 17)
Lovastatin	Antihyperlipidemic: HMG-CoA reductase. inhibitor prototype used for hypercholesterolemia. Acts in liver to reduce synthesis of cholesterol and indirectly increase LDL receptor synthesis. Other "statins": **atorvastatin, fluvastatin, pravastatin, rosuvastatin, simvastatin**. *Tox:* hepatotoxicity (elevated enzymes), muscle damage, teratogen. (35)
Malathion	Organophosphate insecticide cholinesterase inhibitor: prodrug converted to malaoxon. Less toxic in mammals and birds because metabolized to inactive products. Other organophosphates: **parathion** converted to paraoxon, and the nerve gases (eg, **sarin, soman**). (7, 58)
Mannitol	Osmotic diuretic: used short term for reduction of intracranial pressure or to promote excretion of renal toxins in hemolysis, rhabdomyolysis. *Tox:* initial expansion of extracellular fluid volume with resulting hyponatremia, headache, nausea. With excessive use, dehydration and hypernatremia. (15)

Mebendazole	Antihelminthic: important drug for common nematode infections. Inhibits microtubule synthesis and glucose uptake in nematodes. *Tox:* GI distress, caution in pregnancy. **Albendazole** (widely used) and **thiabendazole** (more toxic) are related antihelminthics. (53)
Medroxyprogesterone	Progestin: used in combination with an estrogen for treatment of menopausal symptoms and used as a long-acting injection (Depo-Provera) for contraception. (40)
Mefloquine	Antimalarial: unknown mechanism of action. Used for prophylaxis against and treatment of chloroquine-resistant malaria, but resistance emerging. *Tox:* GI distress, dizziness, seizures in overdose, arrhythmias. (52)
Meperidine	Opioid analgesic: synthetic, equivalent to morphine in efficacy but orally bioavailable. Strong agonist at μ opioid receptors; blocks muscarinic receptors; serotonergic activity. *Tox:* see morphine; normeperidine accumulation may cause seizures, serotonin syndrome with SSRIs. (31)
Metformin	Oral antidiabetic: prototype biguanide; inhibits hepatic and renal gluconeogenesis, minimal hypoglycemia or weight gain. *Tox:* GI distress, lactic acidosis possible but rare. (41)
Methadone	Opioid analgesic: synthetic μ agonist, equivalent to morphine in efficacy but orally bioavailable and with a longer half-life. Used as analgesic, to suppress withdrawal symptoms, and in maintenance programs. *Tox:* see morphine. (31, 32)
Methimazole	Antithyroid drug: inhibits tyrosine iodination and coupling reactions; orally active. *Tox:* rash, agranulocytosis (rare). **Propylthiouracil** is similar. (38)
Methotrexate	Antineoplastic, DMARD, immunosuppressant: cell cycle-specific drug that inhibits dihydrofolate reductase. Major dose reduction required in renal impairment. *Tox:* GI distress, myelosuppression, crystalluria. **Leucovorin** rescue used to reduce toxicity. (36, 54, 55)
Methyldopa	Antihypertensive: prodrug of methylnorepinephrine, a CNS-active α_2 agonist. Reduces SANS outflow from vasomotor center. See also **clonidine**. *Tox:* sedation, positive Coombs test, hemolysis. (11)
Metoclopramide	Prokinetic agent: dopamine D_2 receptor agonist used to stimulate upper GI motility in patients with gastroparesis and used as an antiemetic. *Tox:* restlessness, insomnia, agitation, extrapyramidal effects, elevated prolactin. (59)
Metronidazole	Antiprotozoal antibiotic: drug of choice in extraluminal amebiasis and trichomoniasis (**tinidazole** is equivalent); effective against bacterial anaerobes, including *B fragilis* and in antibiotic-induced colitis resulting from *C difficile*. *Tox:* peripheral neuropathy, GI distress, ethanol intolerance, mutagenic potential. (50, 52)
Mifepristone	Progestin and glucocorticoid receptor antagonist: used in combination with prostaglandin analogs for medical abortion in early pregnancy. (39, 40)
Misoprostol	Prostaglandin E_1 derivative: orally active prostaglandin used to prevent GI ulcers caused by NSAIDs. Also used with **mifepristone** as abortifacient. *Tox:* diarrhea. (18, 40, 59)
Montelukast	Leukotriene receptor blocker (especially LTD_4) used for prophylaxis in asthma. Orally active; once daily administration. **Zafirlukast** is similar. *Tox:* minimal. (20)
Morphine	Opioid analgesic prototype: strong μ receptor agonist. Poor oral bioavailability. *Tox:* constipation, emesis, sedation, respiratory depression, miosis, and urinary retention. Tolerance may be marked; high potential for psychological and physiologic dependence. Additive effects with other CNS depressants. (31, 32)
Nafcillin	Penicillinase-resistant penicillin: narrow spectrum, used for suspected or known staphylococcal infections; not active against methicillin-resistant *S aureus* (MRSA). *Tox:* penicillin allergy. Others in group include **methicillin** (the prototype, rarely used), **oxacillin, cloxacillin**, and **dicloxacillin**. (43, 51)
Naloxone	Opioid μ receptor antagonist: used to reverse CNS depressant effects of opioid analgesics (overdose or when used in anesthesia). **Naltrexone** (orally active), a related compound, is used in ethanol dependency states. (23, 31, 58)
Neostigmine	Cholinesterase inhibitor: prototype synthetic quaternary nitrogen carbamate with little CNS effect. *Tox:* excess cholinomimetic effects. **Pyridostigmine** is similar but longer-acting. **Physostigmine** is a lipid-soluble plant alkaloid. **Echothiophate** is a rarely used organophosphate cholinesterase inhibitor for topical ophthalmic use. (7, 27)
Niacin	Antihyperlipidemic: inhibits VLDL synthesis and release of fatty acids from adipose tissue. Lowers LDL cholesterol and triglycerides and raises HDL cholesterol. *Tox:* flushing, pruritus, liver dysfunction, increased risk of myopathy when combined with statins. (35)
Nifedipine	Dihydropyridine calcium channel blocker prototype: less cardiac depression than **verapamil**, **diltiazem**; used in angina, HTN. *Tox:* constipation, headache, tachycardia, arrhythmias (avoid rapid-onset forms). Others in the dihydropyridine group include **amlodipine, felodipine, nicardipine**. (11, 12)

Nitric oxide (NO)	Endogenous vasodilator released from vascular endothelium; neurotransmitter. Mediates vasodilating effect of acetylcholine, histamine, and hydralazine. Active metabolite of nitroprusside and of nitrates used in angina. Used as pulmonary dilator in neonatal hypoxia, pulmonary HTN. *Tox:* excessive vasodilation, hypotension. (19)
Nitroglycerin	Antianginal vasodilator prototype: releases nitric oxide (NO) in veins, less in arteries, and causes smooth muscle relaxation. Standard of therapy in angina (both atherosclerotic and variant). *Tox:* tachycardia, orthostatic hypotension, headache. Oral nitrates: **isosorbide dinitrate, isosorbide mononitrate.** (12, 13)
Norepinephrine	Adrenoceptor agonist prototype, neurotransmitter: acts at all α adrenoceptors and β_1 adrenoceptors; used as vasoconstrictor. Causes reflex bradycardia. *Tox:* ischemia, arrhythmias, HTN. (6, 9)
Olanzapine	Atypical antipsychotic: high-affinity antagonist at 5-HT$_{2a}$ receptors with minimal extrapyramidal side effects; improves both positive and negative symptoms of schizophrenia. Other atypicals: **quetiapine** (short half-life), **risperidone** (possible EPS dysfunction), **sertindole** (QT prolongation), **clozapine** (agranulocytosis). (29)
Omeprazole	Proton pump inhibitor prototype: irreversible blocker of H$^+$/K$^+$ ATPase proton pump in parietal cells of stomach. Used in GI ulcers, Zollinger-Ellison syndrome, gastroesophageal reflux disease (GERD). Other "prazoles": **esomeprazole, dexlansoprazole, lansoprazole, pantoprazole, rabeprazole.** *Tox:* hypergastrinemia. (59)
Ondansetron	5-HT$_3$ receptor blocker prototype: very important antiemetic for cancer chemotherapy; also used postoperatively to reduce vomiting. *Tox:* extrapyramidal effects. Other "setrons": **dolasetron, granisetron, palonosetron.** (16, 59)
Oseltamivir	Antiviral: neuraminidase inhibitor blocking release of mature virions of influenza A and B and decreasing their infectivity. Prophylactic and shortens duration of flu symptoms. **Zanamivir** is similar in action and use. (49)
Oxybutynin	Muscarinic cholinoceptor blocker: used to relieve bladder spasm and incontinence. **Tolterodine**, weaker but more selective for M$_3$ receptors, has similar uses. (8)
Paclitaxel	Antineoplastic plant alkaloid cell cycle (M phase)-specific agent; inhibits mitotic spindle disassembly. *Tox:* hematotoxicity, peripheral neuropathy, hypersensitivity reactions. **Docetaxel** is similar. (54)
Penicillamine	Chelator, immunomodulator: treatment of copper poisoning and Wilson's disease, and formerly used in rheumatoid arthritis. (36, 57)
Penicillin G	Penicillin prototype: active against common streptococci, gram-positive bacilli, gram-negative cocci, spirochetes (drug of choice in syphilis), and enterococci (if used with an aminoglycoside); penicillinase susceptible. *Tox:* penicillin allergy. (43, 51)
Phenelzine	Irreversible nonselective MAO inhibitor. Backup drug for atypical depression. *Tox:* Malignant hypertension with indirect-acting sympathomimetics and tyramine, serotonin syndrome with serotonergic drugs. (30)
Phenobarbital	Long-acting barbiturate: used as a sedative and for tonic-clonic seizures. Facilitates GABA-mediated neuronal inhibition (by increasing *duration* of channel opening) and may block excitatory neurotransmitters. Partial renal clearance that can be increased by urinary alkalinization. Chronic use leads to induction of liver drug-metabolizing enzymes and ALA synthase. *Tox:* psychological and physiologic dependence; additive effects with other CNS depressants. (22, 24)
Phenoxybenzamine	Alpha-blocker prototype (nonselective): irreversible action. **Phentolamine**: similar with competitive action. Used in pheochromocytoma. *Tox:* excess hypotension; GI distress. (10)
Phenytoin	Anticonvulsant: used for tonic-clonic and partial seizures; blocks Na$^+$ channels in neuronal membranes. Serum levels variable because of first-pass metabolism and nonlinear elimination kinetics. *Tox:* sedation, diplopia, gingival hyperplasia, hirsutism, teratogenic potential (fetal hydantoin syndrome). Drug interactions via effects on plasma protein binding or induction of hepatic metabolism. (24)
Pilocarpine	Muscarinic receptor partial agonist prototype: tertiary amine alkaloid. May cause paradoxic hypertension by activating muscarinic excitatory postsynaptic receptors in postganglionic sympathetic neurons. Used in Sjögren's syndrome, xerostomia, glaucoma. *Tox:* muscarinic excess. (7)
Piperacillin	Extended-spectrum penicillin active against selected gram-negative bacteria, including *Pseudomonas aeruginosa* (synergistic with aminoglycosides). Susceptible to penicillinases unless used with tazobactam. *Tox:* penicillin allergy. (43)
Pralidoxime	Acetylcholinesterase regenerator: antidote (with atropine) for organophosphate poisoning; chemical antagonist with very high affinity for phosphorus in organophosphates. *Tox:* neuromuscular weakness. (8, 58)

Pramipexole	Dopamine D_3 receptor agonist in CNS (**ropinirole** similar): often a first-line drug in parkinsonism. *Tox:* postural hypotension, dyskinesias (both drugs less toxicity than the ergot **bromocriptine**). (28)
Praziquantel	Antihelminthic: important drug for trematode (fluke) and cestode (tapeworm) infections. Increases membrane permeability to Ca^{2+} causing muscle contraction followed by paralysis. *Tox:* headache, dizziness, GI distress, fever; potential abortifacient. (53)
Prazosin	Alpha$_1$-selective blocker prototype: used in HTN and benign prostatic hyperplasia. *Tox:* first-dose orthostatic hypotension but less reflex tachycardia than nonselective α blockers. Other "osins": **terazosin, doxazosin**. **Tamsulosin** similar, but used only in benign prostatic hyperplasia. (10, 11)
Prednisone	Glucocorticoid prototype: potent, short acting; less mineralocorticoid activity than cortisol but more than **dexamethasone, betamethasone,** or **triamcinolone**. (20, 36, 39, 54, 55)
Probenecid	Uricosuric: inhibitor of renal weak acid secretion and reabsorption in proximal tubule; prolongs half-life of some antimicrobial drugs, accelerates clearance of uric acid. Used in gout. **Sulfinpyrazone** is similar. (36)
Procainamide	Group 1A antiarrhythmic drug prototype: short half-life, metabolized by *N*-acetyltransferase. *Tox:* may cause a lupus-like syndrome and torsades de pointes arrhythmia. Similar to **quinidine** but more cardiodepressant. (14)
Propranolol	Nonselective β-blocker prototype: local anesthetic action but no partial agonist effect. Used in HTN, angina, arrhythmias (group 2), migraine, hyperthyroidism, tremor. *Tox:* asthma, AV block, HF. (8, 11, 14, 28, 38)
Prostacyclin	PGI_2: endogenous prostaglandin vasodilator and inhibitor of platelet aggregation. An analog, **epoprostenol**, is used in primary pulmonary HTN. (18)
Pyrimethamine	Antiprotozoal: antifolate that inhibits DHF reductase and synergistic, via sequential blockade, with sulfadiazine against *Toxoplasma gondii*. Folinic acid is needed to offset hematologic toxicity. (46, 52)
Quinine	Antimalarial: blood schizonticide; no effect on liver stages. Interferes with nucleic acid metabolism in plasmodium. Isomer of **quinidine**. *Tox:* cinchonism, GI upset. (52)
Ramelteon	Hypnotic: agonist at brain melatonin receptors; not a controlled substance. *Tox:* fatigue, increased prolactin and decreased testosterone. (22)
Reserpine	Antihypertensive (rarely used): selective inhibitor of vesicle catecholamine-H^+ antiporter (VMAT); obsolete use in HTN, causes depletion of catecholamines and 5-HT from their stores. *Tox:* severe depression, suicide, ulcers, diarrhea. (6, 11)
Rifampin	Antimicrobial: inhibitor of DNA-dependent RNA polymerase used in drug regimens for tuberculosis and the meningococcal carrier state. *Tox:* hepatic dysfunction, induction of liver drug-metabolizing enzymes (drug interactions), flu-like syndrome with intermittent dosing. **Rifabutin** similar but associated with fewer drug interactions. (47)
Ritonavir	Antiviral: HIV protease inhibitor (PI) used at low dose as a component of combination regimens in AIDS to inhibit metabolism of other drugs (See **indinavir**). *Tox:* implicated in many drug interactions when used as sole PI. (49)
Rosiglitazone	Oral antidiabetic: thiazolidinedione stimulator of peroxisome proliferator-activator receptors (PPAR) and enhances target tissue sensitivity to insulin. Less hypoglycemia and weight gain than secretagogue antidiabetics. *Tox:* fluid retention, heart failure, fractures in women. **Pioglitazone** is similar. (41)
Rivaroxaban	Oral factor X inhibitor: used for prevention of deep venous thrombosis (DVT), pulmonary embolism (PE), postsurgery, and stroke in atrial fibrillation. Fixed dose, no routine monitoring. Side effect: bleeding. No specific reversal agent. (34)
Selegiline	MAO-B inhibitor: selective inhibitor of the enzyme that metabolizes dopamine (no tyramine interactions at normal dosage). Used in Parkinson's disease. *Tox:* GI distress, CNS stimulation, dyskinesias, serotonin syndrome if used with selective serotonin reuptake inhibitors. **Rasagiline** similar and used more commonly. (28)
Sildenafil	Inhibits phosphodiesterase (PDE)-5, preventing breakdown of cyclic guanosine monophosphate (cGMP), which promotes vasodilation and smooth muscle relaxation. Used for erectile dysfunction and pulmonary hypertension. **Tadalafil, vardenafil** are similar. *Tox:* severe hypotension when combined with nitrates, impaired blue-green color vision. (12)
Sotalol	Group 3 antiarrhythmic prototype: blocks I_K channels and β receptors. Used for atrial and ventricular arrhythmias. *Tox:* torsades de pointes arrhythmias. Others in group: **ibutilide, dofetilide**. (14)
Spironolactone	Aldosterone receptor antagonist: K^+-sparing diuretic action in the collecting tubules; used in aldosteronism, HTN, and female hirsutism (androgen receptor-blocking action). *Tox:* hyperkalemia, gynecomastia. **Eplerenone**, used in HTN and heart failure, is a more selective aldosterone antagonist. (13, 15, 39, 40)

Streptogramins	Antibiotics: Synercid is the combination of quinupristin and dalfopristin; bactericidal inhibitors of protein synthesis. Intravenous use for drug-resistant gram-positive cocci including MRSA (methicillin-resistant *S aureus*), VRE (vancomycin-resistant enterococci), and pneumococci. *Tox:* infusion-related pain, arthralgia, myalgia. **Linezolid** is another inhibitor of protein synthesis used for drug-resistant gram-positive cocci, including PRSP (penicillin-resistant *S pneumoniae*) strains. (44)
Succinylcholine	Depolarizing neuromuscular relaxant prototype: short duration (5 min) if patient has normal plasma cholinesterase (genetically determined). No antidote (compare with tubocurarine). Implicated in malignant hyperthermia. (7, 27)
Sulfasalazine	5-Aminosalicylate (5-ASA) anti-inflammatory drug: used for inflammatory bowel disease (IBD) and rheumatoid arthritis. *Tox:* rash, GI disturbances, leukopenia. Other 5-ASA drugs used for IBD are **mesalamine, balsalazide, olsalazine.** (36, 59)
Sumatriptan	5-HT$_{1D}$ receptor agonist: used to abort migraine attacks. *Tox:* coronary vasospasm, chest pain or pressure. Six other "triptans" are currently available. (16)
Tamoxifen	Selective estrogen receptor modulator (SERM): blocks estrogen receptors in breast tissue; activates endometrial receptors. Used in estrogen receptor-positive cancers, possibly prophylactic in high-risk patients. **Toremifene** is similar. **Raloxifene**, approved for osteoporosis, activates bone estrogen receptors but is an antagonist of breast and endometrial receptors. (40, 54)
Terbinafine	Antifungal: fungicidal inhibitor of squalene epoxidase. Most effective agent in onychomycosis, oral and topical forms. *Tox:* GI upsets, headache, and rash. (48)
Tetracycline	Antibiotic: tetracycline prototype; bacteriostatic inhibitor of protein synthesis (30S). Broad spectrum, but many resistant organisms. Used for mycoplasmal, chlamydial, rickettsial infections, chronic bronchitis, acne, cholera; a backup drug in syphilis. *Tox:* GI upset and superinfections, Fanconi's syndrome, photosensitivity, dental enamel dysplasia. Other tetracyclines include **doxycycline** (see above) and **tigecycline** (IV) used for multidrug-resistant nosocomial pathogens. (44)
Theophylline	Methylxanthine derivative found in tea; used in asthma. Bronchodilator, mild CNS stimulant. **Caffeine** (coffee), **theobromine** (cocoa) are similar. *Tox:* seizures. (20)
Trimethoprim-sulfamethoxazole (TMP-SMZ)	Antimicrobial drug combination: causes synergistic sequential blockade of folic acid synthesis. Active against many gram-negative bacteria, including *Aeromonas, Enterobacter, H influenzae, Klebsiella, Moraxella, Salmonella, Serratia,* and *Shigella. Tox:* mainly due to sulfonamide; includes hypersensitivity, myelotoxicity, kernicterus, and drug interactions caused by competition for plasma protein binding. (46, 52)
Tubocurarine	Nondepolarizing neuromuscular blocking agent prototype: competitive nicotinic blocker. Analogs: pancuronium, atracurium, vecuronium, and other "-curiums" and "-oniums." *Tox:* respiratory paralysis. Releases histamine and may cause hypotension, therefore rarely used. *Antidote:* cholinesterase inhibitor, for example, neostigmine. (8, 26)
Tyramine	Indirect-acting sympathomimetic prototype: releases or displaces norepinephrine from stores in nerve endings. Presence in certain foods may cause potentially lethal hypertensive responses in patients taking MAO inhibitors. (6, 27)
Valproic acid	Anticonvulsant: primary drug in absence, clonic-tonic, and myoclonic seizure states. Also used commonly for bipolar disorder. *Tox:* GI distress, hepatic necrosis (rare), teratogenic (spina bifida), inhibits drug metabolism. (24, 29)
Vancomycin	Glycopeptide bactericidal antibiotic: inhibits synthesis of cell wall precursor molecules. A drug of choice for methicillin-resistant staphylococci and effective in antibiotic-induced colitis. Dose reduction required in renal impairment (or hemodialysis). *Tox:* ototoxicity, hypersensitivity, renal dysfunction (rare). (43, 51)
Verapamil	Calcium channel blocker prototype: blocks L-type channels; cardiac depressant and vasodilator; used in HTN, angina, and arrhythmias (group 4). *Tox:* AV block, HF, constipation. **Diltiazem**, like verapamil, has more depressant effect on heart than dihydropyridines (eg, **nifedipine**). (11, 12, 14)
Vincristine	Antineoplastic: cell cycle (M phase)-specific plant alkaloid; inhibits mitotic spindle formation. *Tox:* peripheral neuropathy. **Vinblastine**, a congener, causes myelosuppression. (54)
Warfarin	Oral anticoagulant prototype: causes synthesis of nonfunctional versions of the vitamin K-dependent clotting factors (II, VII, IX, X). *Tox:* bleeding, teratogenic. *Antidote:* vitamin K, fresh plasma. (34)
Zidovudine (ZDV)	Antiviral: prototype NRTI used in combinations for HIV infections and in prophylaxis for needlesticks and vertical transmission. *Tox:* severe myelosuppression. Other NRTIs: **abacavir**, **didanosine** (ddI), **lamivudine** (3TC), **stavudine** (d4T), and **zalcitabine** (ddC). (49)
Zolpidem	Nonbenzodiazepine hypnotic: acts via the BZ$_1$ receptor subtype and is reversed by flumazenil; less amnesia and muscle relaxation and lower dependence liability than benzodiazepines. **Zaleplon** and **eszopiclone** are similar. (22)

Examination 1

The following examination consists of 100 questions, mostly in the format ("single best answer") used in USMLE examinations. As in an actual examination, clinical descriptions, tables, or graphs are provided in many of the question stems.

It is suggested that you time yourself in taking this examination; in current USMLE examinations, the time allotted is approximately 1 min per question; thus, 1 h 40 min would be appropriate for this examination.

DIRECTIONS: Each numbered item or incomplete statement in this section is followed by answers or by completions of the statement. Select the ONE lettered answer or completion that is BEST in each case.

1. Phase 3 clinical trials typically involve
   (A) Collection of data regarding late-appearing toxicities from patients previously studied in phase 1 trials
   (B) Double-blind, closely monitored evaluation of the new drug in hundreds of patients with the target disease by specialists in academic centers
   (C) Evaluation of the new drug under conditions of actual use in 1000–5000 patients with the target disease
   (D) Measurement of the pharmacokinetics of the new drug in normal volunteers
   (E) Postmarketing surveillance of drug toxicities

2. A patient is admitted to the emergency department for treatment of a drug overdose. The identity of the drug is unknown, but it is observed that when the urine pH is alkaline, the renal clearance of the drug is much greater than when the urine pH is acidic. The drug is probably a
   (A) Strong acid
   (B) Weak acid
   (C) Nonelectrolyte
   (D) Weak base
   (E) Strong base

3. A 66-year-old woman is in the coronary care unit after an acute myocardial infarction. She has developed signs of pulmonary edema of rapidly increasing severity and several drugs have been suggested. Furosemide, dobutamine, and digoxin can each
   (A) Decrease conduction velocity in the atrioventricular node
   (B) Decrease venous return
   (C) Reduce pulmonary edema
   (D) Increase peripheral vascular resistance
   (E) Increase the amount of cAMP in cardiac muscle cells

4. A 45-year-old man presents with pulmonary hypertension. Which of the following cause–treatment pairs is most relevant to this patient?
   (A) Angiotensin II–minoxidil
   (B) Atrial natriuretic peptide–losartan
   (C) Bradykinin–furosemide
   (D) Endothelin–ambrisentan
   (E) Substance P–capsaicin

5. A 45-year-old man with a duodenal ulcer and laboratory evidence of *Helicobacter pylori* infection was treated with omeprazole, clarithromycin, and amoxicillin. Which of the following is the most accurate description of the mechanism of omeprazole's therapeutic action?
   (A) Activation of prostaglandin E receptors
   (B) Formation of protective coating over the ulcer bed
   (C) Inhibition of bacterial protein synthesis
   (D) Inhibition of H_2 histamine receptors
   (E) Irreversible inactivation of an H^+/K^+ ATPase

6. A patient discharged from the hospital after a myocardial infarction had been receiving small doses of procainamide to suppress a ventricular tachycardia. One month later, his local physician prescribed high-dose hydrochlorothiazide therapy for ankle edema, which was ascribed to congestive heart failure. Three weeks after beginning thiazide therapy, the patient was readmitted to the hospital with a rapid multifocal ventricular tachycardia. The most probable cause of this arrhythmia is
   (A) Procainamide toxicity caused by inhibition of procainamide metabolism by the thiazide
   (B) Direct effects of hydrochlorothiazide on pacemaker cells of the heart
   (C) Direct effects of procainamide on pacemaker cells of the heart
   (D) Block of calcium current by the combination of procainamide plus thiazide
   (E) Reduction of serum potassium caused by the diuretic action of hydrochlorothiazide

7. A 54-year-old woman presented with angina of effort. Laboratory assessment of her serum revealed elevated total and LDL cholesterol. The patient was placed on atorvastatin. This drug lowers serum cholesterol by
(A) Activating endothelial cell-associated lipoprotein lipase
(B) Increasing the shunting of hepatic cholesterol into the biochemical pathway of bile acid synthesis
(C) Indirectly increasing hepatic production of LDL receptors
(D) Inhibiting the uptake of cholesterol in epithelial cells that line the small intestine
(E) Stimulating hepatic fatty acid oxidation

8. While on vacation, a 35-year-old man with a 10-year history of myasthenia gravis loses his supply of medications. He is now admitted to the emergency department complaining of diplopia, dysarthria, and difficulty swallowing. The most appropriate drug from the following list for reversing myasthenic crisis in this patient is
(A) Calcium
(B) Neostigmine
(C) Pralidoxime
(D) Succinylcholine
(E) Vecuronium

9. A 4-year-old child was brought to an emergency department after ingesting a product found in the home. Her symptoms included an elevated temperature; hot, dry skin; moderate tachycardia; and mydriasis. The most likely cause of these symptoms is
(A) Acetaminophen overdose
(B) Amphetamine-containing diet pills
(C) Exposure to an organophosphate-containing insecticide
(D) Ingestion of a medication containing atropine
(E) Ingestion of phenylephrine-containing eye drops

10. A patient is admitted to a hospital emergency department 2 h after taking an overdose of diazepam. The plasma level of the drug at time of admission is 40 mg/L, and the apparent volume of distribution, half-life, and clearance of diazepam are 80 L, 40 h, and 35 L/day, respectively. The ingested dose was approximately
(A) 1.3 g
(B) 2.4 g
(C) 3.2 g
(D) 4.8 g
(E) 6.4 g

11. A semiconscious patient in the intensive care unit is being artificially ventilated. Random spontaneous respiratory movements are rendering the mechanical ventilation ineffective. A useful drug to reduce the patient's ineffective spontaneous respiratory activity is
(A) Baclofen
(B) Dantrolene
(C) Pancuronium
(D) Neostigmine
(E) Succinylcholine

12. A child with strabismus ("wandering eye") is to be treated pharmacologically for a prolonged period. Which of the following drugs is used by the topical route in ophthalmology and causes mydriasis and cycloplegia lasting more than 24 h?
(A) Atropine
(B) Echothiophate
(C) Edrophonium
(D) Pilocarpine
(E) Timolol

13. A 55-year-old surgeon has developed symmetric early morning stiffness in her hands. She wishes to take a nonsteroidal anti-inflammatory drug to relieve these symptoms. Which drug is an NSAID that is appropriate for chronic therapy of her arthritis?
(A) Colchicine
(B) Hydroxychloroquine
(C) Ibuprofen
(D) Indomethacin
(E) Sulfasalazine

14. A 50-year-old man has macrocytic anemia and early signs of neurologic abnormality. Which of the following drugs will probably be required in this case?
(A) Erythropoietin
(B) Filgrastim
(C) Folic acid
(D) Iron dextran
(E) Vitamin B_{12}

15. A patient in the coronary care unit has received warfarin for 2 wk. As a result of this therapy, the patient will exhibit which of the following?
(A) Reduced plasma prothrombin (factor II) activity
(B) Reduced plasma factor VIII activity
(C) Reduced plasma plasminogen activity
(D) Increased tissue plasminogen activator activity
(E) Increased platelet adenosine stores

16. A 55-year-old man with a strong family history of cardiovascular disease has moderate hypertension and angina pectoris. Blood pressure is 160/109 mm Hg, and the ECG shows left ventricular hypertrophy. The rest of his physical examination and laboratory results are normal. His angina is precipitated by exercise. You have been asked to recommend a drug regimen for both conditions. The antihypertensive drug most likely to *aggravate* angina pectoris is
(A) Captopril
(B) Clonidine
(C) Hydralazine
(D) Methyldopa
(E) Propranolol

17. A patient presents to the hematology clinic with a previously unknown clotting abnormality in which platelets aggregate extremely rapidly. Several relatives manifest the same abnormality. Laboratory investigation indicates that their platelets contain a very high eicosanoid concentration. The eicosanoid that stimulates platelet aggregation most strongly is
(A) Leukotriene C_4
(B) Prostacyclin
(C) Prostaglandin E_2
(D) Prostaglandin F_2
(E) Thromboxane A_2

18. A 46-year-old man consults you regarding his sexual performance issues. A drug that is used in the treatment of male erectile dysfunction and inhibits a phosphodiesterase is
(A) Finasteride
(B) Fluoxetine
(C) Mifepristone
(D) Sildenafil
(E) Timolol

19. A physician was considering erythromycin for treatment of a 47-year-old man with an upper respiratory tract infection. However, the physician noted that the patient was taking simvastatin for treatment of hypercholesterolemia and realized that erythromycin, an inhibitor of cytochrome enzymes, would inhibit the metabolism of simvastatin. The physician opted for a different class of antibiotic to avoid exposing the patient to higher concentrations of simvastatin and a risk of dose-dependent toxicity. Which of the following is the primary dose-dependent toxicity of simvastatin?
    (A) Abdominal pain secondary to gallstone formation
    (B) Blurred vision secondary to optic neuritis
    (C) Elevated serum creatinine, possibly progressing to renal failure
    (D) Increased serum uric acid concentration and increased risk of gout
    (E) Muscle pain and weakness, possibly progressing to rhabdomyolysis

20. Although it does not act at any histamine receptor and has no effect on histamine's metabolism, epinephrine reverses many effects of histamine. Epinephrine is a
    (A) Chemical antagonist of histamine
    (B) Competitive inhibitor of histamine
    (C) Metabolic inhibitor of histamine
    (D) Noncompetitive antagonist of histamine
    (E) Physiologic antagonist of histamine

21. Most drug receptors are
    (A) Small molecules with a molecular weight between 100 and 1000
    (B) Lipids arranged in a bilayer configuration
    (C) Proteins located on cell membranes or in the cytosol
    (D) DNA molecules
    (E) RNA molecules

22. The graph below shows the serum insulin level that results from a 2-injection regimen given to a child with type 1 diabetes. Assume that both injections (indicated by arrows along the time line) contain the same medication(s). The drug or drug combination that is most likely to generate the levels of insulin depicted in the figure is

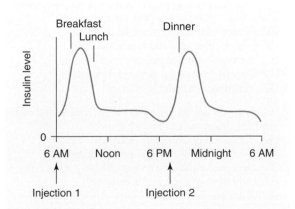

    (A) 100% Regular insulin
    (B) 100% Lispro insulin
    (C) 70% NPH insulin plus 30% regular insulin
    (D) 100% NPH insulin
    (E) 100% Insulin glargine

23. In a laboratory demonstration of the interactions of drugs, an anesthetized dog is given several agents intravenously. Intravenous administration of norepinephrine in a subject already receiving an effective dose of atropine often
    (A) Decreases blood sugar
    (B) Decreases total peripheral resistance
    (C) Increases heart rate
    (D) Increases skin temperature
    (E) Reduces pupil size

24. A 26-year-old woman comes to the outpatient clinic with a complaint of rapid heart rate and easy fatigability. Laboratory workup reveals low hemoglobin and microcytic red cell size. Which of the following is the most suitable therapy?
    (A) Ferrous sulfate
    (B) Folic acid
    (C) Iron dextran
    (D) Pyridoxine
    (E) Vitamin B_{12}

25. The graph below shows a quantal dose-response graph of the results of a study of a new drug in patients with hypertension. The label on the Y-axis (vertical axis) should be

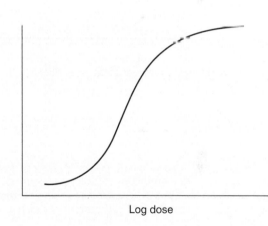

Log dose

    (A) Cumulative maximal efficacy of the experimental drug in the patients
    (B) Cumulative dose of the experimental drug in the patients
    (C) Percentage of patients with a specified response to the drug
    (D) Percentage of receptors bound to the drug
    (E) Percentage of the maximal response to the drug that occurs at each dosage level

26. Mr. Q has been given an intravenous dose of isoproterenol and is now manifesting an undesirably strong heart rate response. Which of the following most effectively blocks the heart rate response to a moderate dose of isoproterenol in conscious patients?
(A) Atropine
(B) Atenolol
(C) Phenoxybenzamine
(D) Pancuronium
(E) Propranolol

27. An accepted clinical use of antimuscarinic drugs is for treatment of
(A) Alzheimer's disease
(B) Chronic obstructive pulmonary disease
(C) Glaucoma
(D) Hypertension
(E) Prostatic hyperplasia

28. Which of the following is an anticlotting drug that binds to and inhibits the platelet glycoprotein IIb/IIIa protein?
(A) Aspirin
(B) Clopidogrel
(C) Enoxaparin
(D) Fondaparinux
(E) Tirofiban

29. A 70-year-old man has severe urinary hesitancy associated with benign prostatic hyperplasia. He has tried α blockers with little relief. His physician recommends a drug that blocks 5α-reductase in the prostate. Which of the following drugs did the physician most likely prescribe?
(A) Finasteride
(B) Flutamide
(C) Ketoconazole
(D) Leuprolide
(E) Oxandrolone

30. A 54-year-old contractor complains of anginal pain that occurs at rest. On examination, his blood pressure is 145/90 and his heart rate is 90. A treatment of angina that often decreases the heart rate and can prevent vasospastic angina attacks is
(A) Diltiazem
(B) Nifedipine
(C) Nitroglycerin
(D) Propranolol
(E) Timolol

31. Which of the following drugs is a partial agonist and can cause vasoconstriction in the absence of other drugs?
(A) Atropine
(B) Ergotamine
(C) Neostigmine
(D) Phentolamine
(E) Verapamil

32. In a study of new diuretics, an investigational drug was given daily for 8 d and urine output was analyzed. The following data were obtained.

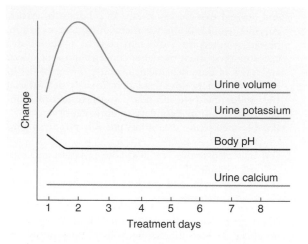

Which mechanism best explains the effects shown on the graph?
(A) Carbonic anhydrase inhibition
(B) Blockade of a $Na^+/K^+/2Cl^-$ transporter in the ascending limb of the loop of Henle
(C) Blockade of a NaCl transporter in the distal convoluted tubule
(D) Osmotic diuresis
(E) Block of aldosterone in the cortical collecting tubule

Questions 33 and 34. A 65-year-old man with cardiomyopathy has recurrent congestive heart failure. Addition of digitalis to his regimen is being considered.

33. In a patient receiving digoxin for congestive heart failure, conditions that may facilitate the appearance of toxicity include
(A) Hyperkalemia
(B) Hypernatremia
(C) Hypocalcemia
(D) Hypomagnesemia
(E) Hypophosphatemia

34. The cellular cause of digitalis toxicity is
(A) Intracellular calcium overload
(B) Intracellular potassium overload
(C) Increased parasympathetic activity
(D) Increased adrenocorticosteroid levels
(E) Impaired sympathetic activity

35. Which of the following effects are characteristic of methylxanthine drugs such as theophylline?
(A) Activation of adenosine receptors
(B) Blockade of the enzyme phosphodiesterase
(C) Decrease in the amount of cAMP in mast cells
(D) Inhibition of cardiac β receptors
(E) Sedation

36. Which of the following drugs often causes tachycardia and tremor when used in asthma?
(A) Albuterol
(B) Cromolyn sodium
(C) Ipratropium
(D) Montelukast
(E) Prednisone

37. Angioneurotic edema precipitated by exposure to an allergen can cause life-threatening laryngeal edema. A probable mediator of such reactions is
(A) Angiotensin II
(B) Epinephrine
(C) Histamine
(D) Norepinephrine
(E) Serotonin

38. A 30-year-old patient in the intensive care unit is to receive a β-agonist drug. Typical responses to β-receptor blockade include
(A) Bradycardia
(B) Decreased renin secretion
(C) Decreased skeletal muscle tremor
(D) Glycogen synthesis
(E) Lipolysis

39. A patient has been taking aspirin for rheumatoid arthritis for 8 yrs. Exacerbations are becoming worse, and she asks the physician about drugs that might stop the progression of the disease. Which of the following is a disease-modifying antirheumatic drug (DMARD)?
(A) Colchicine
(B) Epoprostenol
(C) Leflunomide
(D) Naproxen
(E) Zafirlukast

40. A neuronal cell body located in the substantia nigra has axonal projections to the striatum. The neurotransmitter that it releases, which exerts only inhibitory actions, is most likely to be
(A) Acetylcholine
(B) Dopamine
(C) Glutamic acid
(D) Norepinephrine
(E) Serotonin

Questions 41 and 42. A 40-year-old man had been consuming alcoholic beverages at lunch and in the evenings all his adult life. During the last 2 yr, his alcohol consumption had steadily increased, continuing throughout the day. In response to family pressures, he abruptly stopped drinking alcohol, and within a few hours he became increasingly anxious and agitated and showed symptoms of autonomic hyperexcitability. At this point, he was brought to the hospital.

41. In the emergency department, the symptoms increased in severity, with hyperreflexia progressing to seizures. He was given an intravenous injection of a drug that controlled the seizure activity and was then hospitalized. During the recovery period, the same agent was used in oral form with gradual dose tapering. The drug he received as an injection and then as an oral pill was which of the following?
(A) Acamprosate
(B) Amitriptyline
(C) Diazepam
(D) Ramelteon
(E) Thiamine

42. In the first week of this patient's recovery, he is at risk of a syndrome that is characterized by which of the following?
(A) Ascites, mental confusion, and elevated serum transaminases
(B) Headache, hypotension, and widespread petechiae
(C) Hyperglycemia, acidosis, and stupor
(D) Respiratory depression, miosis, and mental confusion
(E) Tremor, delusions, and visual hallucinations

43. The pharmacokinetic characteristics of several hydantoin derivatives, each with anticonvulsant activity equivalent to that of phenytoin, were examined in phase 1 clinical trials. The rationale was to identify a drug with more desirable kinetic properties than those of phenytoin.

Drug	Oral Bioavailability (%)	Plasma Protein Binding (%)	Elimination Kinetics	Cytochrome P450 Induction
ABC	10	90	First order	++
DEF	90	50	First order	++
GHI	50	98	Zero order	None
JKL	85	10	First order	None
MNO	95	10	First order	++

Based on the data shown in the table above, which drug has the optimum pharmacokinetic properties for oral use in the management of patients with seizure disorders?
(A) ABC
(B) DEF
(C) GHI
(D) JKL
(E) MNO

44. The speed of induction of anesthesia with halogenated hydrocarbons (eg, halothane, isoflurane) is *not* affected by
(A) Arteriovenous concentration gradient
(B) Inspired gas partial pressure
(C) Minimal alveolar anesthetic concentration
(D) Pulmonary blood flow
(E) Ventilation rate

45. A patient is to undergo surgery, and a short-acting anesthetic with a fast onset will be used. Recovery, unhampered by postoperative nausea, will be rapid because the clearance of the drug is greater than hepatic blood flow. The drug to be used is
(A) Enflurane
(B) Halothane
(C) Midazolam
(D) Phenobarbital
(E) Propofol

46. A patient with an incurable cancer is suffering from pain that is gradually increasing in intensity and levorphanol (a strong μ-receptor agonist) is prescribed. With chronic use of the drug, tolerance is not likely to develop to constipation or to
(A) Euphoria
(B) Nausea and vomiting
(C) Pupillary constriction
(D) Sedation
(E) Urinary retention

47. A wide range of receptor types and receptor mechanisms mediate the effects of endogenous signaling molecules and the drugs that mimic or block their effects. Which of the following drugs mediates its effects by binding to and activating an intracellular receptor that, when activated, acts as a transcription factor?
(A) Albuterol
(B) Captopril
(C) Erythropoietin
(D) Morphine
(E) Prednisone

48. The primary clinical application of the 5-HT$_2$ receptor antagonist trazodone is the treatment of
(A) Bipolar disorder
(B) Chronic pain
(C) Insomnia
(D) Major depressive disorder
(E) Premenstrual dysphoric disorder

49. The following data concern the relative activities of hypothetical investigational drugs as blockers of the membrane transporters (reuptake systems) for 3 CNS neurotransmitters.

	Blocking Actions on CNS Transporters for		
Drug	**Dopamine**	**Serotonin**	**Norepinephrine**
UCSF 1	+++	None	None
UCSF 2	+++	++++	++
UCSF 3	None	++	++
UCSF 4	None	+++	++
UCSF 5	+	+	None

Key: Number of + signs denotes intensity of blocking actions

Which drug is likely to be effective in the treatment of major depressive disorders but may also cause marked adverse effects, including thought disorders, delusions, hallucinations, and paranoia?
(A) UCSF 1
(B) UCSF 2
(C) UCSF 3
(D) UCSF 4
(E) UCSF 5

50. Of the following drugs, which has established clinical uses that include attention deficit hyperkinetic disorder, enuresis, and the management of chronic pain?
(A) Bupropion
(B) Citalopram
(C) Imipramine
(D) Risperidone
(E) Sertraline

51. The selective serotonin reuptake inhibitors fluoxetine and paroxetine are potent inhibitors of hepatic CYP2D6 drug-metabolizing enzymes. This action may lead to changes in the intensity of the effects of
(A) Benztropine
(B) Codeine
(C) Gentamicin
(D) Lithium
(E) Methotrexate

52. A 45-year-old woman was suspected of having Cushing's syndrome. To confirm the diagnosis, the patient was given an oral medication late in the evening and had blood drawn the following morning for laboratory testing. The oral medication was which of the following?
(A) Dexamethasone
(B) Fludrocortisone
(C) Glucose
(D) Ketoconazole
(E) Propylthiouracil

53. The reason why clozapine causes less extrapyramidal dysfunction than haloperidol when used in schizophrenia is that in the CNS, clozapine
(A) Activates GABA receptors
(B) Blocks dopamine release
(C) Has greater antagonism at muscarinic receptors
(D) Has a low affinity for dopamine D$_2$ receptors
(E) Is an α-receptor agonist

54. A patient taking medications for a psychiatric disorder develops a tremor, thyroid enlargement, edema, and acneiform eruptions on the face. The drug he is taking is most likely to be
(A) Carbamazepine
(B) Haloperidol
(C) Lamotrigine
(D) Lithium
(E) Sertraline

55. The mechanism of action of the hypnotic drug zolpidem is
(A) Activation of GABA$_B$ receptors
(B) Antagonism of glycine receptors in the spinal cord
(C) Blockade of the action of glutamic acid
(D) Increased GABA-mediated chloride ion conductance
(E) Inhibition of GABA aminotransferase

56. After a very large overdose of diazepam a 2-year-old child is admitted to the hospital. Along with general supportive care, the administration of which of the following is most likely to be used to reverse the action of the benzodiazepine?
(A) Acetylcysteine
(B) Atropine
(C) Flumazenil
(D) Fomepizole
(E) Naloxone

57. If an aerobic gram-negative rod causing bacteremia proves to be resistant to aminoglycosides, the mechanism of resistance is most likely due to
(A) Changed pathway of bacterial folate synthesis
(B) Decreased intracellular accumulation of the drug
(C) Formation of drug-trapping thiol compounds
(D) Inactivation by bacterial group transferases
(E) Induced synthesis of beta-lactamases

58. A 54-year-old woman with a recent history of deep vein thrombosis had been stable on warfarin therapy for the last 2 mos. However, her most recent prothrombin time (PT) test revealed a markedly reduced INR. When asked about changes in diet or medication during the last several weeks, the woman said that she had recently begun taking a dietary supplement recommended by a friend. Based on this information, the supplement is most likely to contain which of the following?
(A) Ginkgo
(B) Ginseng
(C) Kava
(D) Ma huang
(E) St. John's wort

59. Beta-lactamase production by strains of *Haemophilus influenzae* and *N gonorrhoeae* confers resistance against penicillin G. Which of the following drugs is most likely to be effective against resistant strains of these organisms?
(A) Amoxicillin
(B) Ceftriaxone
(C) Clindamycin
(D) Gentamicin
(E) Vancomycin

60. A 24-year-old woman is to be treated with levofloxacin for a urinary tract infection. A contraindication to the use of the antibiotic in this patient is a history of
(A) Deep vein thrombosis
(B) Glucose-6-phosphate dehydrogenase (G6PD) deficiency
(C) Gout
(D) Q-T prolongation
(E) Use at the present time of a combined hormonal contraceptive

61. A 39-year-old woman with recurrent sinusitis has been treated with different antibiotics on several occasions. During the course of one such treatment, she developed a severe diarrhea and was hospitalized. Sigmoidoscopy revealed colitis, and pseudomembranes were confirmed histologically. Which of the following drugs, administered orally, is most likely to be effective in the treatment of colitis caused by *Clostridium difficile*?
(A) Ampicillin
(B) Cefazolin
(C) Metronidazole
(D) Tetracycline
(E) Trimethoprim-sulfamethoxazole

62. In the management of patients with AIDS, trimethoprim-sulfamethoxazole is commonly used to prevent infection resulting from
(A) *Campylobacter jejuni*
(B) *Mycobacterium avium-intracellulare*
(C) *Neisseria gonorrhea*
(D) *Pneumocystis jiroveci*
(E) *Treponema pallidum*

63. In a cancer cell, decreased ability to phosphorylate pyrimidines could result in resistance to the anticancer action of which of the following?
(A) Cisplatin
(B) Etoposide
(C) Fluorouracil
(D) Mercaptopurine
(E) Methotrexate

64. A 65-year-old woman with endometrial cancer came to an outpatient cancer treatment center for her first cycle of platinum-based chemotherapy. To prevent chemotherapy-induced nausea and vomiting, this patient is likely to be given which of the following?
(A) Famotidine
(B) Leucovorin
(C) Mesalamine
(D) Ondansetron
(E) Sumatriptan

65. A 20-year-old foreign exchange student attending college in California is to be treated for pulmonary tuberculosis. Because drug resistance is anticipated, the proposed antibiotic regimen includes ethambutol, isoniazid (with supplementary vitamin B_6), pyrazinamide, and rifampin. Provided that his disease responds well to the drug regimen and that the microbiology laboratory results show sensitivity to the drugs, it would be appropriate after 2 mo to
(A) Change his drug regimen to prophylaxis with isoniazid
(B) Discontinue pyrazinamide
(C) Establish baseline ocular function
(D) Monitor amylase activity
(E) Stop the supplementary vitamin B_6

66. An antifungal drug that binds to ergosterol forming "pores" that disrupt fungal membrane integrity is
(A) Amphotericin B
(B) Caspofungin
(C) Fluconazole
(D) Flucytosine
(E) Terbinafine

Questions 67 and 68. A 20-year-old college student is brought to the emergency department after taking an overdose of a non-prescription drug. The patient is comatose. He has been hyperventilating and is now dehydrated with an elevated temperature. Serum analyses demonstrate that the patient has an anion gap metabolic acidosis.

67. Toxic exposure to which of the following drugs is the most likely cause of these signs and symptoms?
(A) Aspirin
(B) Acetaminophen
(C) Dextromethorphan
(D) Diphenhydramine
(E) Ethanol

68. In the management of this patient, it would be *most* appropriate to
(A) Administer acetylcysteine
(B) Administer fomepizole
(C) Administer glucagon
(D) Alkalinize the urine
(E) Induce vomiting with syrup of ipecac

69. This drug is prophylactic in meningococcal and staphylococcal carrier states. Although the drug eliminates a majority of meningococci from carriers, highly resistant strains may be selected out during treatment.
(A) Ciprofloxacin
(B) Clofazimine
(C) Dapsone
(D) Rifampin
(E) Streptomycin

70. Chemoprophylaxis for travelers to geographic regions where chloroquine-resistant *Plasmodium falciparum* is endemic is effectively provided by
(A) Doxycycline
(B) Malarone (atovaquone-proguanil)
(C) Mefloquine
(D) None of the drugs listed above
(E) Any of the drugs listed above

71. A cardiac Purkinje fiber was isolated from an animal heart and placed in a recording chamber. One of the Purkinje cells was impaled with a microelectrode, and action potentials were recorded while the preparation was stimulated at 1 stimulus per second. A representative control action potential is shown in red in the graph. After equilibration, oxygenation was reduced, and a drug was added to the perfusate while recording continued. A representative action potential obtained at the peak of drug action is shown as the superimposed action potential (*blue*). Identify the drug from the following list.

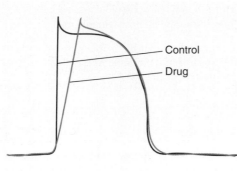

(A) Adenosine
(B) Amiodarone
(C) Diltiazem
(D) Flecainide
(E) Fluoxetine
(F) Lidocaine
(G) Nitroglycerin
(H) Propranolol
(I) Sotalol
(J) Verapamil

72. A 24-year-old man with a 7-year history of Crohn's disease was suffering from persistent diarrhea, abdominal pain, and signs of systemic inflammation that were poorly controlled by first-line agents. The patient's physician proposed treatment with an immunoglobin-based agent that inhibits tumor necrosis factor (TNF). Which of the following drugs fits this description?
(A) Aldesleukin
(B) Cyclosporine
(C) Filgrastim
(D) Infliximab
(E) Interferon-γ

73. A 43-year-old woman was brought to a hospital emergency department by her brother. Visiting the halfway house in which she lived, he had found her to be lethargic, with slurred speech. The patient had a long history of treatment for depression, and the brother feared that she might have overdosed on 1 or more of her prescription drugs. Physical examination revealed hypotension, tachycardia, decreased bowel sounds, dilated pupils, hyperthermia, and mild parkinsonian symptoms. If this patient had taken a drug overdose, the most likely causative agent was
(A) Amitriptyline
(B) Celecoxib
(C) Lithium
(D) Ramelteon
(E) Zaleplon

Questions 74 and 75. A 30-year-old hospitalized patient with AIDS has a CD4 cell count of 50/μL. He is being treated with a highly active antiretroviral therapy (HAART) regimen consisting of zidovudine (ZDV), lamivudine (3TC), and indinavir. Other drugs being administered to this patient include ganciclovir, clarithromycin, rifabutin, and trimethoprim-sulfamethoxazole.

74. The drug in this patient's regimen that inhibits posttranslational modification of viral proteins is
(A) Acyclovir
(B) Indinavir
(C) Lamivudine
(D) Rifabutin
(E) Zidovudine

75. None of the drugs being administered to this patient are useful for prevention or treatment of opportunistic infections caused by
(A) *Candida albicans*
(B) Cytomegalovirus
(C) *Mycobacterium avium-intracellulare*
(D) *Pneumocystis jiroveci*
(E) *Toxoplasma gondii*

76. A 62-year-old woman who presented with pain in her hips, knees, and several vertebrae was diagnosed with Paget's disease. She had been mostly immobile lately due to bone pain and presented with lethargy, fatigue, muscle weakness, anorexia, and constipation. Her serum calcium concentration was found to be 14 mg/dL (normal 9–10 mg/dL). In addition to the bisphosphonates, another drug that has proved useful in reducing bone pain and lowering serum calcium in female patients with Paget's disease is which of the following?
(A) Calcitonin
(B) Fluoride
(C) Hydrochlorothiazide
(D) Raloxifene
(E) Teriparatide (recombinant form of PTH)

77. A 46-year-old man has hypertension of 155/95. His cardiac and kidney function is normal. Losartan has been suggested as therapy. This drug provides an antihypertensive effect by which of the following effects?
    (A) Accelerating the rate of enzymatic inactivation of amine neurotransmitters in the CNS
    (B) Activating α_2-adrenoceptors located in the presynaptic membranes of CNS neurons that regulate peripheral SANS activity
    (C) Blocking the transport of amine neurotransmitters from the cytoplasm to the inside of synaptic transmitter storage vesicles
    (D) Inhibiting the uptake of amine neurotransmitters from the extracellular fluid into the cytoplasm in the presynaptic nerve terminus
    (E) Interfering with the combination of angiotensin II with its receptor

78. Which vasodilator acts on vascular smooth muscle to block calcium influx via L-type channels?
    (A) Diazoxide
    (B) Diltiazem
    (C) Hydralazine
    (D) Minoxidil
    (E) Nitroprusside

79. In anesthesia protocols that include succinylcholine, which of the following is a premonitory sign of malignant hyperthermia?
    (A) Acidosis
    (B) Bradycardia
    (C) Hypotension
    (D) Transient hypothermia
    (E) Trismus

80. Diners at a popular seafood restaurant became ill after consuming clams and mussels. Consultation with the local coastal authorities revealed that the area from which the seafood had been harvested had recently had a major "red tide." The consumption of shellfish harvested during a red tide (resulting from a large population of a dinoflagellate species) is not recommended because of contamination with saxitoxin, a drug that resembles tetrodotoxin. These toxins cause which of the following effects?
    (A) Clonic-tonic seizures
    (B) Malignant hypertension
    (C) Nerve transmission blockade
    (D) Renal failure
    (E) Ventricular torsades de pointes arrhythmias

81. A 66-year-old patient is diagnosed with hypertension and angina. A drug with benefits in both conditions is suggested. Which of the following drugs has both nonselective β-blocking and α_1-selective blocking action?
    (A) Atenolol
    (B) Carvedilol
    (C) Nadolol
    (D) Pindolol
    (E) Timolol

82. A 35-year-old woman who has never been pregnant suffers each month from pain, discomfort, and mood depression at the time of menses. She may benefit from the use of this selective inhibitor of the reuptake of serotonin in a form that can be taken once weekly.
    (A) Amoxapine
    (B) Bupropion
    (C) Fluoxetine
    (D) Mirtazapine
    (E) Tranylcypromine

83. Which one of the following drugs is considered a first-line treatment for post-traumatic stress disorder?
    (A) Citalopram
    (B) Diazepam
    (C) Imipramine
    (D) Nefazodone
    (E) Selegiline

84. Adverse effects of the opioid analgesics do not include
    (A) Diarrhea
    (B) Emesis
    (C) Increased intracranial pressure
    (D) Respiratory depression
    (E) Urinary retention

85. Drugs that selectively inhibit D_2 dopamine receptors in the CNS have efficacy in the treatment of schizophrenia. Efficacy in the treatment of schizophrenia is also seen with drugs that block
    (A) α-Adrenoceptors or D_1 dopamine receptors
    (B) D_4 dopamine receptors or 5-HT_{2A} serotonin receptors
    (C) $GABA_A$ receptors or 5-HT_3 serotonin receptors
    (D) H_1 histamine receptors or β-adrenoceptors
    (E) β-Adrenoceptors or NMDA receptors

86. A 44-year-old patient suffering from an alcohol-use disorder enters a residential treatment program that emphasizes group therapy and also uses pharmacologic agents adjunctively. The patient is given a drug that decreases the craving for alcohol. Because the drug will not cause adverse effects if the patient consumes alcoholic beverages, it can be identified as which of the following?
    (A) Bupropion
    (B) Disulfiram
    (C) Olanzapine
    (D) Naltrexone
    (E) Sertraline

87. A 22-year-old woman presents with left lower quadrant abdominal pain and a purulent vaginal discharge that, on Gram stain, revealed gram-negative rods. A diagnosis is made of pelvic inflammatory disease possibly involving both *N gonorrhoeae* and *C trachomatis*. A drug or drug combination that provides adequate empiric coverage of the organisms involved in this infection is
    (A) Azithromycin
    (B) Ceftriaxone plus doxycycline
    (C) Metronidazole
    (D) Norfloxacin plus ampicillin
    (E) Trimethoprim-sulfamethoxazole

88. A 28-year-old man was diagnosed with Hodgkin's lymphoma, and chemotherapy with multiple anticancer drugs was initiated. Which of the following agents is an agonist of a hormone receptor and is used in the treatment of Hodgkin's lymphoma?
(A) Dacarbazine
(B) Doxorubicin
(C) Prednisone
(D) Procarbazine
(E) Vinblastine

89. Which of the following is a tyrosine kinase enzyme inhibitor that is used to treat chronic myelogenous leukemia?
(A) Anastrozole
(B) Doxorubicin
(C) Imatinib
(D) Rituximab
(E) Vincristine

90. A 17-year-old high school student presents with headache, fever, and cough of 2 days' duration. Sputum is scant and nonpurulent, and a Gram stain reveals many white cells but no organisms. Because this otherwise healthy patient appears to have a community-acquired pneumonia, you should initiate treatment with
(A) Amoxicillin-clavulanate
(B) Clindamycin
(C) Doxycycline
(D) Erythromycin
(E) Quinupristin-dalfopristin

91. Relative to ciprofloxacin, levofloxacin has improved activity against
(A) *Bacteroides fragilis*
(B) *Escherichia coli*
(C) *Haemophilus influenzae*
(D) *Mycoplasma pneumoniae*
(E) *Streptococcus pneumoniae*

92. Which of the following is the drug of choice for the management of osteoporosis caused by high-dose use of glucocorticoids?
(A) Alendronate
(B) Anastrozole
(C) Ethinyl estradiol
(D) Omeprazole
(E) Oxandrolone

93. A 45-year-old man who received an allogenic liver transplant received an immunosuppressive regimen containing prednisone, azathioprine, and cyclosporine. Which of the following most accurately describes the mechanism of anti-inflammatory activity of cyclosporine?
(A) Activation of phospholipase A_2
(B) Block of interleukin-2 receptors
(C) Competitive inhibition of inosine monophosphate dehydrogenase
(D) Inhibition of enzymes involved in purine metabolism
(E) Inhibition of the cytoplasmic phosphatase calcineurin

94. Which one of the following drugs is appropriate for treating a patient with moderate to severe rheumatoid arthritis but is not appropriate for treating a patient with moderate to severe osteoarthritis?
(A) Acetaminophen
(B) Etanercept
(C) Ibuprofen
(D) Interferon α
(E) Fentanyl

Questions 95 and 96. An anesthetized subject was given an intravenous bolus dose of a drug (**Drug 1**) while the systolic and diastolic blood pressures (*blue*) and the heart rate were recorded, as shown on the left side of the graph below. While the recorder was stopped, **Drug 2** was given (center). **Drug 1** was then administered again, as shown on the right side of the graph.

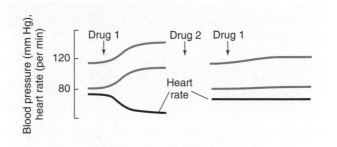

95. Identify Drug 1 from the following list
(A) Atropine
(B) Diphenhydramine
(C) Echothiophate
(D) Endothelin
(E) Epinephrine
(F) Histamine
(G) Isoproterenol
(H) Norepinephrine
(I) Phentolamine
(J) Phenylephrine
(K) Terbutaline

96. Identify Drug 2 from the following list
(A) Angiotensin II
(B) Atropine
(C) Bethanechol
(D) Diphenhydramine
(E) Endothelin
(F) Epinephrine
(G) Isoproterenol
(H) Norepinephrine
(I) Phentolamine
(J) Phenylephrine
(K) Terbutaline

97. In the treatment of hypothyroidism, thyroxine is preferred over liothyronine because thyroxine
(A) Can be made more easily by recombinant DNA technology
(B) Has a longer half-life
(C) Has higher affinity for thyroid hormone receptors
(D) Is faster acting
(E) Is more likely to improve a patient's mood

98. A 29-year-old G1P1 (gravida-1, para-1) woman presents with infertility of 12 months' duration. Questioning reveals that the patient has had only 4 menstrual periods in the last year and that she sometimes notices breast nipple discharge. She has not been taking any prescription medications during the last year. A serum prolactin measurement reveals a concentration of 90 ng/mL (normal for a nonpregnant woman is <25 ng/mL). Based on these findings, which of the following drugs is most likely to help make this woman's ovulation more regular and restore her fertility?
    (A) Bromocriptine
    (B) Desmopressin
    (C) Leuprolide
    (D) Prochlorperazine
    (E) Spironolactone

99. A young woman seeks advice because she had unprotected sexual intercourse 12 hr earlier. Based on her menstrual cycle, she believes that conception is possible. Which drug should she use as a postcoital contraceptive?
    (A) Clomiphene
    (B) Diethylstilbestrol plus raloxifene
    (C) Flutamide
    (D) Letrozole plus finasteride
    (E) Levonorgestrel

100. A 55-year-old woman with type 2 diabetes was going to be started on metformin. Before initiating therapy, it is important to confirm that the patient has normal renal function because patients with unrecognized renal insufficiency who take normal doses of metformin are at increased risk of which of the following?
    (A) Hypoglycemia
    (B) Interstitial nephritis
    (C) Lactic acidosis
    (D) Liver failure
    (E) Torsades de pointes cardiac arrhythmia

ANSWER KEY FOR EXAMINATION 1*

1. **C** (5) Phase 3 trials are carried out under the conditions of proposed use in (usually) several thousand patients.

2. **B** (1) According to the Henderson-Hasselbalch principle (Chapter 1), weak acids are less protonated (and more charged) in alkaline media, and weak bases are more protonated (and more charged) in acidic media. Since the clearance of the unknown drug is greater in alkaline urine, the drug must be a weak acid.

3. **C** (9, 13, 15) Digoxin *decreases* atrioventricular conduction. Furosemide does not increase vascular resistance. Of the agents listed, only dobutamine increases cAMP. All 3 drugs reduce pulmonary edema, albeit probably by different mechanisms.

4. **D** (17) Endothelin is the peptide most closely associated with pulmonary hypertension, and ambrisentan is an orally active ET_A receptor antagonist.

5. **E** (16, 59) Omeprazole, a proton pump inhibitor, very effectively reduces gastric acid secretion by being converted to an active metabolite that irreversibly inhibits the parietal cell H^+/K^+ ATPase that is responsible for acid secretion. Misoprostol activates prostaglandin E receptors. Sucralfate forms a protective coating over an ulcer bed, and cimetidine inhibits H_2 histamine receptors.

6. **E** (14, 15) Cardiac automaticity is enhanced by hypokalemia. Thiazides, loop diuretics, and even carbonic anhydrase inhibitors can reduce serum potassium levels because they present more sodium to the cortical collecting tubules, which attempt to compensate by wasting potassium in exchange for sodium.

7. **C** (35) The statins inhibit de novo cholesterol synthesis through inhibition of HMG-CoA reductase. This forces the liver to upregulate LDL receptors and replenish the cholesterol stores through uptake from the bloodstream. LPL is activated by fibrates. The resins lower cholesterol by shunting more cholesterol into the bile acid pathway. Ezetimibe inhibits uptake of cholesterol in the small intestine. Fibrates enhance fatty acid oxidation.

8. **B** (7) The appropriate treatment for myasthenic crisis is an indirect-acting cholinomimetic, the same medication used for chronic therapy of this condition. Neostigmine is the only cholinesterase inhibitor in the list of choices.

9. **D** (8, 58) The patient has characteristic signs of antimuscarinic (also known as anticholinergic) toxicity, caused by drugs such as atropine. Children are especially susceptible to the hyperthermia caused by antimuscarinic drug overdose.

10. **C** (3) Two hours after an overdose of a drug with a 40-hr half-life, the plasma concentration will approximate that immediately after a loading dose. Using the loading dose equation (dose = $V_d \times C_p$), we obtain dose = 80 L × 40 mg/L, or 3200 mg, or 3.2 g.

11. **C** (27) A drug that antagonizes nicotinic receptors at skeletal neuromuscular junctions (pancuronium) is required to inhibit spontaneous respiratory movements. Succinylcholine is not appropriate partly because it may initially stimulate N-receptors and also because its duration of action is very short.

12. **A** (8) Atropine has a very long duration of action in the eye (>72 hr). By interfering with accommodation in the dominant eye, atropine can sometimes prevent amblyopia. Timolol has no significant effect on accommodation, whereas the other drugs listed cause miosis and cyclospasm.

13. **C** (36) Ibuprofen and indomethacin are the only NSAIDS listed here. Indomethacin is more potent and has more adverse effects compared with ibuprofen and is not the first NSAID of choice for milder symptoms. Colchicine exerts its anti-inflammatory effects by prevention of tubulin polymerization, and it is used predominantly in acute gout attacks. Hydroxychloroquine is an antimalarial with anti-inflammatory effects, and sulfasalazine inhibits the release of inflammatory cytokines (IL-1, IL-6, IL-12, and TNF-α).

14. **E** (33) The most common cause of macrocytic anemia is deficiency of folic acid or vitamin B_{12}. The additional finding of neurologic abnormality suggests vitamin B_{12} deficiency, which is treated with vitamin B_{12} replacement.

15. **A** (34) Warfarin inhibits vitamin K-dependent gamma-carboxylation of the clotting factors X, IX, VII, and II (mnemonic "1972"). Warfarin acts through inhibition of vitamin K epoxide reductase in the liver. It does *not* interact with plasminogen or platelets.

16. **C** (11, 12) Angina pectoris can be precipitated by tachycardia; vasodilators such as hydralazine typically cause increased heart rate.

17. **E** (18, 34) All of the choices listed are eicosanoids, but only thromboxane is associated with enhanced platelet aggregation. Thromboxane A_2 is the pro-aggregation eicosanoid produced by platelets, whereas endothelial cells produce the prostaglandins that inhibit aggregation. Upon irreversible inhibition by aspirin, platelets (without a nucleus) cannot synthesize new COX enzyme to generate thromboxane A_2, whereas the endothelial cell can replace the enzymes and continue to produce prostaglandins that prevent aggregation.

18. **D** (12, 19) Inhibitors of phosphodiesterase, isoform 5, are useful in enhancing erection. Note: Because the mechanism involves increased cGMP in vascular smooth muscle, these drugs also potentiate the hypotensive action of nitrates.

19. **E** (35) Rhabdomyolysis is a serious side effect that can occur with statins. Gallstones are a side effect of the fibrates; uric acid elevation is a side effect of niacin.

20. **E** (2) A physiologic antagonist opposes the action of other drugs by acting at a different receptor; histamine acts at H_1 and H_2 in the periphery, while epinephrine opposes histamine by acting at α_1 and β_2 adrenoceptors.

21. **C** (1) As described in Chapter 1, receptors are usually regulatory molecules or enzymes; proteins constitute the vast majority of regulatory and enzyme molecules.

22. **C** (41) In order to replicate the physiological situation with a baseline and mealtime peaks, one needs to combine insulin preparations with different durations of action. Review duration of action of different insulin formulations in Figure 41–1.

---

*Numbers in parentheses are chapters in which more information about the answers is found.

23. **C** (6, 8, 9) Atropine blocks vagal and other parasympathetic pathways. Norepinephrine causes vasoconstriction and increased blood pressure. The increase in blood pressure usually evokes a reflex bradycardia that is mediated by the vagus nerve. When vagal slowing is blocked, the beta-agonist action of norepinephrine is unmasked, resulting in tachycardia.

24. **A** (33) The most common cause of microcytic anemia is iron deficiency, which can be treated in most patients with an oral iron supplement such as ferrous sulfate.

25. **C** (2) Quantal dose-response curves plot the percentage of the subjects that show a specified response (Y axis) at each increment of dosage (X axis); see Chapter 2.

26. **B** (6, 8, 10) Isoproterenol causes tachycardia and facilitates arrhythmias through its β action. A β antagonist such as propranolol can prevent this action.

27. **B** (8, 20) Antimuscarinic drugs are contraindicated in Alzheimer's disease, glaucoma, and prostatic hyperplasia. They have no useful effect in hypertension. They can produce useful bronchodilation in COPD and appear to cause less cardiac toxicity than sympathomimetics.

28. **E** (34) Aspirin exerts its antiplatelet effect through irreversible inhibition of COX-1 and COX-2. Clopidogrel is a prodrug, and its metabolite irreversibly binds ADP receptors. Enoxaparin is LMW heparin and acts through antithrombin III. Fondaparinux is a small portion of LMW heparin with similar actions. Tirofiban is the only IIb/IIIa protein ligand in the list of options.

29. **A** (40) Finasteride is a 5α-reductase inhibitor. Flutamide is an androgen receptor antagonist. Ketoconazole is a cytochrome P450 inhibitor (also used as an antifungal agent). Leuprolide is a GnRH agonist used in depot form for prostate carcinoma. Oxandrolone is an anabolic androgenic steroid.

30. **A** (12) Beta blockers usually decrease heart rate but are of no value in vasospastic angina. Nitrates usually increase heart rate. Calcium channel blockers such as diltiazem and verapamil decrease heart rate and are valuable in vasospastic angina, but nifedipine can increase heart rate.

31. **B** (16) Ergotamine is a potent vasoconstrictor but is a partial agonist at α adrenoceptors; as such, it can cause epinephrine reversal.

32. **A** (15) The graph shows a self-limited diuresis, potassium wasting, and metabolic acidosis. This is most consistent with a carbonic anhydrase inhibitor like acetazolamide.

33. **D** (13) Digitalis toxicity is associated with hypokalemia and hypomagnesemia (and hypercalcemia). Hyperkalemia (choice A) is a trap for careless readers.

34. **A** (13) Cardiac glycosides act primarily by inhibiting Na^+/K^+-ATPase and thus increase intracellular Na^+. This in turn reduces Ca^{2+} expulsion by the Na^+-Ca^{2+} exchanger. Excess digitalis results in an excess of intracellular Ca^{2+}.

35. **B** (20) The methylxanthines block phosphodiesterase and increase the concentration of cAMP. They may also *block* adenosine receptors.

36. **A** (20) Skeletal muscle tremor is a common adverse effect of beta-adrenoceptor agonists such as albuterol when used in asthma. Even when administered via inhalation, this side effect as well as tachycardia can occur.

37. **C** (16) Several autacoids may be involved in the edema of angioneurotic allergic reactions. Histamine and bradykinin are probable contributors.

38. **E** (9) Beta antagonists typically increase PR interval. Renin secretion and tremor are decreased. Beta *agonists* increase lipolysis.

39. **C** (36) Colchicine is used predominantly in acute gout attacks and exerts its anti-inflammatory effects by prevention of tubulin polymerization. Epoprostenol is a prostacyclin (PGI_2), and it is used in the treatment of pulmonary hypertension. Naproxen is an NSAID with a relatively long half-life, and zafirlukast is a LT_4 receptor antagonist used in the treatment of asthma.

40. **B** (21) Dopamine exerts slow inhibitory actions at synapses in specific neural systems including the nigrostriatal projections via G protein-coupled activation of postsynaptic potassium channels or by inhibition of presynaptic calcium channels.

41. **C** (22, 23, 58) The patient appears to be suffering from the alcohol withdrawal syndrome, which is treated with a long-acting sedative-hypnotic such as diazepam. Diazepam is available in parenteral and oral formulations.

42. **E** (23) This patient is at risk for delirium tremens, which is characterized by tremors, delusions, and hallucinations.

43. **D** (24) Compared with phenytoin, favorable characteristics of a new anticonvulsant would include good oral bioavailability, minimal plasma protein binding, first-order elimination kinetics, and no induction (or inhibition) of cytochromes P450.

44. **C** (25) All of the factors listed influence the rate of induction of the anesthetic state except the minimal alveolar anesthetic concentration. MAC reflects **potency** and is defined as the minimum alveolar anesthetic concentration that eliminates response to a standard painful stimulus in 50% of patients.

45. **E** (25) The onset of anesthesia with propofol is more rapid than intravenous barbiturates. Its clearance is greater than hepatic blood flow, which suggests extrahepatic elimination. The drug has antiemetic actions, and recovery is not delayed after prolonged infusion.

46. **C** (31) Although miosis is characteristic of all opioids except meperidine, which has a muscarinic blocking action, little or no tolerance occurs. Pupillary constriction due to opioids can be blocked by atropine and by naloxone.

47. **E** (2, 39) Prednisone is a steroid and acts via binding the cytoplasmic steroid receptors, followed by a translocation of the receptor-ligand complex into the nucleus, altering gene transcription. All other agents listed in this question bind to membrane-bound extracellular receptors.

48. **C** (30) Nefazodone and trazodone are 5-HT$_2$ receptor antagonists with both anxiolytic and antidepressant actions. In addition, at a relatively low dose, trazodone is a widely used and effective hypnotic with minimal dependence liability compared with most of the sedative-hypnotic drugs used in sleep disorders.

49. **B** (29, 30) Enhancement of the actions of norepinephrine and/or serotonin via inhibition of reuptake transporters is characteristic of many antidepressants including the tricyclics and the SSRIs. However, inhibition of the reuptake of dopamine leading to enhancement of its CNS effects has been equated with thought disorders, delusions, hallucinations, and paranoia.

50. C (30) Enuresis is an established indication for tricyclic antidepressants including imipramine, and they are also used as backup drugs to methylphenidate in attention deficit disorder. Chronic pain states that may be unresponsive to conventional analgesics often respond to the tricyclics.

51. B (30, 31) Codeine, oxycodone, and hydrocodone are all metabolized by cytochrome CYP2D6, which can be inhibited by certain SSRIs including fluoxetine and paroxetine. This may lead to a decreased analgesic effects of codeine which is normally metabolized in part via CYP2D6 forming the more active compound morphine.

52. A (39) Cushing's syndrome is a consequence of too much steroid production and is most commonly due to an ACTH-secreting pituitary adenoma. Dexamethasone will suppress ACTH production and thus can be used diagnostically to separate pituitary Cushing's from those with ectopic ACTH-producing tumors. Fludrocortisone acts on mineralocorticoid receptors only. Glucose is already elevated as a consequence of the disease, and adding more will not be diagnostic. Ketoconazole will inhibit male hormone synthesis but will not provide differential diagnostic information. PTU (propylthiouracil) inhibits thyroid hormone signaling.

53. D (29) Clozapine has greater muscarinic and alpha-blocking activity than haloperidol, but neither of these is the primary reason why the drug is less likely to cause extrapyramidal dysfunction. The main reason is that clozapine has very low affinity for the dopamine D_2 receptor in the striatum.

54. D (29) Edema and thyroid enlargement are common adverse effects of lithium, although the latter does not usually involve hypothyroidism. Neurologic side effects of lithium include tremor, ataxia, and aphasia.

55. D (21, 22) Though not benzodiazepines, zolpidem, zaleplon, and eszopiclone exert their hypnotic effects via interaction with benzodiazepine receptors in the CNS, leading to an increase in GABA-mediated chloride ion conductance.

56. C (22, 58) Diazepam is a benzodiazepine sedative-hypnotic drug whose action can be competitively inhibited by flumazenil. Acetylcysteine is used for acetaminophen overdose. Atropine is used in organophosphate poisoning, fomepizole is used for methanol or ethylene glycol poisoning, and naloxone is used for opioid overdose.

57. D (45) In gram-negative bacteria, the primary mechanism of resistance to aminoglycosides involves the plasmid-mediated formation of inactivating enzymes that acetylate, adenylate, or phosphorylate the drug molecule. Such enzymes are called group transferases.

58. E (3, 34, 60, 61) Warfarin is metabolized by CYP3A4 (and CYP1A and CYP2C). The patient's INR is reduced; her plasma level of warfarin is subtherapeutic. This means the metabolism of warfarin is *induced*. St. John's wort is a potent inducer of CYP3A4. The other drugs do not appear to affect the CYP enzyme family.

59. B (43, 50) The third-generation cephalosporins ceftriaxone and cefotaxime (not listed) are currently the most active beta-lactam antibiotics against beta-lactamase-producing strains of *H influenzae* and *Neisseria*. However, some resistance has been reported recently.

60. D (46) Patients with a history of cardiac irregularities should avoid certain fluoroquinolones including levofloxacin and moxifloxacin since they are known to cause QT prolongation.

61. C (43, 50) The anaerobic bacterium *Clostridium difficile* is a cause of life-threatening pseudomembranous colitis. The primary drugs used in management of such infections are vancomycin (not listed) or metronidazole.

62. D (46, 52) One double-strength tablet of sulfamethoxazole-trimethoprim three times weekly is prophylactic against *P jiroveci* infection in AIDS patients but may cause rash, fever, and leukopenia.

63. C (54) The question asks about antimetabolites. The two options in this class are mercaptopurine and fluorouracil. Mercaptopurine is a purine affecting purine metabolism leaving FU, which is a suicide substrate for thymidylate synthase.

64. D (16, 59) Ondansetron, a serotonin 5-HT_3 receptor antagonist, is a highly effective antiemetic. Famotidine is a H_2 receptor antagonist used for acid-peptic disease. Leucovorin is a form of tetrahydrofolate that can be used to reverse the effects of the anticancer drug methotrexate. Mesalamine is a form of 5-aminosalicylic acid (5-ASA) used for inflammatory bowel disease, and sumatriptan is a serotonin 5-$HT_{1D/1B}$ agonist used for migraine headache.

65. B (47) A 4-drug initial regimen would be appropriate in this case, and if the laboratory reports show sensitivity to the drugs, it would be appropriate to discontinue pyrazinamide, maintaining the 3-drug regimen that includes both isoniazid and rifampin. Pyrazinamide has a high incidence of adverse effects including polyarthralgia as well as hepatic dysfunction, porphyria, and photosensitivity reactions.

66. A (48) The amphipathic character of amphotericin B following its interaction with ergosterol in fungal cell membranes leads to artificial "pores" that disrupt membrane integrity. Nystatin, another polyene, acts similarly but is too nephrotoxic for systemic use.

67. A (36, 58) An overdose of aspirin will cause anion gap metabolic acidosis, as described here. Ethanol can also cause anion gap acidosis as ethanol metabolism generates NADH, leading to conversion of pyruvate to lactate, but the condition is often mild even without treatment. Acetaminophen causes liver failure in overdose, whereas dextromethorphan, an opioid, will cause respiratory depression and not hyperventilation. Diphenhydramine, an antihistamine, causes sedation through its effect on central histamine receptors but does not generally cause acidosis.

68. D (1, 58) Aspirin is a weak acid with a pKa of 3.5. Urinary alkalinization to a pH of 7.5 or above by administration of sodium bicarbonate will enhance urinary excretion of aspirin and other salicylates. Urinary alkalinization traps the charged, polar form of the salicylates in the renal tubule fluid. Hemodialysis is also very effective at removing salicylates.

69. D (47) Resistance emerges rapidly when rifampin is used as a single agent in the treatment of bacterial infections. When used in the meningococcal carrier state, highly resistant strains may be selected out during treatment.

70. E (52) Doxycycline, atovaquone-proguanil (Malarone), and mefloquine are all prophylactic against chloroquine-resistant strains of *P falciparum*.

71. D (14) The action potential has a markedly slowed upstroke and unchanged duration. These effects are characteristic of group 1C drugs, including flecainide.

72. D (55) Infliximab is a humanized monoclonal antibody that binds to tumor necrosis factor-alpha (TNF-α). Anti-TNF-α antibody-based drugs (etanercept, adalimumab) are increasingly used to treat inflammatory disorders such as rheumatoid arthritis.

73. A (30) Adverse effects of the tricyclic antidepressant amitriptyline include sedation, hypotension, tachycardia, and symptoms of muscarinic blockade such as decreased bowel sounds and pupillary dilation. In severe overdose, watch for the "3 Cs"—coma, convulsions, and cardiotoxicity.

74. B (49) Protease inhibitors such as indinavir act at the post-translational step of HIV at which the viral enzyme cleaves precursor molecules to form the final structural proteins of the mature virion core.

75. A (48, 49) Prophylactic drugs used in this AIDS patient provide coverage against most opportunistic infections, including cytomegalovirus (ganciclovir), but there is no coverage against fungal infections commonly due to *Candida albicans.*

76. A (42) Paget's is a condition of too much bone resorption leading to elevated serum calcium. Both the bisphosphonates ("dronates") and calcitonin will inhibit this. Calcitonin is the drug of choice for the acute lowering of serum calcium. Fluoride and raloxifene affect bone formation. PTH and HTZ increase serum calcium.

77. E (6, 11) Losartan is a member of the angiotensin receptor-blocking group. It is a competitive antagonist of angiotensin II at its receptor.

78. B (11) Diltiazem, as well as nifedipine and verapamil, act as vasodilators by reducing calcium influx via L type channels. Hydralazine and nitroprusside act through release of nitric oxide. Diazoxide and minoxidil facilitate potassium channel opening.

79. E (25) Trismus, or masseter hypertonia, that results from the use of succinylcholine during induction of anesthesia is a rare and dangerous phenomenon. It presents to the anesthesiologist the immediate problem of airway management but it also must be recognized by the physician as a harbinger of malignant hyperthermia.

80. C (6) Dinoflagellates secrete saxitoxin, a blocker of voltage-gated Na$^+$ channels in nerves. Exposure to this toxin results in block of transmission initially in sensory nerves (causing numbness and tingling) but may extend to block of motor nerves with paralysis of voluntary muscle, including the diaphragm.

81. B (10) Carvedilol is the only β-blocker in the list that also has α-blocking action.

82. C (30) Approximately 5% of women of child-bearing age experience symptoms during the late luteal phase of the menstrual cycle that are more serious than PMS. It is referred to as premenstrual dysphoric disorder (PMDD). SSRIs, including a long-acting form of fluoxetine given weekly, are approved for this indication.

83. A (30) SSRIs are considered first-line treatment of PTSDs and can benefit a number of symptoms including anxious thoughts and hypervigilance. Psychotherapeutic interventions are usually required in addition to antidepressants.

84. A (31) With the exception of diphenoxylate and loperamide, which are used for the treatment of diarrhea, constipation is considered an adverse effect of the opioid analgesics.

85. B (29) Although all effective antipsychotic drugs block D$_2$ receptors, some are more potent inhibitors of D$_4$ dopamine receptors (eg, clozapine) or 5-HT$_{2A}$ serotonin receptors (eg, olanzapine).

86. D (23, 31, 32) Naloxone, a nonselective opioid receptor antagonist, is used by individuals recovering from alcohol-use disorders.

87. B (43, 44) Ceftriaxone (or cefixime) is a drug of choice for treatment of gonococcal infections, and chlamydial infections usually respond to a tetracycline. Though not listed, azithromycin as a single agent is considered a co-drug of choice for chlamydial infections and an alternative drug for gonococcal infections.

88. C (39, 54) Hodgkin's lymphoma is a cancer of lymph tissue found in the lymph nodes, spleen, liver, bone marrow, and other sites. It responds well to prednisone. Prednisone acts via binding the cytoplasmic steroid receptors followed by a translocation of the receptor-ligand complex into the nucleus, binding to DNA, and altering gene transcription. All other agents listed in this question are cytotoxic agents.

89. C (54) Note that kinase inhibitors have names ending in "nib." Anastrozole is an aromatase inhibitor. Doxorubicin is an antitumor antibiotic. Imatinib (Gleevec) targets bcr-abl kinase. Rituximab is a monoclonal antibody against CD20. Vincristine is an alkaloid affecting microtubules.

90. C (46) With respect to microbial etiology, the most likely organisms in community-acquired pneumonia (CAP) are *S pneumoniae, H influenzae,* and *M catarrhalis.* Depending on resistance patterns in the community, it is possible to treat CAP with a single antibiotic, and doxycycline is one of the antibiotics commonly used.

91. E (46) In the case described in question 90, though not listed, levofloxacin is also used both as a single drug and in drug combinations in CAP, precisely because the drug has much greater activity than ciprofloxacin against likely organisms, especially the pneumococcus.

92. A (42) "Dronates" inhibit bone resorption. Anastrozole is an aromatase inhibitor used for treatment of breast cancer. Ethinyl estradiol is an estrogen stimulating bone resorption. Omeprazole is a proton pump inhibitor. Oxandrolone is an androgen used when its anabolic action is needed (wasting due to illness: cancer, HIV, etc.)

93. E (55) Cyclosporine exerts its immunosuppressive effect by binding to the immunophilin cyclophilin and forming a complex with the cytosolic phosphatase calcineurin, which is necessary for activation of the T-cell nuclear factor of activated T-cell (NF-AT) transcription factor. As a result, cyclosporine inhibits the synthesis of interleukins such as IL-2 by activated T cells.

94. B (36) Etanercept is not appropriate for osteoarthritis because it binds to and inactivates TNF-α. Thus, it will only be of use in inflammatory disorders that are mediated through TNF-α such as rheumatoid arthritis, juvenile-onset arthritis psoriasis, psoriatic arthritis, and ankylosing spondylitis.

95. J (9) This question and the following one require a combined knowledge of agonist and antagonist actions. Note that systolic and diastolic blood pressures are increased, but heart rate is decreased. This is compatible with a strong α-agonist drug such as norepinephrine (choice **H**) or phenylephrine (choice **J**). The final choice must be withheld until the actions of drug 2 are evaluated. Following drug 2, there is no change in heart rate, suggesting that the bradycardia seen previously was a reflex response to the pressor effect. Thus, drug 1 lacks β-agonist effect; it is a "pure" α agonist.

96. **I** (10) As noted in the answer to the previous question, the agonist drug (drug 1) is probably a strong α-agonist sympathomimetic. Drug 2 markedly reduces the pressor action of drug 1 (compatible with α blockade) and also suppresses the change in heart rate. If drug 1 was norepinephrine, its β-agonist effect on heart rate would have been unmasked. Thus, drug 2 is a simple α blocker.

97. **B** (38) Thyroxine (T_4) is preferred over liothyronine (T_3) because it has a longer half-life. It is less expensive and has a slower onset of action. It is converted into T_3 in the tissues; thus, the affinity for the receptor or the effects on the patient's mood will be the same.

98. **A** (37) This patient has signs and symptoms of hyperprolactinemia, which is caused by prolactin-secreting pituitary adenomas. Dopamine D_2 receptor agonists such as bromocriptine can be used to suppress the excessive prolactin secretion.

99. **E** (40) Levonorgestrel is a progestin. Progestins used within 72 hr are effective as emergency contraception either alone or in combination with estrogens. "Progestin-only" emergency contraceptives have fewer side effects than those containing estrogens.

100. **C** (41) Metformin carries a black box warning for lactic acidosis. Note that metformin is a "euglycemic agent" (ie, it does not cause hypoglycemia).

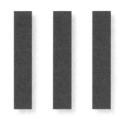

Examination 2

DIRECTIONS: Each numbered item or incomplete statement in this section is followed by answers or by completions of the statement. Select the ONE lettered answer or completion that is BEST in each case.

1. A patient is admitted to the emergency department with signs and symptoms that could be due to either a muscarinic stimulant or an opioid. Which of the following is a common effect of both muscarinic stimulant drugs and opioids?
   (A) Decreased peristalsis
   (B) Decreased secretion by salivary glands
   (C) Hypertension
   (D) Inhibition of thermoregulatory sweat glands
   (E) Miosis

2. Which statement about nitric oxide is most correct?
   (A) Nitric oxide is synthesized in vascular endothelium and the brain
   (B) Nitric oxide is released from storage vesicles by acetylcholine
   (C) Nitric oxide synthase is stimulated by nitroprusside
   (D) Nitric oxide synthase is inhibited by histamine
   (E) Nitric oxide causes pulmonary vasoconstriction

3. A 35-year-old patient is brought to the emergency department in a drug-induced coma. Blood samples taken over the next several hours show a declining drug concentration, as shown in the graph below. Which of the following drugs is the most likely cause of this patient's coma?

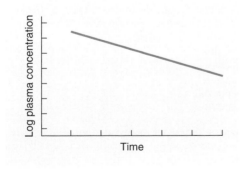

   (A) Aspirin
   (B) Diazepam
   (C) Ethanol
   (D) Phenytoin

4. In a laboratory study of a new agent, the activity of a membrane-bound enzyme was found to be increased by the drug. Analysis of this enzyme molecule revealed that it is an integral tyrosine kinase, the extracellular domain of which binds ligands while the intracellular domain phosphorylates tyrosine residues. Which of the following receptors communicate their activation by turning on an integral intracellular tyrosine kinase domain?
   (A) Acetylcholine nicotinic receptors
   (B) G protein-coupled receptors
   (C) Insulin receptors
   (D) Steroid receptors
   (E) Vitamin D receptors

5. A patient with a myocardial infarction, heart failure, and an arrhythmia is to receive lidocaine by constant IV infusion. The target plasma concentration is 3 mg/L. The pharmacokinetic parameters for lidocaine in the general population are V_d 70 L, CL 35 L/h, and $t_{1/2}$ 1.4 h. An infusion is begun. The plasma concentration of lidocaine is measured 2.8 h later and reported to be 2.4 mg/L. This indicates that the final steady state plasma concentration in this patient will be
   (A) 1.5 mg/L
   (B) 2.4 mg/L
   (C) 3.2 mg/L
   (D) 4.6 mg/L
   (E) 6.9 mg/L

6. A new drug for the prophylaxis of asthma is under development in a pharmaceutical company. Before human trials are begun, FDA regulations require that
   (A) All acute and chronic animal toxicity data be submitted to the FDA
   (B) The drug be shown to be free of carcinogenic effects
   (C) The drug be shown to be safe in animals with the target disease
   (D) The drug be studied in 3 mammalian species
   (E) The effect of the drug on reproduction be studied in at least 2 animal species

7. Ms. B, a 40-year-old woman, has been receiving a slow IV infusion of phenylephrine. She is currently showing an excessive heart rate effect from this drug. A drug that blocks the heart rate effect of a slow IV infusion of phenylephrine is
   (A) Atropine
   (B) Echothiophate
   (C) Neostigmine
   (D) Pilocarpine
   (E) Propranolol

8. A patient admitted to the emergency department is vomiting blood. Her supine blood pressure is 100/60 mm Hg; sitting up, her BP is 50/0. Which of the following most accurately describes the probable autonomic response to the bleeding?
   (A) Slow heart rate, dilated pupils, damp skin
   (B) Rapid heart rate, dilated pupils, damp skin
   (C) Slow heart rate, dry skin, increased bowel sounds
   (D) Rapid heart rate, dry skin, constricted pupils, increased bowel sounds
   (E) Rapid heart rate, constricted pupils, warm skin

9. A 65-year-old man has chronic open-angle glaucoma. The drug that is most likely to have therapeutic value for this condition is
   (A) Ephedrine
   (B) Isoproterenol
   (C) Latanoprost
   (D) Mannitol
   (E) Propranolol

10. A new drug was administered to a group of normal volunteers in a phase 1 clinical trial. Intravenous bolus doses produced the changes in blood pressure and heart rate shown in the graph below. The most probable receptor affinities of this new drug are
    (A) α_1, α_2, and β_1
    (B) α_1 and α_2 only
    (C) β_1 and β_2 only
    (D) Muscarinic M_3 only
    (E) Nicotinic N_N only

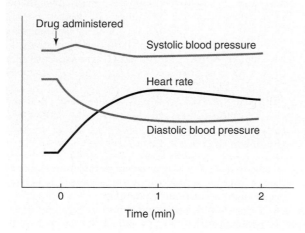

11. Persons who ingest three or more alcoholic drinks daily can develop severe hepatotoxicity after doses of acetaminophen that are not toxic to individuals with normal liver function. This increased sensitivity to acetaminophen's toxicity is due to which of the following mechanisms?
    (A) Decreased availability of acetaldehyde dehydrogenase
    (B) Decreased hepatocellular stores of NADPH
    (C) Increased extraction of acetaminophen by the cirrhotic liver
    (D) Increased activity of cytochrome P450 mixed function oxidase isozymes
    (E) Increased liver blood flow

12. An example of a phase I drug-metabolizing reaction is
    (A) Acetylation
    (B) Glucuronidation
    (C) Hydroxylation
    (D) Methylation
    (E) Sulfation

Questions 13 and 14. A 52-year-old plumber comes to the office with a complaint of periodic onset of chest pain, described as a sensation of heavy pressure over the sternum that comes on when he exercises and disappears within 15 min when he stops. After a full physical examination and further evaluation, you make the diagnosis of angina of effort.

13. In considering medical therapy for this patient, which of the following best describes the beneficial action of nitroglycerin in this condition?
    (A) Dilation of coronary arterioles reduces resistance and increases coronary flow through ischemic tissue
    (B) Dilation of peripheral arterioles increases cardiac work
    (C) Dilation of systemic veins results in decreased diastolic cardiac size
    (D) Increased sympathetic outflow increases coronary flow
    (E) Tachycardia increases diastolic coronary flow

14. A drug that is useful in angina but causes constipation, edema, and increased cardiac size is
    (A) Atenolol
    (B) Hydralazine
    (C) Isosorbide dinitrate
    (D) Nitroglycerin
    (E) Verapamil

15. A 15-year-old girl is admitted complaining of palpitations and shortness of breath. An ECG reveals sinus tachycardia with a heart rate of 160 bpm. A drug suitable for producing a brief (5- to 15-min) increase in cardiac vagal effects is
    (A) Digoxin
    (B) Edrophonium
    (C) Ergotamine
    (D) Pralidoxime
    (E) Pyridostigmine

16. A patient with a 30-yr history of type 1 diabetes comes to you with a complaint of bloating and sour belching after meals. On several occasions, vomiting has occurred after a meal. Evaluation reveals delayed emptying of the stomach, and you diagnose diabetic gastroparesis. Which drug would be most useful in this patient?
    (A) Famotidine
    (B) Metoclopramide
    (C) Misoprostol
    (D) Omeprazole
    (E) Ondansetron

17. An important difference between nonselective α-receptor antagonists and α_1-selective antagonists is that α_1-selective antagonists
    (A) Are more likely to cause hypoglycemia
    (B) Are more likely to precipitate bronchoconstriction in patients with asthma
    (C) Have greater efficacy in relaxing smooth muscle in the urinary tract
    (D) Produce less reflex tachycardia
    (E) Reduce mean arterial blood pressure to a greater extent

18. A 70-year-old woman with mild to moderate hypertension fell 2 yr ago during a spell of dizziness and broke her hip. During the last 18 mo, her blood pressure has increased. Now she is to be treated for a blood pressure of 170/100 mm Hg. When treating hypertension chronically, orthostatic hypotension is greatest with
    (A) ACE inhibitors
    (B) Arteriolar dilators
    (C) Centrally acting α_2 agonists
    (D) Peripherally acting α_1 antagonists
    (E) Beta blockers

19. A 52-year-old woman is admitted to the emergency department with a history of drug treatment for several conditions. Her serum electrolytes are found to be as follows (normal values in parentheses):

    Na^+ 140 mEq/L (135–145) K^+ 6.5 mEq/L (3.5–5.0)
    Cl^- 100 mEq/L (98–107)   pH 7.3 (7.31–7.41)

    This patient has probably been taking
    (A) Acetazolamide
    (B) Atenolol
    (C) Digoxin
    (D) Furosemide
    (E) Spironolactone

20. A 40-year-old woman was being treated for chronic moderate hypertension. When she went on vacation and forgot her pills, her blood pressure rose markedly and she was admitted to the emergency service with blurred vision, severe headache, and retinal hemorrhages. A drug that is most likely to be followed by rebound hypertension if stopped suddenly is
    (A) Atenolol
    (B) Clonidine
    (C) Labetalol
    (D) Losartan
    (E) Prazosin

21. Ventricular muscle from a cardiac biopsy was prepared for transmembrane potential recording in an isolated muscle chamber. Action potentials were recorded before and after application of drug X.

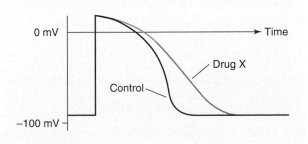

    Identify drug X from the following list.
    (A) Adenosine
    (B) Amiodarone
    (C) Procainamide
    (D) Sotalol
    (E) Verapamil

22. Propranolol and hydralazine have which of the following effects in common?
    (A) Decreased cardiac force
    (B) Decreased cardiac output
    (C) Decreased mean arterial blood pressure
    (D) Increased systemic vascular resistance
    (E) Tachycardia

23. A 54-year-old farmer has a 5-yr history of frequent, recurrent, and very painful calcium-containing kidney stones. The patient has hypercalciuria caused by a primary defect in proximal tubule calcium reabsorption. Which of the following is the most appropriate chronic therapy for this man?
    (A) Aldosterone antagonist
    (B) Loop diuretic
    (C) NSAID
    (D) Strong opioid
    (E) Thiazide diuretic

24. A 55-year-old executive has cardiomyopathy and congestive heart failure. He is being treated with diuretics. The mechanism of action of furosemide is best described as
    (A) Interference with H^+/HCO_3^- exchange
    (B) Blockade of a $Na^+/K^+/2Cl^-$ transporter
    (C) Blockade of a Na^+/Cl^- cotransporter
    (D) Blockade of carbonic anhydrase
    (E) Inhibition of genetic expression of DNA in the kidney

25. A 56-year-old woman has arthritis of the knees that limits her activity and post herpetic neuralgia on her torso after an episode of herpes zoster. Which of the following drugs is used topically to control arthritic pain and post-herpetic neuralgia?
    (A) Aliskiren
    (B) Bosentan
    (C) Capsaicin
    (D) Losartan
    (E) Nesiritide

26. In your pursuit of a Nobel Prize, you have been studying several intracellular enzymes. You recall that cyclooxygenase-1 and -2 are responsible for the
    (A) Conversion of GTP to cyclic GMP (cGMP)
    (B) Conversion of ATP to cyclic AMP (cAMP)
    (C) Metabolic degradation of cAMP
    (D) Synthesis of leukotrienes from arachidonate
    (E) Synthesis of prostaglandins from arachidonate

Questions 27 and 28. A 16-year-old student has had asthma for 8 yr. The number of episodes of severe bronchospasm has increased recently, and you have been asked to review the therapeutic plan.

27. Which of the following agents is most likely to be of immediate therapeutic value in relieving an acute bronchospastic attack?
    (A) Albuterol
    (B) Atenolol
    (C) Formoterol
    (D) Metoprolol
    (E) Theophylline

28. A long-acting β_2-selective agonist that is used as an inhaled therapy for moderate or severe asthma is
(A) Ipratropium
(B) Montelukast
(C) Salmeterol
(D) Theophylline
(E) Zafirlukast

29. Lidocaine is commonly used as a local anesthetic. If a patient mistakenly receives a toxic dose of lidocaine intravenously, the patient is likely to exhibit
(A) Cardiovascular stimulation
(B) Excessive salivation, mydriasis, and diarrhea
(C) Hyperthermia and hypertension
(D) No effects immediately but then delayed, massive hepatocellular damage
(E) Seizures and coma

30. Early in an anesthesia procedure, which includes the use of succinylcholine and halothane, a surgical patient develops severe muscle rigidity, hypertension, and hyperthermia. Management of this patient will almost certainly include the administration of
(A) Baclofen
(B) Dantrolene
(C) Fentanyl
(D) Naloxone
(E) Tubocurarine

31. A 34-year-old woman in her second trimester of pregnancy presented with a tender, red, swollen calf that was diagnosed as a deep vein thrombosis (DVT) and was treated successfully. However, because of the high risk of recurrence of the DVT, she was treated with an anticoagulant for the remainder of her pregnancy. The drug used most likely was which of the following?
(A) Aspirin
(B) Clopidogrel
(C) Enoxaparin
(D) Lepirudin
(E) Warfarin

32. Which of the following, an inhibitor of fungal cell membrane synthesis, is effective intravenously in the management of disseminated infections due to *Aspergillus* or *Candida* species?
(A) Amphotericin B
(B) Caspofungin
(C) Flucytosine
(D) Nystatin
(E) Voriconazole

33. Which of the following statements about acyclovir is accurate?
(A) A pro-drug converted to valacyclovir by hepatic enzymes
(B) Active versus cytomegalovirus
(C) Bioactivated by viral thymidine kinase
(D) Highly active against papilloma virus (HPV)
(E) Toxic to bone marrow

34. A 5-year-old boy was diagnosed as having an intestinal infection with *Enterobius vermicularis* (pinworm). He should be treated with
(A) Ivermectin
(B) Mebendazole
(C) Mefloquine
(D) Praziquantel
(E) Quinine

35. Which antimalarial drug can cause a dose-dependent toxic state that includes blurred vision, dizziness, flushed and sweaty skin, nausea, diarrhea, and tinnitus?
(A) Artesunate
(B) Atovaquone-proguanil
(C) Mefloquine
(D) Quinidine
(E) Primaquine

36. Which of the following is an oral antidiabetic drug that inhibits an enzyme in the gastrointestinal tract that converts polysaccharides to monosaccharides and thereby reduces postprandial hyperglycemia?
(A) Acarbose
(B) Glipizide
(C) Metformin
(D) Rosiglitazone
(E) Sitagliptin

37. A young patient with end-stage kidney disease receives a transplant from a living related donor who is HLA-identical and red blood cell ABO matched. To prevent rejection, the transplant recipient is treated with cyclosporine. Two years after initiating cyclosporine therapy, the patient developed evidence of cyclosporine-induced nephrotoxicity and hypertension. He was switched to an immunosuppressant that lacks renal toxicity and produces its immunosuppressant effect by inhibiting the de novo pathway of guanosine monophosphate (GTP) synthesis. The new immunosuppressant is which of the following drugs?
(A) Azathioprine
(B) Etanercept
(C) Mycophenolate mofetil
(D) Sulfasalazine
(E) Prednisone

38. The mechanism of high-level isoniazid (INH) resistance of *M tuberculosis* is
(A) Changed pathway of mycolic acid synthesis
(B) Decreased intracellular accumulation of isoniazid
(C) Formation of drug-inactivating N-methyltransferase
(D) Mutation in the *inhA* gene
(E) Reduced expression of the *katG* gene

39. A 2-year-old girl was brought to the emergency department because of vomiting, bloody diarrhea, and hypotension. An abdominal x-ray film showed multiple radiopaque pills, and a relative at the child's home reported the discovery of an open bottle of iron pills behind a large piece of furniture. In addition to supportive care, treatment of the child is most likely to include which of the following actions?
(A) Intravenous administration of acetylcysteine
(B) Intravenous administration of deferoxamine
(C) Intravenous administration of pralidoxime
(D) Oral administration of activated charcoal
(E) Oral administration of edetate (EDTA)

40. A 55-year-old man being treated with a monoamine oxidase inhibitor for resistant major depressive disorder is admitted to the emergency department with a stroke after consuming a large meal in a restaurant. His blood pressure on admission is 180/110 mmHg. When monoamine oxidase inhibitors are used as antidepressant drugs, some patients may suffer hemodynamic effects caused by tyramine in their diet. Which of the following is the primary site of action of tyramine?
(A) Ganglionic receptors
(B) Gut and liver catechol-*O*-methyltransferase
(C) Postganglionic sympathetic nerve terminals
(D) Preganglionic sympathetic nerve terminals
(F.) Vascular smooth muscle cell receptors

41. A 57-year-old contractor with hypertension has been treated by 2 different physicians. He now comes to the emergency department with a severe reaction. Questioning reveals that he has been taking captopril and spironolactone. This combination is usually ill-advised because of the risk of
(A) Bone loss and osteoporosis
(B) Calcium-containing kidney stones
(C) Hyperkalemia
(D) Metabolic acidosis
(E) Postural hypotension

42. The research division of a pharmaceutical corporation has characterized the receptor-blocking actions of 5 new drugs, each of which may have potential therapeutic value. The relative intensities of their blocking actions are shown in the following table. Because each of these drugs is lipophilic and can cross the blood-brain barrier, they are expected to have CNS effects.

Based on the data shown in the table below, which drug is most likely to exacerbate the symptoms of Parkinson's disease?

	Blocking Action on CNS Receptors			
Drug	Adrenergic (Beta)	Cholinergic (M)	Dopaminergic (D2)	GABAergic (A)
A	++	+++	+++	None
B	None	None	None	++++
C	None	++++	+	None
D	+	None	+++	+
E	None	+	+	+

Key: Number of + signs denotes intensity of blocking actions.

(A) Drug A
(B) Drug B
(C) Drug C
(D) Drug D
(E) Drug E

43. Which statement is accurate?
(A) Alprazolam is effective in obsessive-compulsive disorders
(B) Clonazepam is a useful antiseizure drug
(C) Diazepam is a drug of choice for bipolar affective disorder
(D) Ramelteon is used in status epilepticus
(E) Symptoms of alcohol withdrawal may be alleviated by buspirone

44. An individual who ingested an antifreeze solution containing ethylene glycol was brought to a hospital emergency department. In an attempt to prevent severe acidosis and renal damage, the patient was given fomepizole. Fomepizole is useful in ethylene glycol poisoning because it inhibits which of the following?
(A) Alcohol dehydrogenase
(B) Aldehyde dehydrogenase
(C) Enzymes in the microsomal ethanol-oxidizing system (MEOS)
(D) Enzymes that require thiamin as a cofactor
(E) Glutathione transferase

45. A young patient has a seizure disorder with recurrent contractions starting in muscles of the right hand that spread through the arm and the right side of the face. The attacks last for only a minute or two with no loss of consciousness. Which of the following drugs is least likely to be useful in the treatment of this patient?
(A) Carbamazepine
(B) Ethosuximide
(C) Lamotrigine
(D) Phenobarbital
(E) Phenytoin

46. A young woman suffering from myoclonic seizures was receiving effective single-drug therapy. Because she was planning a pregnancy, her physician switched her to an alternative medication with much less potential for teratogenicity. The original antiseizure drug prescribed for this patient was most likely to have been
(A) Baclofen
(B) Diazepam
(C) Ethosuximide
(D) Olanzapine
(E) Valproic acid

47. The mechanism of local anesthetic action of cocaine is
(A) Activation of G protein-linked membrane receptors
(B) Block of the reuptake of norepinephrine at sympathetic nerve endings
(C) Competitive pharmacologic antagonism of nicotinic receptors
(D) Inhibition of blood and tissue enzymes that hydrolyze acetylcholine
(E) Use-dependent blockade of voltage-gated sodium channels

48. A patient is brought to the emergency department suffering from an overdose of an illicit drug. She is agitated, has disordered thought processes, suffers from paranoia, and "hears voices." Her physical symptoms include tachycardia, hyperreflexia, and hyperthermia. The drug most likely to be responsible for her condition is
(A) Gamma-hydroxybutyrate (GHB)
(B) Hashish
(C) Heroin
(D) Marijuana
(E) Methamphetamine

49. Regarding drugs that relax skeletal muscle which one of the following statements is accurate?
    (A) Baclofen blocks the release of calcium from skeletal muscle fibers.
    (B) Dantrolene is an activator of specific GABA receptors in the spinal cord.
    (C) Halothane decreases the action of skeletal muscle relaxants.
    (D) Muscle relaxation caused by succinylcholine is not reversed by acetylcholinesterase inhibitors.
    (E) Tubocurarine prevents histamine release via a stabilizing action on mast cells.

50. Although fentanyl or one of its congeners is usually administered in the early stages of a general anesthesia procedure, it is likely that the patient will receive an injection of morphine during the last phase. The rationale for switching to morphine is that the drug has
    (A) A longer duration of action
    (B) Greater analgesic efficacy
    (C) More of a "ceiling effect" and less tendency to cause respiratory failure
    (D) Opioid receptor agonist activity, whereas fentanyl is a selective kappa receptor agonist
    (E) The advantage of being more completely reversed by naloxone

51. Mental retardation, microcephaly, and underdevelopment of the midface region in an infant is associated with chronic heavy maternal use during pregnancy of which of the following?
    (A) Cocaine
    (B) Diazepam
    (C) Ethanol
    (D) Heroin
    (E) Methylenedioxymethamphetamine (MDMA)

52. After ingestion of a meal that included sardines, cheese, and red wine, a patient taking phenelzine experienced a hypertensive crisis. The most likely explanation for this untoward effect is that phenelzine
    (A) Acts to release tyramine from these foods
    (B) Inhibits MAO type B
    (C) Inhibits the metabolism of catecholamines
    (D) Is an activator of tyrosine hydroxylase
    (E) Promotes the release of norepinephrine from sympathetic nerve endings

53. Which one of the following is characteristic of succinylcholine?
    (A) Actions in phase I block are reversed by neostigmine
    (B) Is an antagonist at muscarinic receptors
    (C) Blocks the release of histamine
    (D) May cause hyperkalemia
    (E) Is primarily metabolized by acetylcholinesterase

54. A 48-year-old surgical patient was anesthetized with an intravenous bolus dose of propofol, then maintained on isoflurane with vecuronium as the skeletal muscle relaxant. At the end of the surgical procedure, she was given pyridostigmine and glycopyrrolate. The rationale for use of glycopyrrolate was to
    (A) Antagonize the skeletal muscle relaxation caused by vecuronium
    (B) Counter emetic effects of the inhaled anesthetic
    (C) Counter the potential cardiac effects of the acetylcholinesterase inhibitor
    (D) Prevent muscle fasciculations
    (E) Provide postoperative analgesia

55. A woman taking haloperidol developed a spectrum of adverse effects that included the amenorrhea-galactorrhea syndrome and extrapyramidal dysfunction. Another, newer, antipsychotic drug was prescribed which however caused weight gain and hyperglycemia due to a diabetogenic action. The drug prescribed was
    (A) Bupropion
    (B) Chlorpromazine
    (C) Fluoxetine
    (D) Lithium
    (E) Olanzapine

56. Naloxone will not antagonize or reverse
    (A) Analgesic effects of morphine in a cancer patient
    (B) Drug actions resulting from activation of μ opioid receptors
    (C) Opioid-analgesic overdose in a patient on methadone maintenance
    (D) Pupillary constriction caused by levorphanol
    (E) Respiratory depression caused by overdose of nefazodone

57. Several drugs used in patients with advanced Parkinson's disease allow patients to lower their dose of L-dopa/carbidopa, and thus reduce the incidence of L-dopa-induced dyskinesias. These drugs also decrease the amount of "off" time for the patient. Which drug is used in this way but does not, if used alone, ameliorate the symptoms of early Parkinson's disease or enhance CNS dopaminergic activity?
    (A) Amantadine
    (B) Bromocriptine
    (C) Entacapone
    (D) Pramipexole
    (E) Selegiline

58. Ramelteon, a drug prescribed for insomnia, is thought to act in the CNS via
    (A) Activation of benzodiazepine receptors
    (B) Activation of melatonin receptors
    (C) Block of the GABA transporter
    (D) Inhibition of GABA metabolism
    (E) Stimulation of glutamate receptors

Questions 59 and 60. A young man comes to a community clinic with a urogenital infection that, based on the Gram stain, appears to be due to *Neisseria gonorrhoeae*. Questioning suggests that the patient acquired the infection while vacationing abroad. The physician is concerned about drug resistance of the gonococcus.

59. Which drug is least likely to be effective in the treatment of gonorrhea in this patient?
    (A) Amoxicillin
    (B) Azithromycin
    (C) Cefixime
    (D) Ceftriaxone
    (E) Ciprofloxacin

60. The physician is also concerned about the possibility of a nongonococcal urethritis in this patient. Several antibiotics in the list below are active in, nongonococcal urethritis, However, these infections, including those caused by *C trachomatis*, can usually be eradicated by the administration of a *single* dose of
    (A) Azithromycin
    (B) Doxycycline
    (C) Erythromycin
    (D) Levofloxacin
    (E) Trimethoprim-sulfamethoxazole

61. The antibacterial action of aminoglycosides is due to their ability to
    (A) Activate autolytic enzymes
    (B) Bind to the 30S ribosomal subunit and block initiation of bacterial protein synthesis
    (C) Inhibit bacterial topoisomerases II and IV
    (D) Inhibit the synthesis of precursors of the linear peptido glycan chains of the bacterial cell wall
    (E) Interfere with the synthesis of tetrahydrofolate

62. A 26-year-old woman with chronic bronchitis lives in a region of the country where winter conditions are harsh. Her physician recommends prophylactic use of oral doxycycline, to be taken once daily, during the winter season. Which statement about the characteristics and use of doxycycline in this patient is accurate?
    (A) Absorption from the gastrointestinal tract is enhanced by yogurt.
    (B) Elimination of doxycycline is predominantly via cytochrome P450-mediated hepatic metabolism.
    (C) Formation of drug-metabolizing enzymes is a primary mechanism of resistance to tetracyclines.
    (D) The patient should discontinue the tetracycline if she becomes pregnant.
    (E) The tetracyclines have no value in prophylaxis against infections in patients with chronic bronchitis.

63. The long-term daily oral administration of therapeutic doses of prednisone results in which of the following?
    (A) Anemia
    (B) Decreased bone density
    (C) Elevated serum calcium concentration
    (D) Hyperplasia of cells in the zona fasciculata and zona reticularis of the adrenal cortex
    (E) Increased male-pattern hair growth in women

64. A 67-year-old man with osteoporosis was being treated with once-weekly alendronate. This medication has the potential to cause which of the following unusual adverse effects?
    (A) A bluish hue to skin color
    (B) Esophageal irritation
    (C) Impairment of blue-green color vision
    (D) Priapism
    (E) Tendinitis

65. Which of the following drugs is approved for primary prophylaxis in AIDS patients with low CD4 counts against infections due to *Mycobacterium avium-intracellulare*?
    (A) Amoxicillin
    (B) Ceftriaxone
    (C) Clarithromycin
    (D) Doxycycline
    (E) Nafcillin

66. A 30-year-old male patient who is HIV positive has a CD4 T lymphocyte count of 450 cells/μL (normal, 600–1500 cells/μL) and a viral RNA load of 11,000 copies/mL. His treatment involves a 3-drug antiviral regimen (HAART) consisting of zidovudine, didanosine, and efavirenz. Efavirenz limits HIV infection by
    (A) Binding to the active site of HIV reverse transcriptase
    (B) Blocking the binding of HIV virions to the CD4 receptor on T cells
    (C) Inhibiting the HIV enzyme that cleaves sialic acid residues from the surface of HIV virions
    (D) Inhibiting the HIV protease
    (E) Serving as an allosteric inhibitor of HIV reverse transcriptase

Questions 67 and 68. A 73-year-old patient has chronic pulmonary dysfunction requiring daily hospital visits for respiratory therapy. She is hospitalized with pneumonia, and it is not clear whether the infection is community or hospital acquired.

67. If she has a community-acquired pneumonia, coverage must be provided for pneumococci and atypical pathogens. In such a case, the most appropriate drug treatment in this patient is
    (A) Ampicillin plus gentamycin
    (B) Ceftriaxone plus erythromycin
    (C) Penicillin G plus gentamicin
    (D) Ticarcillin-clavulanic acid
    (E) Trimethoprim-sulfamethoxazole

68. If she has a hospital-acquired pneumonia, coverage must be provided for gram-negative bacteria (especially *Pseudomonas aeruginosa*) and for *Staphylococcus aureus,* many of which can be multiple drug-resistant organisms. In such a case, empiric treatment is likely to involve
    (A) Amoxicillin-clavulanic acid
    (B) Cefazolin plus metronidazole
    (C) Doxycycline
    (D) Imipenem
    (E) Vancomycin plus piperacillin/tazobactam

69. Resistance to acyclovir is most commonly due to mutations in a viral gene that encodes a protein that
(A) Converts viral single-stranded RNA into double-stranded DNA
(B) Phosphorylates acyclovir
(C) Synthesizes glutathione
(D) Transports acyclovir into the cell
(E) Transports acyclovir out of the cell

70. A male patient with AIDS has a CD4 T lymphocyte count of 50 cells/μL (normal, 600–1500 cells/μL). He is being maintained on a multidrug regimen consisting of acyclovir, clarithromycin, dronabinol, fluconazole, lamivudine, indinavir, trimethoprim, sulfamethoxazole, and zidovudine. The drug that provides prophylaxis against cryptococcal infections of the meninges is
(A) Acyclovir
(B) Clarithromycin
(C) Fluconazole
(D) Lamivudine
(E) Trimethoprim-sulfamethoxazole

Questions 71 and 72. A patient with diffuse non-Hodgkin's lymphoma is treated with a combination drug regimen that includes bleomycin, cyclophosphamide, vincristine, doxorubicin, and prednisone.

71. The patient's cumulative dose of bleomycin will be carefully monitored because high cumulative doses are associated with which of the following?
(A) Cardiotoxicity
(B) Hemorrhagic cystitis
(C) Hypoglycemia
(D) Peripheral neuropathy
(E) Pulmonary fibrosis

72. Dexrazoxane is thought to protect against the distinctive toxicity of which drug in this patient's regimen?
(A) Bleomycin
(B) Cyclophosphamide
(C) Doxorubicin
(D) Prednisone
(E) Vincristine

73. After delivery of a healthy infant, a young woman begins to bleed extensively because her uterus has failed to contract. Which drug should be administered to this woman?
(A) Prednisone
(B) Desmopressin
(C) Leuprolide
(D) Oxytocin
(E) Prolactin

74. Adding a progestin to the estrogenic component of hormone replacement therapy for postmenopausal women provides which of the following effects?
(A) Prevents thromboembolic events
(B) Provides better control of problematic hot flushes
(C) Reduces the risk of endometrial cancer
(D) Restores regular vaginal bleeding
(E) Slows bone loss

75. You are on the Hospital Pharmacy Committee and revising the formulary. Relative to loratadine, diphenhydramine is more likely to
(A) Be used for treatment of asthma
(B) Be used for treatment of gastroesophageal reflux disease
(C) Cause cardiac arrhythmias in overdose
(D) Have efficacy in the prevention of motion sickness
(E) Increase the serum concentration of warfarin

76. Chronic heart failure is commonly treated with a combination of drugs that both improve symptoms and provide long-term benefits. Three drugs or drug groups that have been shown in clinical trials to provide benefits in patients with chronic heart failure are
(A) ACE inhibitors, carvedilol, and spironolactone
(B) Alpha$_1$-selective antagonists, digoxin, and hydrochlorothiazide
(C) Digoxin, β-agonists, and nitroglycerin
(D) Dobutamine, propranolol, and furosemide
(E) Verapamil, isosorbide dinitrate, and furosemide

77. Which of the following is a drug that inhibits the synthesis of thyroid hormone by preventing coupling of iodotyrosine molecules?
(A) Dexamethasone
(B) Levothyroxine
(C) Lithium
(D) Methimazole
(E) Propranolol

78. Long-term use of meperidine for analgesia is avoided because the accumulation of a metabolite, normeperidine, is associated with risk of
(A) Constipation
(B) Dependence
(C) Neutropenia
(D) Renal impairment
(E) Seizures

79. A 60-year-old man with a history of a mild myocardial infarction was discovered to have low serum HDL cholesterol and moderately high serum triglyceride level. His serum total and LDL cholesterol concentrations were well below the upper limit of normal. Which of the following drugs is likely to result in the greatest lowering of this patient's serum triglyceride concentration and elevation of his serum HDL cholesterol concentration?
(A) Cholestyramine
(B) Ezetimibe
(C) Gemfibrozil
(D) Lovastatin
(E) Rosiglitazone

80. Protamine can be used to reverse the anticoagulant effect of which of the following?
(A) Abciximab
(B) Clopidogrel
(C) Lepirudin
(D) Unfractionated heparin
(E) Warfarin

81. In a patient with familial combined hyperlipidemia that is associated with increased VLDL and LDL, which of the following drugs is most likely to *increase* plasma triglycerides while also decreasing plasma LDL?
 (A) Cholestyramine
 (B) Ezetimibe
 (C) Gemfibrozil
 (D) Niacin
 (E) Lovastatin

82. A 31-year-old premenopausal woman has been using a combined oral contraceptive for 10 yr. As a result of this contraceptive use, she has a reduced risk of which of the following?
 (A) Deep vein thrombosis
 (B) Episodes of migraine headache
 (C) Ischemic stroke
 (D) Ovarian cancer
 (E) Pituitary adenoma

83. Hypercoagulability and dermal vascular necrosis resulting from protein C deficiency is known to be an early-appearing adverse effect of treatment with which of the following drugs?
 (A) Alteplase
 (B) Aspirin
 (C) Clopidogrel
 (D) Heparin
 (E) Warfarin

84. A 45-year-old woman suffers from abdominal pain and bloody diarrhea that has been diagnosed as Crohn's disease. Which of the following is a first-line drug for treatment of Crohn's disease that acts locally in the gastrointestinal tract to provide an anti-inflammatory effect?
 (A) Aluminum hydroxide
 (B) Metoclopramide
 (C) Misoprostol
 (D) Mesalamine
 (E) Ranitidine

85. A 24-year-old man with a history of partial seizures has been treated with standard anticonvulsants for several years. He is currently taking valproic acid, which is not fully effective, and his neurologist prescribes another drug approved for adjunctive use in partial seizures. Unfortunately, the patient develops a toxic epidermal necrolysis. The second drug prescribed was
 (A) Diazepam
 (B) Ethosuximide
 (C) Felbamate
 (D) Lamotrigine
 (E) Phenobarbital

86. Drugs classified as selective serotonin reuptake inhibitors have minimal clinical efficacy in the treatment of patients who suffer from
 (A) Bulimia
 (B) Diminished sexual function and interest
 (C) Obsessive-compulsive disorder (OCD)
 (D) Panic attacks
 (E) Premenstrual dysphoric disorder (PMDD)

87. A 29-year-old accountant has recurrent episodes of tachycardia that sometimes convert to sinus rhythm spontaneously but more often require medical treatment. A drug that is commonly given as an intravenous bolus for the purpose of converting AV nodal tachycardias to normal sinus rhythm is
 (A) Adenosine
 (B) Amiodarone
 (C) Lidocaine
 (D) Quinidine
 (E) Sotalol

88. Which one of the following pairs of drug and indication is accurate?
 (A) Amphetamine: Alzheimer's dementia
 (B) Bupropion: acute anxiety
 (C) Fluoxetine: insomnia
 (D) Pramipexole: Parkinson's disease
 (E) Ramelteon: attention deficit disorder

89. Which of the following toxic compounds is correctly paired with an antidote that is used in the treatment of a patient poisoned with the toxic compound?
 (A) Acetaminophen: vitamin K
 (B) Beta-blocker: dobutamine
 (C) Ethanol: methanol
 (D) Cyanide: hydroxocobalamin
 (E) Tricyclic antidepressants: neostigmine

90. This cell cycle-nonspecific agent is commonly used as a component of cancer chemotherapy regimens, including those for non-Hodgkin's lymphoma and for breast cancers; administration of mercaptoethanesulfonate (mesna) decreases the risk of hematuria.
 (A) Cyclophosphamide
 (B) Azathioprine
 (C) Fluorouracil
 (D) Methotrexate
 (E) Vinblastine

91. A 64-year-old recipient of a kidney transplant was being treated with immunosuppressants. After several episodes of gout, the decision was made to treat his gout with the xanthine oxidase inhibitor allopurinol. The dose of which of the following of his immunosuppressant drugs should be reduced to avoid excessive bone marrow suppression due to a drug-drug interaction?
 (A) Azathioprine
 (B) Cyclosporine
 (C) Hydroxychloroquine
 (D) Methotrexate
 (E) Tacrolimus

92. A 57-year-old man presented with signs and symptoms of acute gout that included intense pain in the first metatarsophalangeal joint of his right big toe of 1 day's duration and a joint that was swollen, tender, and red. Examination of synovial fluid removed from the joint revealed crystals of uric acid. The patient had a serum uric acid concentration of 10 mg/dL (normal 3.0–8.2 mg/dL). This was the patient's first episode of gout. He did not have any other medical illnesses and was not taking any medications. Which of the following is the most appropriate drug for immediate treatment of this acute attack of gout?
(A) Allopurinol
(B) Indomethacin
(C) Methotrexate
(D) Morphine
(E) Probenecid

93. A 57-year-old woman with moderately severe rheumatoid arthritis was treated with etanercept. Which of the following proteins is the direct target of etanercept?
(A) Cyclophilin
(B) Granulocyte colony-stimulating factor (G-CSF)
(C) Interferon α
(D) Interleukin-11 (IL-11)
(E) Tumor necrosis factor-α (TNF-α)

94. A 42-year-old woman developed a syndrome of polyuria, thirst, and hypernatremia after surgical removal of part of her pituitary gland. These signs and symptoms will be treated with which of the following?
(A) Bromocriptine
(B) Desmopressin
(C) Octreotide
(D) Prednisone
(E) Somatropin

95. Relative to Lugol's solution, propylthiouracil has
(A) A faster onset of antithyroid action
(B) A greater inhibitory effect on the proteolytic release of hormones from the thyroid gland
(C) Increased likelihood of causing exophthalmos during the first week of treatment
(D) Increased risk of fetal toxicity
(E) More sustained antithyroid activity when used continuously for several months

96. A 54-year-old woman was found to have node-positive breast cancer. Following her surgery, she was treated with a drug that prevents the conversion of testosterone to estradiol. The drug used for her treatment most likely was which of the following?
(A) Anastrozole
(B) Ethinyl estradiol
(C) Finasteride
(D) Spironolactone
(E) Tamoxifen

97. Which of the following drugs is most likely to cause hypoglycemia when used as monotherapy in the treatment of a patient with type 2 diabetes?
(A) Acarbose
(B) Glipizide
(C) Metformin
(D) Miglitol
(E) Rosiglitazone

98. Anticoagulation is needed immediately in a patient with deep vein thrombosis. The patient has a history of heparin-induced thrombocytopenia. Which of the following is the most appropriate drug for parenteral administration in this patient?
(A) Eptifibatide
(B) Lepirudin
(C) Clopidogrel
(D) Unfractionated heparin
(E) Warfarin

Questions 99 and 100. A drug (Drug 1) was given as an IV bolus to a subject while blood pressure and heart rate were recorded as shown on the left side of the graph below. After recovery from the effects of Drug 1, a long-acting dose of Drug 2 was given. After the recorder was turned back on, Drug 1 was repeated with the results shown on the right side of the graph.

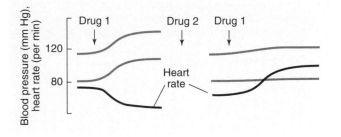

99. Identify Drug 1 from the following list.
(A) Albuterol
(B) Angiotensin II
(C) Endothelin
(D) Epinephrine
(E) Hexamethonium
(F) Isoproterenol
(G) Norepinephrine
(H) Phenylephrine
(I) Prazosin
(J) Propranolol

100. Identify Drug 2 from the following list.
(A) Albuterol
(B) Angiotensin II
(C) Endothelin
(D) Epinephrine
(E) Hexamethonium
(F) Isoproterenol
(G) Norepinephrine
(H) Phenylephrine
(I) Prazosin
(J) Propranolol

ANSWER KEY FOR EXAMINATION 2[*]

1. **E** (7, 31) Neither opioids nor muscarinic agonists decrease salivation, decrease sweating, or raise blood pressure. Opioids decrease peristalsis; muscarinics increase it. Both drug groups can cause miosis.

2. **A** (19) Nitric oxide (NO) is not stored, it is synthesized on demand in response to acetylcholine and histamine in several tissues, including brain and endothelium. NO is released from the nitroprusside molecule.

3. **B** (1) The graph shows first-order elimination of the drug in question. Aspirin, ethanol, and phenytoin are eliminated mainly by zero-order kinetics. Diazepam is the only drug in the list that is eliminated by first-order kinetics.

4. **C** (2) Membrane-bound tyrosine kinase receptors are activated by peptides such as insulin and epidermal growth factor, see Table 2–1.

5. **C** (3) During a continuous IV infusion, the plasma concentration approaches steady state according to the algorithm: 50% at 1 half-life, 75% at 2, etc. Since the sample was taken at two half-lives, the steady state concentration will be in the range of four-thirds the measured concentration (2.4/0.75) or 3.2 mg/L.

6. **E** (5) Before clinical trials can be carried out with a new drug, reproductive toxicity data must be provided for at least 2 species.

7. **A** (6, 8, 9) The increase in blood pressure caused by pressor drugs such as phenylephrine evokes a reflex slowing of heart rate that is mediated by the vagus nerve acting on muscarinic receptors in the sinoatrial node. This slowing can be blocked by antimuscarinic agents such as atropine.

8. **B** (6) Questions about the baroreceptor reflex are common; Figure 6–4 is very high yield. The major responses to hypotension are sympathetic discharge (choice B) and activation of the renin-angiotensin-aldosterone system.

9. **C** (10, 18) Mannitol is sometimes used to rapidly reduce intraocular pressure in acute angle-closure glaucoma. Of the drugs listed, only latanoprost is used in chronic glaucoma.

10. **C** (9) The graph shows a marked decrease in diastolic BP and heart rate, with only a small, transient increase in systolic BP. These effects are characteristic of isoproterenol and similar β_1, β_2 agonists.

11. **D** (4, 23, 36) Chronic alcohol use induces hepatic cytochrome (CYP) P450 mixed oxidase isozymes enzymes. Elevated CYP activity converts more acetaminophen into a toxic intermediate, which requires inactivation by glutathione (GSH). This alcohol-induced increase in CYP increases the risk of reaching a level of toxic acetaminophen metabolite that can overwhelm the liver's detoxification capacity and result in severe hepatotoxicity.

12. **C** (4) Acetylation, glucuronidation, methylation, and sulfation are phase 2 conjugation reactions.

13. **C** (12) Although nitrates may dilate large and medium coronary vessels, they have little effect on the arterioles in ischemic tissue, which are already dilated maximally by local ischemia. A major beneficial effect is venodilation, leading to reduction in cardiac size, which decreases diastolic fiber tension and reduces myocardial oxygen demand.

14. **E** (12) Verapamil (and diltiazem) is useful for prophylaxis of both effort and vasospastic angina. Calcium blockers reduce cardiac work and oxygen demand. They also cause constipation and sometimes peripheral edema that is not associated with heart failure.

15. **B** (7) Symptomatic paroxysmal sinus tachycardia often occurs in young patients and can sometimes be converted to normal sinus rhythm with increased vagal discharge. Brief amplification (5–15 min) of the vagal effects on heart rate can be accomplished with a short-acting cholinesterase inhibitor such as edrophonium. Pyridostigmine (E) would have a much longer action (4–6 hr).

16. **B** (59) Metoclopramide, a dopamine D_2 receptor antagonist, is a prokinetic drug that can be used to increase gastric emptying and intestinal motility in patients with diabetes-associated gastric paresis. Famotidine is a histamine H_2 receptor antagonist used for acid-peptic disease. Misoprostol is a prostaglandin E_1 analog used for acid-peptic disease and for medical abortions. Omeprazole is a proton pump inhibitor used for acid-peptic disease, and ondansetron is a serotonin 5-HT_3 receptor antagonist used as an antiemetic.

17. **D** (10) Reflex tachycardia is a major disadvantage of nonselective α blockers in the treatment of hypertension because the tachycardia is exaggerated by the α_2 blockade of nonselective agents. The α_1-selective blockers are much less likely to evoke this reflex.

18. **D** (11) ACE inhibitors, arteriolar dilators, and β blockers do not ordinarily cause orthostatic hypotension; venodilators do. Peripheral α_1 antagonists block sympathetic effects on both arterioles and veins and thus may cause orthostatic hypotension, especially with the first few doses.

19. **E** (15) This patient is hyperkalemic and slightly acidotic. These changes are typical of a K^+-sparing diuretic such as spironolactone.

20. **B** (11) Of the drugs listed, only clonidine, an α_2 agonist, is associated with severe rebound hypertension if stopped suddenly. It is speculated that this effect is due to down-regulation of α_2 receptors.

21. **D** (14) The action potential is prolonged without significant slowing of the upstroke, so the drug effect is mainly on potassium channels (group 3 action) and not on both sodium and potassium channels (group 1a action).

22. **C** (10, 11) Hydralazine reduces blood pressure by direct vasodilation. Propranolol has indirect effects on vascular tone but (at least initially) reduces pressure by reducing cardiac output. Hydralazine thus evokes reflex sympathetic discharge and increases cardiac force, output, and rate.

23. **E** (15, 42) Thiazides increase calcium absorption from the urine into blood, whereas loop diuretics increase calcium excretion from the blood into the urine. None of the other options listed here affects serum calcium. Opioids are indicated for management of severe pain due to kidney stones.

---

[*]Numbers in parentheses are chapters in which answers are found.

24. **B** (15) Furosemide acts on the ascending limb of the loop of Henle and inhibits the major transporter in this segment, a $Na^+/K^+/2Cl^-$ transporter.

25. **C** (17) Substance P is the endogenous peptide closely associated with peripheral pain transmission, and capsaicin (the "hot" component from hot peppers) is an antagonist.

26. **E** (18) The cyclooxygenase enzymes are responsible for cyclizing arachidonate to prostaglandin precursors.

27. **A** (20) Albuterol, metaproterenol, and terbutaline are rapid-onset, selective β_2 agonists used as first-line therapy for acute asthma.

28. **C** (20) Salmeterol and formoterol are slow-onset, long-acting, selective β_2 agonists usually used by inhalation with corticosteroids in asthma prophylaxis. Indacaterol is similar but approved only for COPD.

29. **E** (26) Intravenous lidocaine causes typical local anesthetic toxicity including central nervous system stimulation with possible seizures. Cardiovascular *depression* may occur, but it is usually minor.

30. **B** (25, 27) Malignant hyperthermia is a rare disorder characterized by massive calcium release within skeletal muscle triggered by use of succinylcholine in anesthesia protocols. Dantrolene is given to block calcium release.

31. **C** (34) Deep vein thromboses are located in the venous side of the circulation, making them less responsive to the antiplatelet agents (aspirin, clopidogrel). Warfarin is teratogenic and is contraindicated in pregnancy. Lepirudin is the thrombin inhibitor that can be used parenterally only. A low-molecular-weight (LMW) heparin is the drug of choice to treat and prevent deep vein thromboses and is safe to use during pregnancy.

32. **E** (48) Amphotericin B and caspofungin are active against many systemic fungal infections, but they interfere with fungal cell *wall* functions. Voriconazole, an azole antifungal, like fluconazole and itraconazole, interferes with cell membrane permeability by inhibiting ergosterol synthesis.

33. **C** (49) Acyclovir is a guanosine analog activated by viral thymidine kinases of HSV and VZV to form acyclovir triphosphate, a competitive substrate for DNA polymerase resulting in chain termination when incorporated into viral DNA.

34. **B** (53) Mebendazole is the primary drug for treatment of pinworm, roundworm, and whipworm infections. The drug is contraindicated in pregnancy. Mebendazole and thiabendazole (a more toxic azole) are inhibitors of microtubule synthesis in nematodes.

35. **D** (52) These dose-related symptoms are characteristic adverse effects of the alkaloids (eg, quinine, quinidine) derived from the bark of the cinchona tree and are termed cinchonism.

36. **A** (41) Acarbose inhibits polysaccharide breakdown. Glipizide is a secretagogue. Metformin acts in the liver. Rosiglitazone is a PPAR-γ activator, and sitagliptin is a DPP-IV inhibitor.

37. **C** (55) Mycophenolate mofetil is an immunosuppressant whose active metabolite inhibits de novo production of guanosine monophosphate (GMP). Lymphocytes are particularly sensitive to the antimetabolite effect of mycophenolate mofetil because they lack the alternative salvage pathway for GMP synthesis that is present in most cells.

38. **E** (47, 61) Mutations in the *katG* gene result in the underproduction of mycobacterial catalase-peroxidase, an enzyme that bioactivates INH, facilitating its interaction with its "target" ketoacyl carrier protein sythetase. The result is high level resistance to INH. Mutations in the *inhA* gene result in low-level resistance with cross-resistance to pyrazinamide.

39. **B** (57, 58) Deferoxamine, a chelator with high selectivity and affinity for iron, is used intravenously for acute iron poisoning. Activated charcoal does not bind iron. Acetylcysteine is used for acetaminophen poisoning. Pralidoxime is used for organophosphate poisoning. Intravenous EDTA is used for lead poisoning; oral EDTA does not significantly reduce iron absorption after an oral iron overdose.

40. **C** (6, 9) Tyramine ingested in food is normally metabolized rapidly in the liver by monoamine oxidase. When MAO inhibitors are used in patients, this first-pass effect is blocked and high tyramine concentrations circulate to the tissues. Tyramine acts on noradrenergic nerves (postganglionic sympathetic fibers) to release stores of norepinephrine and may precipitate a hypertensive emergency.

41. **C** (11, 15) Spironolactone inhibits potassium excretion in the kidney by blocking aldosterone. Captopril reduces angiotensin II levels and secondarily reduces aldosterone. The combination may increase serum potassium to dangerous levels.

42. **D** (21, 28) Antagonism at dopamine D_2 receptors in the CNS is equated with parkinsonian symptoms (Drugs A and D). However, in the case of Drug A, this action would be offset by its ability to block muscarinic receptors. M blockers, like benztropine, improve tremor and rigidity in parkinsonism but have little effect on bradykinesia.

43. **B** (22, 32) Clonazepam, a benzodiazepine, is effective in the management of absence seizures and is also used in the treatment of bipolar disorder.

44. **A** (23) Fomepizole, an antidote for ethylene glycol and methanol poisoning, inhibits alcohol dehydrogenase, which converts ethylene glycol and methanol to toxic metabolites.

45. **B** (24) Simple partial seizures can have the characteristics of the "jacksonian march." Many drugs are used in management including those listed, with the exception of ethosuximide, which is not effective in partial seizures or generalized tonic-clonic seizure states.

46. **E** (24) Myoclonic seizure syndromes are usually treated with valproic acid. Neural tube defects (spina bifida) are associated with the use of valproic acid during pregnancy. Lamotrigine is approved for adjunctive use but is often used as a sole agent, and several backup drugs are available including topiramate and zonisamide.

47. **E** (26) Local anesthetics block voltage-dependent sodium channels in excitable tissues including nerves, decreasing action-potential conduction. Rapidly firing fibers are more sensitive than slowly firing nerve fibers. Cocaine has this action and also blocks the reuptake of norepinephrine at sympathetic neuroeffector junctions with effects on both the heart and the CNS.

48. **E** (32) The signs and symptoms are those of high-dose abuse of dextroamphetamine or methamphetamine. There is no specific antidote, and supportive measures are directed toward protection against cardiac arrhythmias and seizures and control of body temperature.

49. **D** (27) Baclofen activates GABA receptors, dantrolene blocks the release of calcium from skeletal muscle fibers, halothane enhances skeletal muscle relaxants, and tubocurarine causes histamine release. Acetylcholinesterase inhibitors do not reverse skeletal muscle relaxation caused by succinylcholine.

50. **A** (31) Fentanyl is much shorter acting than morphine. Both drugs are μ-receptor activators, equivalent in terms of analgesic activity and reversible by naloxone. Both drugs cause respiratory depression at high doses.

51. **C** (23) Mental retardation, microcephaly, and facial dysmorphia are characteristics of fetal alcohol syndrome, caused by excessive use of ethanol during pregnancy.

52. **C** (9, 30, 61) Phenelzine, a rarely used antidepressant, is a potent MAO-B inhibitor and increases the amount of catecholamine transmitter stored in sympathetic nerve endings. When an indirectly acting sympathomimetic such as tyramine (found in some foods) avoids first-pass metabolism (due to MAO inhibition) and reaches the nerve endings, it can release large amounts of norepinephrine and cause a hypertensive crisis.

53. **D** (27) In phase I block, the action of succinylcholine is not reversed by acetylcholinesterase inhibitors. The drug is metabolized by pseudocholinesterases. It may cause histamine release, and it can cause hyperkalemia.

54. **C** (7, 8, 27) The acetylcholinesterase inhibitor pyridostigmine can reverse skeletal muscle relaxation (caused by vecuronium) but may also cause bradycardia. The later effect can be prevented by use of glycopyrrolate, which has muscarinic receptor blocking action.

55. **E** (29) Significant weight gain and hyperglycemia due to a diabetogenic action occur with several atypical antipsychotics, especially clozapine (not listed) and olanzapine. Neurologic dysfunctions are less common with the atypical agents.

56. **E** (30, 31) Naloxone is an opioid μ-receptor antagonist and will oppose the actions of opioids at this class of receptors including analgesia, miosis, and symptoms of opioid overdose including respiratory depression. However, respiratory depression due to nefazodone is not exerted via the μ-opioid receptor.

57. **C** (28) Entacapone is a catechol-O-methyltransferase inhibitor that enhances the action of levodopa by preventing its metabolism in the blood and peripheral tissues. It does not cross the blood-brain barrier and if used alone will not ameliorate symptoms of Parkinson's disease.

58. **B** (22) The hypnotic action of ramelteon is thought to be due to its activation of melatonin receptors in the suprachiasmatic nuclei of the CNS.

59. **A** (43, 46) The drugs of choice for treatment of gonorrhea currently are the cephalosporins ceftriaxone and cefixime. Azithromycin and spectinomycin are alternatives. Resistance to amoxicillin is common.

60. **A** (44) The only drug likely to be effective in nongonococcal urethritis in a single dose is azithromycin, which has an elimination half-life of several days. Other drugs used in nongonococcal urethritis include clindamycin, ofloxacin, and the tetracyclines.

61. **B** (45) The aminoglycoside antibiotics are bactericidal inhibitors of protein synthesis. You may recall that their actions continue well beyond their short half-lives because they exert a "postantibiotic action."

62. **D** (44) Tetracycline use during pregnancy is discouraged since fetal exposure to these antibiotics may ultimately lead to irregularities in bone growth and dentition. In addition, gastrointestinal effects and the potential for hepatic dysfunction are increased in the pregnant patient.

63. **B** (39) Long-term use of prednisone has several side effects such as growth inhibition, diabetes, muscle wasting, and osteoporosis. Regarding the other options: Excess steroid use results in baldness. Corticosteroids (such as prednisone) can be used to treat some hemolytic anemias. Choice D is incorrect because it describes congenital adrenal hyperplasia, a condition in which the adrenal gland fails to make the hormones cortisol and aldosterone. Treatment would be to provide these hormones to restore physiological levels.

64. **B** (42) The bisphosphonates can cause esophageal irritation, which is managed by drinking lots of fluids and staying upright after taking the drug. Blue skin is an adverse effect of amiodarone. Color vision can be affected by anti-TB treatment. Priapism can be caused by sildenafil in combination with nitrates, and tendinitis is a side effect for fluoroquinolones.

65. **C** (44, 47) Azithromycin (not listed) or clarithromycin with or without rifabutin is recommended for primary prophylaxis against *Mycobacterium avium* complex (MAC) in patients with AIDS.

66. **E** (49) Efavirenz is used in highly active antiretroviral therapy (HAART) regimens against HIV. The drug is an allosteric inhibitor of HIV reverse transcriptase and does not bind to the active site of the enzyme.

67. **B** (43, 44, 46) In a community-acquired pneumonia, the wider spectrum cephalosporin ceftriaxone would cover typical organisms, and erythromycin would be active against the atypical organisms.

68. **E** (43, 44, 46) Single antimicrobial drug therapy would be inadequate coverage in a hospital-acquired pneumonia that could include possible infection due to multidrug-resistant staphylococci as well as gram-negative bacilli such as *Pseudomonas aeruginosa*. Vancomycin should cover gram-positive organisms, and piperacillin plus the penicillinase inhibitor would be active against most strains of likely gram-negative pathogens.

69. **B** (49) Many resistant strains of HSV commonly lack thymidine kinase, the enzyme involved in the viral-specific activation of acyclovir.

70. **C** (48) Fluconazole is the only antifungal drug listed. It is the drug of choice for treatment and secondary prophylaxis against cryptococcal meningitis.

71. **E** (54) Bleomycin is one of the 4 drugs for which myelosuppression is not dose-limiting. The 3 others are cisplatin for nephrotoxicity, doxorubicin for cardiotoxicity, and vincristine for peripheral neuropathy.

72. **C** (54) The toxicity of doxorubicin (one of the 4 drugs with unique dose-limiting toxicity; see Question 71) can be mitigated by dexrazoxane.

73. **D** (37) The posterior pituitary hormone oxytocin contracts uterine smooth muscle. It is used to augment labor and, in this case, to treat postpartum uterine atony.

74. **C** (40) Progestin acts on the endometrium, where estrogen agonists can induce proliferation and endometrial cancer. Progestin has been shown to reduce this risk. Progestin

toxicity includes increased blood pressure and a decrease in HDL. Long-term use of progestin can lead to a reduction in bone density.

75. **D** (16) Diphenhydramine is a first-generation anti-H_1 blocker with significant anti-motion sickness and sedative actions. Loratadine is a second-generation antihistamine with neither of these effects. Neither drug is effective in asthma or GERD, and neither blocks drug-metabolizing enzymes.

76. **A** (13) While therapeutic strategies in chronic heart failure include use of several different drug classes including diuretics and positive inotropics, only 3 drugs or drug groups have been shown to provide benefits in terms of survival: ACE inhibitors, certain β blockers including carvedilol, and the aldosterone antagonists spironolactone and eplerenone.

77. **D** (38) Methimazole [and propylthiouracil (PTU)] is a small sulfur-containing thioamide that inhibits thyroid hormone synthesis by blocking peroxidase catalyzed reactions, iodination of thyroglobulin, and coupling of DIT and MIT (see Figure 38–1). Dexamethasone is an orally active corticosteroid, lithium is a mood stabilizer, and propranolol is a β-blocker capable of inhibiting the peripheral conversion of T_4 to T_3.

78. **E** (31) Meperidine is a strong opioid agonist with analgesic efficacy equivalent to that of morphine. The drug has a muscarinic blocking action and does not cause miosis or contraction of biliary smooth muscle. With long-term use, its metabolite normeperidine accumulates and may cause seizures.

79. **C** (35) Fibrates are the main triglyceride-lowering drugs. Cholestyramine, ezetimibe, and lovastatin mainly lower LDL cholesterol, whereas rosiglitazone is an antidiabetic drug that increases insulin sensitivity through PPAR-γ activation.

80. **D** (34) Heparin is negatively charged and will be effectively reversed with the positively charged protamine. There is no antidote for options A through C. If the dose of warfarin is too high, vitamin K_1 supplements or parenteral phytonadione (vitamin K_1) can be added. For urgent reversal of anticoagulation by any drug, fresh frozen plasma may be used.

81. **A** (35) Resins increase triglycerides (TGs), particularly in patients who are genetically predisposed to high TGs. Ezetimibe has no effect on TGs, but fibrates and niacin both lower TGs and lovastatin mostly lowers LDL cholesterol.

82. **D** (40) Combination hormonal contraceptives have clinical uses and beneficial effects in treatment of acne, hirsutism, and dysmenorrhea. In addition, with long-term use, they have been shown to reduce the risk of ovarian and endometrial cancer.

83. **E** (34) Warfarin interferes with gamma carboxylation of clotting factors IX, X, VII, and II, and the anticlotting factors protein C and protein S. Alteplase carries the risk of bleeding and not thrombosis. Aspirin can cause gastrointestinal ulcers and bleeding. Heparin is the only drug on this list that can also cause thrombosis, but in the case of heparin, it is mediated not through protein C but rather through an immunologic reaction against heparin-platelet complexes.

84. **D** (59) Mesalamine is a form of 5-aminosalicylic acid (5-ASA) used as first-line treatment for inflammatory bowel disease. Aluminum hydroxide is an antacid used for symptomatic relief of heartburn. Metoclopramide is a prokinetic agent. Misoprostol and ranitidine are used for acid-peptic disease.

85. **D** (24) A number of antiseizure drugs have caused serious toxicities including hepatotoxicity with both valproic acid and felbamate. In the case of lamotrigine, which has been commonly used in the myoclonic seizures, toxic epidermal necrolysis (Stevens-Johnson syndrome) has occurred.

86. **B** (30) The selective serotonin reuptake inhibitor (SSRI) class of antidepressants has been shown to have therapeutic value in a wide range of psychiatric dysfunctions ranging from bulimia to obsessive compulsive disorder. One of the *adverse* effects of the use of SSRIs is diminished sexual function and interest.

87. **A** (14) Adenosine is favored for the prompt conversion of atrioventricular nodal rhythms to normal sinus rhythm. Adenosine has a very short duration of action (seconds) and good efficacy.

88. **D** (28) Pramipexole is a non-ergot dopamine agonist with high affinity for the D_3 receptor. It is used as monotherapy in mild parkinsonism and together with levodopa in more advanced disease. Mental disturbances such as confusion, delusions, and impulsivity are more common with pramipexole than with levodopa.

89. **D** (33, 58) In cyanide poisoning, the vitamin B_{12} analog hydroxocobalamin reacts with cyanide to form a nontoxic metabolite that is eliminated by the kidney.

90. **A** (54) Cyclophosphamide is converted into acrolein, which damages the kidney. mesna can bind to and detoxify acrolein. Note that the dose-limiting toxicity of cyclophosphamide is bone marrow suppression.

91. **A** (54, 55) Allopurinol interferes with the metabolism of azathioprine, increasing plasma levels of 6-mercaptopurine, which may result in potentially fatal blood dyscrasias. Concomitant use requires the dose of azathioprine to be reduced to 25%.

92. **B** (36) Treatment of gout falls into 2 categories: 1) to treat the acute attack where the goal is to reduce pain and inflammation, and 2) to prevent attacks by reducing the uric acid pool through inhibition of uric acid buildup (allopurinol) or by enhanced elimination (probenecid). Indomethacin is an NSAID that can reduce pain and inflammation. Morphine will reduce only the pain but not the inflammation, and methotrexate is more effective for immuno-inflammatory disorders.

93. **E** (33, 36, 55) Etanercept is a recombinant fusion protein consisting of 2 soluble TNF-α receptor moieties linked to human IgG. It binds to TNF-α and inhibits its action.

94. **B** (37) This woman's central diabetes insipidus is due to insufficient posterior pituitary production of vasopressin. Desmopressin, a selective vasopressin V_2 receptor agonist, can be administered orally, nasally, or parenterally to treat central diabetes insipidus.

95. **E** (38) Iodide salts inhibit iodination of tyrosine and thyroid hormone release. The salts also decrease vascularity and size of the hyperplasic thyroid gland. Onset of effect is rapid since both release and synthesis of hormones are inhibited. The effects are transient as the gland "escapes" from the iodide block after several weeks of treatment. Choice D is incorrect; propylthiouracil is the preferred treatment in pregnancy because it is *less* likely to cross the placenta and into breast milk.

96. A (40, 54) Anastrozole prevents conversion of testosterone to estradiol. Ethinyl estradiol is an orally available form of estradiol. Finasteride is a 5-α-reductase inhibitor. Spironolactone is an androgen receptor antagonist (also known as K-sparing diuretic), and tamoxifen is a selective estrogen receptor modulator.

97. B (41) Glipizide is the only agent in this list that can stimulate insulin secretion, potentially leading to hypoglycemia.

98. B (34) Deep vein thromboses are located in the venous side of the circulation, making them less responsive to the antiplatelet agents (eptifibatide, clopidogrel). Unfractionated heparin carries the risk of triggering more heparin-induced thrombocytopenia. Warfarin will take several days to achieve a therapeutic effect. Lepirudin (direct thrombin inhibitor) is the drug of choice for fast anticoagulation in patients with heparin-induced thrombocytopenia.

99. G (9, 10) See answers to questions 95 and 96 in Examination 1 (Appendix II). Drug 1 evokes a strong pressor effect and a bradycardia that is probably a reflex compensatory response. Thus, both norepinephrine and phenylephrine are possible answers. However, the effect of Drug 2 unmasks a tachycardia produced by Drug 1, so this agonist must be norepinephrine; phenylephrine does not have β agonist action.

100. I (10) See answers to the preceding question and to questions 95 and 96 in Examination 1. Drug 2 is an α blocker without β-blocking action.

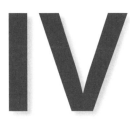

Strategies for Improving Test Performance

There are many strategies for studying and exam taking, and decisions about which ones to use are partly a function of individual habit and preference. However, basic study rules may be applied to any learning exercise; test-taking strategies depend on the type of examination. For those interested in test-*writing* strategies, the Case and Swanson reference is strongly recommended (see References).

FIVE BASIC STUDY RULES

1. When studying dense textual material, stop after a few pages to write out the gist of it from memory. If necessary, refer to the material just read. After finishing a chapter, construct your own tables of the major drugs, receptor types, mechanisms, and so on, and fill in as many of the blanks as you can. Refer to tables and figures in the book as needed to complete your notes. Create your own mnemonics if possible. Look up other mnemonics in books if you can't think of one yourself. These are all active learning techniques; mere reading is passive and far less effective unless you happen to have a photographic memory. Your notes should be legible or typed on a computer, and saved for ready access when reviewing for exams.

2. Experiment with other study methods until you find out what works for you. This may involve solo study or group study, flash cards, or text reading. You won't know how effective these techniques are until you have tried them.

3. Don't scorn "cramming," but don't rely on it either. Some steady, day-by-day reading and digestion of conceptual material is usually needed to avoid last-minute indigestion. Similarly, don't substitute memorization of lists (eg, the Key Words list, Appendix I) for more substantive understanding.

4. If you are preparing for a course examination, make every effort to attend all the lectures. The lecturer's view of what is important may be different from that of the author of a course textbook, and chances are good that exam questions will be based on the instructor's own lecture notes.

5. If old test questions are legitimately available (as they are for the USMLE and courses in most medical schools), make use of these guides to study. By definition, they are a strong indicator of what the examination writers have considered core information in the recent past (also see Point 4).

STRATEGIES APPLICABLE TO ALL EXAMINATIONS

Three general rules apply to all examinations:

1. When starting the examination, scan the entire question set before answering any. If the examination has several parts, allot time to each part in proportion to its length and difficulty. Within each part, answer the easy questions first, placing a mark in the margin by the questions to which you will return. Practice saving enough time for the more difficult questions by scheduling 1 minute or less for each question on practice examinations such as those in Appendices II and III in this book. (The time available in the USMLE examination is approximately 55–60 seconds per question.)

2. Students are often advised to avoid changing their first guess on multiple-choice questions. However, research has shown that students who are unsure of the answer to a question make a change from the incorrect answer to the correct answer about 55% of the time. So if you are unsure of your first choice for a particular question and on further reflection see an answer that looks better, research supports your making one—but only one—change.

3. Understand the method for scoring wrong answers. The USMLE does not penalize for wrong answers; it scores you only on the total number of correct answers. Therefore, even if you have no idea as to the correct answer, make a guess anyway; there is no penalty for an incorrect answer. In other words, *do not leave any blanks on a USMLE answer sheet or computer screen.* Note that this may not be true for some local examinations; some scoring algorithms do penalize for incorrect answers. Make sure you understand the rules for such local examinations.

STRATEGIES FOR SPECIFIC QUESTION FORMATS

A certain group of students—often characterized as "good test-takers"—may not know every detail about the subject matter being tested but seem to perform extremely well most of the time. The strategy used by these people is not a secret, although few instructors seem to realize how easy it is to break down their questions into much simpler ones. Lists of these strategies are widely available (eg, in the descriptive material distributed by the National Board of Medical Examiners to its candidates). A paraphrased compendium of this advice is presented next.

A. Strategies for the "Choose the One Best Answer" (of 5 Choices) Type Question

1. Many of the newer "clinical correlation" questions on the Board exam have an extremely long stem that provides a great deal of clinical data. Much of the data presented may be irrelevant. The challenge becomes one of *finding out what is being asked.* One method for rapidly narrowing the search, especially when confronted with a long stem, is to just read the last sentence of the stem, then scan the answer list. The nature of the last sentence and the answers provide a clue to the parts of the stem that are relevant and those that are not.

2. If 2 statements are contradictory (ie, only 1 can be correct), chances are good that 1 of the 2 is the correct answer (ie, the other 3 choices may be distracters). For example, consider the following:

   1. *In treating quinidine overdose, the best strategy would be to*
      (A) Acidify the urine
      (B) Administer a calcium chelator such as EDTA
      (C) Alkalinize the urine
      (D) Give potassium chloride
      (E) Give procainamide

The correct answer is **A:** acidify the urine.

   In the pair of the correct answer with a contradictory distractor (choices A and C), the instructor revealed what was being tested and then used the other three as "filler." Therefore, if you don't know the answer, you are better off guessing **A** or **C** (a 50% success probability) than **A** or **B** or **C** or **D** or **E** (a 20% success probability). Note that this strategy is valid only if you **must** guess; many instructors now introduce contradictory pairs as distracters. Another "rule" that should be used only if you must guess is the "longest choice" rule. When all the answers in a multiple-choice question are relatively long, the correct answer is often the longest one. Note again that sophisticated question writers may introduce especially long **incorrect** choices to foil this strategy.

3. Statements that contain the words "always," "never," "must," and so on are usually false. For example,

   Acetylcholine always increases the heart rate when given intravenously because it lowers blood pressure and evokes a strong baroreceptor-mediated reflex tachycardia

   The statement is false because, although acetylcholine often increases the heart rate, it can also cause bradycardia. (When given as a bolus, it may reach the sinus node in high enough concentration to cause initial bradycardia.) The use of trigger words such as "always" and "must" suggests that the instructor had some exception in mind. However, be aware that there are a few situations in which the statement with a trigger word is correct.

4. Choices that do not fit the stem grammatically are usually wrong. For example:

   1. *A drug that acts on a β-receptor and produces a maximal effect that is equal to one half the effect of a large dose of isoproterenol is called a*
      (A) Agonist
      (B) Analog of isoproterenol
      (C) Antagonist
      (D) Partial agonist

   The use of the article *a* at the end of the stem rather than *an* implies that the answer must start with a consonant (ie, choice **D**). Similar use may be made of disagreements in number. Note that careful question writers avoid this problem by placing the articles in the choice list, not in the stem.

5. A statement is not false just because changing a few words will make it somewhat more true than you think it is now. "Choose the one best answer" does not mean "Choose the only correct statement."

B. Strategies for "All of the Following Are Accurate Except" Questions

1. This type of question is avoided now on the USMLE because of problems with ambiguity; however, this type still is used in many local examinations because question-writers perceive them to be relatively easier to construct. When faced with this type of question, approach it as a nested set of true/false questions in which (hopefully) only one is true. It may help to mark each choice as either "T" or "F" as you read through them.

2. If 2 statements are contradictory, then 1 of them is certain to be the correct (false) answer because they cannot both be accurate statements, and yet this type of question cannot have 2 false answers. For example, consider the following:

   1. *All of the following may result from the use of thiazide diuretics EXCEPT*
      (A) Hyperglycemia
      (B) Hypernatremia
      (C) Hyponatremia
      (D) Hyperuricemia
      (E) Metabolic alkalosis

The correct answer is **B:** hypernatremia.

   The possibility that thiazide diuretics do not affect serum sodium concentrations is not tenable because that would produce 2 false choices. It is also somewhat unlikely that a drug could cause 2 opposite effects: therefore, the probability that 1 of the opposites is the correct (false) answer is high.

3. If the choices contain 2 drugs that are highly similar, then neither is likely to be the correct (false) answer. For example, consider the following:

1. *A young man who had become physiologically dependent after illicit use of secobarbital is undergoing severe withdrawal symptoms, including nausea, vomiting, delirium, and periodic seizures. Which one of the following drugs will NOT alleviate these symptoms?*
   (A) Buspirone
   (B) Chlordiazepoxide
   (C) Diazepam
   (D) Midazolam
   (E) Phenobarbital

The correct answer is **A:** buspirone.

If you recognize that chlordiazepoxide, diazepam, and midazolam all are benzodiazepine drugs with virtually identical pharmacologic effects, then you can quite safely rule out all three of them.

C. Strategies for Matching Type Questions

Matching questions usually test name recognition, and the most efficient approach consists of reading each stem item and then scanning the list of choices from the start and picking the first clear "hit." This is especially important on extended matching questions in which just reading the list can be time consuming. (Note, however, that the strategy suggested by the National Board of Medical Examiners for the USMLE differs from the above; see their *General Instructions* publication.) Occasionally, the strategies described above for the single best answer type question can be applied to the matching and extended matching type.

D. Strategies for the "Answer A if 1, 2, and 3 Are Correct" Type Question

This type of question, known as the "K type," has been dropped from the USMLE and therefore is no longer represented among the practice questions provided in this *Review*. However, it is still used in many local examinations.

For this type of question, one rarely must know the truth about all 4 statements to arrive at the correct answer. The instructions are to select

   (A) if only (1), (2), and (3) are correct;
   (B) if only (1) and (3) are correct;
   (C) if only (2) and (4) are correct;
   (D) if only (4) is correct;
   (E) if all are correct.

Useful strategies include the following:

1. If statement 1 is correct and 2 is wrong, the answer must be **B** (ie, 1 and 3 are correct). You don't need to know anything about 3 or 4.

2. If statement 1 is wrong, then answers **A, B,** and **E** are automatically excluded. Concentrate on statements 2 and 4.

3. The converse of 1 above: If choice 1 is wrong and 2 is correct, the answer must be **C** (ie, 2 and 4 are correct).

4. If statement 2 is correct and 4 is wrong, the answer is **A** (ie, 1 and 3 must be correct and you need not even look at them). (See example below.)

5. If statements 1, 2, and 4 are correct, the answer must be **E.** You need not know anything about 3.

6. Similarly, if statements 2 and 3 are correct and 4 is wrong, the answer must be **A,** and statement 1 must be correct.

7. If statements 2, 3, and 4 are correct, then the answer must be **E,** and statement 1 must be correct.

No doubt, more of these rules exist. In general, if you know whether 2 or 3 of the 4 statements in each question are right or wrong (ie, 50–75% the material), you should achieve a perfect score on this kind of question. The best way to learn these rules is to apply them to practice questions until the principles are firmly ingrained.

Consider the following question. Using the above rules, you should be able to answer it correctly even though there is no reason why you should know anything about the information contained in 2 of the 4 statements. The answer follows.

Which of the following statements is (are) correct?

1. The "struck bushel" is equal to 2150.42 cubic inches.

2. Medicine is one of the health sciences.

3. The fresh meat of the Atlantic salmon contains 220 IU of vitamin A per 100 g edible portion.

4. Hippocrates was the founder of modern psychoanalysis

The answer is **A.** Because statement 2 is clearly correct and 4 is just as patently incorrect (let's give Freud the credit), the answer can only be **A,** and statements 1 and 3 must be correct. (The data are from Lentner C, editor: *Geigy Scientific Tables,* 8th ed. Vol. 1. Ciba-Geigy, 1981.)

REFERENCES

Karpicke JD et al: Retrieval practice produces more learning than elaborative studying with concept mapping. *Science* 2011;331:772.

Le T et al: *First Aid for the USMLE STEP 1 2012*. McGraw-Hill, 2012.

Case SM, Swanson DB: *Constructing Written Test Questions for the Basic and Clinical Sciences,* 2nd ed. National Board of Medical Examiners, 1998. Available only from the World Wide Web (www.nbme.org/Publications; Item-Writing Manual).

Fischer MR, Herrmann S, Kopp V: Answering multiple-choice questions in high-stakes medical examinations. *Medical Education* 2005;39:890.

Step 1 content description and sample test materials. National Board of Medical Examiners. Available annually from the USMLE World Wide Web page at www.usmle.org.

Index

NOTE: Page numbers in **boldface** indicate a major discussion. Page numbers followed by *f* and *t* indicate figures and tables, respectively. A *b* following a page number indicates a boxed feature.